Dr. T. Derek V. Cooke
La Salle Building
146 Stuart Street
Kingston, Ont. K7L 3N6
Tel: 549-6414

Anatomy
of the Foot and Ankle

Anatomy
of the

Shahan K. Sarrafian, M.D.

Assistant Professor of Orthopedic Surgery, Northwestern University Medical School;
Chief, Orthopedic Section, Grant Hospital; Attending Orthopedic Surgeon, Northwestern Memorial Hospital;
Consulting Orthopedic Surgeon, Lakeside V.A. Hospital and Rehabilitation Institute of Chicago, Chicago, Illinois

Foot and Ankle

Descriptive, Topographic, Functional

J. B. Lippincott Company
Philadelphia
London
Mexico City
New York
St. Louis
São Paulo
Sydney

Sponsoring Editor: Richard Winters
Manuscript Editor: Delois Patterson
Indexer: Eleanor Kuljian
Art Director: Maria S. Karkucinski
Designer: Patrick Turner
Production Supervisor: N. Carol Kerr
Production Assistant: Charles W. Field
Compositor: Ruttle, Shaw & Wetherill, Inc.
Printer/Binder: Halliday Lithograph

The author and publisher have exerted every effort to ensure that drug selection and dosage set forth in this text are in accord with current recommendations and practice at the time of publication. However, in view of ongoing research, changes in government regulations, and the constant flow of information relating to drug therapy and drug reactions, the reader is urged to check the package insert for each drug for any change in indications and dosage and for added warnings and precautions. This is particularly important when the recommended agent is a new or infrequently employed drug.

Copyright © 1983, by J. B. Lippincott Company. All rights reserved. No part of this book may be used or reproduced in any manner whatsoever without written permission except for brief quotations embodied in critical articles and reviews. Printed in the United States of America. For information write J. B. Lippincott Company, East Washington Square, Philadelphia, Pennsylvania 19105.

Library of Congress Cataloging in Publication Data

Sarrafian, Shahan K.
    Anatomy of the foot and ankle.

    Bibliography.
    Includes index.
    1. Foot—Anatomy.   2. Ankle—Anatomy.   I. Title.
[DNLM: 1. Foot—Anatomy.   2. Ankle—Anatomy.   WE 880 S247a]
QM549.S27   1983   611'.98   82-17305
ISBN 0-397-50517-5

To the memory of my father, with admiration.
To my wife, Suzy, and our sons, Shahan, Jr., Raffi, and Armen, with love.

Foreword

The study of the foot has long been regarded as the stepchild of anatomical teaching. As medical students we began by dissecting the head and ended with the foot. At the end of 3 or 6 months (in my time it was 6 months), when we reached the foot we found it dried out, gnarled, and so hard that it could not be cut with a scalpel, to say nothing about dissecting it. For some reason standard textbooks of anatomy devote relatively limited space to the foot, and what is written hardly benefits the practicing surgeon. Dr. Sarrafian mentions the text, *Structure and Function as Seen in the Foot*. The author of this book, following the tradition of his predecessor, Sir Arthur Keith, gave surgeons a friendly wink and went on meandering in his wanted territory: comparative anatomy. Wood Jones said very little of value to practicing surgeons who need detail and more detail and no pontifical remarks or generalizations.

I am aware of no book in anatomy that has supplied as much detail about the structure of the ankle and foot than the present one by Dr. Sarrafian. He has not taken the words of his predecessors for granted. He has put their findings to test by numerous dissections of fetal as well as postnatal ankles. I have seen him virtually compare 100 tali, measure their facets, note their configuration, and their disposition or axis as he prefers to call it. Besides his section about the talus, I am fascinated by his discussion of collateral ligaments of the ankle (especially the medial or deltoid ligament), Lisfranc's articulation, and the first metatarsophalangeal joint. These are only a few nuggets. *Anatomy of the Foot and Ankle* abounds with equally brilliant ones. If any book deserves the epithet "classical," this one does. It will be read and used for reference for many years to come.

HAMPAR KELIKIAN, M.D.
Emeritus Professor of Orthopedic Surgery
Northwestern University Medical School
Chicago, Illinois

Preface

Also we can affirm, without fear of being taxed for exaggeration, that it is at the school of anatomy, particularly in topographic anatomy, that the best surgeons are formed.

TESTUT AND JACOB★

The knowledge of anatomy is essential for the treating surgeon and physician. As stated by Testut and Jacob, for the surgeon "the human body should be transparent like crystal" and the study of the topographic or surgical anatomy determines the regional knowledge to guide the scalpel, avoiding vital structures and interfering with other structures as specifically indicated. The practical concept of "down to bone" without due attention to the surrounding fine soft tissue structures is a primitive one and invites complications in foot and ankle surgery.

Five years ago I was invited to write a book on the anatomy and function of the foot. After 6 weeks of soul searching I accepted the great responsibility of undertaking the gigantic project. The excellent book of F. W. Jones, "Structure and Function as Seen in the Foot" was then 28 years old. Thus, it became evident that there was a great need to update the knowledge in the field, particularly since the advent of the rapid progress in the surgery of the foot and ankle.

A unified source of anatomical knowledge was set as a goal, bringing forth the classic and often forgotten works of giants of anatomy, combined with the recent comprehensive anatomical investigations. At no time was this approach intended to be encyclopedic but remained highly selective. This phase of the work required the translation of French, German, and Japanese works, the latter when written in German.

The personal investigative interest of the anatomy of the foot dates back to 1961. It was triggered by Dr. J. Boyes as he was explaining—at the end of a working day—the anatomy of the transverse lamina of the finger and the retention of the common extensor tendon. The explanation and his diagrams were lucid and I decided to investigate, on my return to Chicago, the same retention mechanism in the toes. I undertook the anatomical investigation of the intrinsic muscles of the toes with my colleague, Dr. L. K. Topouzian and the data was presented as an exhibit in 1965 and published in 1969. My personal anatomical and functional studies of the foot and ankle continued as dictated by various teaching responsibilities. The dissections were carried out primarily on the ankle and the hindfoot.

For the past 5 years all the dissections were personally done in a systematic manner. All specimens were fresh or preserved as fresh–frozen. No embalmed material was used. Each anatomical dissecting session was carried out in a continuous fashion for a period of 8 to 10 hours. Occasionally, the same foot and ankle were used a second time for another 6 to 8 hours. The documentation was done at each significant step through immediate photography, supplemented by pencil diagram during or immediately after the dissection. The pertinent phases were further documented by dictation and recording while dissecting. This methodology allowed me to remain as accurate as possible.

The cross sections of the foot and ankle were obtained by slicing the frozen specimens, followed by thawing and dissection. The latter was done under magnification and lasted 4 to 5 hours for each section. The arterial dissections were done after injecting the arterial tree with micropaque. The measurements on the tali and the calcanei were obtained from 100 dry tali and 50 dry calcanei from my own collection.

The osteo-anatomy and the syndesmology were emphasized as it became apparent that the knowledge of the geometry of the articular surfaces and the direction and tension of the various binding ligaments are essential to the understanding of the functional behavior of the

---

★Testut L, Jacob O: Traite d'Anatomie Topographique avec applications Médico-Chirurgicales, Vol 1, p 3. Paris, Doin, 1909

joints. Skeletal coalition was added to the study of osteology because of its important clinical implications. I did not economize energy in bringing forth data related to variations. Unifying such information from many rare sources under one cover may be beneficial to colleagues, especially if they are not versed in other languages. The advent of microsurgery as related to the foot necessitated obtaining details on the vascular anatomy, and the works of Adachi, Huber, Edwards, and more recently, the works of Gilbert, Murakami, Man, and Acland were referred to extensively. The arterial blood supply of the skeletal element was dealt with in a comprehensive manner.

The topographic or surgical anatomy was presented in four regions. The first region includes the anterior aspect of the ankle and the dorsum of the foot. The second region includes the posterolateral aspect of the ankle and foot. The third region incorporates the posteromedial aspect of the ankle and the tibiotalocalcaneal tunnel. The subdivision of the latter into two distinct neurovascular compartments is emphasized. The fourth region is represented by the sole of the foot. Practical landmarks and guidelines are provided to localize the neurovascular bundles and the compartments. The ball of the foot and the big toe are dealt with separately.

In the study of the functional anatomy of the foot, the contributions of Hicks and MacConnail are enormous in the appreciation of the functional relationship of the forefoot and hindfoot. Most of the recent orthopaedic literature refers to Hicks' windlass mechanism of tightening of the plantar aponeurosis through the hyperextension of the big toe, but I think that his explanation of the interrelationship of the forefoot and hindfoot deserves as much, if not more, attention. MacConnail's concept of the foot as a twisted plate—supination meaning untwisting and pronation meaning more twisting of the plate—is expressing the same relationship as defined by Hicks from a different angle. This also deserves much attention especially when untwisting or supination (forefoot supination and hindfoot valgus) renders the foot plate rigid and subject to fracture, and twisting or pronation (forefoot pronation and hindfoot varus) renders the foot pliable. These facts, very easily verifiable on ones own foot or on specimens, seem contrary to the present, common understanding of the relationship of the hindfoot and forefoot as presented in the orthopaedic biomechanical literature. The works of Elftman and Huson deserve due consideration. The subluxation of the talus at the midtarsal joint during supination, immediately reduced by midtarsal combined motion of adduction–supination–flexion, as described by Huson, is expressing Elftman's explanation that in supination the major axes of the calcaneocuboid and the talonavicular joints do not coincide and require the intervention of the subtalar axis for adjustment. The recent anatomical and functional investigations of Bojsen–Møller are also most interesting and are referred to extensively.

The effort invested in the preparation of this book has been gigantic but the learning process has been a most rewarding experience. If *Anatomy of the Foot and Ankle* offers useful information to my colleagues and provides a new platform of knowledge from which others can advance the frontier of knowledge of the anatomy and function of the foot and ankle, I will have then reached my goal.

Shahan K. Sarrafian, M.D.

Acknowledgments

To write a book of anatomy in a "home environment" requires the full support of a very unusual team. The root of the involvement has been dedication, true friendship, and a high degree of professionalism.

Without hesitation, I would like to single out the great contribution of Mrs. **Betsy** Addison, my research secretary. She searched the literature old and new, provided **unusual** rare documents, and corrected and typed the manuscript. Without her constant support **this** work would never have seen the light and I am greatly indebted to her.

I am grateful to my partner, Dr. James H. Breihan, for making possible, in a subtle **way,** the "extra times" and for listening to, with patience, my anatomical "exposés."

My gratitude goes to my friend, Dr. Fedor Banuchi, who in a truly dedicated manner provided the majority of the anatomical specimens and my appreciation goes to Dr. James Milgram for providing some unusually good fresh specimens.

For the process of recovery of some of the anatomical specimens I would like to thank Mrs. Margo Kissane, Mrs. Darlene Lewis, and also Mr. Tony McKeehan and Mr. Bob Bylina, for their skill in doing rapid above-the-ankle amputations at the morgue.

All the dissections were carried out in a surgical environment created in my home basement and my thanks to Ms. Sandra Richie for providing the necessary surgical facilities.

My family was deeply involved in the project. The topographic anatomy required the step-by-step photographic documentation during a given session of dissection. I could only impose the unpredictable moments on my family and I would like to express my sincere thanks to my wife Suzy and my son Armen for taking all the photographs of the dissected specimens; for them, this was not a pleasant task. My thanks also to my son Raffi for developing and printing some of the photographs at the early phase of the work and to Shahan, Jr., for helping me to understand the recent biomechanical investigations.

I am very appreciative of Dr. M. B. Rodney's generosity in providing the embryo feet. This was possible through the graciousness of Dr. H. Hasson and Dr. L. Keith. The photographic documentation played a great role in the presentation of the anatomical facts. I wish to express my thanks to Mr. H. Sheklanian for the professional osteophotography. To Mrs. G. Sharp, my profound gratitude for her superb expertise and artistic touch in preparing and printing most of the photographs in *Anatomy of the Foot and Ankle*. Mr. E. Beck, an excellent medical illustrator, prepared the outstanding anatomical plates which became the backbone of the book and for this I express my thanks and gratitude.

I know of no man whose unselfish dedication could surpass that of my good friend Dr. H. Schlecht, who for a period of at least three years, twice a week, one to two hours at each session, translated the excellent German documents of anatomy. No words could ever express my gratitude. My appreciation is also extended to my friend Mr. G. Martin for translating the extensive work of Zchakaja.

The initiation, development, and completion of a book requires an intuitive feel, subtle guidance, and final systematization. I wish to thank Mr. Stuart Freeman, Editor-in-Chief at Lippincott, for his understanding when the work was delayed as his only concern was the quality of the work. His periodic visits, gentle guidance, and support were most appreciated. He allowed the dream of the author to become a reality.

My great appreciation and gratitude is extended to Mr. Richard Winters, Ms. Delois Patterson, and the entire Lippincott team for their dedicated work and their enormous effort invested in the conversion of the manuscript into the final printed form.

Contents

1

Development of the Foot and Ankle

Prenatal Development

The embryonic period is divided into 23 horizons or stages. Each horizon corresponds to a developmental stage of the embryo based on a system of point scores.

This method of classification and identification of the embryo advocated by Streeter has brought greater precision to embryologic descriptions.[1] Embryos of different crown-to-rump (C-R) lengths might belong to the same horizon. The growth curve of the embryo, correlating the C-R length with the fertilization or menstrual age of the embryo, as presented by Patten (Fig. 1-1), is used throughout this study.[2]

The use of a growth curve in terms of one linear measurement correlated with age is still of value for the interpretation of embryologic information predating Streeter's classification.

MORPHOGENESIS OF THE FEET

Morphogenesis of the feet is illustrated in Figures 1-2 and 1-3.[1] The embryo of 2 weeks post fertilization is curved irregularly in a semicircle and presents no external evidence of a lower limb bud in the caudal area (Fig. 1-4).

Horizons or Stages of Development

At 3 weeks, a slight longitudinal swelling is discernible opposite the five lumbar and first sacral myotomes. Once initiated, the ontogeny of the lower limb progresses in a rapid sequential fashion, and definite morphologic changes are recognizable at 2-day intervals. At 4 weeks, in horizon 13 (3 mm–6 mm), a minute lower limb bud germinates at the site of the previous swelling. Within the next 2 days (horizon 14, 5 mm–7 mm), the bud increases in size and springs laterally from the trunk. It exhibits a flat ventral and a rounded dorsal surface united by a convex margin (Figs. 1-2 and 1-5). In horizon 15 (6 mm–9 mm), the bud extends its base distally toward the sacral myotomes and further increases in length. The lumbar segment retains a round

contour, whereas the sacral part tapers. A differentiation is initiated and is well evident in horizon 16 (8 mm–11 mm). Three regions are visible, corresponding to the thigh, the leg, and the foot anlage. All three regions are more or less located in the same transverse plane, perpendicular to the plane of the lower trunk.

A rounded foot disk is recognized in horizon 17 (11 mm–13.5 mm), at the fifth embryonic week. The surface of the foot plate is located in the transverse plane, and the ventral surface, the future plantar surface, faces the head. An inward

Fig. 1-1. Crown-to-rump (C-R) length as compared with age of embryo. (After Patten BM: Human Embryology, 2nd ed, p 185. New York, McGraw-Hill, 1953)

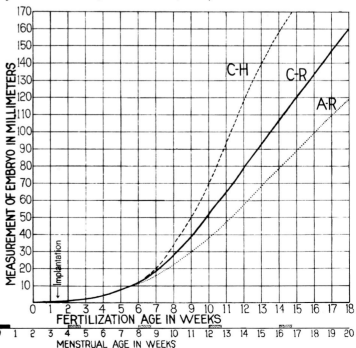

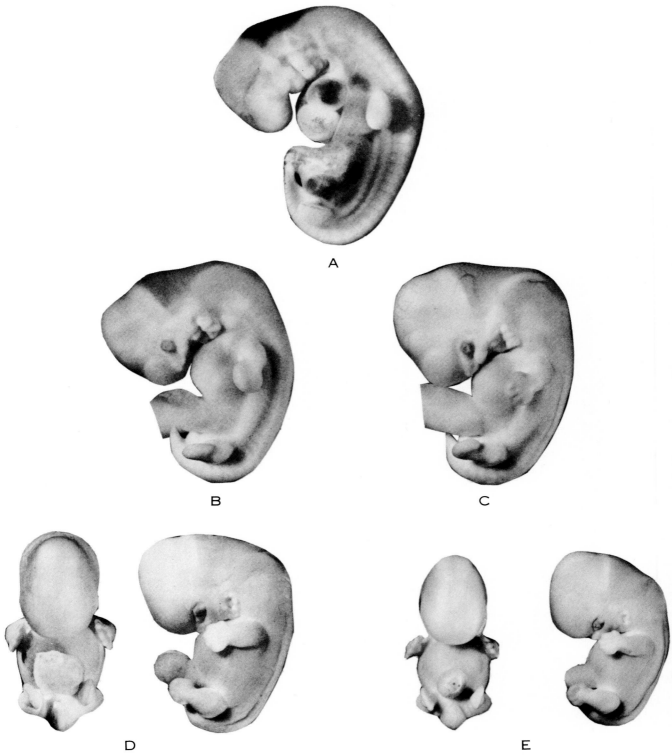

Fig. 1-2.   Embryos. (*A*) Horizon 14 (4.9 mm–8.2 mm). (*B*) Horizon 16 (8 mm–11 mm). (*C*) Horizon 17 (11 mm–13.5 mm). (*D*) Horizon 18 (14 mm–16 mm). (*E*) Horizon 19 (16.5 mm–20 mm). (Assembled after Streeter GL: Developmental horizons in human embryos. In Contributions to Embryology, Vols. 21, 32, 34. Washington, DC, Carnegie Institution of Washington, 1945, 1948, 1951)

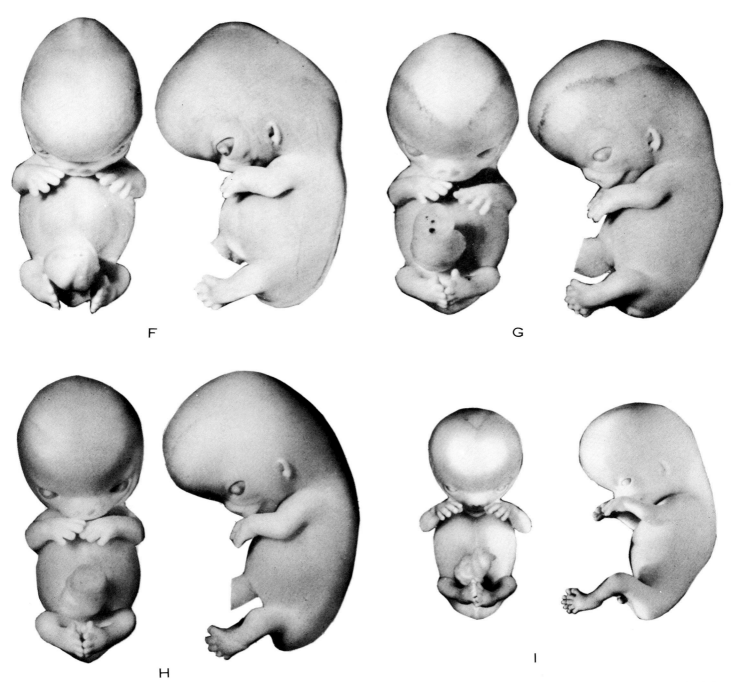

Fig. 1-3. Embryos. (*F*) Horizon 20 (21 mm–23 mm). (*G*) Horizon 21 (21 mm–24 MM). (*H*) Horizon 22 (25 mm–27 mm). (*I*) Horizon 23 (28 mm–30 mm). (Assembled after Streeter GL: Developmental horizons in human embryos. In Contributions to Embryology, Vols. 21, 32, 34. Washington, DC, Carnegie Institution of Washington, 1945, 1948, 1951)

rotation occurs, and the future flexor surface obliquely faces the median sagittal plane of the trunk (Figs. 1-2 and 1-6). When viewed from the ventral aspect of the embryo, the rotation of the foot plate—a fundamental change—is counterclockwise on the left and clockwise on the right; the leg segment participates in this inward rotation. Morphologically, no toe rays are present in the foot plate. However, the older embryos of this group have an indication of the great toe on the tibial or preaxial border. Within the next 2

days (horizon 18, 14 mm–16 mm; see Fig. 1-2), the sixth embryonic week, the inward rotation of the foot–leg segment continues. The medial surface of the foot plate faces more toward the median plane of the trunk, and this surface, when extended distally, makes with its counterpart an acute angle, open proximally. When the embryo is viewed from the lateral aspect, the future dorsal surface of the foot plate can be seen. An inward rotation of nearly 90° has occurred. The preaxial or tibial border is cephalad and the postaxial

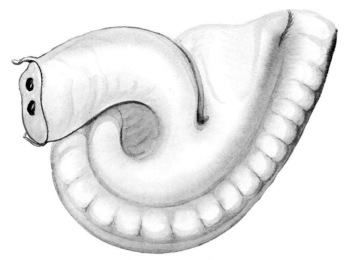

Fig. 1-4. Embryo of 4.2 mm.

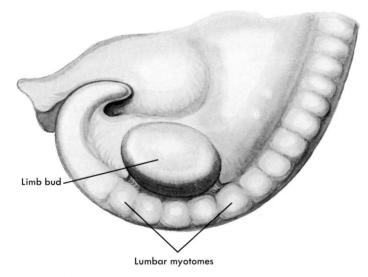

Fig. 1-5. Embryo of horizon 14 (6.3 mm).

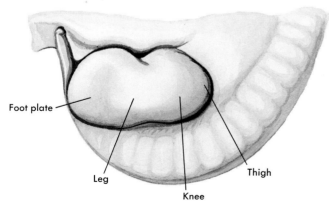

Fig. 1-6. Embryo of horizon 17 (11 mm–13.5 mm).

or peroneal border is caudad. Digital rays are clearly visible, and some interdigital notching is present. In horizon 19 (16.5 mm–20 mm), the features of the previous stage are accentuated. The digital notching is deeper (Figs. 1-2 and 1-7). The foot plates are converted to a more recognizable foot structure in horizon 20 (21 mm–23 mm) (Figs. 1-3 and 1-8), and by horizon 21 (22 mm–24 mm; see Fig. 1-3), the seventh embryonic week, the orientation of the parts is as follows:

Both feet face each other and are located in a nearly sagittal plane.

The preaxial or tibial border of the leg–foot is cephalad.

The postaxial or fibular border of the leg–foot is caudad.

The extensor surface (future anterior surface of the leg and dorsum of the foot) faces laterally.

The flexor surface (future posterior surface of the leg and plantar of the foot) faces medially.

The toes are well delineated and spread apart. The big toe is on the tibial border of the foot.

The foot surface is in continuity with the leg surface. There is no angulation of the foot relative to the leg. The foot is in an equinus position relative to the leg.

The entire lower extremity is in a position of marked external rotation.

Horizon 23 marks the end of the embryonic period proper (Figs. 1-3 and 1-9). It corresponds to the end of the eighth embryonic week and an average C–R length of 30 mm. The feet touch each other at their soles or medial aspects and are in a praying position. The toes are still fanning out.

During the fetal period, important rotational changes take place that alter the leg–foot relationship. Initially the feet, their soles facing each other, are in equinus relative to the leg. A progressive internal rotation of the thigh–leg occurs, and the foot is then in equinus, supination, and external rotation relative to the leg. Subsequently, the foot dorsiflexes and pronates, bringing the foot close to the adult neutral position; the toes do not diverge.

Böhm, describing the developmental phases of the foot in the embryo–fetus, ascribes four stages to the morphologic determinism:[5]

Stage one (second month): The foot is in 90° equinus and adducted.

Stage two (beginning of third month): The foot is in 90° equinus, adducted, and markedly supinated.

Stage three (middle of third month): The foot dorsiflexes at the ankle, but a mild degree of equinus is still present. The marked supination persists. The first metatarsal remains adducted. This stage corresponds to the fetal period of development.

Stage four (beginning of fourth month): The foot pronates and reaches a position of midsupination. A slight metatarsus varus remains. The equinus is not present.

The pronation "continues during the remainder of foetal development and is not yet complete in the newborn."[5]

The division of the development of the foot into four stages brings schematic clarity, but in reality, as mentioned by Böhm, "the changes do not actually occur within the exact limits of four stages, but by means of gradual, continuous transformations."[5]

Digital Formula

The study of the position and relative length of the toes presents another interesting aspect of the morphogenesis of the foot (Fig. 1-10).

The pedal digits make their clear appearance in horizon 20 (21 mm–23 mm). They diverge from the convex border of the foot plate. The third toe arises from the apex of the convexity, and is therefore the longest. Within a few days, the preaxial side of the foot grows more rapidly, and the second toe surpasses the third.[6] It is later in fetal life that the first toe might take the lead. According to Jones, in the very early embryo, the pedal digit formula may be 3>2>1>4>5 or 3>2>4>1>5 for a brief period.[6] When the embryo reaches horizon 22 (25 mm–27 mm), the second toe takes the lead with the 2>3>1>4>5 distribution; later, the adult formula is reached in the form of 1>2>3>4>5 or its variant 2>1>3>4>5.

I have analyzed the pedal digital formula in 29 embryo feet. The feet were classified according to their length into three developmental groups: group 1, feet 5mm in length; group 2, feet 5 mm to 9 mm in length; group 3, feet 10 mm in length. The following distribution was present: group 1 (5 feet): 3>2>4>1>5, 4 feet (3 mm, 4 mm, 4 mm, 4.5 mm); 2>3>4>1>5, 1 foot (4 mm); group 2 (19 feet): 3>4>2>1>5, 1 foot (5.5 mm); 3>2>4>1>5, 7 feet (5 mm, 5.5 mm, 5.5 mm, 6 mm, 6 mm, 6 mm, 6 mm); 2>3>4>1>5, 6 feet (6 mm, 6 mm, 6 mm, 7 mm, 8 mm, 8 mm); 2>3>1>4>5, 4 feet (5 mm, 6.5 mm, 7 mm, 9.5 mm); 2>1>3>4>5, 1 foot (8 mm); group 3 (5 feet):

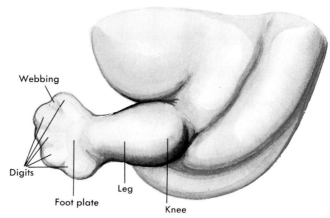

Fig. 1-7. Embryo of horizon 19 (17.5 mm).

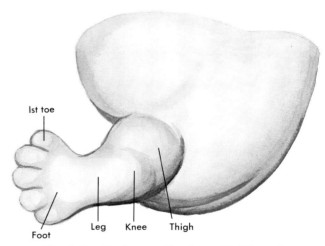

Fig. 1-8. Embryo of horizon 20 (20 mm).

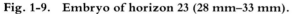

Fig. 1-9. Embryo of horizon 23 (28 mm–33 mm).

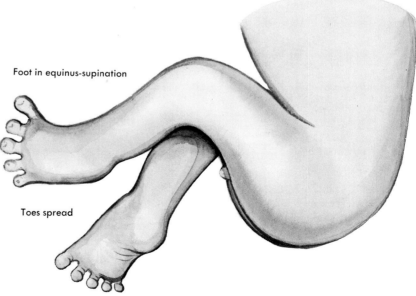

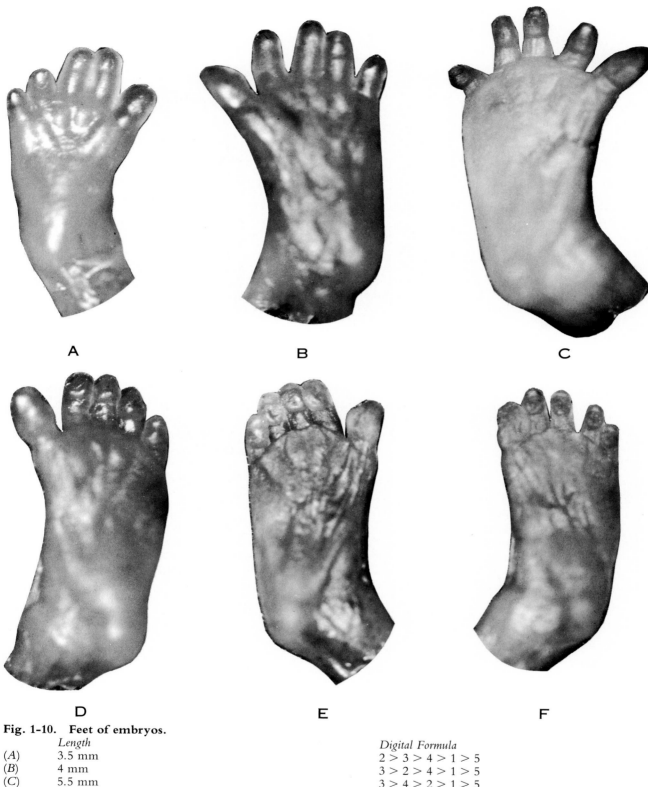

A B C

D E F

Fig. 1-10. Feet of embryos.

	Length	*Digital Formula*
(*A*)	3.5 mm	2 > 3 > 4 > 1 > 5
(*B*)	4 mm	3 > 2 > 4 > 1 > 5
(*C*)	5.5 mm	3 > 4 > 2 > 1 > 5
(*D*)	5 mm	2 > 3 > 1 ≧ 4 > 5
(*E*)	6 mm	2 > 3 > 4 > 1 > 5
(*F*)	6mm	2 > 3 > 1 ≧ 4 > 5

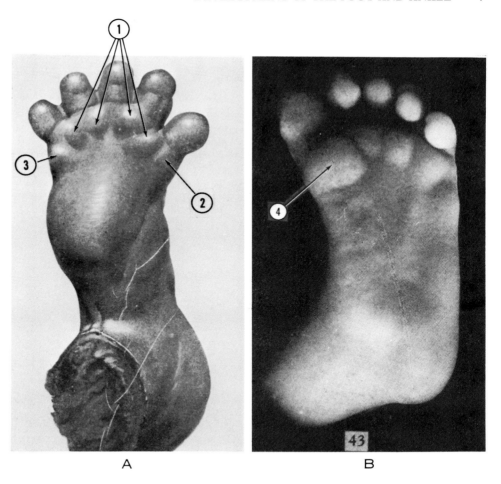

Fig. 1-11. Plantar pads. (*A*) Foot of 24-mm embryo. (1, Interdigital pads; 2, tibial pad; 3, fibular pad.) (*B*) Foot of 62.5-mm embryo. (4, Hallucal pad formed by fusion of tibial pad and first interdigital pad.) (From Cummins H: The topographic history of the volar pads [walking pads, tastballen] in the human embryo. Contrib Embryol 20:105, 1929)

A   B

2>1>3>4>5, 2 feet (11 mm, 12 mm); 2>3>1>4>5, 1 foot (10 mm); 1>2>3>4>5, 2 feet (11 mm, 14 mm).

It is apparent, based on these measurements that the third toe is the longest in the very young embryo. As the embryo grows, the third toe loses its place to the second. Later the first toe moves next to the second, thus reaching one variation of the adult digital formula (2>1>3>4>5), and in the oldest embryo of this group (14 mm) the first toe takes the lead with the most common adult distribution (1>2>3>4>5).

Metatarsal Formula

In the embryo the metatarsal formula initially is 3>2>1>4>5 or 3>2>4>5>1. In the fourth and fifth month of fetal life the rule is 2>3>1>4>5, already resembling the common adult formula. From the sixth to the ninth month the metatarsal formula is 2>1>3>4>5 or the occasional variant 2>3>1>4>5.[7]

Plantar or Walking Pads

Plantar or walking pads are soft-tissue elevations produced by localized accumulation of subcutaneous connective tissue and fat (Fig. 1-11).[8]

In the embryo of horizon 20, four distal plantar pads appear, corresponding to the interdigital spaces. A tibial pad and a fibular pad are also separately indicated. The proximal region of the sole of the foot shows no distinct pads. By horizon 22, five apical pads appear on the plantar aspect of the toes distally. The distal interdigital pads become more prominent in horizon 23, and on the tibial side the first interdigital pad and the tibial pad merge to form the "hallucal pad." The interdigital pads are reduced to three. A central sole pad now makes its appearance, and the heel region is also slightly elevated. In the embryo of 40 mm, the central pad is nearly level. A general regression of the pads occurs when the fetus is 100 mm in C-R length or older. The pads become gradually lower and discrete. These pads persist during the remaining period of the gestation in discrete regressed form.

In the last fetal weeks, the feet are swollen and the pads are temporarily masked. In the postnatal phase, the hallucal and interdigital pads are demonstrable, and the fibular pads are not noticeable.

Foot Growth

Foot measurement is possible only after the embryo reaches a C-R length of 24 mm, that is, after horizon 21.[9,10]

In the early fetal stage (30 mm–60 mm), the foot grows less rapidly than the body (sitting height). After 70 mm, until term, there is a retardation in the increase of sitting height, whereas the foot maintains its growth rate and displays a relative acceleration of growth. This increase in foot length is slow from the 8th to the 14th week, then becomes more rapid until the 26th week, then slows down slightly until term. The average increase in length from the 14th week on is about 3 mm/week, with only slight variation.[9] The tabulated data of Scammon and Calkins, when converted into a growth curve, give a pattern as indicated in Figure 1-12.[10] At the end of the third month the foot measures 0.8 cm (average) and at term 7.6 cm (maximum, 8.7 cm; minimum, 7.1 cm). These dimensions are measured as

a straight line from the posterior margin of the heel to the tip of the extended big toe.

The fetal foot narrows gradually with growth and remains longer than the adult foot when compared with the corresponding leg length. The ratio greatest foot length/leg length is 1.41 at 8 weeks, 0.9 at birth, and 0.6 in the adult.[7]

INTERNAL STRUCTURES

Skeleton

The lower limb bud makes its appearance in horizon 13 (3 mm–6 mm) at 4 weeks post fertilization. The bud is filled with blastemic tissue. An ectodermal thickening forms on

Fig. 1-12.   Prenatal foot growth and length. (Curves based on data from Scammon RE, Calkings LA: The Development and Growth of the External Dimensions of the Human Body in the Fetal Period, pp 245–246. Minneapolis, University of Minnesota Press, 1929)

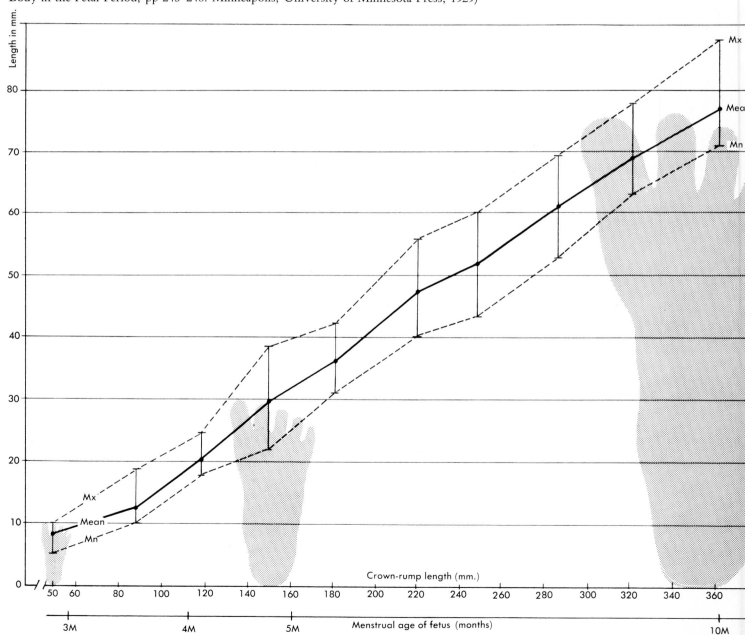

the ventral aspect, and within 4 days (horizon 15), it is converted into an ectodermal ridge on its lateral part. This ridge is transient, disappearing within a week (horizon 19). Its importance seems primordial, as it induces the differentiation of the future limb components and determines their directional (proximodistal) formation.[4]

Stages of Skeletal Development.   There are three stages in the formation of the skeletal elements: mesenchymal, cartilaginous, and osseous.

Mesenchymal.   The mesenchymal stage is illustrated in Figure 1-13.[11,12] In horizon 17 (11 mm–13 mm) and 18 (14 mm–16 mm), the footplate is already present. The axial mesenchyme condenses, differentiates, and forms the anlage of the foot. The metatarsals differentiate later. When the phalangeal models are formed, for a short time a thick web remains between the digital rays. The metatarsal rays are spread apart, but they will gradually approximate.

The differentiation of the tarsus follows that of the metatarsals. Within the areas of condensation tissue, procartilage soon makes its appearance. The lower ends of the tibia and fibula are still formed of condensed blastemic tissue in horizon 20.

Cartilaginous.   The cartilaginous stage is illustrated in Figure 1-14, *A, B*). Cartilage cells form in the mesenchymal–prochondral anlage. As the process of chondrification advances, the skeletal elements become clearly identifiable; morphogenesis, aiming to the adult form, occurs. The chronologic sequence of chondrification was reported by Senior.[13] The process occurs in 14 stages (Fig. 1-15). The central three metatarsals chondrify first, followed by the fifth metatarsal and the cuboid. The chondrification of the tarsus continues with the calcaneus, the talus, and the third and second cuneiforms. The first cuneiform and the first metatarsal follow. The navicular is the last tarsal element to chondrify. The phalanges are next, and the process occurs here in a proximodistal sequence.

The proximal phalanges of the second, third, and fourth toes chondrify, followed by the proximal phalanx of the fifth toe. The proximal phalanx of the big toe is next to be followed by the middle phalanges of the central toes, two, three, and four. Next in sequence is the chondrification of the middle phalanx of the little toe, the distal phalanx of the big toe, and the distal phalanges of the second, third, and fourth toes. The last element to chondrify is the distal phalanx of the little toe.

The chondrification of the foot is initiated in horizon 18 (14 mm–16 mm), and the last element, except for the sesamoids, chondrifies in horizon 23 (28 mm–32 mm), which represents the end of the embryonic period proper.

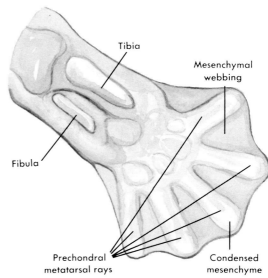

Fig. 1-13.   Foot plate of embryo in horizon 18 (14 mm–16 mm). Skeleton in mesenchymal stage. (After Bardeen CR: Studies of the development of the human skeleton. Am J Anat 4:265, 1905)

Fig. 1-14.   (A) Foot and leg of embyro in horizon 19 (20 mm). Skeleton in cartilaginous stage. **(B) Foot and ankle of 33-mm fetus.** Skeleton in cartilaginous stage. (After Bardeen CR: Studies of the development of the human skeleton. Am J Anat 4: 265, 1905)

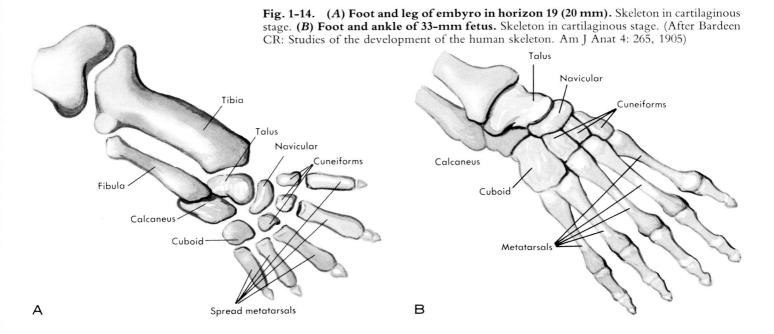

A

B

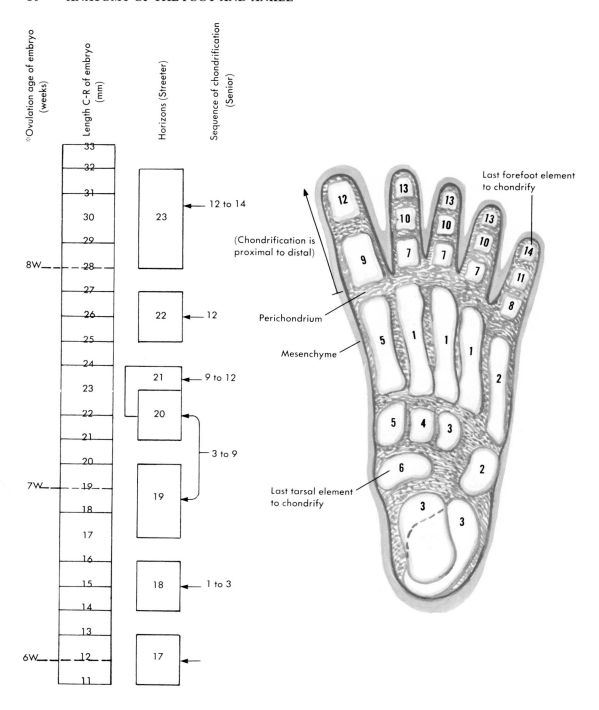

*Ovulation age (wk) = Menstrual age (wk) minus 2 weeks

Fig. 1-15.   Chronologic sequence of chondrification of the foot in the embryo.
(Based on data from Senior HD: The chondrification of the human hand and foot skeleton
(abstr). Anat Rec 42:35, 1929. Correlation between sequence of chondrification and Streeter's
horizons based on O'Rahilly R, Gray DJ, Gardner E: Chondrification in the hands and feet
of staged human embryos. Contrib Embryol 36:185, 1957)

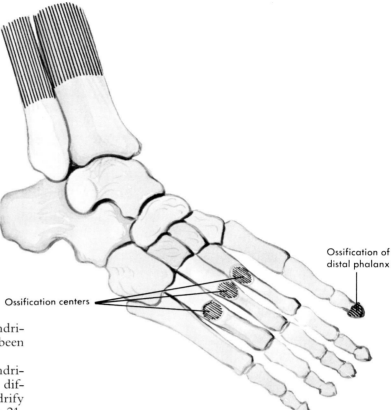

Ossification of distal phalanx

Ossification centers

Fig. 1-16.   Foot of 50-mm fetus. Skeleton at onset of ossification. (After Bardeen CR: Studies of the development of the human skeleton. Am J Anat 4: 265, 1905)

The relationship between Senior's sequence of chondrification and Streeter's horizons (see Fig. 1-15) has been reported by O'Rahilly and co-workers.[12]

Within a given condensed mesenchymal unit, chondrification of the future anatomic components occurs at different times. The body of the calcaneus begins to chondrify centrally in horizon 18, the tuber calcanei in horizon 21, and the sustentaculum tali in horizon 23.[14]

By the end of the embryologic period proper, the morphology and relationship of the cartilaginous skeletal components are determined and resemble closely those of the adult. The future articular surfaces acquire their definite contour at this early stage, prior to the formation of a joint space.[11]

Chondrification is present in the distal tibia and fibula in horizon 21.

Osseous.   The osseous stage is shown in Figure 1-16 and 1-17.[11,14,15] The forefoot ossifies before the hindfoot. The general sequence of ossification is distal phalanx of the big toe, metatarsals, distal phalanges of lesser toes, proximal phalanges, and finally middle phalanges. The last element to ossify in the forefoot is the middle phalanx of the little toe. The ossification of the forefoot takes place between the third and fifth prenatal lunar months.

In the hindfoot, the calcaneus is the first to ossify. Gardner and associates describe periosteal bone formation on the inferolateral aspect of the calcaneus in a 93-mm fetus.[14] At 125 mm, the endochondral center of ossification appears. The talus may begin to ossify during the eighth lunar month, but an ossification center is not always present at birth. An extensive study correlating roentgenographic findings in the newborn with the body weight indicates that regardless of the weight of the newborn, the calcaneus is always ossified; the talus is also ossified except in infants weighing less than 2000 g.[16] In this group the talar ossification was absent at birth in an average of 13.3%. The cuboid is the last tarsal element that can exhibit prenatal ossification.

The histologic process of ossification is periosteal and endochondral in the metatarsals and proximal and middle phalanges. A bone collar forms first around the middle of the cartilaginous diaphysis, followed by invasion of the cartilaginous shaft by a periosteal bud, thus initiating the endochondral ossification that extends in a proximal and distal direction.

The distal phalanx differs in this regard from the other phalanges. The intramembranous and endochondral ossification starts at the tip and extends proximally. Dixey describes clearly the process as a "cap" of intramembranous bone formed at the distal end of the cartilaginous phalanx.[17] This cap is then converted into a bony "thimble fitting over the cartilaginous phalanx and enclosing it almost up to its base."[17]

Morphologic Development of the Skeletal Elements of the Foot

Embryonic phase and early fetal phase.   Bardeen and, more recently, Olivier provided a detailed morphologic study of the skeletal elements of the foot in the embryonic phase.[11,18] In the embryo of 13.5 mm, Olivier describes a foot with three rays: a principal median ray and two lateral rudimentary rays.[18] This tridactylic stage suggests a fanlike growth from the median axis. This primitive foot is digitigrade, in acute plantar flexion, and there is no evidence of angulation of the foot relative to the leg.

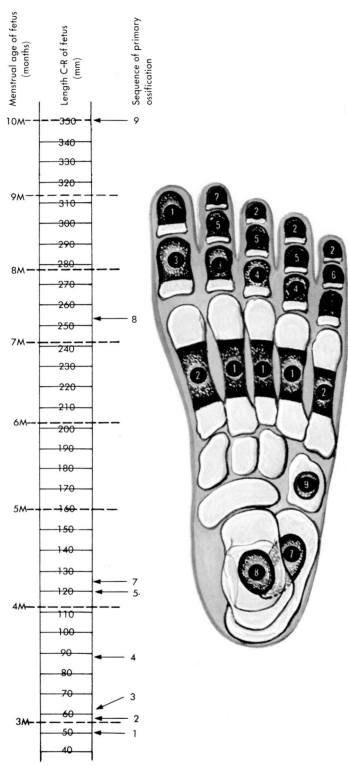

Menstrual age of fetus (months)

Length C-R of fetus (mm)

Sequence of primary ossification

Fig. 1-17. Chronologic sequence of ossification of fetal foot. (Correlation of menstrual age and C-R length based on Arey LB: Developmental Anatomy, 7th ed, p 104. Philadelphia, WB Saunders, 1965)

The interosseous slit of the leg is extended onto the ventral aspect by a groove and divides the foot into two parts: preaxial (cranial), comprising the second ray, a rudiment of the first ray, the tarsal elements corresponding to the talus, the navicular, and the cuneiforms, and postaxial (caudal), comprising the third ray, the beginning of the fourth ray, and the tarsal elements corresponding to the cuboid and the calcaneus.[18] The fibula is extended by the calcaneus and the three lateral rays.

In embryos of 14.2 mm and 17 mm (horizon 18), the foot presents five rays separated fanlike from each other. The foot is sagittal in orientation, the medial border being cranial and the lateral border caudal. The mesenchymal anlages of the distal end of the tibia and fibula in horizon 18 (14 mm) are separated, and the talar element is wedged in between.[18] The distal end of the tibia is oblique and concave. Due to the obliquity of the tibial surface, the medial malleolus projects more distally than the end of the fibula (Fig. 1-18). In horizon 19 (17 mm) and 20 (21 mm), the malleoli are at the same level; it is only after horizon 22 (27 mm) that the lateral malleolus extends more distally than the medial. The fibulocalcaneal contact has been established early and is clearly present at horizon 20 (21 mm). The tip of the lateral malleolus loses contact with the calcaneus at horizon 22 (27 mm). It is during this period that the distal tibia and fibula come close and establish contact for the formation of a distal tibiofibular joint; this is of relatively late occurrence.

The talus is delineated at horizon 18 (14.2 mm; Fig. 1-18).[18] The contour is irregular. The element is angled at 90°, with a transverse segment, corresponding to the body and future trochlea, and a sagittal segment located inward and inferiorly, corresponding to the neck and head. The superior surface is located between the tibia and the fibula. The element of the talar neck is directed toward the second metatarsal. The lower surface establishes contact with the calcaneus only in the lateral third (Fig. 1-19). The anterior surface is in continuity with the navicular. The posterior part of the lateral surface has a surface corresponding to the lateral malleolus. The posterior part of the medial surface presents a convex surface (see Fig. 1-18) corresponding to the tibial plafond and the medial malleolus. At this stage "the talus is low, large located on the medial flank of the calcaneum over which it overlaps slightly; there is yet no torsion of the head, nor clear declination of the neck."[18]

Sudden rapid changes occur in horizon 22 (27 mm). The sustentaculum tali appears, and the talus passes nearly entirely over the calcaneus (Fig. 1-19). The talus "narrows transversely, elongates but does not elevate yet."[18] The superior talar surface is flat, descending medially and articulating with the tibia. No true trochlea is present yet. At 34 mm the talus more or less resembles the adult structure (Fig. 1-19). The foot has pronated. The declination angle of the talar neck–head has increased to 25°. The cephalic torsion has not occurred. The trochlea is narrow; the lateral process is well developed, supporting the articular surface for the lateral malleolus. The talus is still a relatively flat structure. The navicular has separated from the talar head.

The calcaneus is initially short, with a narrow superior surface.[18] The anteromedial segment of this surface corre-

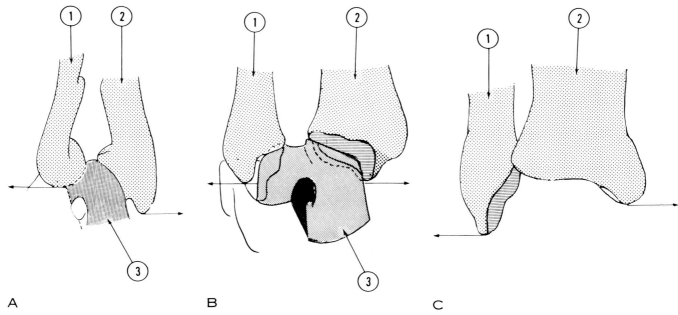

Fig. 1-18. (*A*) **Ankle of embryo in horizon 18 (14 mm).** The talus is wedged between the tibia and the fibula. The distal end of the tibia is oblique and concave. The distal ends of the fibula and tibia are separated, and the former is proximal to the medial malleolus. (*B*) **Ankle of embryo in horizon 19 (17 mm).** The distal tibia and fibula are still separated, and the talus is wedged between the two. The fibular and tibial malleoli are at the same level. The talus is angled at 90°. (*C*) **Ankle of embryo in horizon 22 (27 mm).** The lateral malleolus is more distal than the medial malleolus. 1, Fibula; 2, tibia; 3, Talus. (Adapted from Olivier G: Formation du Squelette des Membres. Paris, Vigot Frères, 1962)

sponds to the talar overlapping segment; the posterolateral segment gives support to the distal end of the fibula. This small fibular supportive surface, still seen early in horizon 22 (27 mm), fades away, the lateral malleolus retaining only the talar relationship. The sustentaculum tali, clearly present at horizon 22, extends farther medially, and by 34 mm it nears the medial border of the talus. The inferior calcaneal surface presents a large posterolateral tuberosity in horizon 19 (17 mm), and by horizon 20 (21 mm) a posteromedial tuberosity emerges.

The navicular is isolated at horizon 20 (21 mm).[18] It is flat and enters in contact laterally with the cuboid.

The cuboid is slightly distinct at horizon 20.[18] An anteromedial extension wedges between the bases of the third and fourth metatarsals. A medial extension meets the navicular. At 34 mm the cuboid resembles the cuneiforms and articulates obliquely with the anterior surface of the calcaneus.

The lateral and middle cuneiforms are not distinct at horizon 20.[18] The medial cuneiform is present and voluminous, and the anterior surface is oriented anteriorly and medially.[18] The cuneiforms 2 and 3 appear in horizon 22 (27 mm). The second cuneiform is the smallest and the highest; "The anterior surface is at the level of the lateral cuneiform and even of the 4th metatarsal, therefore without any evidence of posterior retreat."[18]

Fetal phase. During the fetal period of development, morphologic changes continue. A comprehensive study has been conducted by Straus.[7]

Bones. The *talus* does not grow uniformly in all directions (Fig. 1-20 *A, B*). The talar body increases more rapidly in height than in length. The width of the posterior talar segment increases slightly more rapidly than the length.

The talar neck–trochlea declination angle narrows steadily during fetal development (Fig. 1-20, *A, B*). Furthermore, the angle formed by the long axis of the talar head and the transverse axis of the talar body increases gradually as the head turns more and more laterally (Fig. 1-21). The lateral shift and the lateral torsion of the talar head–neck are some of the factors explaining the correction of the pedal supination.

The *calcaneus* of the fetus has a very short body, but subsequently, this segment grows faster relative to the total calcaneal length. A gradual increase of the posterior segment of the calcaneus results, contributing to the mechanical efficiency of the triceps surae (Fig. 1-22). It is also of interest to note that at 3 months the calcaneus of the fetus represents an average of 25.3% (range, 22.7%–27.9%) of the total foot length; in the adult its contribution is 35% (33.2%–38.5%).

The long axes of the calcaneal tuber and of the tibial diaphysis determine the angle of torsion of the calcaneus (Fig. 1-22). At 3 months, the supination–varus angle of the calcaneus is 36.8° (35–38°). This angle decreases gradually, and by 9 months, it is 26.3° (24.5°–29.5°), and in the adult it measures 3.5° (1°–6°).[7] The calcaneus is overlapped by the talus, and during fetal growth the collum tali and calcaneal angle narrows from 42° at 4 months to 30° at birth. The

(Text continues on p. 16.)

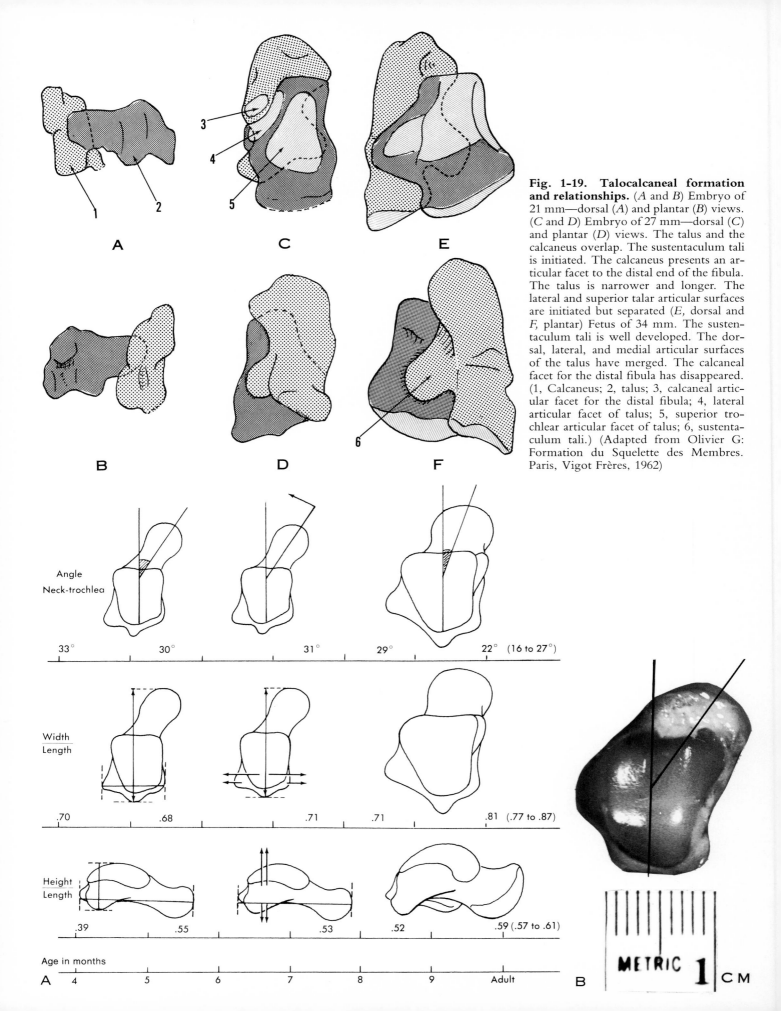

Fig. 1-19. Talocalcaneal formation and relationships. (*A* and *B*) Embryo of 21 mm—dorsal (*A*) and plantar (*B*) views. (*C* and *D*) Embryo of 27 mm—dorsal (*C*) and plantar (*D*) views. The talus and the calcaneus overlap. The sustentaculum tali is initiated. The calcaneus presents an articular facet to the distal end of the fibula. The talus is narrower and longer. The lateral and superior talar articular surfaces are initiated but separated (*E*, dorsal and *F*, plantar) Fetus of 34 mm. The sustentaculum tali is well developed. The dorsal, lateral, and medial articular surfaces of the talus have merged. The calcaneal facet for the distal fibula has disappeared. (1, Calcaneus; 2, talus; 3, calcaneal articular facet for the distal fibula; 4, lateral articular facet of talus; 5, superior trochlear articular facet of talus; 6, sustentaculum tali.) (Adapted from Olivier G: Formation du Squelette des Membres. Paris, Vigot Frères, 1962)

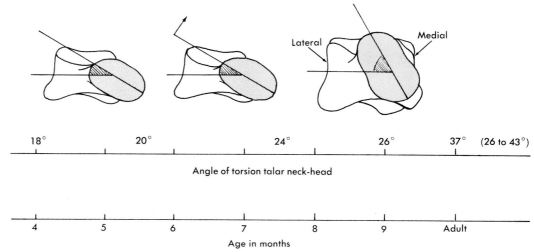

Angle of torsion talar neck-head

Age in months

Fig. 1-21.   Lateral rotation of the talar head in the fetus and in the postnatal phase. The rotation contributes to the prone position of the foot. (Diagrammatic representation based on data from Straus WL Jr: Growth of the human foot and its evolutionary significance. Contrib Embroyol 19:95, 1927)

Fig 1-22.   Morphologic changes and growth of the calcaneus. The posterior aspect of the calcaneal body grows faster than the anterior segment. In the fetus the os calcis is in varus torsion, which gradually diminishes. (Diagrammatic representation based on data from Straus WL Jr: Growth of the human foot and its evolutionary significance. Contrib Embryol 19:95, 1927)

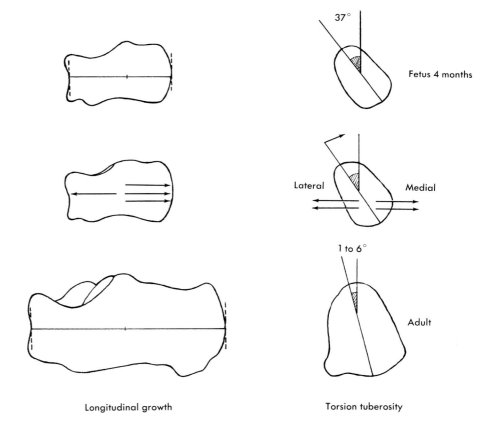

Longitudinal growth

Torsion tuberosity

Fig. 1-20.   (A) Morphologic changes and growth of the talus in fetus. (Diagrammatic representation based on data from Straus WL Jr: Growth of the human foot and its evolutionary significance. Contrib Embryol 19: 95, 1927) **(B) Declination angle between the trochea and the neck of the tatlus in 7-month fetus.**

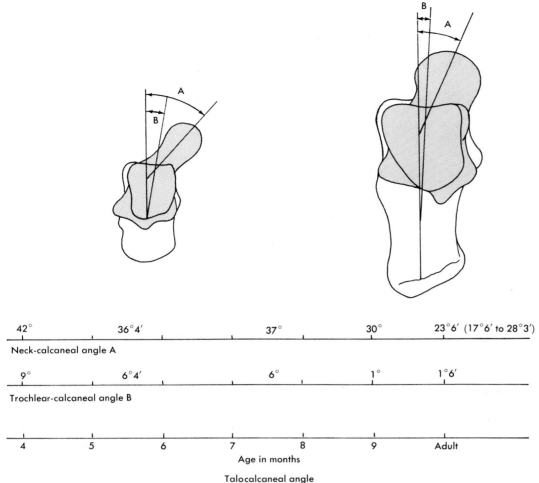

42°	36°4'	37°	30°	23°6' (17°6' to 28°3')

Neck-calcaneal angle A

9°	6°4'	6°	1°	1°6'

Trochlear-calcaneal angle B

4	5	6	7	8	9	Adult

Age in months

Talocalcaneal angle

Fig. 1-23. Talar neck and calcaneal angle (*A*) and talar trochlear and calcaneal angle (*B*) in the fetus and in postnatal phase. Both angles diminish with growth, and this contributes to the correction of the adducted position of the forefoot. (Diagrammatic representation based on data from Straus WL Jr: Growth of the human foot and its evolutionary significance. Contrib Embryol 19:95, 1927)

talar trochlear–calcaneal angle diminishes from 9° at 4 months to 1° at 9 months (Fig. 1-23).

In the fetus, the first metatarsal is shorter and thicker than the second metatarsal (Fig. 1-24).[7] Until birth, the first metatarsal grows faster than the second metatarsal; subsequently, they develop at about the same rate. The metatarsal 1/metatarsal 2 length ratio is 0.73 (0.63–0.81) at 3 months, 0.83 (0.80–0.85) at 9 months, and 0.83 (0.79–0.88) in the adult. The angle of divergence of the first two metatarsals is 32° at 2 months. Gradually the divergence of the first metatarsal decreases, and at 9 months the angle is 8.9° (3°–19.5°) and it is 6.2° (3°–9°) in the adult.

Early in fetal life there is a torsion of the first and second metatarsals, which gradually decreases and reaches 13° for the first metatarsal and 5° for the second metatarsal in the adult. The first metatarsal presents a lateral twist and the second a medial twist.

During early fetal life, the lateral *phalanges* are longer than in the adult, indicating a phalangeal reduction.[7] Si-

multaneously as the lesser toes reduce, the hallux reaches its dominant position. The reduction in the lesser toes occurs at the distal phalanges; the middle phalanges retain the same proportionate length, whereas the proximal phalanges become relatively longer with growth.

Fusion of the distal and middle phalanges of the little toe is common. Hasselmander reports this symphalangia to be present in 50% of fetuses and children; Straus reports a 9.4% occurrence in a corresponding group.[7,19] Pfitzner gives a figure of a 37% occurrence in the adult, whereas Adachi reports an 80% occurrence in the Japanese.

The *sesamoids* appear as condensed blastemic tissue at 8 weeks and as definite cartilage at 12 weeks.[20] They remain cartilaginous during the entire prenatal period.

Two sesamoids are regularly present at the metatarsophalangeal joint of the big toe. The lateral sesamoid appears first in the third month, followed in a week by the medial sesamoid, which may be bipartite.[21]

Sesamoids are also found sometimes at the metatarso-

Fig. 1-24. Intermetatarsal $M_1 - M_2$ angle and rotation of the metatarsal heads M_1 and M_2 during growth. The intermetatarsal angle (A) decreases with time. The first metatarsal grows faster than the lesser metatarsals to reach its adult length. (Diagrammatic representation based on data from Straus WL Jr: Growth of the human foot and its evolutionary significance. Contrib Embryol 19:95, 1927)

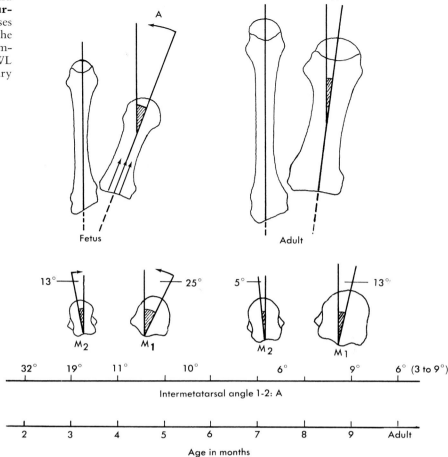

phalangeal joint of the little toe but rarely at the other metatarsophalangeal joints. Interphalangeal sesamoids are frequently seen in the big toe and are occasionally present in the little toe.[14]

A cartilaginous anlage of the *os trigonum* has been demonstrated in the 2 month fetus by Bardeleben.[22] Harris has described a cartilaginous anlage for the same skeletal element in a 12-week embryo (80.5 mm).[23] At birth the development center of the os trigonum is cartilaginous.[24]

Joints. A joint is formed initially by a homogenous cellular condensation in the interzone, which then becomes a three-layered zone, followed by the apparition of a cavity in its middle.[14] Synovial tissue then lines the cavity.

The homogenous interzones appear in the foot in horizon 20 at the metatarsophalangeal joint. By the end of the embryonic period (horizon 23), most of the interzones are still homogenous. The three-layered interzones occur subsequently during the fetal period of development. Cavitation is present in most of the joints between the seventh and ninth postovulation weeks. The time of initial appearance of the three-layered interzone and of the process of cavitation is, however, variable. Cavitation of the ankle occurs earlier, at horizon 23, 8 weeks post ovulation.

Leboucq attributes the abduction of the big toe in the embryo not only to the tibial deviation of the talar head but also to the obliquity of the distal articular surface of the first cuneiform.[25] "This surface, rather than to be located sensibly in the frontal plane, makes an angle of more than 45° [Fig. 1-25]. As the evolution progresses, the tibial surface of the cuneiform develops more rapidly than the peroneal surface and the position of the distal articular surface approximates that of the adult. The obliquity of the facet has nearly completely disappeared already in the fetus of 40 mm in length."[25]

Barlow, in a cross sectional study of the first metatarsocuneiform joint in 52 embryos and fetuses, indicates that the curvature of the joint is different in the upper and lower halves.[20] He makes, more specifically, the following observations (Fig. 1-26): *In the upper part of the joint* the articular surface of the metatarsal is always larger than that of the cuneiform, and in the majority of the sections, it is flatter than the corresponding cuneiform surface. The joint faces anteromedially up to 48 mm and slightly anteromedially at 75 mm, but at 86 mm it faces anteriorly. *In the lower part of the joint* the articular surface of the metatarsal coincides in size and curvature with that of the cuneiform, and the obliquity is not noticeable after 48 mm.

Leboucq reports on a calcaneonavicular fusion in an embryo of 25 mm, and a talocalcaneal fusion in a fetus of 80 mm.[26] Harris describes the occurrence of a talocalcaneal bridge in 4 (25 mm, 27.8 mm, 60.9 mm, and 72.3 mm) of

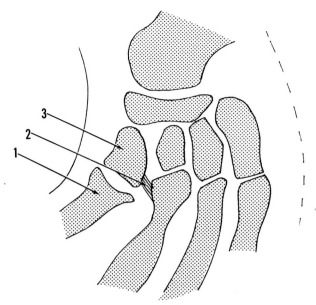

Fig. 1-25.   First metatarsocuneiform joint and Lisfranc's ligament in a cross section of an embryo foot measuring 2.3 mm. The embryo measures 21 mm. The distal surface of the first cuneiform makes a 45° angle with the frontal plane, and this contributes to the adducted position of the first metatarsal. (1, First metatarsal; 2, Lisfranc's ligament; 3, first cuneiform.) (Adapted from Leboucq G: Le développement du premier métatarsien et de son articulation tarsienne chez l'homme. Arch Biol 3:335, 1882)

20 embryos.[23] The union extends from the posterior aspect of the sustentaculum tali to the talus. This bridge could be bilateral or unilateral. According to Harris, the talocalcaneal bridge could resorb, remain cartilaginous, or ossify.[23] When the center ossifies only, an os sustentaculi results. Instances of calcaneonavicular fusion in fetuses are reported by O'Rahilly and co-workers.[27] Fusions involving the plantar aspect of the third metatarsal and third cuneiform or that of the fourth metatarsal with the cuboid are also reported by Harris.[23]

Ligaments and Tendon Sheaths. Ligaments differentiate during the fetal period of development prior to the formation of the joint space or the capsule. Specific studies are reported relative to the ligaments of the ankle and subtalar joints, extensor retinaculum or anterior annular ligament, medial annular ligament or flexor retinaculum, interosseous ligaments of Lisfranc's joint, fibrous tunnel of peronei, long plantar ligament, transverse metatarsal ligament.[20,28–33]

Beau studied the sequential development of the *ligaments of the ankle and subtalar joints* in fetuses from 33 mm to 85 mm.[28]

In the 33-mm fetus, the posterior talofibular ligament is first to appear and extends transversely from the inner surface of the lateral malleolus to the posterior border of the talus. The posterior tibiofibular ligament is present as a layer of fibrous tissue uniting the tibia and fibula. Slightly below, another tibiofibular ligament differentiates; this represents the future ligamentum transversum or inferior transverse tibiofibular ligament. This ligament is triangular and originates from the lower fibular extremity. Directed trans-

versely, it inserts along the posterior border of the tibia, reaching its inferomedial corner. The calcaneofibular ligament is clearly recognized. The anterior tibiofibular ligament is formed, but the anterior talofibular ligament is hardly seen. The deep layer of the deltoid or posterior talotibial ligament is already present and differentiates prior to the superficial layer, which is not clearly distinguishable at this stage. No ligaments are visible in the subtalar joint. With subsequent development, the posterior talofibular ligament bulges into the posterior ankle joint, depressing the capsule and thus forming two transverse cul-de-sacs. This arrangement gives the appearance of an intra-articular ligament.

In the 40-mm fetus, the superficial layer of the deltoid is well delineated. It originates from the medial malleolus, partly covers the posterior talotibial ligament, and inserts on the superomedial corner of the calcaneus, the sustentaculum tali, and the tuberosity of the navicular, forming a continuous fibrous envelope. Ligaments now also appear in the sinus tarsi. With further development, the origin of the extensor digitorum brevis is seen in the sinus tarsi. The heads of this muscle are separated by three fibrous septa. The most lateral septum enters in contact with the sheath of the peronei. The inner septum extends to form the sling for the extensor digitorum communis in front of the talus, and the deep surface of this sling attaches to the perichondrium of the talus.

In the 85-mm fetus, a well-organized talocalcaneal interosseous ligament is present, located in the mid portion between the articular capsules of the two subastragalar joints.

The peroneotalocalcaneal ligament of Rouvière and Canela Lazaro, the superomedial calcaneonavicular ligament (ligamentum neglectum), and the cervical talocalcaneal ligament have been demonstrated in the foot of a 7-month fetus (Fig. 1-27, *A, B, C*).

Lucien analyzed the development of the *anterior annular ligament* (extensor retinaculum) in fetuses measuring 30 mm to 70 mm (Fig. 1-28).[29]

Initially in the 30-mm embryo, the superior extensor retinaculum is recognized as a narrow cellular band extending from the inner border of the tibial epiphysis to the anterior border of the fibula. In this chondrocellular tunnel, the tendons of the tibialis anterior, extensor digitorum communis, and extensor hallucis longus are united with embryonic connective tissue. In the 40-mm fetus the inferior extensor retinaculum differentiates. The two extremities of this retinaculum arise (vaguely at this stage) from the sinus tarsi and form a distinct sling or frondiform ligament surrounding the extensor digitorum communis tendons. A second sling corresponding to the extensor hallucis longus is also recognized, but its limits are less precise. In the 65-mm fetus the two extremities of the inferior extensor retinaculum are clearly seen arising from the sinus tarsi. The sling of the extensor hallucis longus, which arises from the medial malleolus, fuses with the sling of the extensor digitorum communis. A third fibrous band is recognized distally over the second row of the tarsal bones. This retinaculum extends from the medial border of the scaphoid to the third cuneiform. It passes over the tendons of the tibialis anterior and extensor hallucis longus and enters in close relationship with the aponeurosis of the extensor digitorum brevis.

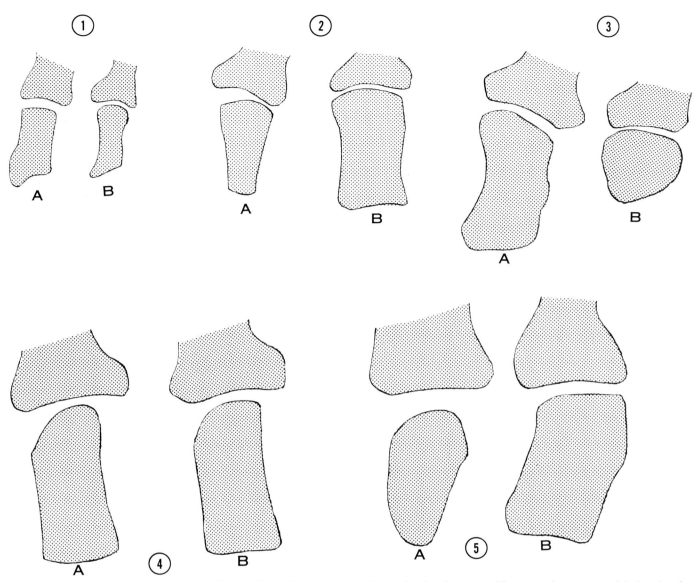

Fig. 1-26. Cross section through the first cuneiform and metatarsal joint in the embryo and the fetus. (*A*) Cross section at the level of Lisfranc's ligament. (*B*) Cross section at the level of the peroneus longus tendon. The curvatures of the surfaces are different in the upper (*A*) and lower (*B*) sections. In the upper part of the joint the articular surface of the first metatarsal is larger and flatter than that of the first cuneiform. The first cuneiform surface in the upper part is initially inclined anteromedially up to 48 mm and faces anteriorly by 86 mm. In the lower segment the articular surfaces of the first metatarsal–first cuneiform coincide in size and curvature. (1, 25-mm embryo; 2, 30-mm embryo; 3, 48-mm fetus; 4, 90-mm fetus; 5, 200-mm fetus.) (Adapted from Barlow TE: Some observations on the development of the human foot. Thesis University of Manchester, 1943)

The three fibrous bands sequentially determined in a proximodistal direction are completely independent intially from the superficial aponeurosis of the leg and the foot. Ultimately these structures blend and determine the architecture of the extensor retinaculum in the adult. The frondiform ligament is demonstrated in the dissected foot of a 7-month fetus in Figure 1-29.

The *medial annular ligament,* also known as laciniate ligament or flexor retinaculum, was also studied by Lucien in embryos measuring 30 mm to 70 mm.[30]

The deep component of the medial annular ligament forms first. Initially, three fibrous semirings appear around the tendons of the tibialis posterior, flexor digitorum longus, and flexor hallucis longus, anchoring the tendons against the skeletal elements (Fig. 1-30). Subsequently, the fibrous tunnels of the tibialis posterior and flexor digitorum longus are united by an expansion from the inferior extensor retinaculum. The leg aponeurosis differentiates next and unites the previous two tunnels to the aponeurosis of the abductor of the big toe. A fourth tunnel is thus formed,

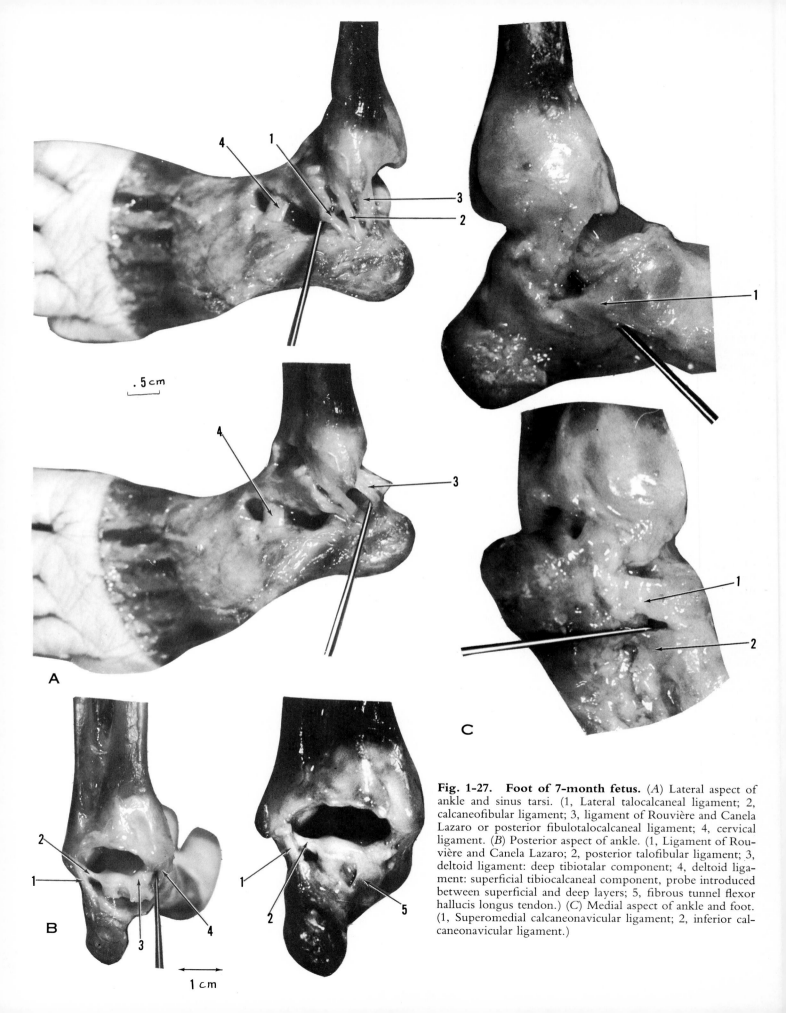

Fig. 1-27. **Foot of 7-month fetus.** (*A*) Lateral aspect of ankle and sinus tarsi. (1, Lateral talocalcaneal ligament; 2, calcaneofibular ligament; 3, ligament of Rouvière and Canela Lazaro or posterior fibulotalocalcaneal ligament; 4, cervical ligament. (*B*) Posterior aspect of ankle. (1, Ligament of Rouvière and Canela Lazaro; 2, posterior talofibular ligament; 3, deltoid ligament: deep tibiotalar component; 4, deltoid ligament: superficial tibiocalcaneal component, probe introduced between superficial and deep layers; 5, fibrous tunnel flexor hallucis longus tendon.) (*C*) Medial aspect of ankle and foot. (1, Superomedial calcaneonavicular ligament; 2, inferior calcaneonavicular ligament.)

.5 cm

1 cm

Fig. 1-28. Morphogenesis of the extensor retinaculum. (*A*) Embryo of 30 mm. (*B*) Fetus of 40 mm. (*C*) Fetus of 65 mm. The extensor retinaculum is formed in a proximal-to-distal direction. First to differentiate is the superior extensor retinaculum, followed by the frondiform ligament; this is followed by formation of the tunnel for the extensor hallucis longus. The tunnel of the tibialis anterior is the last to form at the level of the inferior extensor retinaculum. (1, Superior extensor retinaculum; 2, inferior extensor retinaculum—frondiform ligament of extensor digitorum communis [6]; 3, tunnel for extensor hallucis longus [7]; 4, tunnel for tibialis anterior tendon [8]; 5, distal extensor retinaculum for [7] and [8].) (Diagrammatic representation based on data from Lucien M: Notes sur le développement du ligament annulaire anterieur du tarse. Comptes Rendus Hebd Soc Biol 2:253, 1908)

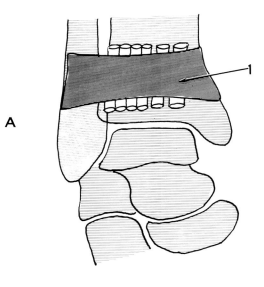

A

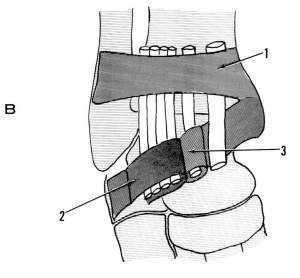

B

through which passes the neurovascular bundle. The tunnel of the flexor hallucis longus is deep in location and does not participate in the architecture of the annular ligament (Fig. 1-30). It thus becomes apparent that the laciniate ligament has a deep layer formed by arciform fibers representing the vestiges of the primitive peritendinous sheaths. These fibers correspond to the frondiform ligaments of the peronei and extensors. The superficial layer of this ligament is formed by oblique fibers arising from both the anterior annular ligament and the aponeurosis of the leg.

Thomas described the development of the *interosseous ligaments of Lisfranc's joint* in fetuses measuring 15.6 to 47 cm crown to heel.[31]

Initially, a transverse lamina formed of connective tissue is present, extending proximally from the cuneoscaphoid interline to the intermetatarsal zone at the base. In each intercuneiform, intermetatarsal region, the continuous layer of fibrous tissue is transversely oriented (Fig. 1-31). With subsequent growth of the chondral elements, the intercuneiform ligaments and the intermetatarsal ligaments are formed and retain their transverse direction. The middle fibers are obliquely oriented. In the first space the oblique fibers extend from the first cuneiform to the second metatarsal, forming Lisfranc's ligament (Fig. 1-31). Gradually the transverse intermetatarsal ligament M^1-M^2 disppears. Only the superior fibers persist, and these blend with the oblique cuneo$_1$-metatarsal$_2$ ligament. The first interspace is thus occupied only by Lisfranc's ligament.

No interosseous ligament is present between the cuboid and the fourth and fifth metatarsals (Fig. 1-31).

Lucien analyzed the formation of the *fibrous tunnels of the peronei tendons* in embryos and fetuses from 23 mm to 70 mm C-R length.[32]

The fibrous tunnel of the lateral peronei appears first in the form of a half-ring, cellular structure attached to the outer and inner borders of the retromalleolar canal. One tunnel results for the two peronei. Next to be differentiated is a double tunnel at the level of the lateral aspect of the calcaneus. The fibers of the cellular rings originate from the external calcaneal apophysis, separately encircle each tendon, and return to their point of origin. These two structures form the superior and inferior peronei retinaculum but are in continuity without a precise line of demarcation. The intermediary portion, however, remains very thin.

At the level of the sole of the foot, the sheath of the peroneus longus appears, attached posteriorly to the pos-
(Text continues on p. 24.)

C

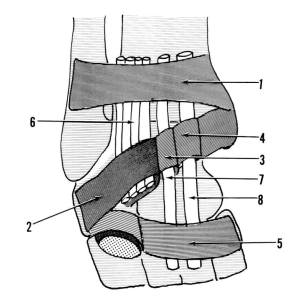

Fig. 1-29.   Frondiform ligament of the inferior extensor retinaculum in the foot of a 7-month fetus. (1, Frondiform ligament; 2, extensor digitorum communis tendons.)

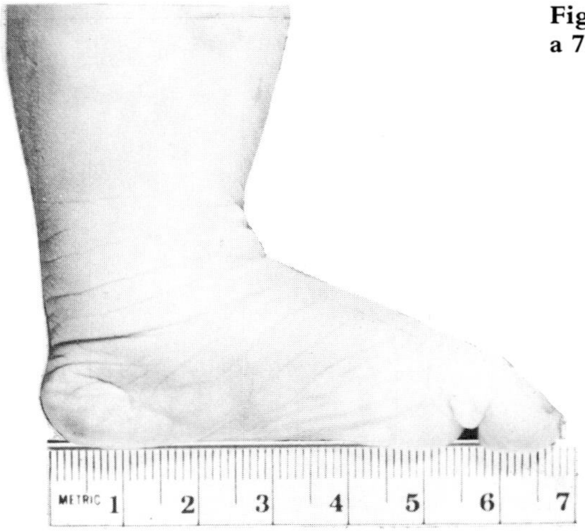

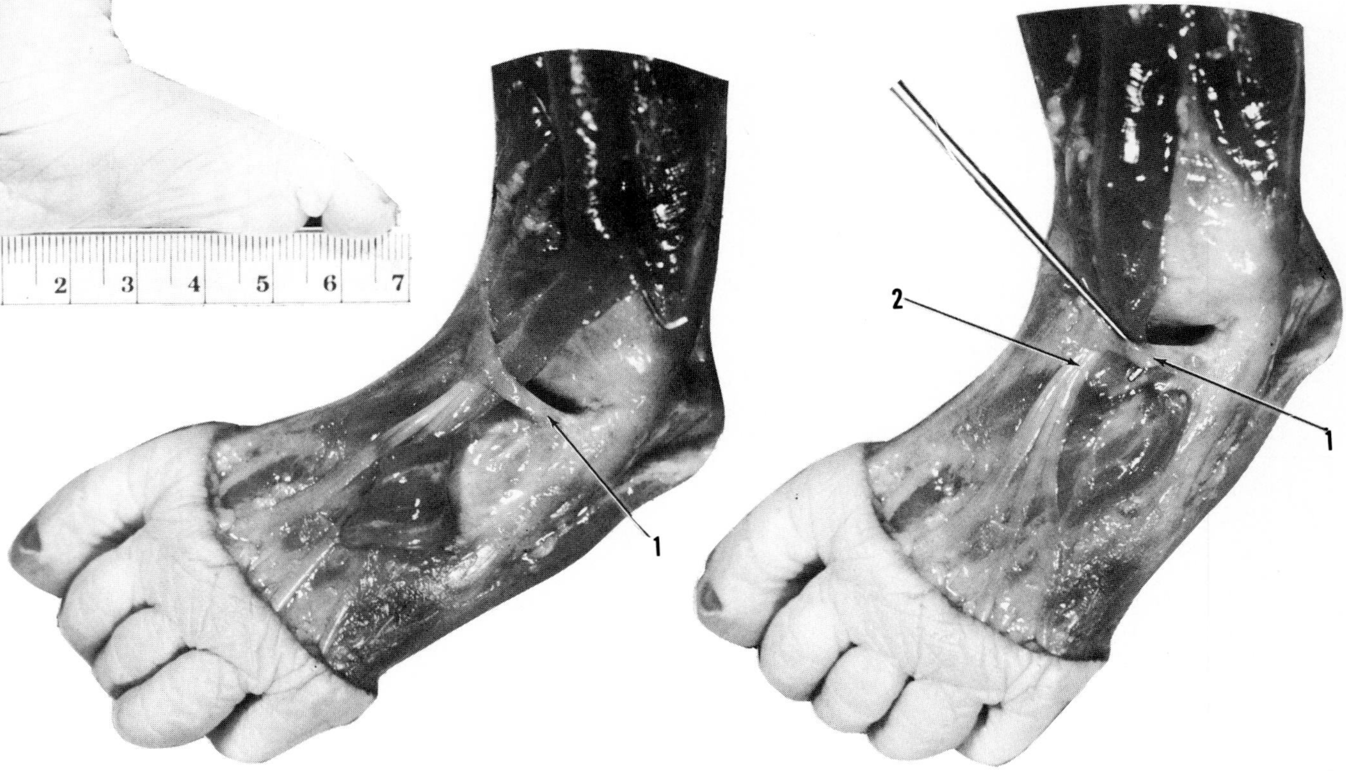

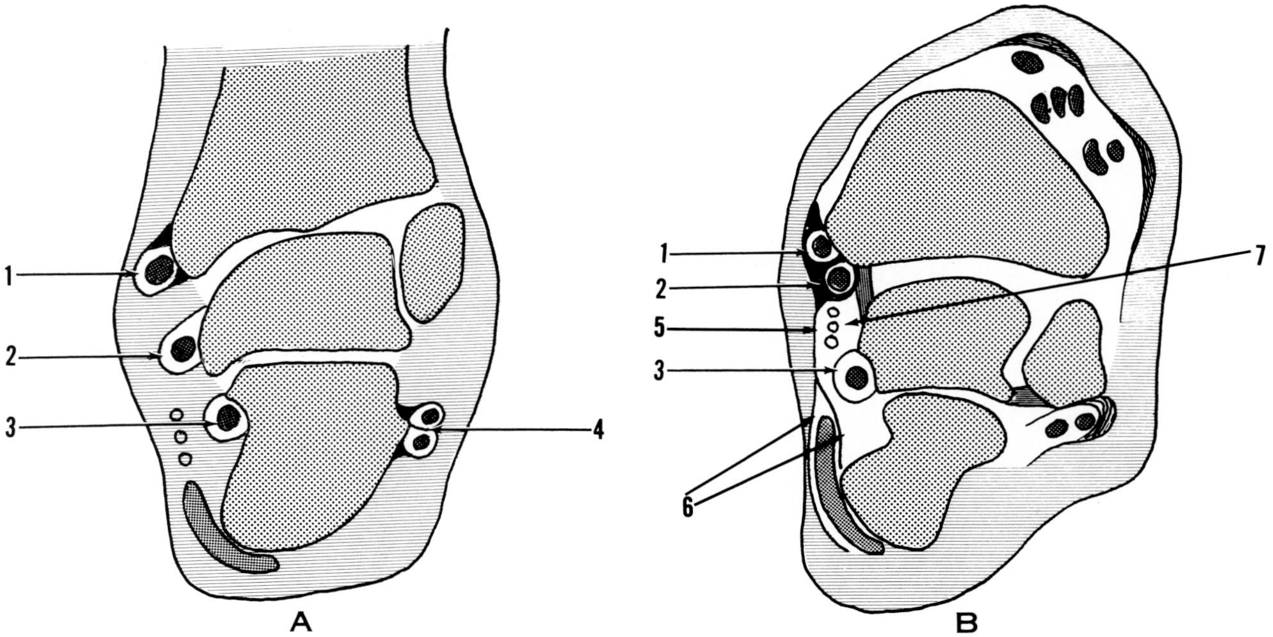

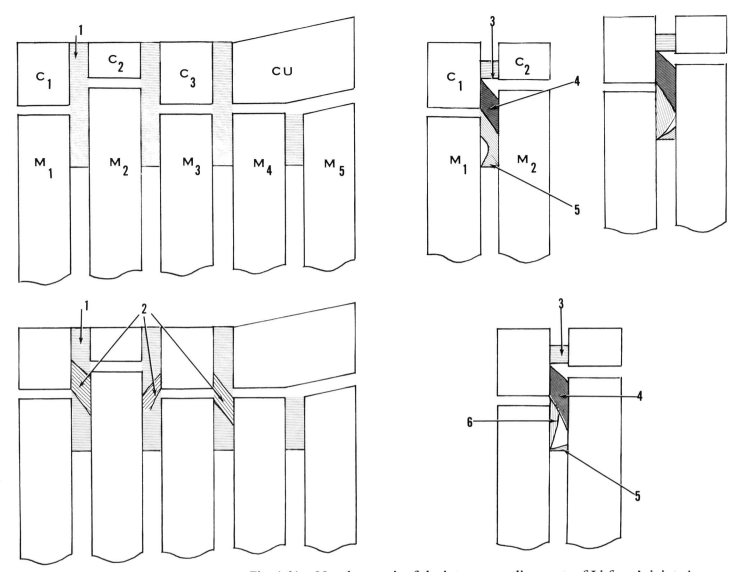

Fig. 1-31. Morphogenesis of the interosseous ligaments of Lisfranc's joint. A transverse homogenous lamina is formed initially. Within this lamina are next differentiated oblique cuneometatarsal ligaments. A regression of some fibers occurs, and in the first space are delineated the intercuneiform $C_1 - C_2$ ligament and Lisfranc's ligament. The intermetatarsal $M_1 - M_2$ ligament becomes very atrophic or may disappear completely. (C_1, first cuneiform; C_2, second cuneiform; C_3, third cuneiform; CU; cuboid; M_1 to M_5, metatarsals one to five; 1, homogenous transverse lamina; 2, differentiation of oblique cuneometatarsal ligaments; 3, intercuneiform $C_1 - C_2$ ligament; 4, Lisfranc's ligament; 5, intermetatarsal $M_1 - M_2$ ligament; 6, longitudinal remnant of intermetatarsal ligament $M_1 - M_2$.) (Adapted from Thomas L: Recherches sur les ligaments interosseux de l'articulation de Lisfranc. Arch Anat Histol Embryol 5:104, 1926)

Fig. 1-30. Morphogenesis of the flexor retinaculum or laciniate ligament. Frontal cross section of the ankle in (*A*) 49-mm embryo and (*B*) 65-mm embryo. The tunnels of the tibialis posterior, flexor digitorum longus, and flexor hallucis longus are formed first. Subsequently appears the flexor retinaculum, which adheres to the tunnels of the tibialis posterior and the flexor digitorum longus; splits into two layers, incorporating the abductor hallucis longus; unites with the extensor retinaculum; and forms the cover to the tarsal tunnel. It thus becomes apparent that the tendinous compartments at the level of the tarsal tunnel are not formed by deep expansions from the flexor retinaculum; instead, they antedate the latter. (1, Tunnel of tibialis posterior; 2, tunnel of flexor digitorium longus; 3, tunnel of flexor hallucis longus; 4, tunnel of peronei longus, brevis; 5, flexor retinaculum; 6, split layers of flexor retinaculum covering abductor hallucis; 7, medial neurovascular bundle.) (Adapted from Lucien M: Développement et signification anatomique du ligament lateral interne du cou-du-pied. Comptes-Rend Assoc Anat 10–11:182, 1908–1909)

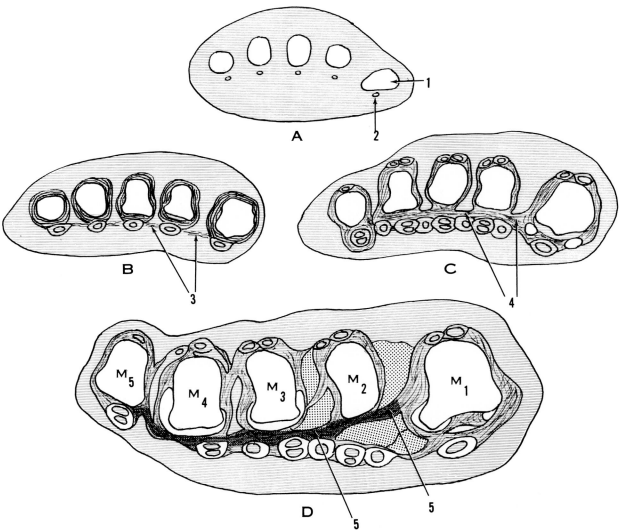

Fig. 1-32. Morphogenesis of the deep transverse metatarsal ligament—cross section of the foot. (*A*) Embryo of 22 mm. (*B*) embryo of 32 mm. (*C*) Fetus of 40 mm. (*D*) Fetus of 110 mm. (1, $M_1 - M_5$, Metatarsals one to five; 2, flexor hallucis longus tendon; 3, early formation of transverse metatarsal ligament; 4, further structuring of transverse metatarsal ligament; 5, transverse metatarsal ligament connecting plantar plates.) (Adapted from Barlow TE: Some observations on the development of the human foot. Thesis University of Manchester, 1943)

terior border of the cuboid groove and anteriorly to the base of the last metatarsal.[33] This tunnel is independent of the inferior calcaneocuboid ligament.

The lateral annular ligament is the last to appear and results from the fusion of the fibrous tunnel of the lateral peroneus to the superficial and middle aponeuroses of the leg.

The synovial sheath corresponding to the plantar segment of the peroneus longus tunnel differentiates first. A synovial cavity forms, with the mesotenon attached superiorly. Two synovial cavities are next formed, corresponding to the double portion of the peronei tendons, and these synovial cavities extend upward and penetrate the superior retromalleolar segment of the peronei tunnel. With further

development in the fetus, all three synovial cavities fuse and establish continuity.

Lucien and Bleicher analyzed the development and anatomy of the *long plantar ligament*.[33] In the fetus prior to 6 months, the calcaneocuboid component of the long plantar ligament and the fibrous sheath of the peroneus longus are clearly separate. The inferior calcaneocuboid ligament inserts on the crest of the cuboid and is well developed as a fibrous lamina, whereas at this stage the sheath of the peroneus longus tendon is much thinner and transparent. After 6 months, the distinction between these two structures becomes even more evident.

The embryologic development of the *transverse metatarsal ligament* has been studied by Barlow.[20] At 22 m, there is no evidence of this ligament in the region of the metatarsals (Fig. 1-32). At 23 mm, the beginnings of the transverse metatarsal ligament are seen. From 40 mm to 110 mm, the transverse metatarsal ligament is differentiated as an addition to the thick plantar portion of the capsule of the metatarsophalangeal joints. "There is no evidence in this series that there is a stage when the ligament includes the four lateral toes and not the great toe."[20]

Muscles and Nerves. Bardeen and Lewis have researched the development of muscles and nerves.[3, 34] At 9 mm the limb bud is filled with mesenchymal tissue. A capillary network connected with the umbilical artery and the cardinal vein soon make their appearance (Fig. 1-33). The nerves to the limb arise from the lumbosacral plexus and penetrate the bud (Fig. 1-33). During this process the skeletal and muscular anlages begin to differentiate *in situ*. At 11 mm the very condensed mesenchymal tissue or scleroblastema marks the development of the skeleton of the leg and, to a lesser degree, of the foot. An area of less-condensed tissue differentiates into a myogenous zone, the myoblastoma (Fig. 1-34, *A, B*). During this very early stage of development the true muscle tissue cannot be clearly distinguished from the skeletal anlage or scleroblastoma. The myoblastoma is not a homogenous zone. Anlages of muscle group are recognized early, separated more or less clearly from regions representing intermuscular spaces. The chief nerve trunks grow first in the regions where intermuscular spaces will develop. As the muscle group differentiates, the nerve trunk sends muscular branches into the muscle mass.

At 14 mm, the anlage of the ankle and foot is well differentiated. The main nerve trunks grow a considerable distance ino the limb, and multiple muscular and cutaneous branches arise. The differentiation of muscular tissue from the skeletal anlage is well marked (Fig. 1-35, *A*). The peroneal nerve extends over the dorsal aspect of the limb bud

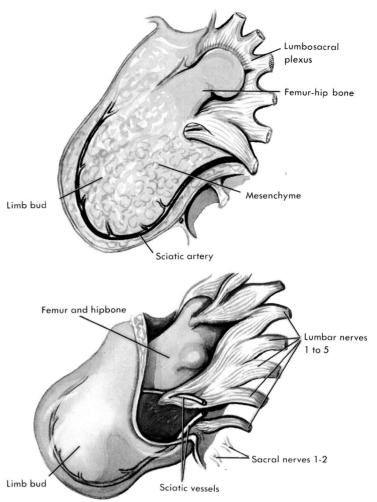

Fig. 1-33. Limb bud in 9 mm embryo, about 44 weeks. The five lumbar and the first two sacral nerves form a plexus, and the main four nerves enter the limb. The sciatic vessels are present in the bud. (After Bardeen CR, Lewis WH: Development of the limbs, body wall and back in man. Am J Anat 1:1, 1901–1902)

Fig. 1-34. Limb bud in 11-mm embryo about 5 weeks. (*A*) Flexor surface. Dense mesenchymal skeletal anlage is seen. The tibial nerve extends distally from the sciatic nerve and terminates in the flexor musculature anlage of the foot. The sciatic vessels are located at the periphery. (*B*) Extensor surface. Dense mesenchymal skeletal anlage is present. The extensor musculature anlage differentiates around the peroneal branches of the sciatic nerve. The peroneal musculature has not differentiated from the mesenchyme. (After Bardeen CR, Lewis WH: Development of the limbs, body wall and back in man. Am J Anat 1:1, 1901–1902)

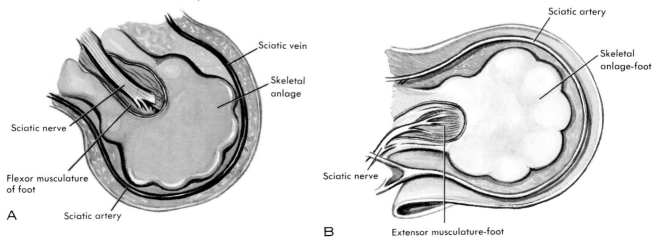

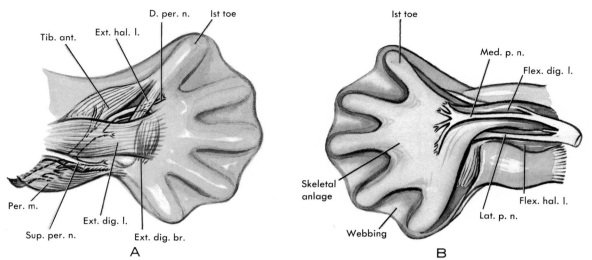

Fig. 1-35.   Foot plate in 14-mm embyro, 54 weeks. (*A*) Extensor surface. The peroneal and extensor muscles are differentiating. The superficial and deep peroneal nerves are recognized. The digital rays are well delineated with the connecting interdigital webbing. (*B*) Flexor surface. The medial and lateral plantar nerves are differentiated, including the flexor digitorum longus, the flexor hallucis longus, and the tibialis posterior muscles. (After Bardeen CR: Development and variation of the nerves and the musculature of the inferior extremity and of the neighboring regions of the trunk in man. Am J Anat 6:263, 1906–1907)

Fig. 1-36.   Foot in 20-mm embryo, about 7 weeks. (*A*) Extensor surface. The superficial peroneal nerve innervating the 34 medial digitis, the sural nerve innervating the lateral 14 digits, and the saphenous nerve are well defined. The peroneus longus and brevis muscles, the tibialis anterior, the extensor digitorum longus, and the extensor hallucis longus are well delineated. The extensor digitorum brevis is also present. (*B*) Extensor surface, deep layer. The anterior tibial nerve and the deep peroneal nerve are demonstrated. *D.p.n.,* deep peroneal nerve; *Sup.p.n.,* superficial peroneal nerve; *Sur.n.,* sural nerve; *Ant.tib.n.,* anterior tibial nerve.) (After Bardeen CR, Lewis WH: Development of thr limbs, body wall and back in man. Am J Anat 1:1, 1901–1902)

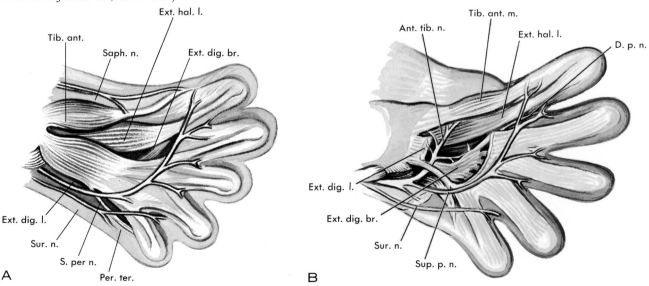

and ends in a slightly differentiated myogenous zone representing the anlage of the extensor muscles of the leg and foot. The anlage of the peroneal muscles is separated from the myogenous zone of the extensor group, and the superficial peroneal nerve runs between the two groups. The tibialis nerve is recognized with the medial plantar nerve on the tibial side and the lateral plantar nerve on the fibular side (Fig. 1-35, B). The former reaches the tarsus, whereas the latter does not yet reach as far distally. The muscles of the calf are very evident.

In the subsequent development, the muscle units are further delineated. Their anlages are often connected with the corresponding skeletal anlage at one end (less frequently, at both ends). The tendons are developed in continuity with the myogenous zones.

The peroneal nerve is divided into a superficial and a deep branch. The latter is clearly traced into the first intermetatarsal space.

The extensor muscle group of the leg and the foot is further differentiated. The anlage of the tibialis anterior is followed by a broad tendon that fades out over the first cuneiform and the first metatarsal base. From the central portion of the myogenous sheet, the extensor digitorum longus and the extensor hallucis longus differentiate simultaneously. An extensor tendon plate forms; initially this plate is connected to the metatarsal scleroblastema, but it gradually separates from the scleroblastema. The extensor digitorum brevis differentiates beneath the extensor tendon plate, which gradually becomes segmented. The tendon of the extensor hallucis longus, fused to this tendinous plate, acquires its independence through further development.

The peroneus longus muscle anlage is continued into a tendon that fades out over the base of the fifth metatarsal. The peroneus brevis lies close to the extensor digitorum brevis, and the tendon is not connected to the extensor tendon plate but independently reaches the base of the fifth metatarsal.

The medial and lateral plantar nerves are seen separately in the foot plate. The medial plantar nerve spreads out superficially to the plantar aponeurosis; the lateral plantar nerve crosses underneath.

The gastrocnemius–soleus group of muscles unites broadly with the scleroblastema of the calcaneus. The anlage of the flexor hallucis longus is distinct, and the flexor digitorum longus differentiates more medially. The anlage of the latter covers that of the tibialis posterior. Both flexor groups end up distally in a flexor tendon plate, a rather flat aponeurosis from which tendinous processes extend to the blastema of the metatarsals and toes. The tibialis posterior is formed from the deep region of the tibial portion of the flexor anlage. The tendon differentiates early and independently and reaches the anlage of the navicular.

In the sole of the footplate the anlage of the quadratus plantae and abductor digiti quinti may be seen, but the other intrinsic muscles are not defined.

At 20 mm, the nerves are well developed and the muscles of the foot are identifiable. The terminal branches of the common peroneal nerve are easily traced (Fig. 1-36, A, B). The superficial branch divides into two main terminal branches above the ankle. The medial branch reaches the

tibial aspect of the first toe and the second web space. It also sends a small anastomotic branch to the cutaneous branch of the first web space arising from the deep branch of the common peroneal nerve. The lateral branch extends to the third and fourth web spaces and the corresponding contiguous surface of the toes dorsally. The sural nerve is visible and supplies the peroneal border of the foot and the fourth web space. The tendon of the peroneous longus, intimately fused to the scleroblastema of the foot, can be partially traced in the sole. The saphenous nerve is continued in one or two main trunks toward the ankle medially. The relationship of the musculotendinous units on the dorsum of the foot closely resembles that in the adult. Tendinous attachments extend from the extensor tendon plate to the digits. The tibialis anterior makes a firm attachment to the first cuneiform and the first metatarsal base. The Achilles tendon is well differentiated. On the plantar aspect the long flexor muscles, continuous with the common plate, send extensions into the digits (Fig. 1-37, A, B). The anlages of most of the muscles can be distinguished but are incompletely differentiated (Fig. 1-37, A, B). The quadratus plate extends from the calcaneus to the deep surface of the plantar aponeurosis. The abductor digiti quinti reaches the base of the fifth metatarsal. The slightly differentiated anlages of the flexor brevis of the fifth toe and of the opponens digit quinti are present. The interossei and lumbricals are ill defined.

The flexor digitorum brevis differentiates on the surface of the flexor plate, and with further development, tendons are extended to the toes. The adductor hallucis is present. The transverse and oblique heads arise from the same anlage. The abductor hallucis can be distinguished but is not well defined. The flexor hallucis brevis begins to appear. It is incompletely divisible into a lateral and a medial portion. With further development, the lateral head approaches the adductor hallucis, whereas the medial head is associated with the abductor hallucis.

The medial plantar nerve reaches the medial aspect of the big toe and the three medial web spaces; the lateral plantar nerve extends to the fibular border of the fifth toe and the fourth web space.

In horizon 23, when the big toe is gradually adducted and the foot is rotated, the peroneus longus tendon attaches to the first cuneiform and the deep transverse metatarsal ligament develops, with its fibers attaching to the soft tissues around the head of the first metatarsal. In this horizon or slightly later, the tendons of the flexor digitorum longus and flexor hallucis longus cross in the tarsal region and are surrounded by a common sheath at the crossing point; a slip of tissue unites them.[23]

Arteries. The arteries during the fetal phase are illustrated in Figure 1-38.[35,36] In the 6-mm embryo, the axial artery arises from the dorsal root of the umbilical artery and ends up in two branches, each of which breaks up into a plexus.

At 8.5 mm, the axial artery passes distally into the posterior aspect of the skeletal anlage of the leg into the sole. Prior to ending in a plantar plexus, it gives origin to two or three branches, which perforate the mesenchymal skel-

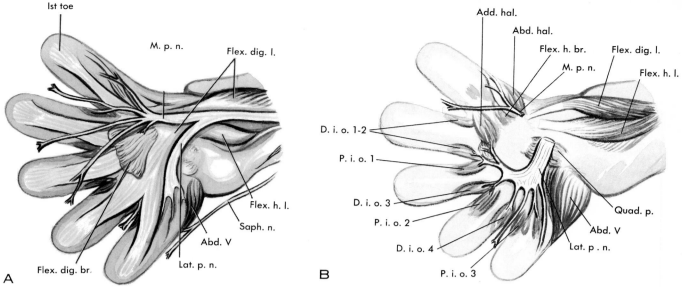

A

B

Fig. 1-37.   Foot in 20-mm embryo about 7 weeks, flexor surface. (*A*) Superficial layer. The medial and lateral plantar nerves and the saphenous nerve are well delineated and in their definitive positions. The tibialis posterior muscle, the flexor digitorum longus, and the flexor hallucis longus muscles are well formed. The flexor digitorum brevis is differentiated. (*B*) Deep layer. The intrinsic muscles are delineated. *D.i.o. 1-4,* dorsal interossei muscles, 1 to 4; *P.i.o. 1-3,* plantar interossei muscles 1 to 3; *Add.hal.,* adductor hallucis muscle; *Flex.h.br.,* flexor hallucis brevis muscle; *Abd.hal.,* abductor hallucis muscle; *Quad.p.,* quadratus plantae muscle; *Abd.V,* abductor digiti quinti; *M.p.n.,* medial plantar nerve; *Lat.p.n.,* lateral plantar nerve.) (After Bardeen CR: Development and variation of the nerves and the musculature of the inferior extremity and of the neighboring regions of the trunk in man. Am J Anat 6:263, 1906–1907)

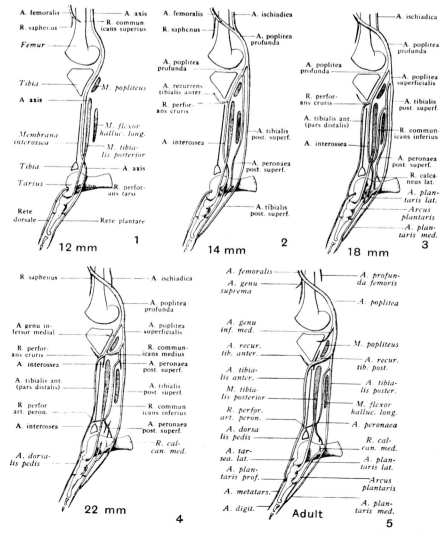

Fig. 1-38.   Morphogenesis of the main arteries of the leg and foot at four stages of development and in the adult. Labels in Roman type refer to embryonic arteries; italics are used for adult arteries and for all other structures. (From Senior HD: An interpretation of the recorded arterial anomalies of the human leg and foot. Anat 53:130, 1919)

Fig. 1-39.   Arteries supplying the foot in 17.8-mm embryo. The medial branch of the artery peronea posterior superficialis divides into two branches and unites the artery tibialis posterior superficialis to the plantar branch of the artery interossea. (1, Artery tibialis anterior; 2, artery interossea dividing into two branches; dorsal, forming artery perforans tarsi [5], and plantar, contributing to formation of lateral plantar artery [7]; 3, artery peronea posterior superficialis dividing into two branches, lateral and medial; 4, artery tibialis posterior superficialis forming the medial plantar artery [6].) (Diagrammatic representation based on data from Senior HD: An interpretation of the recorded arterial anomalies of the human leg and foot. J Anat 53:130, 1919)

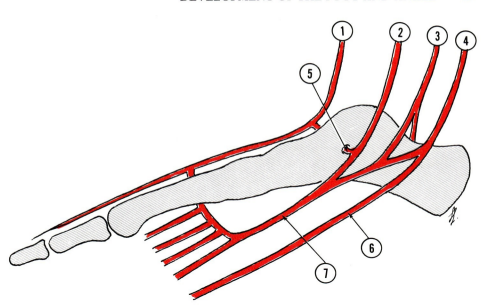

eton and reach the dorsum of the foot, forming a dorsal plexus.

At 12 mm, the dorsal and plantar retia (plexuses) of the foot are richer. The axial artery is now connected to the dorsal rete of the foot through a single vessel of large size, the ramus perforans tarsi.

At 14 mm, major changes occur. The femoral artery participates in the blood supply of the leg and foot. A superior communicating artery unites the femoral artery of the thigh to the axial or sciatic artery. An arterial branch, the ramus perforans cruris, passes through the proximal end of the tibiofibular interspace. The axial artery is now divided into three segments: the ischiatic artery (proximal to the superior communicating artery), the arteria poplitea profundus (between the superior communicating artery and the ramus perforans cruris), and the interosseous artery (distal to the perforans cruris). Two branches arise from the arteria poplitea profundus: the arteria tibialis posterior superficialis and the arteria peronea posterior superficialis. The former penetrates the sole, whereas the latter ends blindly in a medial and a lateral branch. At 17.8 mm, the tibialis anterior artery appears, originating from the ramus perforans cruris and ending in the dorsal foot plexus. In this proliferative stage, four major arterial lines reach the foot: arteria tibialis posterior superficialis, arteria peronea posterior superficialis, arteria interossea (former arteria axis), and arteria tibialis anterior.

The arteria interossea is divided into two branches: plantar and dorsal. The dorsal branch is the arteria perforans tarsi. It passes dorsally through the talocalcaneal mass and is joined by the distal segment of the arteria tibialis anterior to form the dorsal arterial system. The plantar branch of the arteria interossea courses distally and forms the lateral plantar artery and the deep plantar arch after receiving the terminal branch of the arteria peronea superficialis. The latter unites the plantar branch of the arteria interossea to the arteria tibialis posterior superficialis. The medial plantar artery is the terminal branch of the latter (Fig. 1-39).

At 18 mm, the ischiatic artery becomes slender and the femoral artery enlarges. The arterial arrangement is similar to that in the preceding stage except for a new communicating branch, the ramus communicans inferiori, extending from the anterior arteria peronea superficialis to the interosseous artery.

At 22 m, the ischiatic artery is interrupted, and the blood supply to the leg and foot is provided only by the femoral artery. Proximally, a new branch, the ramus communicans medius, connects the anterior tibial artery with the distal part of the anterior arteria poplitea profundus. Regressive changes now occur: The arteria interossea disappears, including the dorsal ramus perforans tarsi and a segment of its plantar branch up to the point of union with the anastomotic branch of the arteria peronea posterior superficialis. The lateral plantar artery is now only a branch of the arteria tibialis posterior superficialis. Also, the arteria peronea posterior superficialis, including its medial division branch, disappears. The lateral terminal branch of this artery unites with the ramus communicans inferioris. The latter now becomes the adult peroneal artery and sends a ramus perforans, the peroneal perforating artery, to the arteria tibialis anterior.

The adult arterial pattern of the foot is achieved by the eighth week.

Postnatal Development of the Foot
GROWTH OF THE NORMAL FOOT

Growth of the normal foot is illustrated in Figure 1-40. The length and growth pattern of the foot during childhood and adolescence, from age 1 to 18 years, has been studied by Anderson and co-workers and Blais and co-workers.[37,38]

The length of the foot is measured from the back of the heel to the tip of the great toe in the standing position. The analyzed group comprised 227 girls and 285 boys.

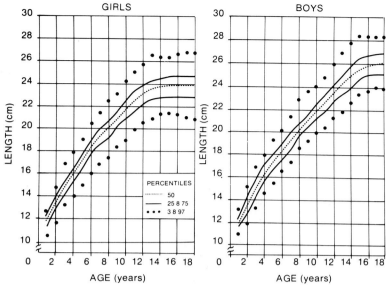

Fig. 1-40. **Length of normal foot.** (From Blais MM, Green WT, Anderson M: Lengths of the growing foot. J Bone Joint Surg 38 [A]:998, 1956)

At age 1 year in girls and 1.5 years in boys, the foot has achieved half the mature or adult dimension. The average annual increase in length is 0.9 cm from age 5 years through 12 years in girls and from 5 years through 14 years in boys, after which time the rate of growth markedly decreases. The mature foot length is reached at the average age of 14 years in girls and 16 years in boys. At all ages through 12 years the average length of the foot is about the same for girls as for boys. At 12 years of age, the average foot length is 23.2 cm for girls and 23.5 for boys. After the age of 12, the foot grows slowly in girls for the next 2 years, with an average increase of 0.8 cm. The foot in boys continues to grow until age 16 and is an average of 2.2 cm longer than the female foot. The foot grows in synchrony with the body rather than with the lower extremity. Adult length is achieved first in the foot, next in the long bones, and last in stature.

In the female the foot increases in size and width during and following pregnancy.[39]

PRIMARY AND SECONDARY OSSIFICATION CENTERS AND EPIPHYSEAL CLOSURES

Primary and secondary ossification centers and epiphyseal closures are shown in Figure 1-41. A comprehensive study of the postnatal appearance of the ossification centers and closure of the epiphyseal plates of the foot has been conducted by Hoerr and associates.[40] Variation ranges are evident when the available data from different sources are compared.[41-43] In the postnatal period the primary ossification center of the lateral cuneiform is first to appear, followed by the secondary ossification center of the distal fibula. The sequence of ossification continues with the medial cuneiform, the intermediary cuneiform, and the navicular in the tarsus. At the level of the forefoot, the ossification center of the distal phalangeal epiphysis of the big toe is first to appear, followed by the ossification of the

basal epiphyses of the proximal phalanges of toes two, three, and four. Subsequently the epiphyseal ossification of the central lesser toes continues in a proximal distal direction. The epiphyseal ossification centers of the distal phalanges of the lesser toes are seen at 3 to 4 years. In the big toe the secondary ossification centers appear in a distal to proximal direction. At the level of the metatarsal heads, the epiphyseal ossification centers appear in a medial to lateral direction (M_2–M_5). The ossification centers—primary or secondary—appear and close at the dates shown in Table 1-1.[40]

POSTNATAL STRUCTURAL CHANGES

The skeletal development changes initiated during the fetal period continue until adulthood; of interest are the structural changes occurring in the distal tibia, talus, os calcis, and metatarsals.

Fig. 1-41. **Postnatal primary and secondary ossification centers and epiphyseal closures.** (*A*) Cluster of ossification centers in cuboid. (*B*) Onset of ossification, lateral cuneiform. (*C*) Onset of ossification, medial cuneiform. Ossification of the great toe phalangeal epiphyses occurs in a distal-to-proximal sequence; in the lesser toes, it is the opposite. (*D*) Ossification of the epiphysis of the first metatarsal base and of the capital epiphysis of the other metatarsals follows a medial-to-lateral sequence. (*E*) Onset of ossification of the navicular is variable (2.7 years to 4 years) and late compared with that of the other tarsal bones. (*F*) Onset of ossification of calcaneal apophysis. (*G*) Onset of ossification of the trigonum. (*H*) Onset of ossification of the apophysis of the fifth metatarsal base and of the lateral sesamoid of the big toe. (*I*) Epiphyseal closure of the apophysis of the base of the fifth metatarsal, occurring before age 15 years for males and 12 years for females. (*J*) Epiphyseal closures occurring around 16 years for males and 14 years for females. (*B*, At birth; letters preceding numbers—*M*, month *Y*, year; letters following numbers—*M*, male, *F*, Female.)

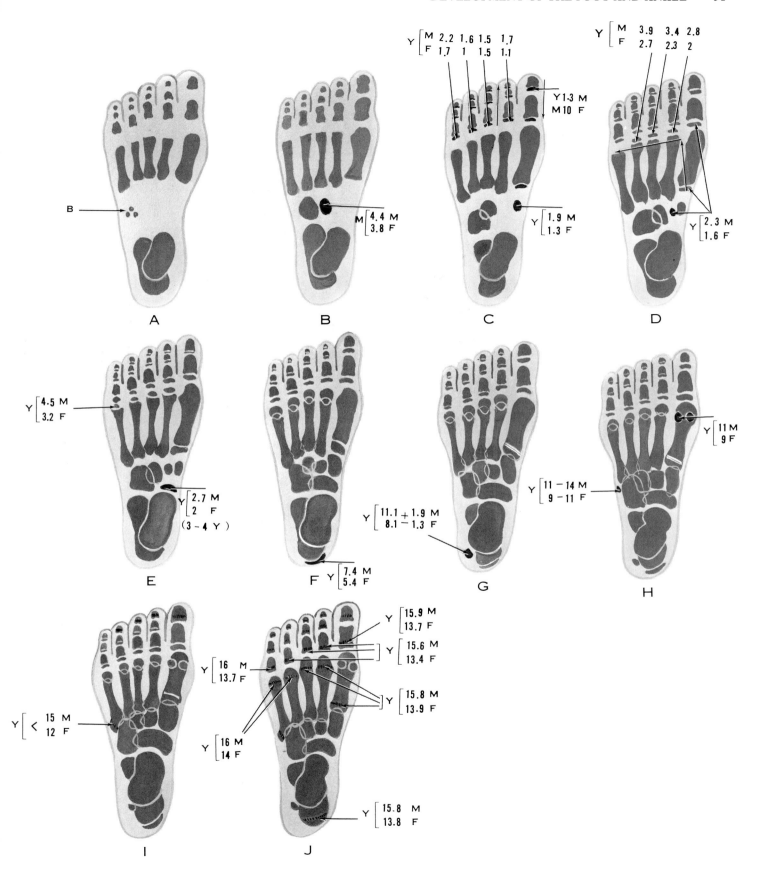

TABLE 1-1. Average Times of Appearance and Closure of Ossification Centers

Site	Ossification Center		Site	Ossification Center	
	Appearance	**Closure**		**Appearance**	**Closure**
Distal tibia–fibiula			**Big toe ray (con't)**		
Distal tibial epiphysis	4.1 mo M, 3.7 mo F	16.4 yr M, 14.4 yr F	Metatarsal 1, head epiphysis‡ (present in 96% of children 4–5 yr)	2–3 yr	10–11 yr
Distal fibular epiphysis	12.5 mo M, 9.1 mo F	16.4 yr M, 14.1 yr F	Sesamoids metatarsophalangeal (lateral precedes the medial)		
Separate accessory centers*†			Lateral	11 yr M, 9 yr F	
Medial malleolus (20%) } Lateral malleolus (1%)	8.7 yr M, 7.6 yr F	12 yr, M F	**Lesser toe rays**		
			Proximal phalanges, epiphysis		
Tarsus			Toe two	1.7 yr M, 1.1 yr F	15.6 yr M, 13.4 yr F
Lateral cuneiform	4.4 mo M, 3.8 mo F		Toe three	1.5 yr M, 1.5 yr F	15.6 yr M, 13.3 yr F
Medial cuneiform	1.9 yr M, 1.3 F		Toe four	1.6 yr M, 1 yr F	15.6 yr M, 13.4 yr F
Intermediary cuneiform	2.3 yr M, 1.6 yr F		Toe five	2.2 yr M, 1.7 yr F	16 yr M, 13.7 yr F
Navicular	2.7 yr M, 2 yr F (ranges up to 3–4 yr)		**Metatarsals, capital epiphysis**		
Calcaneal apophysis	7.4 yr M, 5.4 yr F	15.8 yr M, 13.8 yr F	Metatarsal 2	2.8 yr M, 2 yr F	15.8 yr M, 13.9 yr F
Secondary ossification center posterior border of talus	11.1 ± 1.9 yr M, 8.1 ± 1.3 yr F	12.9 ± 1.3 yr M, 9.8 ± 1.3 yr F	Metatarsal 3	3.4 yr M, 2.3 yr F	15.8 yr M, 13.9 yr F
			Metatarsal 4	3.9 yr M, 2.75 yr F	15.9 yr M, 14 yr F
			Metatarsal 5	4.5 yr M, 3.2 yr F	16 yr M, 14.1 yr F
Os trigonum (14% M, 18% F)	11.1 ± 1.9 yr M, 8.1 ± 1.3 yr F	Remains unfused; ossification completed as in posterior border of talus	Apophysis tuberosity of metatarsal 5§	11–14 yr M, 9–11 yr F	Before 15 yr M, before 12 yr F
Forefoot			**Distal phalanges, epiphysis**		
Big toe ray			Toe two	4.7 yr M, 2.9 yr F	14.7 yr M, 11.8 yr F
Distal phalanx, ephiphysis	1.3 yr M, 10 mo F	16.3 yr M, 13 yr F	Toe three	4.4 yr M, 3.2 yr F	14.7 yr M, 11.7 yr F
Proximal phalanx, epiphysis	2.3 yr M, 1.6 yr F	15.9 yr M, 13.7 yr F	Toe four	4.2 yr M, 2.5 yr F	14.6 yr M, 11.5 yr F
Metatarsal 1, base epiphysis	2.3 yr M, 1.6 yr F	15.8 yr M, 13.7 yr F			

*Powell HDW: Extra centre of ossification for the medial malleolus in children: Incidence and significance. J Bone Joint Surg [Br] 43:107, 1961

†Selby S: Separate centers of ossification of the tip of the internal malleolus. Am J Roentgenol 86:496, 1961

‡Vilaseca RR, Ribes ER: The growth of the first metatarsal bone. Foot Ankle 1:117, 1980

§Dameron TB: Fractures and anatomical variations of the proximal portion of the fifth metatarsal. J Bone Joint Surg [Am] 57:788, 1975

M, male; F, female

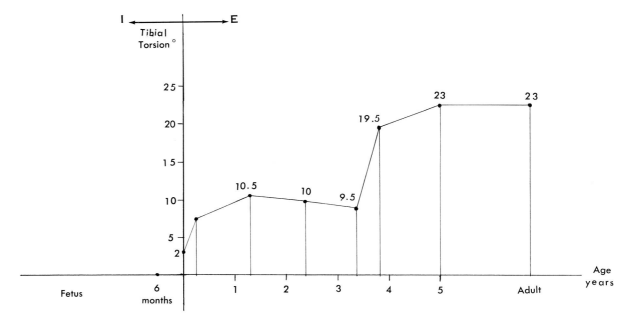

Fig 1-42. External torsion of the tibia during growth. (*E*, external torsion; *I*, internal torsion.) (After Dupuis PV: La Torsion Tibiale: Sa Mesure—Son Intérêt Clinique, Radiologique et Chirurgical. Liège et Paris, Dosoer et Masson, 1951)

Distal Tibia

Le Damany, in an anatomic study of the distal tibia in the fetus, newborn, and adult, has demonstrated that the distal end of the tibia in the fetus and the newborn has no torsion.[44] External torsion of the distal end of the tibia is then acquired and increases gradually, reaching the adult degree of external torsion by age 5 years.

LeDamany's measurements of the external torsion of the distal tibia were in 100 right adult tibias, 23.5° average; in 100 left adult tibias, 20° average.

Dupuis, in a comprehensive study of tibial torsion, has provided more detail about the sequential acquisition of the torsion after birth.[45] In the newborn, there is a minimal degree of external torsion (2°) of the distal tibia in the majority; in about 40%, an internal torsion of 0° to 10° may be present. During the first 3 months of postnatal life, there is a rapid increase in the external torsion, which will reach an average of 10° and remain stationary during the second and third years of life. Between 3.5 years and 4 years, there is again a sudden increase of the external tibial torsion, which will average 20°. From 4 to 5 years the torsion reaches 23°, which is the average external tibial torsion seen in the adult (Fig. 1-42).

Talus

The declination angle between the axis of the trochlea of the talus and that of the talar neck is about 29° at birth and decreases until adulthood, reaching an average value of 22°

(16°–27°).[7] From birth to adulthood the talus grows faster in width and height relative to the talar length. The relative values are as follows: talar width/length is 0.71 in the newborn, 0.81 (0.77–0.87) in the adult; talar height/length is 0.52 in the newborn, 0.59 (0.57–0.61) in the adult. The external rotation of the talar head continues and progresses from 23° at birth to 37° (26°–43°) in adulthood.[7]

Os Calcis

The varus position of the os calcis diminishes after birth until cessation of bone growth.[7] The posterior segment of the calcaneal body maintains its increased rate of growth as compared with the anterior segment. The talar neck–calcaneal angle is 30° at birth and decreases to 23.6° (17.6°to 289.3°) in the adult.

Metatarsals

The intermetatarsal angle M_1-M_2 is 9° (average) in the newborn and decreases to 6° in the normal adult foot.[7]

The longitudinal arch of the foot is not clinically apparent in the newborn, because it is hidden by adipose tissue. It does not shape before 12 months to 16 months, and a definite longitudinal arch is present by 2 years. By 2.5 years, maximum longitudinal arching is attained, with the apex located at the junction of the posterior third and the distal two thirds of the medial longitudinal arch; the apex corresponds to the tuberosity of the navicular.[39]

REFERENCES

1. Streeter, GL: Developmental horizons in human embryos. In Contributions to Embryology, Vols 21, 32, 34. Washington DC: Carnegie Institution of Washington, 1945, 1948, 1951
2. Patten BM: Human Embryology, 2nd ed, p. 185. St Louis, McGraw-Hill, 1953
3. Bardeen CR, Lewis WH: Development of the limbs, body wall and back in man. Am J Anat 1:1, 1901–1902
4. O'Rahilly R, Gardner E, Gray DJ: The ectodermal thickening and ridge in the limbs of staged human embryos. J Embryol Exp Morphol 4:256, 1956
5. Bohm M: The embryologic origin of club-foot. J Bone Joint Surg 11, No. 2:229, 1929
6. Jones WF: Structure and Function as Seen in the Foot, 2nd ed, p 24. London, Baillière, Tindall & Cox, 1949
7. Straus WL, Jr: Growth of the human foot and its evolutionary significance. Contrib Embryol 19, No. 101:95, 1927
8. Cummins H: The topographic history of the volar pads (walking pads, Tastballen) in the human embryo. Contrib Embryol 20, No. 113:105, 1929
9. Streeter GL: Weight, sitting height, head size, foot length and menstrual age of the human embryo. Contrib Embryol 11, No. 55:156, 1920
10. Scammon RE, Calkins LA: The Development and Growth of the External Dimensions of the Human Body in the Fetal Period, pp 245–246. Minneapolis, University of Minnesota Press, 1929
11. Bardeen CR: Studies of the development of the human skeleton. Am J Anat 4: 265, 1905
12. O'Rahilly R, Gray DJ, Gardner E: Chondrification in the hands and feet of staged human embryos. Contrib Embryol 36, No. 250:185, 1957
13. Senior HD: The chondrification of the human hand and foot skeleton (abstr). Anat Rec 42:35, 1929
14. Gardner E, Gray DJ, O'Rahilly R: The prenatal development of the skeleton and joints of the human foot. J Bone Joint Surg [Am] 41, No. 5:847, 1959
15. Noback CR, Robertson GG: Sequences of appearance of ossification centers in the human skeleton during the first five prenatal months. Am J Anat 89, No. 1:16, 1951
16. Christie A: Prevalence and distribution of ossification centers in the newborn. Am J Dis Child 77:355, 1949
17. Dixey FA: On the ossification of the terminal phalanges of the digits. Proc R Soc Lond 31:63, 1881
18. Olivier G: Formation du Squelette des Membres, pp 145–189. Paris, Vigot Frères, 1962
19. Hasselmander: In Straus WL Jr: Growth of the human foot and its evolutionary significance. Contrib Embryol 19:95, 1927
20. Barlow TE: Some observations on the development of the human foot. Thesis, University of Manchester, Manchester, 1943
21. Inge GAL, Ferguson AB: Surgery of sesamoid bones of the great toe. Arch Surg 27:466, 1933
22. Bardeleben, C: Das Intermedium Tarsi beim Menschen. Sitzungsberichte Jenaischen Gesellschaft Medicin Naturwissenschaft 2 März, 37, 1883
23. Harris BJ: Observations on the development of the human foot. Thesis, University of California, 1955
24. Dwight T: Clinical Atlas: Variations of the Bones of the Hand and Foot, p. 15. Philadelphia, JB Lippincott, 1907
25. Leboucq H: Le développement du premier metatarsien et de son articulation tarsienne chez l'homme. Arch Biol 3:335, 1882
26. Leboucq H: De la soudure congénitale de certains os du tarse. Bull Acad, Royale Med Belgique 4, 4, No. 2:1890
27. O'Rahilly R, Gardner E, Gray DJ: The skeletal development of the foot. Clin Orthop 16:7, 1960
28. Beau A: Recherches sur le développement et la constitution morphologiques de l'articulation du cou-du-pied chez l'homme. Arch Anat Histol Embryol 26:205, 1939
29. Lucien M: Notes sur le développement du ligament annulaire anterieur du tarse. Comptes Rendus Hebd Soc Biol 2:253, 1908
30. Lucien M: Développement et signification anatomique du ligament lateral interne du cou-du-pied. Comptes Rendus Assoc Anat 10–11:1908–1909
31. Thomas L: Recherches sur les ligaments interosseux de l'articulation de Lisfranc. Arch Anat Histol Embryol 5:104, 1926
32. Lucien M: Note sur le développement des coulisses fibreuses et des gaines synoviales annexées aux péroniers latéraux. Comptes Rendus Assoc Anat 148, 1908
33. Lucien M, Bleicher M: Le grand ligament de la plante et ses constituants anatomiques. Comptes Rendus Assoc Anat No. 3:285, 1928
34. Bardeen CR: Development and variation of the nerves and the musculature of the inferior extremity and of the neighboring regions of the trunk in man. Am J Anat 6:263, 1906–1907
35. Senior HD: The development of the arteries of the human lower extremity. Am J Anat 25:55, 1919
36. Senior HD: An interpretation of the recorded arterial anomalies of the human leg and foot. J Anat 53:130, 1919
37. Anderson M, Blais M, Green TW: Growth of the normal foot during childhood and adolescence. Am J Phys Anthropol 14:287, 1956
38. Blais MM, Green WT, Anderson M: Lengths of the growing foot. J Bone Joint Surg [Am] 38:998, 1956
39. Giannestras JJ: Foot Disorders, 2nd ed, pp 70–73, 84. Philadelphia, Lea & Febiger, 1973
40. Hoerr LN, Pyle SI, Francis CC: Radiographic Atlas of Skeletal Development of the Foot and Ankle—A Standard of Reference. Springfield, Charles C Thomas, 1962
41. Caffey J: Pediatric X-Ray Diagnosis, Vol 2, 6th ed, p 884. Chicago, Year Book Medical Publishers, 1972
42. Lang J, Wachsmuth W: Praktische Anatomie Erster Band Vierter Teil—Bein und Statik, p 31. Berlin, Springer Verlag, 1972
43. Paturet G: Traité d'Anatomie Humaine. Vol 2, Membres Supérieur et Inférieur, pp 627–629. Paris, Masson et Cie, 1951
44. Le Damany P: La torsion du tibia: Normale, pathologique, expérimentale. J Anat Physiol Normal Patholog 45:598, 1909
45. Dupuis PV: La Torsion Tibiale: Sa Mesure—Son Intérêt Clinique, Radiologique et Chirurgical. Liège et Paris, Dosoer et Masson, 1951

2

Let us begin by reviewing the osteology. No matter how an experienced a surgeon you may be, do not overlook these first pages. They are indispensable but tiresome to read; better to defer it to another day than to undertake it ill disposed.

FARABEUF, 1889

Osteology

Lower Ends of the Fibula and Tibia

The lower ends of the fibula and tibia form an anatomic and functional unit providing the osseoligmantous retention system to the talus and contributing to the ligamentous stabilization of the calcaneus at the subtalar joint. The bimalleolar retaining fork is rigid medially and movable laterally.

LOWER END OF THE FIBULA

The lower end of the fibula is divided into the distal fibular shaft and the lateral malleolus.

Distal Fibular Shaft

The distal one fourth of the fibular shaft terminates at the level of the tibial plafond. It has two surfaces, lateral and medially, separated by an anterior and a posterior border (Fig. 2-1).

Medial Surface. The interosseous crest divides the upper segment of the medial surface into an anterior narrow segment giving attachment to the peroneus tertius and a broader posterior part, flat or markedly convex, for the lower fibers of the flexor hallucis longus muscle. Where the anterior border and the interosseous crest merge, an oblique line originates and is directed downward and posteriorly, delineating a triangular area with a distal base and an antero-superior apex. This triangular surface is covered by rugosities and gives insertion to the tibiofibular interosseous ligament, which is in continuity at the apex with the interosseuous membrane. Distal to the insertion of the interosseous membrane is a triangular smooth surface with an anterior base and a posterior apex. The broader anterior part, 1 cm average height, corresponds to the tibioperoneal recess lined by periosteal synovium. The narrow posterior part gives insertion to a fatty synovial fringe that descends in the ankle joint (Fig. 2-2).

Lateral Surface. At the level of the distal fibula the anterior border divides into two branches, anterior and posterior. The anterior branch remains anterior, merges with the interosseous crest, and continues into the anterior border of the lateral malleolus. The posterior branch or oblique crest is directed downward and posteriorly and continues with the posterior border of the lateral malleolus, forming the lateral border of the peroneal sulcus. This oblique crest delineates two surfaces—anteroinferior and posterosuperior. The anteroinferior segment is limited by the anterior and posterior divisions of the anterior border. The surface is laterally oriented, flat, and subcutaneous. The posterosuperior segment is intially posterolateral in orientation. Farther down, through a twist, it becomes posterior and is in continuity with the posterior aspect of the lateral malleolus. The lower fibers of the peroneus brevis muscle originate from the upper segment of this surface. Both peronei muscle tendons, initially in a lateral position, follow the posterior shift of this segment. The anteroinferior and posterosuperior surfaces are slanted relative to each other along the oblique crest, and this must be taken into consideration during the application of a plate to a fractured fibular shaft at this level.

The anterior border is described above. The posterior border is distinct proximally but loses its definition distally and dissipates toward the medial border of the peroneal groove.

Lateral Malleolus

The lateral malleolus is pyramidal in contour and presents three surfaces: lateral, medial, and posterior (Figs. 2-3 and 2-4). The lateral and medial surfaces converge toward the anterior border. The posterior surface is limited laterally by the oblique fibular crest and medially by the direct extension of the posterior border of the fibular shaft. The apex of the pyramid is inferoposterior. The lateral malleolus is projected outward and descends 1 cm farther than the medial malleolus.

35

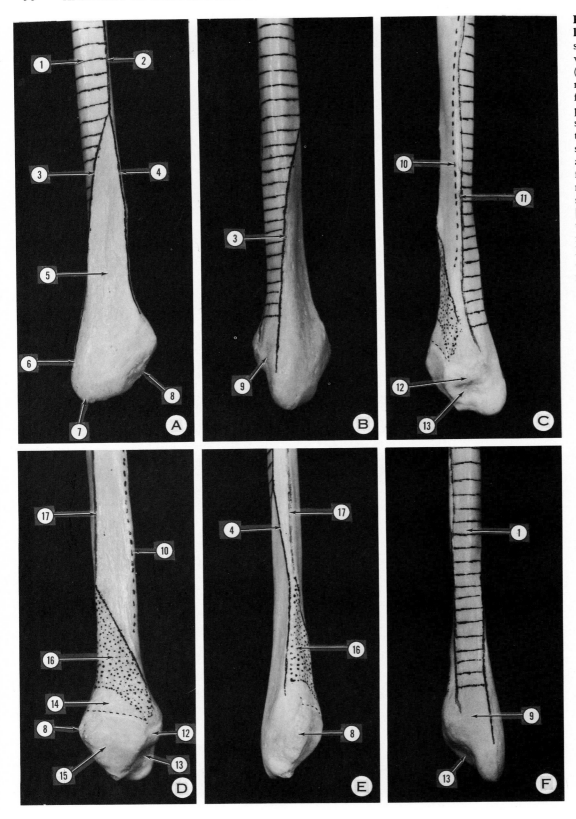

Fig. 2-1. Distal fibula and lateral malleolus. (*A*) Lateral surface. (*B*) Posterolateral view. (*C*) Posteromedial view. (*D*) Medial surface. (*E*) Anterior surface. (*F*) Posterior surface. (1, Surface of origin of peroneus brevis muscle; this surface becomes posterior distally and continues as posterior surface of lateral malleolus; 2, anterior border of fibular shaft for insertion of anterior peroneal septum; 3, posterior division branch of anterior border [2]; it forms a crest and continues as lateral border of posterior surface of lateral malleolus; 4, anterior division branch of anterior border; 5, subcutaneous surface; 6, posterior border of lateral malleolus; 7, tip of lateral malleolus; 8, anterior border of lateral malleolus; 9, sulcus of peronei tendons; 10, line of insertion of deep transverse fascia of leg; 11, line of insertion of posterior peroneal septum; 12, posterior tubercle of medial surface of lateral malleolus; 13, digital fossa; 14, surface corresponding to peroneotibial recess; 15, articular surface corresponding to lateral surface of talus; 16, insertion of tibiofibular interosseous ligament; 17, insertion line of the interosseous membrane.) The anterior division line (4) of the anterior fibular border and the line of the interosseous membrane (17) join distally.

Fig. 2-2. (*A*) **Medial surface of distal fibula and lateral malleolus.** (*B*) **Same view as in** (*A*)**. Distal tibia connected to fibula.** (*C*) **Inferior view of the distal tibiofibular complex.** (1, Anterior tibiofibular ligament; 2, main component of anterior talofibular ligament; 3, secondary band of anterior talofibular ligament; 4, calcaneofibular ligament; 5, tip of lateral malleolus, free of insertion; 6, gliding surface of peronei tendons; 7, posterior talofibular ligament; 8, cribriform fossa; 9, superficial component of posterior tibiofibular ligament; 10, synovial fringe; 11, peroneal surface corresponding to tibioperoneal recess; 12, insertion of tibiofibular interosseous ligament; 13, deep component of posterior tibiofibular ligament; 14, articular surface for the lateral surface of the talus; 15, posterosuperior tuberosity; 16, tibia; 17, tibial plafond; 18, medial malleolus.)

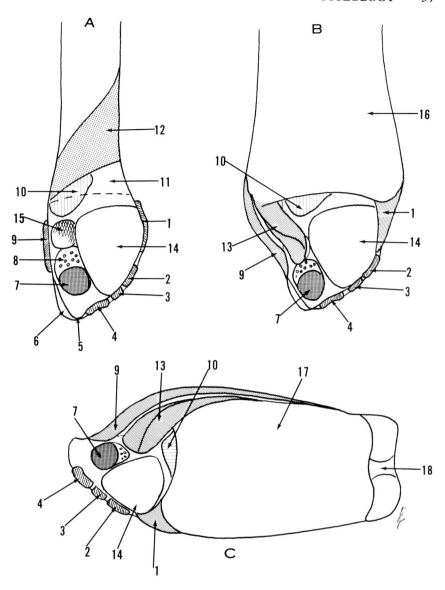

Lateral Surface. The lateral surface of the malleolus is smooth, convex, and subcutaneous and is in continuity with the anteroinferior segment of the fibular lateral surface.

Medial Surface. The medial surface is limited at a level corresponding to the incisura fibularis of the distal tibia. A large triangular articular surface occupies the anterosuperior aspect. The base of the triangle is proximal and convex. The apex is anteroinferior, located on the anterior border of the malleolus. The anterior border is inclined backward, whereas the posterior border is directed anteroinferiorly. The surface is convex along its long axis and corresponds to the lateral articular surface of the talus. Behind the posterosuperior angle of the triangular articular surface is the round posterior fibular tubercle, which gives origin to the deep component of the posterior tibiofibular ligament. Below the tubercle and behind the triangular articular surface is the digital fossa. The upper segment of the fossa is crib-

riform, with multiple vascular foramina. The lower segment gives origin to the posterior talofibular ligament. The superficial components of the posterior tibiofibular ligament originates from the posterior border of the peroneal tubercle and digital fossa (Fig. 2-2).

The lateral malleolus is in contact with the incisura fibularis of the tibia through a minute crescentic cartilage-coated surface that is in continuity with the triangular articular surface of the fibula.

Posterior Surface. The posterior surface is broad proximally and tapers distally. The tendons of the peroneus brevis and peroneus longus follow the twist of the fibular corpus and lie upon the posterior surface. The tendon of the peroneus brevis is against the bone, with the tendon of the longus on top of it. Usually a sulcus is present on this surface. Edwards, in a study of 178 dry fibulas, gives the following data in regard to the contour of the posterior surface:[1] definite sulcus present, 82%; flat surface, 11%;

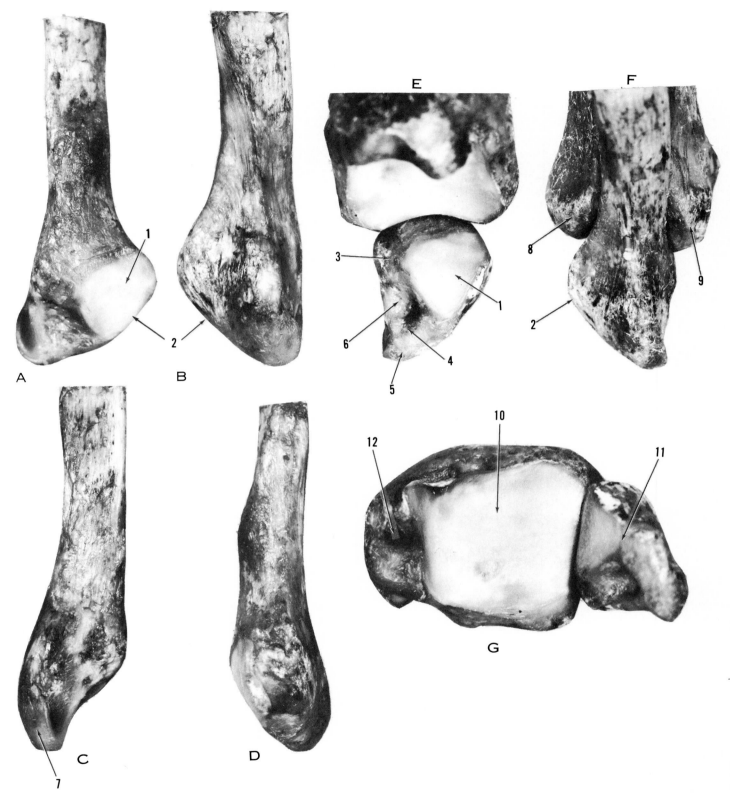

Fig. 2-3. (*A*) **Medial view left fibula.** (*B*) **Lateral view of fibula.** (*C*) **Posterior view fibula.** (*D*) **Anterior view fibula.** (*E*) **Medial view of tibia–lateral malleolus.** (*F*) **Lateral view of distal fibula–tibia.** (*G*) **Inferior view of distal tibia–fibula.** (1, Articular surface; 2, anterior border; 3, posterosuperior tubercle; 4, insertion tubercle of posterior talofibular ligament; 5, tip lateral malleolus; 6, digital fossa; 7, gliding surface for peronei tendon; 8, anterior tibial tubercle; 9, posterior tibial tubercle; 10, tibial plafond; 11, lateral malleolus; 12, medial malleolus.)

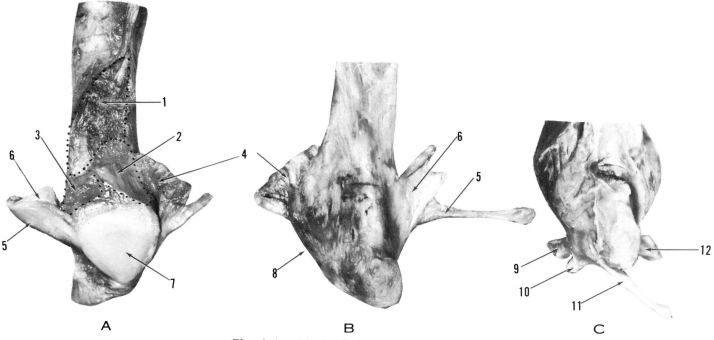

Fig. 2-4. (*A*) **Medial view of left distal fibula and lateral malleolus.** (*B* **and** *C*) **Lateral view of lateral malleolus.** (1, Insertion of tibiofibular interosseous ligament; 2, fibular component of tibiofibular recess; 3, insertion of synovial fringe; 4, anterior tibiofibular ligament; 5, 6, Posterior tibiofibular ligament; 7, articular surface; 8, anterior border; 9, main component of anterior talofibular ligament; 10, secondary component of anterior talofibular ligament; 11, calcaneofibular ligament; 12, posterior talofibular ligament.)

convex surface, 7%. The width of the sulcus is given as the narrowest, 5 mm; the majority (62%), 6 mm to 7 mm; and the widest, 10 mm. The lateral border of the posterior surface may become prominent and form a lateral bony ridge. "It helps to form a flange against which the tendons of the peroneal muscles play, and it gives attachment to some of the fibers of the superior peroneal retinaculum."[1] The occurrence of this lateral bony ridge, based on Edwards' data, is as follows:[1] well-developed lateral bony ridge, 22%; slightly developed lateral bony ridge, 48%; absence of a developed lateral bony ridge, 30%. The majority of the ridges are 2 mm high, but occasionally the ridges may reach an elevation of 4 mm. Cartilage covering may increase the ridge 1 mm to 2 mm, and not infrequently, the ridge is formed by cartilage only.[1]

Edwards further reports on the presence of a prominence on the medial border on the posterior surface that forms, in about 50%, a medial ridge or, in the remaining half, a rounded tubercle.[1] In 4% of the fibulas, an intermediate low ridge is present between the lateral and medial ridges.

The peroneal sulcus, when present, is very shallow.

The anterior border of the lateral malleolus is thin above and thick below. The contour is strongly convex anteriorly. A longitudinal tubercle extending from the level of the anterosuperior angle of the articular surface to the mid segment gives insertion to the anterior tibiofibular ligament. Below this level, the anterior border bears flat tubercles corresponding to the insertion of the two bands of the

anterior talofibular ligament. Farther distally but still anterior in location is the insertion of the calcaneofibular ligament. The apex of the lateral malleolus is free of insertion.

The posterolateral and posteromedial borders of the lateral malleolus are covered in the descriptions of the posterior and medial surfaces.

LOWER END OF THE TIBIA

The lower end of the tibia is formed by five surfaces: inferior, anterior, posterior, lateral, and medial (Fig. 2-5). The latter is prolonged distally by the medial malleolus.

Inferior Surface

The inferior surface is articular and corresponds to the dome of the talus. It is concave anteroposteriorly and slightly convex transversely due to the presence of a slightly elevated ridge dividing the surface into a wider lateral and a narrower inner segment.

The lateral border is larger than the medial and the anterior border longer than the posterior (Fig. 2-6). Geometrically, this surface is a section of a frustum of a cone with an average medial conical angle of $22° \pm 4°$.[2] This angle ranges from $0°$ to $35°$.[2] An angle of $0°$ corresponds to a cylindrical surface. The radius of this cylinder is an average of 2 cm, and the corresponding articular arc measures $60°$.[3] In any position of the talus, the tibial plafond covers only two thirds of the talar surface and one third remains uncov-

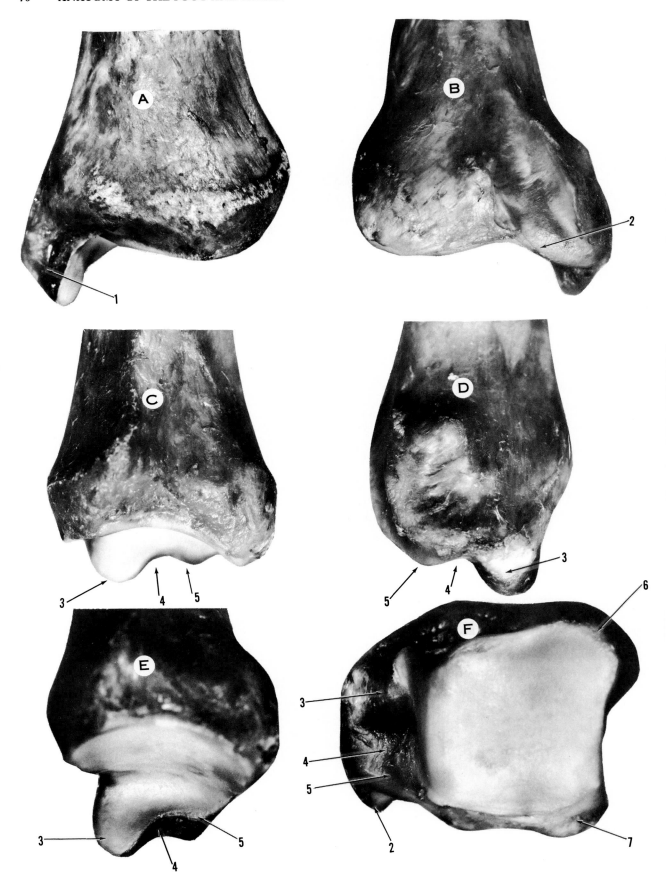

Fig. 2-5. (*A*) **Anterior aspect of left distal tibia.** (*B*) **Posterior aspect of distal tibia.** (*C*) **Lateral aspect of distal tibia.** (*D*) **Medial aspect of distal tibia and medial malleolus.** (*E*) **Lateral aspect of medial malleolus.** (*F*) **Inferior view of distal tibia.** (1, Medial malleolus; 2, sulcus for tibialis posterior tendon; 3, anterior colliculus; 4, intercollicular groove; 5, posterior colliculus; 6, anterior tibial tubercle; 7, posterior tibial tubercle.)

Fig. 2-6.   Distal tibia and medial malleolus. The anterior border of the distal tibia is longer than the posterior border, and the lateral border of the distal tibia is longer than the medial border. The anterior colliculus of the medial malleolus is 0.5 cm longer than the posterior colliculus. (1, Anterior border distal tibia; 2, posterior border distal tibia; 3, lateral border distal tibia—incisura tibialis; 4, tibial plafond; 5, anterior colliculus of medial malleolus; 6, intercollicular groove of medial malleolus; 7, posterior colliculus of medial malleolus; 8, groove for tibialis posterior tendon.)

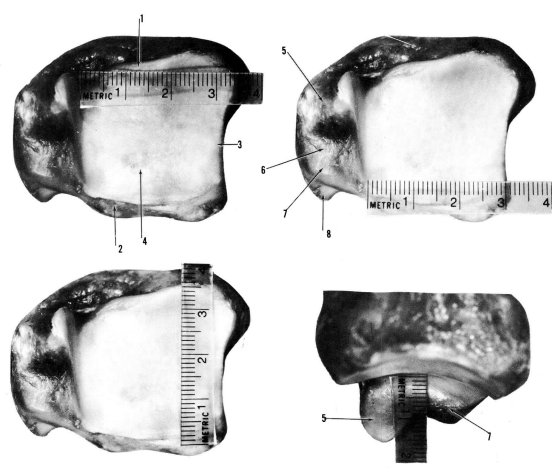

ered (Fig. 2-7). With the long axis of the tibia, the tibial plafond makes an angle of 93.3° ± 3.2°, with a range of 88° to 100°.[2]

The posterior border of the inferior articular surface is lower than the anterior. The direct implantation of the transverse component of the deep posterior tibiofibular ligament on the lateral half of this border forms a true labrum, thus increasing the depth of the containing surface (Fig. 2-7).

Anterior Surface

The anterior surface is in continuity with the lateral surface of the tibial shaft. It is limited laterally by the interosseous border and medially by the anterior border. The surface is narrow proximally and enlarges distally, where it acquires a convexity in both the transverse and vertical directions.

A transverse ridge is present at 0.5 cm to 1 cm proximal to the anterior border and gives insertion to the anterior

articular capsule. The transverse segment of the bone located between the articular border and the transverse ridge recedes posteriorly and is an intra-articular segment. This surface may bear a small articular surface (squatting facet), usually lateral in location and very occasionally medial and lateral. The distribution of these facets is as shown in Table 2-1.

TABLE 2-1.   Distribution of Squatting Facets

Author	Number of Tibias	Lateral Facet (%)	Medial Facet (%)
Wood★	118 European	17	1.7
	236 Australian	80.5	2.1
Singh†	292 Indian	77.4	1.7

★Wood WQ: The tibia of the Australian aborigine. J Anat 54:232, 1920

†Singh I: Squatting facets on the talus and tibia in Indians. J Anat 93:540, 1959

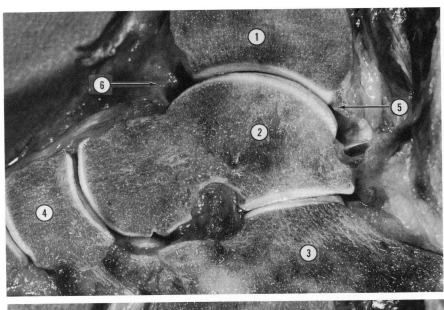

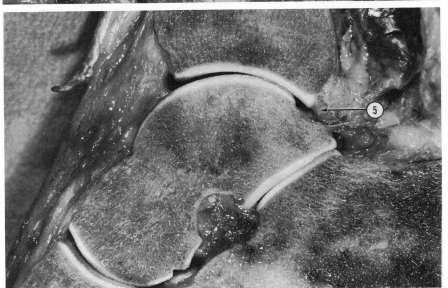

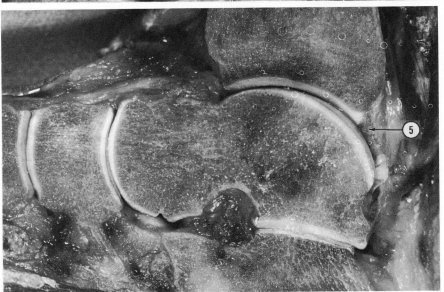

Fig. 2-7.   Sagittal cross section of the ankle. (*A*) Ankle in neutral. (*B*) Ankle in plantar flexion. (*C*) Ankle in dorsiflexion. In any position, the articular surface of the distal tibia covers only two thirds of the corresponding talar articular surface. (1, Tibia; 2, talus; 3, calcaneus; 4, navicular; 5, deep component of tibiofibular ligament forming a labrum; 6, anterior adipose body with large anterior joint cavity.)

Posterior Surface

The posterior surface is in continuity with the posterior surface of the tibial shaft. The proximal segment is smooth and slightly convex. The distal segment bears an oblique groove medially, directed downward and inward, corresponding to the tendon of the tibialis posterior. This segment is in continuity with the posterior surface of the medial malleolus. A second, much less delineated groove may be recognized, corresponding to the tendon of the flexor digitorum longus (see Fig. 2-5).

Lateral Surface

The lateral surface is triangular with an inferior base and a superior apex. It has the contour of a vertical gutter. The apex continues with the lateral border of the tibial shaft. The anterior and posterior borders are continued distally by soft crests that terminate in an anterior and a posterior tubercle.

The anterior tubercle, larger than the posterior, gives attachment to the anterior tibiofibular ligament which extends its fibers into the anterior surface of the distal tibia. The posterior tubercle gives attachment to the deep component of the posterior tibiofibular ligament, which extends its insertion through the transverse band onto the posterior border of the tibia. The superficial component of the posterior tibiofibular ligament has a broad attachment on the posterior tubercle and the posterior surface of the distal tibia, reaching the lateral border of the groove for the tibialis posterior tendon. The anterior tubercle overlaps the fibula, and this relationship is given interpretation in the radiologic study of the tibiofibular syndesmosis.

The tibiofibular interosseous ligament inserts on the rugosities of the upper segment of the lateral surface. The inferior segment presents a smooth small triangular surface (base anterior, apex posterior), corresponding to the tibiofibular recess described above. This segment is limited inferiorly by a minute crescentic cartilage-coated surface corresponding to a similar surface on the fibula.

Medial Surface

The medial surface is smooth, directed obliquely downward and inward. It is larger proximally, narrows progressively distally, and continues with the medial surface of the medial malleolus. It is limited by the anterior and posterior borders of the tibial shaft. This surface gives insertion to the upper arm of the inferior extensor retinaculum and to the flexor retinaculum.

Medial Malleolus

The medial malleolus (see Figs. 2-5 and 2-6) is a strong apophysis implanted at an obtuse angle into the medial aspect of the distal tibia. It is large at the base anteroposteriorly and flat and narrow transversely. It is formed by two segments or colliculi separated by the intercollicular groove. The anterior colliculus descends lower, usually 0.5 cm, than the posterior colliculus. The intercollicular groove is large and measures 0.5 cm to 1 cm in width. The deep talotibial component of the deltoid ligament inserts in the intercollicular groove, the anterior aspect of the posterior colliculus, and the posterior border of the anterior colliculus. The superficial deltoid ligament inserts on the medial surface and anterior border of the anterior colliculus and extends the attachment on the medial subcutaneous surface of the malleolus. The lateral surface of the malleolus is articular with the comma-shaped articular medial surface of the talus. The posterior border of the medial malleolus bears a groove and gives attachment to the fibrous tunnel of the tibialis posterior tendon.

The lateral malleolus, the tibial plafond, and the medial malleolus form a bony unit, the malleolar fork, covering and holding the talus on three sides. The long axis of the ankle mortise is directed posterolaterally in the transverse plane and makes an angle of 23° with the transverse axis of the tibial plateaus (Fig. 2-8, *A, B*). This torsion locates anatomically the medial malleolus anteromedially and the lateral malleolus posterolaterally.

Talus

The talus is an intercalated bone located between the ankle bimalleolar fork and the tarsus. It is moored with strong ligaments but has no tendinous attachments.

The talus is formed by three parts: the body (corpus tali), the neck (collum), and the head (caput). The body is defined as the part of the bone located posterior to an imaginary plane passing through the anterior border of the superior surface of the trochlea tali and the posterior calcaneal surface. The neck is the segment of bone anterior to this plane, located between the body and the head. *The body and the neck are not coaxial.* In the horizontal plane, the neck shifts medially and makes an angle of declination with the long axis of the trochlea tali. This angle is variable (Fig. 2-9), as indicated in Table 2-2.

In the sagittal plane, the neck is deviated downward relative to the talar body and makes an angle of inclination (Fig. 2-10, Table 2-2).

The length and width of the bone measured on 100 dry tali are as follows (Fig. 2-11, *A, B*): length—average, 48 mm; maximum, 60 mm; minimum, 40 mm; width—average, 37 mm; maximum, 45 mm; minimum, 30 mm.

BODY

The body (corpus tali) has five surfaces (Fig. 2-12): superior, lateral, medial, posterior, and inferior.

Superior Surface

The superior surface of the talar body is pulley shaped (Fig. 2-13) and articulates with the distal surface of the tibia and the transverse component of the inferior and posterior tibiofibular ligament. The groove of the pulley runs nearer the medial border, which makes the lateral segment of the surface wider than the medial. The surface is markedly convex anteroposteriorly, with a sagittal radius of convexity of 20 mm (average). It presents a mild concavity transversely.

(Text continues on p. 47.)

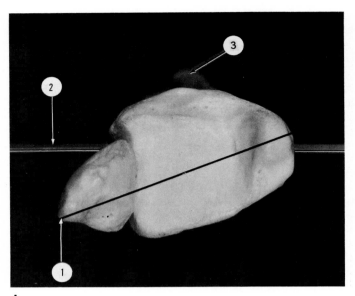

A

Fig. 2-8. (*A*) **Distal tibia-fibula, right ankle, inferior view.** (1, Bimalleolar axis; 2, transverse axis, transtibial plateau; 3, anterior tibial tubercle.) The bimalleolar axis is oriented posterolaterally. The lateral malleolus is posterior, and the medial malleolus is anterior. (*B*) **Cross section of left ankle, lower surface, passing 1 cm above the tip of the medial malleolus.** (*A*, Anterior; *P*, posterior; *L*, lateral; *M*, medial; 1, talus; 2, anterior colliculus of medial malleolus; 3, lateral malleolus; 4, tibialis posterior tendon and tunnel; 5, flexor digitorum longus tendon and tunnel; 6, flexor hallucis longus tendon-muscle; 7, peroneus longus tendon; 8, peroneus brevis, inverted U-shaped tendon; 9, achilles tendon; 10, extensor digitorum longus tendon; 11, extensor hallucis longus tendon; 12, tibialis anterior tendon; 13, dorsalis pedis artery and veins; 14, posterior tibial artery and veins; 15, greater saphenous vein; 16, lesser saphenous vein; 17, sural nerve; 18, deltoid ligament, deep talotibial component. [note relationship of tibialis posterior tendon and deltoid ligament]; *X-Y*, bimalleolar axis oriented posterolaterally.)

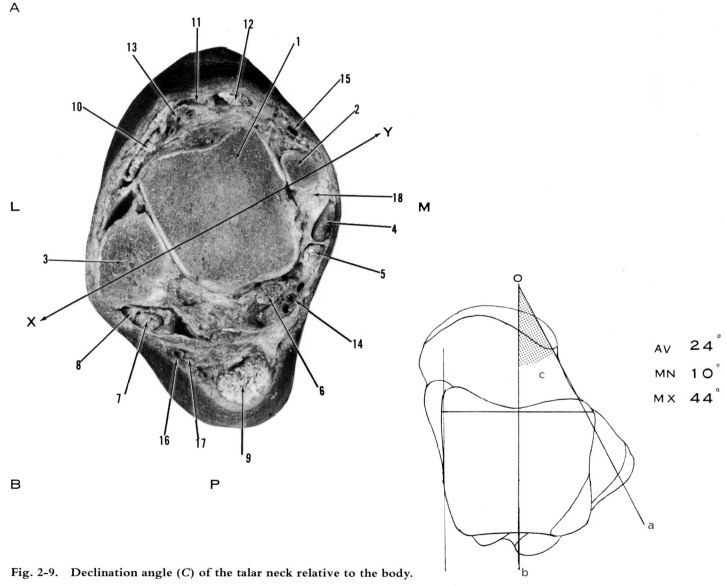

Fig. 2-9. Declination angle (*C*) of the talar neck relative to the body.

TABLE 2-2. Angles of Declination and Inclination of Talus

30	Author	Number of Tali	Declination Angle	Inclination Angle
32	Testut★		22°	115°
33	Paturet†		20°–30°	115°
34	Sewell‡	1006 Egyptian	18° average, 7° minimum, 43° maximum	112° average, 98° minimum, 127° maximum
35	Present series	100	24° average, 10° minimum, 44° maximum	114° average (24° plantar tilt), 95° minimum (5° plantar tilt), 140° maximum (50° plantar tilt)

★Testut L: Traité d'Anatomie Humaine, 7th ed, Vol 1, p 368. Paris, Doin, 1921
†Paturet G: Traité d'Anatomie Humaine, Vol 2, p 573. Paris, Masson, 1951
‡Sewell RBS: A study of the astragalus, Part I. J Anat Physiol 38:233, 1904

Fig 2-10. Inclination angle (*e*) of the talar neck relative to the body. The center *O* of the lateral trochlear arc is determined. The arc is bisected by the radius *OC*. A tangent *a* is drawn at the apex of the navicular articular surface. A perpendicular line *b* is drawn at the tangential point. The line *b* gives the direction of the talar neck and intersects the radius *OC* of the talar trochlear arc. At this point of intersection a perpendicular line *d* is traced, determining the inclination angle *e*.

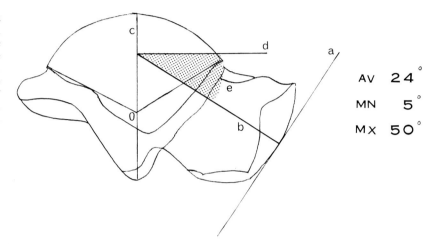

AV 24°
MN 5°
MX 50°

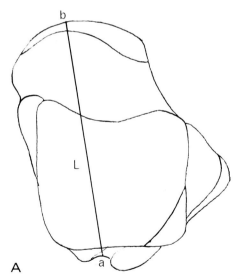

AV 48 mm
MN 40 -
MX 60 -

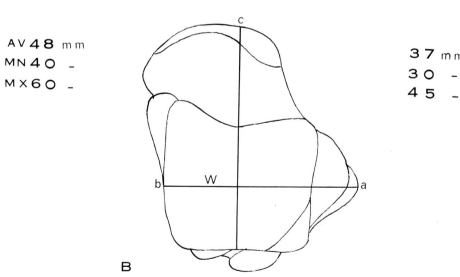

37 mm
30 -
45 -

Fig. 2-11. Measurements of talus. (*A*) Length of talus is determined by a line joining the apex of the navicular articular surface to the flexor hallucis longus groove. (*B*) Width of talus, determined with caliper holding the talus at the tip of the lateral process and the middle of the medial trochlear line. The direction of the caliper is maintained perpendicular to the latter.

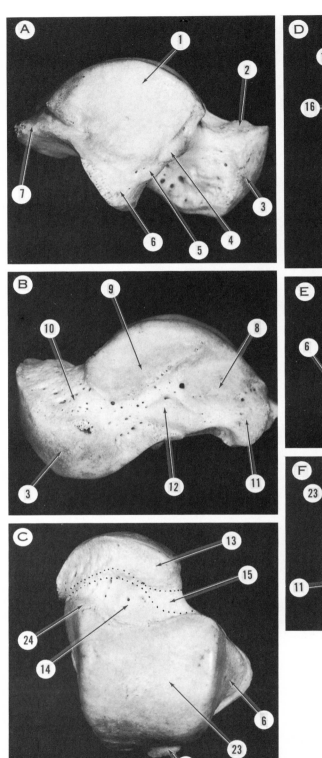
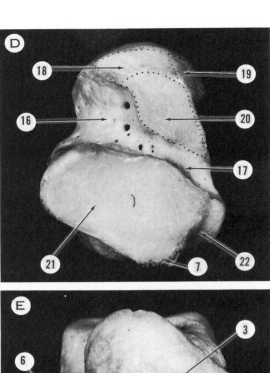
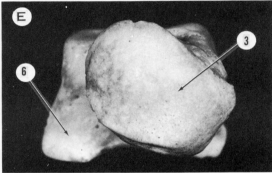
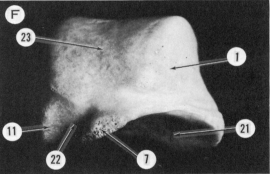

Fig. 2-12. Talus. (*A*) Lateral aspect. (*B*) Medial aspect. (*C*) Superior aspect. (*D*) Inferior aspect. (*E*) Anterior aspect. (*F*) Posterior aspect. (1, Articular surface—facies malleolus lateralis; 2, cervical collar; 3, articular surface—facies articularis navicularis; 4, 5, tubercles for insertions of anterior talofibular ligaments; 6, lateral process; 7, posterolateral tubercle; 8, oval surface for insertion of talotibial component of deltoid ligament; 9, articular surface—facies malleolaris medialis; 10, talar neck; 11, posteromedial tubercle; 12, tubercle of insertion of deltoid ligament; 13, segment of talar neck located within talonavicular joint; 14, segment of talar neck located within talotibial joint; 15, extra-articular segment of talar neck where a bursa may be found against which glides medial root of inferior extensor retinaculum; 16, sinus tarsi; 17, canalis tarsi; 18, anterior calcaneal articular surface of the talar head; 19, articular segment of talar head corresponding to superomedial and inferior calcaneonavicular ligaments; 20, middle calcaneal articular surface of talar neck; 21, posterior calcaneal articular surface of the talar body; 22, canal of the flexor hallucis longus tendon; 23, trochlear surface; 24, anteromedial extension of trochlear surface.)

TABLE 2-3. Difference of Anterior and Posterior Transverse Diameters

Author	Number of tali	Difference
Testut★		5 mm–6 mm
Poirier and Charpy†		4 mm–5 mm
Inman‡	100	2.4 mm ± 1.3 mm average
Present series	100	4.2 mm average, 2 mm minimum, 6 mm maximum

★Testut L: Traité d'Anatomie Humaine, 7th ed, Vol 1, p 632. Paris, Doin, 1921
†Poirier P, Charpy A: Traité d'Anatomie Humaine, Vol 1, p 758. Paris, Masson, 1899
‡Inman VT: The Joints of the Ankle, p 2. Baltimore, William & Wilkins, 1976.

This concavity may be shallow or deep and is the norm in 80% of the tali; in the remaining 20%, the transerse curvature is more complex, with a medial concavity and a lateral convexity. These talar curvatures have their interlocking counterparts in the distal tibias.

The medial border of the trochlear surface is straight, slightly lower than the lateral, and soft in contour. The lateral border is oblique, directed posteromedially, and bevelled in its posterior segment, thus forming a triangular facet (the facies articularis intermedia corporis tali). The lateral border is sharper than the medial in the mid segment. Due to the obliquity of the lateral border, the trochlear surface is wedge shaped and is narrower posteriorly.

The difference in width between the anterior and posterior transverse diameters, including the triangular facet, is shown in Table 2-3.

The anterior border of the trochlear surface is variable in contour: it may be straight, slightly concave, convex in its entirety, or in the shape of an elongated S. Extension facets from the superior articular surface onto the neck are seen both medially and laterally (see Fig. 2-12). A medial extension facet is always accompanied by a forward prolongation of the medial malleolar articular surface of the talus; however, the reverse is not true. The frequency of occurrence of a medial extension facet from the trochlear surface is shown in Table 2-4.

A lateral extension surface is to be differentiated from a squatting facet. The criteria of differentiation are clearly stated by Singh.[4] A lateral extension surface continues the convexity of the trochlear surface. During dorsiflexion, this facet establishes contact with the lower end of the distal tibia and not with its anterior border. In contradistinction, a squatting facet, in continuity with the trochlear surface, is concave anteroposteriorly and is directed upward and occasionally backward. During dorsiflexion of the foot, it establishes contact with the anterior margin of the distal tibia. The frequency of occurrence of these lateral prolongations is shown in Table 2-5.

Lateral Surface

The lateral surface of the talar body is mostly occupied by a large trigonal articular surface, the facies malleolus lateralis. The curved base of this articular surface corresponds to the lateral border of the trochlear surface. The lateral profile of the base is almost an arc of a true circle measuring $106° \pm 13°$.[2, 5] The surface is concave in the vertical direction and slightly convex transversely. The convexity is more pronounced in the apical portion. Rarely, a concavity replaces the convexity in this location. The vertical concavity is determined by the outward projection of the lateral talar process. The angle of projection as measured in 100 tali is 32° average, 55° maximum, 15° minimum (Fig. 2-14).

The lateral talocalcaneal ligament inserts on the apex of the lateral process.

Along the anterior border of the trigonal articular surface are two tubercles for the insertion of the anterior talofibular ligament, the lower tubercle being less pronounced. Sometimes the tubercles are replaced by a depression or notch. Occasionally a small accessory articular surface is seen on

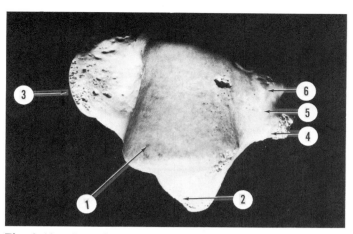

Fig. 2-13.   Superior aspect of talus. (1, Talar pulley; 2, lateral process; 3, talar head; 4, posterolateral tubercle; 5, canal of flexor hallucis longus; 6, posteromedial tubercle.)

TABLE 2-4.   Frequency of Occurrence of Medial Extension Facet

Author	Number of Tali	Occurrence (%)
Singh★	300 Indian	55
Present series	100	36
Sewell★	1006 Egyptian	19
Barnett†	100 European	11

★Singh I: Squatting facets on the talus and tibia in Indians. J Anat 93:540, 1959

†Sewell RBS: A study of the astragalus: III. The collum tali. J Anat Physiol 39:74, 1906

‡Barnett CH: Squatting facets on the European talus. J Anat Physiol 88:509, 1954

TABLE 2-5.   Frequency of Occurrence of Lateral Extension and Squatting Facets

Author	Tali	Lateral Extension Facet	Squatting Facet	Total
		Occurrence (%)		
Singh★	300 Indian	54.6	26.6	81.2
Present series	100	36	33	69
Barnett†	100 European	17	2	19

★Singh I: Squatting facets on the talus and tibia in Indians. J Anat 93:540, 1959

†Barnett CH: Squatting facets on the European talus. J Anat Physiol 88:509, 1954

the anterior segment of the lateral process. This surface, the facies externa accessoria corporis tali, is in continuity with the posterior calcaneal surface. When well developed it is triangular with an inferior base and oriented anteroinferiorly (Fig. 2-15). In 100 Egyptian tali, this accessory surface was present in 10.15%.[6] In the present series of 100 tali, a large accessory surface was present in 4%, and an accessory surface of variable size was present in 34%.

Along the posteroinferior border of the lateral malleolar surface, there is a groove that gives attachment to the pos-

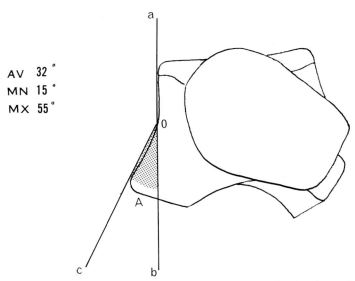

AV 32°
MN 15°
MX 55°

Fig. 2-14. Angle of lateral projection (A) of talar lateral process.

Fig. 2-15. (A) Inferolateral view of tali. (1, Posterior calcaneal articular surface with 2, facies externa accessoria; 3, absent accessory facet.) **(B) Medial view of tali.** (1, 2, Posterior extension of medial articular facet.)

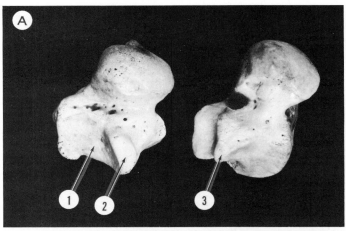

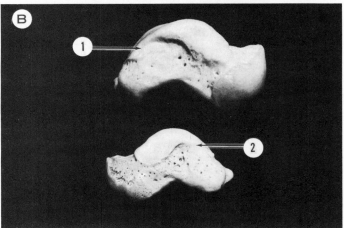

terior talofibular ligament. This groove extends forward, usually up to the midsegment of the posteroinferior border, where it makes a notch. Rarely, it is continued forward to the apex of the facet.

Medial Surface

The medial surface is divided into two fields, superior and inferior.

The superior segment is occupied by the facies malleolaris medialis or the auricular facet. This articular surface is comma shaped, and the long axis is oriented anteroposteriorly. The anterior part is broad and circular; the tail is thin and posterior. The superior border of this surface forms the medial border of the trochlea. This border is convex anteroposteriorly. The anterior third of this curve is part of a circle with a smaller radius than that of the lateral surface. The posterior two thirds is an arc of a circle, the radius of which is larger than that of the lateral profile.[5] Inman, contouring the trochlear surface in planes perpendicular to the functional axis of the ankle, found the medial side of the trochlea to be an arc of a circle in 80% of the tali and to deviate from it in the remaining 20%.[2] The average arc on the medial side is 103° ± 14°.[2]

The medial facet is often extended anteriorly over the medial aspect of the collum tali beyond the level of the anterior border of the trochlea. The frequency of occurrence of this extension was 96% in 300 Indian tali,[4] and in the present series of 100 tali, it was 91% (55% isolated extension, 36% in association with anterior extension of trochlear surface).

When well developed, the anterior extension of the medial articular surface projects medially and downward and articulates in strong dorsiflexion with the corresponding anterior aspect of the medial malleolus, which is then covered with articular cartilage. A posterior extension of the medial articular surface behind the area of attachment of the deep portion of the deltoid ligament is also seen (Fig. 2-15).

The inferior segment is occupied in the anterior half by a depressed surface perforated by numerous vascular foramina. Under the tail of the articular surface, the posterior half is occupied by a large oval surface, flat or elevated, which gives insertion to the talotibial deep component of the deltoid ligament.

Posterior Surface

The posterior surface or processus posterior tali comprises the posterolateral and posteromedial tubercles flanking the sulcus for the flexor hallucis longus tendon.

The posterolateral tubercle is large, more prominent than the medial tubercle. The size varies from a barely perceptible structure to a well-developed tubercle projecting posterolaterally from the talus (Fig. 2-16). This tubercle presents an inferior articular surface in continuity with the posterolateral corner of the posterior calcaneal surface of the talus. The superior surface is irregular and nonarticular and gives insertion on the lateral aspect to the posterior talofibular ligament and the talar component of the fibuloastragalo

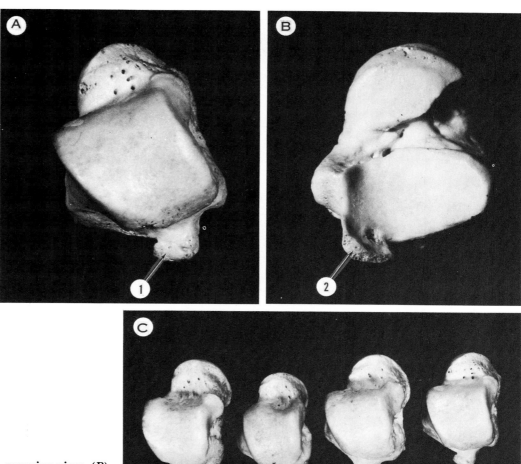

Fig. 2-16. **(A) Trigonal process, superior view. (B) Trigonal process, inferior view.** Its articular surface is in continuity with that of the posterior calcaneal articular surface. **(C) Variations in the size of the trigonal process.** (1, Absent; 2, moderate; 3, medium; 4, large.)

calcaneal ligament of Rouvière and Canela Lazaro.[7] The deep layer of the flexor retinaculum inserts on the medial aspect, whereas the posterior talocalcaneal ligament attaches to its inferior border.

An accessory bone, os trigonum, (Figs. 2-17 and 2-18), may be found in connection with the posterolateral tubercle. This ossicle has three surfaces, anterior, inferior, and posterior. The anterior surface articulates with the posterolateral tubercle or is attached to the latter with fibrous, fibrocartilaginous, or cartilaginous tissue. The inferior surface articulates with the os calcis. The posterior surface is nonarticular. The capsuloligamentous structures attaching on the posterolateral tubercle extend their insertions on this surface. The frequency of occurrence of the os trigonum in adults is shown in Table 2-6.

Sewell found a percentage of "separation" of 10.9% in 1006 tali.[6] "Separation" includes the presence of a notch in the margin of the lateral process, a groove on the articular surface, a combination of both, or a frank separation. The last occurred in 24.1% of the separated group, 3% of the total group.

TABLE 2-6. **Frequency of Occurrence of Os Trigonum in Adults**

Author	Number of Tali	Occurrence (%)
Thomson★	438	2.7
Stieda†	305	5.9
Pfitzner‡	841	6.1
Grant§	558	7.7

★Report of the Committee of Collective Investigation of the Anatomical Society of Great Britain and Ireland for the Year 1899–90. J Anat Physiol 25:98, 1891
†Stieda L: Der Talus und das Os Trigonum Bardelebens beim Menschen. Anat Anz 4:305–319, 336–351, 1899
‡Pfitzner W: Beiträge zur Kenntniss des Menschlichen Extremitätenskelets: VI. Die Variationen in Aufbau des Fussskelets. In Schwalbe (ed): Morphologische Arbeiten, pp 245–527. Jena, Gustav Fischer, 1896
§Grant JCB: Grant's Atlas of Anatomy, 5th ed, p 356. Baltimore, Williams & Wilkins, 1962

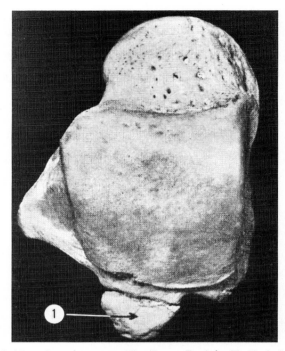

Fig. 2-17.   Os trigonum (1). (From Dwight T: Variations of the Bones of the Hands and Feet: A Clinical Atlas, pp 14–23. Philadelphia, JB Lippincott, 1907)

A fused os trigonum is called a *trigonal process* (see Fig. 2-16). The os trigonum is more often bilateral than unilateral. Very rarely, it is found in two equal or unequal parts. Distinct on one side, it may be present as a trigonal process on the other.

The medial tubercle is of variable size. It is in continuity with the medial talar surface and gives attachment to the deep and superficial layers of the talotibial components of the deltoid ligament, the medial talocalcaneal ligament, and the tunnel of the flexor hallucis longus tendon. Rarely, the tubercle may be very large and may extend downward over the os calcis, contributing to a talocalcaneal coalition (Fig. 2-19).

The sulcus of the flexor hallucis longus tendon is located between the posterolateral and the posteromedial tubercle. It is directed obliquely downward and inward and is curved anteriorly. The angle made by the long axis of the sulcus with the transverse trochlear axis in 100 tali is 68° average, 85° maximum, 55° minimum (Fig. 2-20, *A*).

Inferior Surface

The inferior surface is occupied by the facies articularis calcanea posterior. The long axis of this articular surface is directed anterolaterally. The angle made by this axis with the anterior border of the trochlea in 100 tali is 37° average, 50° maximum, 26° minimum (Fig. 2-20, *B*).

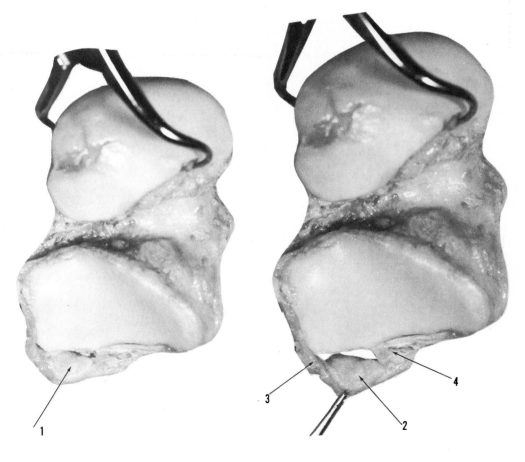

Fig. 12-18.   Os trigonum. (1, 2, Inferior articular surface; 3, 4, ligaments of attachment on each side: thin anterior capsular structure has been removed.)

Fig. 2-19.   Talus. (*A*) Medial aspect. (*B*) Anterior aspect. (*C*) Inferior aspect. (*D*) Posteromedial aspect. Large posteromedial talar tubercle (1 to 4) forming probably a coalition with its corresponding calcaneus.

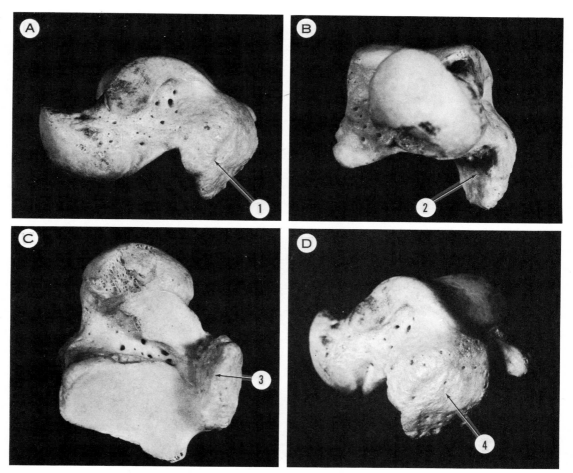

The articular surface is quadrilateral, rectangular medially, and more or less oval laterally. The surface is strongly concave in the long axis and usually flat or very minimally concave transversely. The anteromedial border is usually convex and forms the posterior border of the tarsal canal and the sinus tarsi. This border extends obliquely from the medial tubercle to the anterior surface of the lateral process of the talus. Occasionally the border is straight or has a complex configuration (see Fig. 2-12). The posterolateral border is straight and parallel to the long axis. Of the two short sides, the medial is straight and directed posterolaterally and supports the posterior process of the talus; the lateral border is convex and supports the base of the lateral process of the talus.

Accessory articular surfaces may be present in continuity with the posterior calcaneal surface. Extending from the anterolateral corner is the facies externa accessoria corporis tali (see Fig. 2-15). A small facet may be present in the anteromedial corner, covering the undersurface of the medial tubercle. A trigonal process or a large lateral tubercle prolongs the articular surface posteriorly (see Fig. 2-16).

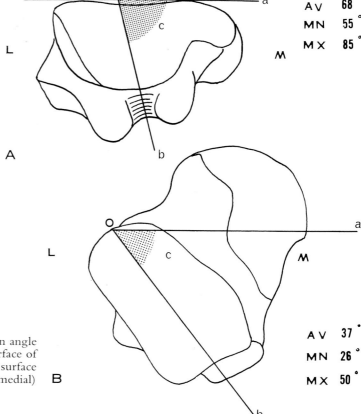

Fig. 2-20.   Angles of talus. (*A*) Posterior aspect of talus. Inclination angle (*c*) of the sulcus for the flexor hallicus longus tendon. (*B*) Inferior surface of talus. Angle (*c*) formed by the long axis *ob* of the posterior calcaneal surface with a line *oa* parallel to the anterior trochlear border. (*L*, lateral; *M*, medial)

The posterior calcaneal surface may establish union with the facies articularis calcanea media, creating a single articulating surface running along the undersurface of the bone and closing the tarsal canal medially. In other instances, these two surfaces fuse through a direct anterior extension from the posterior calcaneal surface, without the medial detour, this extension completely obliterates the tarsal canal and a segment of the sinus tarsi (see Fig. 2-21).

NECK

The neck (collum tali) is the segment of the talus located between the body posteriorly and the head anteriorly (see Fig. 2-12). Its average length is 17 mm, with a maximum of 23 mm and a minimum of 12 mm (Fig. 2-22).

The neck is projected anteromedially and downward, as described previously. The lateral border is slightly concave and well delineated, whereas the medial border is round and at times not discernible. The neck presents four surfaces: superior, lateral, inferior, and medial.

Superior Surface

The superior surface is limited anteriorly by the articular surface corresponding to the navicular and posteriorly by the anterior border of the trochlea. The lateral half of the surface is mostly occupied by a deep, concave cribriform fossa. The remaining anterior part of this surface is occupied by a bony prominence or a smooth, flat bony segment. The medial half of the superior surface is inclined medially due

Fig. 2-21. Variations in size and contour of the inferior articular surfaces of the talus. (*A*) Common configuration of the articular surfaces. (*B*) Posterior extension of the middle calcaneal surface. (*C*) (I) Moderate posterior extension of middle calcaneal surface. (II) Marked posterior extension of middle calcaneal surface. (III) Fusion (5) of all articular surfaces, obliterating the tarsal canal and a segment of the sinus tarsi. (*D*) Fusion (5) of the middle and posterior calcaneal surfaces on the medial aspect of the tarsal canal, which is still maintained. (1, Anterior calcaneal articular surface of talar head; 2, middle calcaneal articular surface of talar neck; 3, articular segment of talar head corresponding to superomedial and inferior calcaneonavicular ligament; 4, posterior calcaneal articular surface of talar body.)

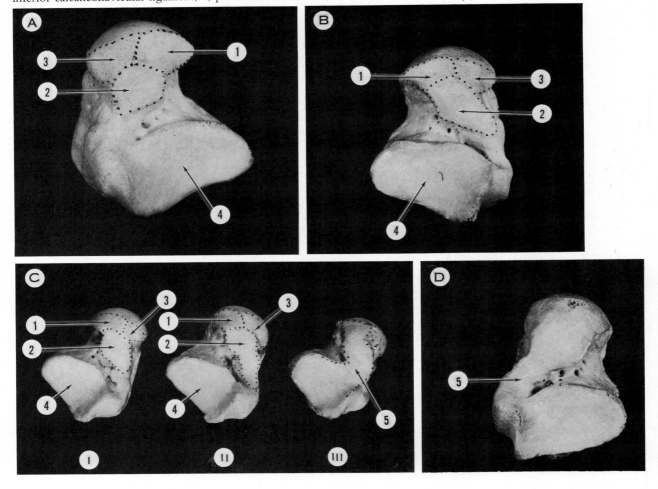

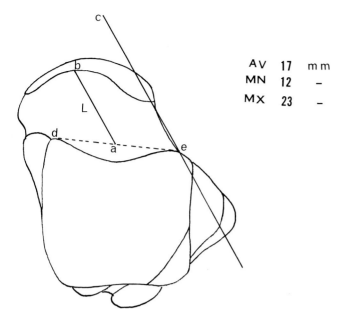

$$\begin{array}{lcc} AV & 17 & mm \\ MN & 12 & - \\ MX & 23 & - \end{array}$$

Fig. 2-22. Length of talar neck *L*. An anterior trochlear line *de* is drawn as indicated. The midpoint *a* is determined. A line *ec* is drawn along the talar neck. From the point *a* a line *ab* is drawn, parallel to line *ec*. The segment *ab* is considered the length of the talar neck, and it terminates where the articular surface is encountered.

to the rotation of the talar head. In certain tali, a transverse cervical ridge or collar runs parallel to the articular surface of the head.[8] The talotibial capsule inserts close to the malleolar facets laterally, medially, and distal to the cribriform fossa, which remains intra-articular. The talonavicular capsule inserts transversely along the articular surface of the head. On the lateral aspect of the neck, the capsules of the talotibial and talonavicular joints are separated by a bare extra-articular bony segment, over which glides the medial root of the inferior extensor retinaculum; a bursa may be found in this location. The superficial talotibial component of the deltoid ligament inserts on the medial aspect of the cervical surface. The articular facets extending from the trochlear surface onto the superior aspect of the neck, the facies articularis interna and externa collae tali, including the squatting facet located laterally, are discussed above.

Lateral Surface

The lateral surface of the neck is converted to a ridge extending from the anterolateral corner of the trochlea and talar body to the articular surface of the head. It is oriented anteromedially and presents a slight concavity. It may give insertion to the medial root of the inferior extensor retinaculum.

Inferior Surface

The inferior surface of the neck is formed by two nonarticulating segments, corresponding to the sinus tarsi and the tarsal canal, and an articular surface. The latter forms the facies articularis calcanea media, which occupies the antero-

medial segment of the cervical surface. It has a variable contour and may be oval, elliptic, pyriform, or pentagonal. It is in continuity with the facies articularis calcanea anterior and the articular segment corresponding to the inferior calcaneonavicular ligament (Figs. 2-21 and 2-23). A ridge may delineate these surfaces. Occasionally a separation notch is seen between the surfaces; if the notch is deep enough, a near-complete separation occurs between the middle and anterior calcaneal surfaces. In rare instances, a complete separation is present.

The bony segment corresponding to the sinus tarsi occupies the lateral half of the cervical surface. It is triangular, with a lateral base and a posteromedial apex continuing in the tarsal canal. Anteriorly, it bears a tubercle (tuberculum cervicis tali) that gives insertion to the cervical ligament.[9] In the present series of 100 tali, the tubercle was identified in 37%. Vascular foramina are distributed on the inner aspect of this surface. The lateral segment bears only a few vascular foramina.

The segment corresponding to the tarsal canal is located between the facies articularis calcanea media and the facies articularis calcanea posterior. It has a narrow, oblique surface oriented posteromedially. Laterally, it communicates with the sinus tarsi. Its medial opening is anterior to the talar posteromedial tubercle. Multiple vascular foramina are distributed along its longitudinal axis. A longitudinal crest may be present, giving insertion to the interosseous talocalcaneal ligament of the canalis tarsi and to the oblique calcaneotalar band of the inferior extensor retinaculum. As previously described, this sulcus interarticularis may be completely obliterated if a fusion occurs between the posterior and middle calcaneal articulating surfaces.

Medial Surface

The medial surface of the neck is higher than the lateral surface. It represents the forward extension of the nonarticular segment of the medial surface of the talar body and provides insertion to the talonavicular capsule and ligaments. Occasionally a posterior extension of the articulating surface of the head or an anterior extension of the medial malleolar articulating surface considerably narrows the medial surface of the neck.

HEAD

The talar head (caput) articulates with the navicular, the calcaneus, and the calcaneonavicular ligaments. These articular fields are usually recognizable (see Fig. 2-21). The head is turned along a longitudinal axis relative to the talar body; the rotation is clockwise on the right and counterclockwise on the left. Due to this rotation, the navicular articular surface is higher laterally and lower medially, and its longitudinal axis is oriented upward and laterally. The longitudinal axis rotation relative to the transverse plane in 1006 Egyptian tali[10] was 45° average, 62° maximum, 25° minimum; in the present series of 100 tali it was 49° average, 65° maximum, 30° minimum (Figs. 2-24 and 2-25).

The facies articularis navicularis is the largest of the three surfaces. It is convex along its long and short axes. The

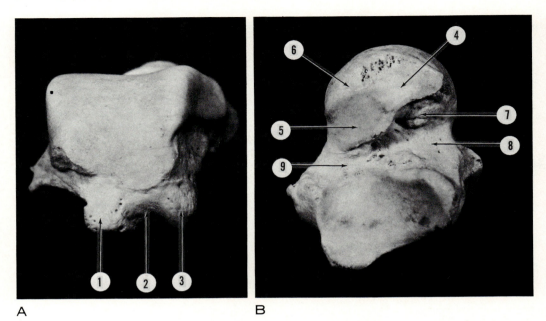

Fig. 2-23. *(A) Posterior aspect of talus. (B) Inferior aspect of talus.* (1, Posterolateral tubercle; 2, sulcus for flexor hallucis longus tendon; 3, posteromedial tubercle; 4, anterior calcaneal articular surface; 5, middle calcaneal articular surface; 6, articular segment of head corresponding to superomedial and inferomedial calcaneonavicular ligaments; 7, tubercle for cervical ligament; 8, sinus tarsi; 9, tarsal canal.)

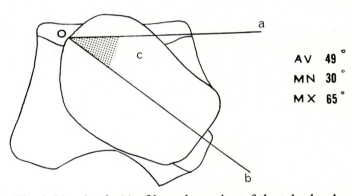

AV 49°
MN 30°
MX 65°

Fig. 2-24. Angle (*c*) of lateral rotation of the talar head.

superolateral and lateral borders are sharply defined from the neck surface; the superomedial border, less defined, may be bevelled. The navicular articular field is in continuity inferiorly with the facies articularis calcanea anterior and the facet for the inferior calcaneonavicular ligament (see Fig. 2-21). A low ridge or a change of direction of the surface demarcates the division.

The medial, inferior segment of the elliptic articular surface corresponds to the deep surface of the superomedial calcaneonavicular ligament and may have a more or less flat contour.

The anterior calcaneal articular surface is nearly quadrilateral or oval, and its surface curvature is clearly different from that of the navicular surface. It is flat and is continuous anteriorly with the navicular surface and posteriorly with the middle articular calcaneal surface, from which it may be separated by a ridge or a notch of variable depth. It is adjacent medially to the articular segment corresponding to the inferior calcaneonavicular ligament. This last surface is wedged between the navicular surface anteriorly and the middle calcaneal articular surface posteriorly.

Calcaneus

The calcaneus is the largest bone of the foot. The long axis is directed anteriorly, upward, and laterally. The upward tilt determines an angle of inclination relative to the horizontal plane—calcaneal pitch—and measures 10° to 30°.[11] The long axis of the calcaneus and of the talar neck normally make an angle of 30° to 35° in the horizontal plane (Fig. 2-26).[12]

The length and width of the calcanei vary (Fig. 2-27): in 750 calcanei, the length was 94 mm maximum and 48 mm minimum; the width was 53 mm maximum and 26 mm minimum.[13] In the present series of 50 calcanei, the length was 75 mm average, 83 mm maximum, and 65 mm minimum; the width was 40 mm average, 46 mm maximum, and 35 mm minimum. The average breadth × 100/length index in the present series is 53 and may range between 50 and 60.[13] The height of the os calcis is close to 50% of the length, in 50 calcanei, the average height was 40 mm, maximum 47 mm, minimum 33.5 mm. The calcaneus is in the form of an irregular rectangle solid and presents six surfaces: superior, inferior, lateral, medial, posterior, and anterior.

SUPERIOR SURFACE

The superior surface is divided into three parts: posterior, middle, and anterior (Fig. 2-28).

Posterior Third

The posterior third of the superior surface is nonarticular, narrow, transversely convex, and longitudinally concave. It is perforated by multiple vascular foramina, and the surface corresponds to the pre-Achilles corpus adiposum. Posterolaterally, it gives insertion to the calcaneal component of the ligament of Rouvière and Canela Lazaro.[7] The anterior segment gives attachment to the posterior talocalcaneal ligament and to the deep crural aponeurosis.

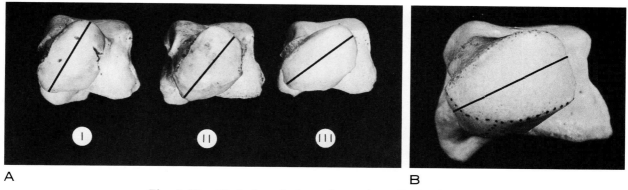

Fig. 2-25. Variations in lateral rotation of talar head. (*A*) (I) Marked rotation. (II) Moderate rotation. (III) Minimal rotation. (*B*) Minimal rotation.

Fig. 2-26. Talotibial relationship. (*A*) Superior view—angle between long axis of calcaneus and axis of talar neck, 30° to 35°. (*B*) Lateral view. (*C*) Medial view (1, Sinus tarsi; 2, medial opening of tarsal canal between posterior border of sustentaculum tali and anterior border of talar posteromedial tubercle; 3, sustentaculum tali.)

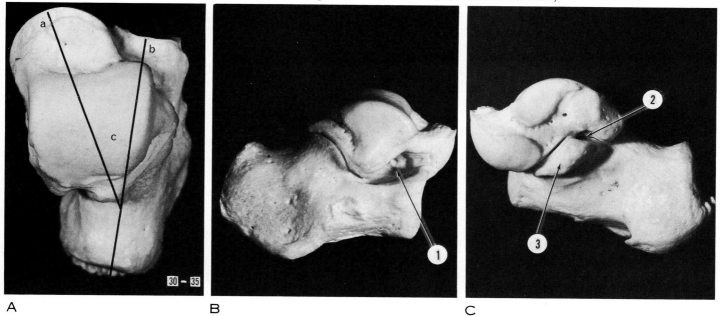

Middle Third

The middle third of the superior surface supports the large facies articularis talaris posterior. This articular surface makes a sharp change in orientation relative to the posterior segment. It inclines anteriorly and creates a step contour. The angle of inclination in 50 calcanei was average 65.5°, maximum 75°, minimum 55° (Fig. 2-29, see Fig. 2-32).

Boehler has determined roentgenographically an angle expressing the height of the posterior talar surface.[14] This "tuber-joint angle" (Fig. 2-29) measures 30° to 35°. This angle, measured anatomically, yields the following distribution in the present series of 50 calcanei: 17° to 20°, 2 calcanei; 21° to 30°, 25 calcanei; 31° to 40°, 20 calcanei; 41° to 44°, 3 calcanei; average 32°.

The long axis of the posterior articular surface is directed forward, downward, and outward. The surface is convex along the longitudinal axis and represents a segment of a cone. The apex of the cone is directed toward the sustentaculum tali and the axis of the cone—the axis of revolution of the surface or the axis of motion along this surface—points anteromedially, intersecting the sustentaculum tali on the inner side at a nearly right angle in the adult.[3] The radius of the curvature along the greatest diameter (at the base of the cone) is 30 mm in average, with a minimum of 12 mm and a maximum of over 40 mm.[13]

Manter considers the posterior talar articular surface as an oblique helicoid or screw-shaped surface inasmuch as sections made perpendicular to the joint surface axis reveal "spiral rather than circular arcs."[15] Inman, contouring the posterior talar articular surface with a dial indicator, demonstrated a screwlike behavior of the surface only in 58%

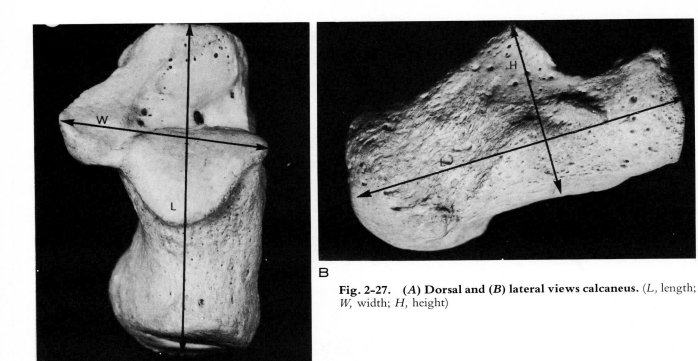

B

Fig. 2-27. (*A*) Dorsal and (*B*) lateral views calcaneus. (*L*, length; *W*, width; *H*, height)

A

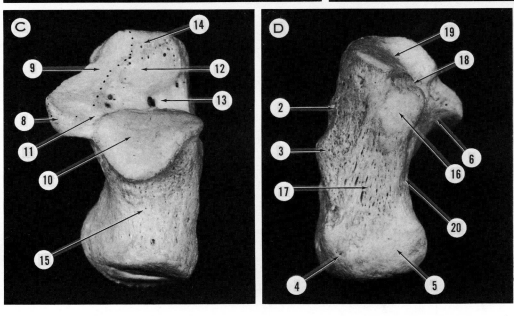

Fig. 2-28. Calcaneus. (*A*) Lateral surface. (*B*) Medial surface. (*C*) Superior surface. (*D*) Inferior surface. (*E*) Anterior surface. (*F*) Posterior surface. (1, Great apophysis; 2, trochlear process; 3, eminentia retrotrochlearis; 4, lateral tuberosity; 5, medial tuberosity; 6, canal for flexor hallucis longus tendon; 7, medial surface of sustentaculum tali; 8, posterior border of sustentaculum tali; 9, fused anterior and middle talar articular surfaces; 10, posterior talar articular surface; 11, canalis tarsi; 12, sinus tarsi—bony eminence; 13, sinus tarsi—fossa calcanei; 14, sinus tarsi—insertion surface of bifurcate ligament; 15, posterior third of superior surface; 16, anterior tuberosity of inferior surface; 17, longitudinally striated inferior surface; 18, coronoid fossa; 19, cuboidal articular surface; 20, (*continued*)

of 42 specimens and concluded that "the remarkable variation is the important factor" in considering the geometry of this surface.[2]

Three accessory or extension facets may be present relative to the facies articularis talaris posterior: anterior, posterior, and medial. The anterior facet is seen in the anterolateral corner, extending onto the floor of the calcaneal fossa in a tonguelike projection. The counterpart to this surface on the talar side is the facies externa accessoria. The posterior facet is a trianglelike projection over the posterior third of the superior surface, corresponding to the presence of a trigonal process or to an os trigonum. The medial extension is directed toward the facies articularis talaris media and at times may succeed in establishing a union, thus obliterating the posterior end of the sulcus calcanei. The frequency of occurrence of these accessory facets is as shown in Table 2-7.

TABLE 2-7. Frequency of Occurrence of Accessory Facets

	Laidlaw*	Present Series
Number of calcanei	750	50
Anterior extension facet		
	Tonguelike 4%	6%
	Minor degree 4.5%	
Posterior extension facet		6%
	Triangular area 3.5%	
	Less definite triangular area 5%	
Medial extension facet		5%
Union with middle surface	1.5%	2%

*Laidlaw PP: The varieties of the os calcis. J Anat Physiol 38:133, 1904

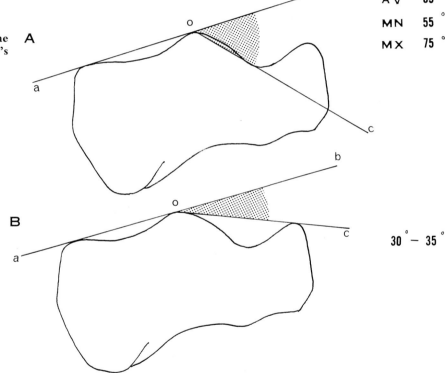

Fig. 2-29. *(A)* Angle of inclination boc of the posterior talar articular surface. *(B)* Boehler's tuber-joint angle *boc.*

A∨ 65° MN 55° MX 75° 30°–35°

Fig. 2-28. *(continued)*
medial calcaneal canal; 21, upper third of posterior surface, corresponding to pre-achilles bursa; 22, 23, middle and lower thirds of posterior surface, corresponding to insertion of achilles tendon.)

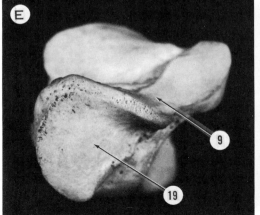
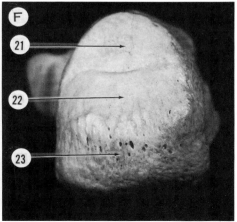

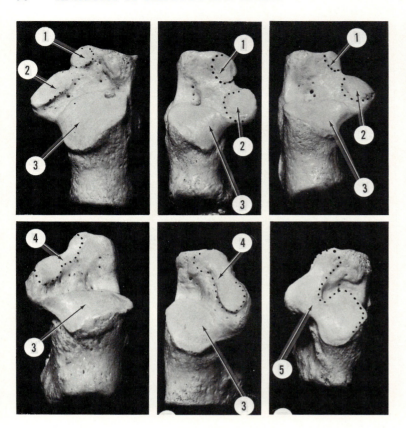

Fig. 2-30.　Variations of the articular surfaces on the superior aspect of the os calcis. (1, Anterior talar articular surface; 2, middle talar articular surface; 3, posterior talar articular surface; 4, fused anterior and middle talar anticular surfaces; 5, fused anterior, middle, and posterior talar articular surfaces.)

Anterior Third

The surface of the anterior third is formed by the sinus tarsi, the sulcus calcanei, and the facies articularis talaris anterior and media (see Figs. 2-26 and 2-28). The long axes of these last two articular surfaces and of the facies articularis talaris posterior make a diverging angle open anterolaterally.

The facies articularis talaris media and anterior form a continuous supportive surface located on the medial aspect of the sinus tarsi and sinus canal. The long axis of the surface is directed forward and laterally. These two surfaces form a concavity along the long axis, corresponding to the convexity of the talar head. The anterior surface is supported by the beak of the os calcis, and the middle surface is supported by the sustentaculum tali. Variations are present in the contour and the degree of separation of these two surfaces. Bunning and Barnett classify the calcanei into three types: A, B, and C.[16] In type A, the anterior and middle surfaces are separate, and in type B they are confluent. In type C, the anterior, middle, and posterior facets are united into a single surface. The distribution of these variations is shown in Table 2-8 (Fig. 2-30).

The degree of confluence of the anterior and middle facets is variable, being partial or complete. A constriction of the continuous surface determines two equal parts in 34% of the calcanei and a small anterior facet in association with a large middle surface in 18%. Trace of constriction is present in 12%, whereas nearly complete separation of the surfaces is seen in 2% of the calcanei of the present series. When a complete division of the surfaces is the norm, the two surfaces are of equal size in 12%, and in 20%, the middle facet

is larger than the anterior; in only 2% of the calcanei is the facies articularis talaris anterior larger than the facies articularis talaris media.

The canalis tarsi separates the middle and the posterior articular facets. It is narrow and oriented obliquely forward, laterally, and inferiorly. It is at a higher level than the floor of the sinus taris and has the same inclination as the sustentaculum tali. This angle of inclination relative to the lower border of the os calcis is 46° in average. This canal is not as deep as its counterpart on the talus, and it opens abruptly into the sinus tarsi. The interosseous talocalcaneal ligament or ligament of the tarsal canal makes its insertion on the floor of the canal, joined by the inward extension of the medial root of the inferior extensor retinaculum. Occasionally a bony crest is seen in the canal, corresponding to this ligamentous insertion. The axis of motion of the talotarsal joint also passes through the canal. Both from the anatomic and the physiologic point of view, the canalis tarsi and its contents are of prime importance.

The sinus tarsi, located on the anterior segment of the superior calcaneal surface, is limited posteriorly by the facies articularis talaris posterior and anteriorly by the anterior border separating the superior calcaneal surface from the anterior cuboidal articular surface. Laterally, the sinus tarsi is limited by the crista lateralis; medially, by the lateral border of the facies articularis talaris anterior. The posteromedial corner of the sinus tarsi continues with the calcaneal or tarsal canal.

In front of the posterior talar surface is the fossa calcanei, perforated by multiple foramina leading to the antrum cal-

TABLE 2-8. Frequency of Occurrence of Variations in Calcanei

Author	Number of calcanei	Occurrence (%)		
		Type A	Type B	Type C
Laidlaw★†	750	32	69	
Bunning and Barnett‡	Veddah 10	0	60	40
	African 492	36	63	1
	British 194	67	33	0
	Indian 78	22	78	0
Present series	50	34	64	2

★Laidlaw reports complete absence of the anterior facet in 0.9%.
†Laidlaw PP: The os calcis, Part II. J Anat Physiol 33:168, 1905
‡Bunning PSC, Barnett CH: A comparison of adult and foetal talocalcaneal articulations. J Anat 99:71, 1965

canei, an interior space free of cancellous trabeculae. Occasionally a large, funnel-shaped foramen is seen in the fossa.

The anterolateral segment of the sinus tarsi is occupied by a bony eminence of variable configuration. This surface may be flat, covered only by rugosities, or it may be slightly elevated like a small plateau; occasionally, it is quite prominent in the form of a high tubercle.

The sinus tarsi gives attachment to the following structures:

The extensor digitorum brevis, arising from the anterolateral bony eminence and partially from the fossa calcanei

The intermediate and medial roots of the inferior extensor retinaculum, located medial to the origin of the extensor digitorum brevis

The cervical ligament, located between the anterior talar articular surface and the origin of the extensor digitorum brevis. A tubercle may indicate the origin.

The dorsal lateral calcaneonavicular and the medial calcaneocuboid ligaments, arising from the anteromedial corner of the surface

The lateral calcaneocuboid ligament, originating from the anterolateral corner of the surface

The crista lateralis is a beamlike bony segment limiting the sinus tarsi laterally. It extends from the posterior articular surface to the anterolateral corner of the superior calcaneal surface, where it becomes less distinct.

INFERIOR SURFACE

The inferior surface of the calcaneus is triangular, with the base posterior and the apex anterior (see Fig. 2-28). Two tuberosities occupy the base: the medial (which is the larger) and the lateral. The width of the bony heel as measured from the inner border of the medial tuberosity to the outer border of the lateral tuberosity is, on the average, 3 cm in the present series of 50 calcanei (maximum, 3.5 cm; minimum, 2.5 cm).

The width of the posterior tuberosities in the present series of 50 calcanei is medial—average 2 cm, maximum 2.4 cm, minimum 1.6 cm; lateral—average 1 cm, maximum 1.4 cm, minimum 0.6 cm.

The medial tuberosity is the main weight-bearing bony segment. Rarely is the lateral tuberosity absent. In most of the calcanei, a triangular space separates the two tubercles; this space is directed anteromedially, with the apex located posterolaterally. At times the apical separation takes the form of a groove. Occasionally there is no intertubercular space and both tubercles are united with a common anterior (nearly) transverse border. Both tubercles have an anteroposterior convex contour.

The mid segment of the inferior calcaneal surface is covered by longitudinal bony striations. The lateral border is oblique and directed anteromedially and many times is less distinct than the rounder medial border, which presents a shallow medial concavity.

An anterior tuberosity is located near the apex of the triangular inferior surface. It is a round eminence measuring 1.5 cm width in average (maximum 2 cm, minimum 1.2 cm).

On the posterior tuberosities, the aponeurosis plantaris and the flexor digitorum brevis muscle are inserted transversely in a posteroanterior sequence. The medial tuberosity gives origin to the abductor hallucis muscle and the lateral tuberosity to the abductor digiti minimi (which also reaches the medial tuberosity). The triangular surface interposed between the anterior and posterior tubercles gives attachments to the ligamentum plantaris longus. The anterior tuberosity provides insertion to the deep fibers of the longitudinal plantar ligament and to the short plantar calcaneocuboid ligament.

Between the anterior tuberosity and the anterior apex of the sustentaculum tali is located a small depression, the coronoid fossa, that gives origin to the inferior calcaneonavicular ligament. A small articular surface in continuity with the anterior cuboidal articular surface is located on the lateral aspect of this fossa and receives the beak or coronoid process of the cuboid.

In the present series of 50 os calcis. a "heel spur" or shelflike anterior bony projection originating from the medial tubercle occurred in 36%.

LATERAL SURFACE

The lateral surface is shown in Figure 2-28. It is high posteriorly and low anteriorly. The posterior third is subcutaneous and is flat, except at the supper segment, where it is slightly convex in the vertical dimension. The middle third presents a tubercle, the eminentia retrotrochlearis, in its lower segment. This is nearly always present.[13] It is a large oval eminence of very variable dimensions. Edwards, in a study of 150 dry calcanei, found this eminence to be present in 98% and absent only in 2%.[1] Anterior to the retrotrochlear eminence is another tubercle, the processus trochlearis (Fig. 2-31). When present and well delineated, this process is a ridgelike structure located below the angle formed by the lateral border of the sinus tarsi and the lateral border of the facies articularis talaris posterior. This tro-

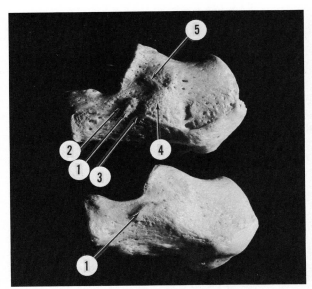

Fig. 2-31. Lateral aspect, calcanei. (1, Trochlear process; 2, sulcus for peroneus brevis tendon; 3, sulcus for peroneus longus tendon; 4, eminentia retrotrochlearis; 5, tubercle for calcaneofibular ligament.)

chlear process is oriented downward and anteriorly, and the long axis makes an angle of 45° with the horizontal.[13]

The frequency of occurrence of the processes trochlearis in various series is as follows: Gruber,[17] 39.1%; Stieda,[18] 33%; Pfitzner,[19] 39.9%; Laidlaw,[13] 36.5% (prominent, 20.5% less marked, 16%); Edwards,[1] 44%; present series (50 calcanei), 32%.

The dimensions of the trochlear process are as follows:[1] length—maximum 17 mm, minimum 2 mm; breadth at base—maximum 10 mm, minimum 2 mm; height—maximum 7 mm, minimum 1 mm.

On the inferior surface of this process glides the peroneus longus tendon. The superior surface is smooth and corresponds to the peroneus brevis tendon. The groove of the peroneus longus tendon leaves a landmark on the lateral aspect of the os calcis in 85%.[1] This groove may be present in the absence of a trochlear process, located then on the anterior aspect of the retrotrochlear eminence or on the lateral aspect of the os calcis.

A cartilage-covered gliding facet may be present on the os calcis along the course of the peroneus longus tendon. Edwards found such facets in 44% of his series, and of these, 10.6% were present in the absence of a trochlear process.[1] These gliding facets are oval, usually not elevated, and located on the posterior slope of the trochlear process or partly on this slope and partly on the lateral surface of the calcaneus.

A definite groove for the peroneus brevis tendon is present in only 2.6%.[1] The inferior peroneal retinaculum, bridging both peroneal tendons, attaches to the os calcis above and below the trochlear process and sends a septum to the crest of the process.

The tuberculum ligamenti calcaneofibularis is a small tubercle situated behind the mid segment of the facies artic-

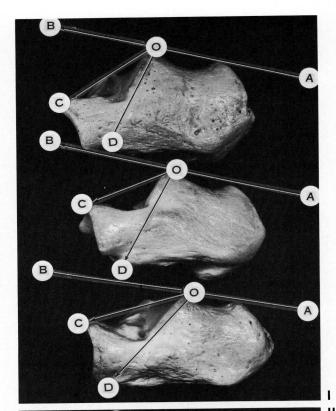

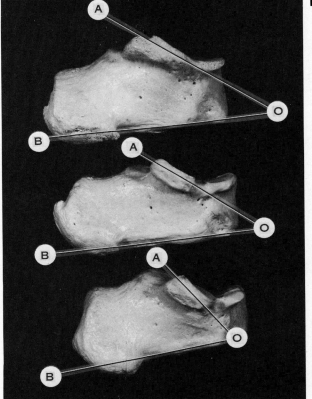

Fig. 2-32. (I) Variable inclination of sustentaculum tali—angle *AOB*. (II) Variations of inclination angle *BOD* and of tuber-joint angle (Boehler's) *BOC*. Top, marked inclination; center, moderate inclination; bottom, minimal inclination.

ularis talaris posterior and is posterosuperior to the eminentia retrotrochlearis. It is present as a well-defined tubercle in 43%.[13] The location of this tubercle for the insertion of the calcaneofibular ligament is typical in 64.5% and varies in the remaining 35.5% (anterior location, 25.5%; downward location, 4.5%; posterior location, 5.5%).[13]

The calcaneal component of the fibulocalcaneoastragalar ligament of Rouvière and Canela Lazaro extends its insertion on the superior aspect of the lateral surface behind the insertion of the calcaneofibular ligament in an oblique linear fashion; the lateral talocalcaneal ligament inserts anterior to it.[7] A tubercle (tuberculum ligamenti talicalcanei) may be present for this attachment. Occasionally a small tubercle for the attachment of the lateral calcaneocuboid ligament is seen in the superior segment of the anterior third of the lateral surface. Morestin describes a second trochlear gliding facet for the tendon of the peroneus longus, located at the anteroinferior corner of the external calcaneal surface.[20] He recognizes two varieties: intra- and extra-articular. The intra-articular facet is at the extreme anterior portion of the calcaneus, and the capsule–synovium of the calcaneocuboid joint inserts at its periphery. The extra-articular type is at a distance from the calcaneocuboid articulation and is oval or circular, cartilage covered, and somewhat elevated above the surrounding parts. When well developed, a sesamoid is found in the substance of the peroneus longus tendon; this sesamoid is different than the sesamoid found in the same tendon farther distally as it passes over the tuberosity of the cuboid.

The frequency of occurrence of this second trochlear facet in various series is as follows: Morestin,[20] 5%; Edwards,[1] 6.6%; present series (50 os calcis), 4%.

MEDIAL SURFACE

The medial surface of the os calcis, similar to the lateral surface, is high posteriorly and low anteriorly (Figs. 2-28 and 2-32). This surface forms a large oblique canal directed downward and anteriorly. It accepts the width of two fingers. The configuration is determined by the medial projection of the sustentaculum tali and the medial extension of the medial calcaneal tubercle. This calcaneal canal is the port of entry from the posteromedial aspect of the ankle to the plantar aspect of the foot.

The sustentaculum tali is a bracketlike projection, triangular with a posterior base and an anterior apex. This surface projects anteromedially and is inclined downward and anteriorly at an angle of 46° average (maximum 60°, minimum 30°) (Fig. 2-32). The superior surface corresponds to the facies articularis talaris media, described above. The inferior surface is carved into a groove for the gliding of the flexor hallucis longus tendon and provides attachment to the fibrous tunnel of the tendon. A crest may be present at the attachment site posteriorly. The medial surface of the sustentaculum tali is triangular, with a posterior base and an anterior apex. This surface corresponds to the flexor digitorum longus tendon and its fibrous tendon sheath. The tibiocalcaneal components of the deltoid ligament and the superomedial calcaneonavicular ligament insert on the upper border of the medial surface. The recurrent band of

the tibialis posterior tendon inserts on the lower border of the same surface.

The posterior border of the sustentaculum tali corresponds to the medial entrance of the canalis tarsi and gives insertion to the medial talocalcaneal ligament. On rare occasions when the posterior talar articular surface extends medially over the superior surface of the sustentaculum, the opening of the canalis tarsi is on the medial border of the sustentaculum tali (see Fig. 2-30).

The sustentaculum tali has a variable width and length. The width of the sustentaculum tali, as measured at the base (see Fig. 2-27), was average 13 mm, maximum 18 mm, minimum 8 mm in the present series of 50 dry calcanei. The ratio of the sustentacular width to the total width of the os calcis at the same level is average 0.33, maximum 0.47, minimum 0.23. These values may be correlated with the supportive function of the sustentaculum tali relative to the talar head. An "incompetent" sustentaculum tali may fall into a group with minimum value or lower.

The sustentaculum tali may also be classified by length as long or short. A long sustentaculum is continuous through its medial border with the processus anterior, which is then in association with a fusion of the facies articularis media and anterior. A short sustentaculum ends suddenly anteriorly, and a notch separates the two articular surfaces (see Figs. 2-30 and 2-32).[21] The frequency of occurrence of these varieties, including the intermediary forms, in Laidlaw's series is long, about 40%; short, 32%; intermediary, 28%.[21] In the present series the frequency is long, 60%; short, 34%; intermediary, 6%.

The medial surface of the os calcis gives insertion on its inferior two thirds to the medial head of the quadratus plantae. This field of insertion is triangular, with the base posterior. The transverse interfascicular ligament inserts above the quadratus plantae and below the tunnel of the flexor hallucis longus.

POSTERIOR SURFACE

The posterior surface is triangular, with the apex superior and the base inferior (see Fig. 2-28). The medial and lateral borders are well delineated, but the inferior border is ill defined, as the surface is continuous with the plantar aspect. The overall contour of the surface is convex. The upper segment is directed upward and anteriorly and is divided into two fields. The lower field is transverse and trapezoidal with an irregular, striated, crenated lower border and a soft and regular superior border. This surface corresponds to the insertion of the Achilles tendon. The upper field is free from tendinous insertion. It is triangular and smooth and corresponds to the pre-Achilles bursa. The lower surface is broad, directed downward and anteriorly; it is striated due to the insertion of the Achilles tendon.

ANTERIOR SURFACE

The anterior surface is almost entirely articular (see Fig. 2-28). It is saddle shaped, convex transversely and concave vertically. The contour of the surface forms a spiral-type groove directed downward and inward. At the postero-

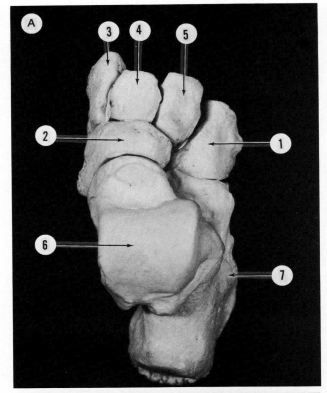

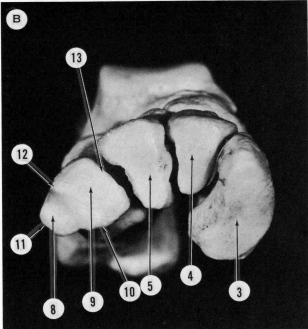

Fig. 2-33. *(A)* **Dorsal aspect, tarsus.** *(B)* **Transverse arch formed by the cuneiforms and the cuboid, which is also wedge shaped.** (1, Cuboid; 2, navicular; 3, medial cuneiform; 4, middle cuneiform; 5, lateral cuneiform; 6, talus; 7, calcaneus; Cuboid. 8, 9, lateral and medial aspect of anterior articular surface; 10, inferior border; 11, apex; 12, dorsolateral border; 13, medial border.)

medial end of this groove is the calcaneal coronoid fossa, which receives the beak of the cuboid.

The superomedial corner of the articular surface makes a shelflike projection anteromedially. This beak or rostrum of the os calcis overhangs the cuboid.

Cuboid

The cuboid is intercalated between the calcaneum and the base of metatarsals 4 and 5. It gives support to the lateral cuneiform and may enter in contact with the scaphoid.

The bone is wedge shaped or cuneiform rather than cuboid, as the dorsal and plantar surfaces slope toward the narrow lateral surface or border (Fig. 2-33). It presents five surfaces; dorsal, plantar, medial or base, posterior, and anterior, and a lateral border or apex.

DORSAL SURFACE

The dorsal surface is markedly inclined outward and is in continuity with the lateral surface of the calcaneum (Figs. 2-34 and 2-35). Tranversely, it continues the curvature of the dorsal surface of the cuneiforms, contributing to the formation of the transverse arch of the midfoot (see Fig. 2-33).

The surface is trapezoidal, covered by rugosities, and crossed by the extensor digitorum brevis and the peroneus tertius tendon. This surface has four borders:

Medial, which represents the base of the trapezoid. The distal segment has a medial projection. It corresponds to the navicular and the third cuneiform.
Lateral, which represents the apex of the trapezoid. This border is short and slightly concave, corresponding to the crossing of the peroneus longus tendon.
Proximal and convex, corresponding to the os calcis
Distal and obtuse, corresponding to the base of the fourth and fifth metatarsals

The dorsal surface provides attachment to the following:

Dorsomedial calcaneocuboid ligament, which attaches on a small tubercle located on the posteromedial corner of the surface
Dorsolateral calcaneocuboid ligament, which attaches at least 0.5 cm distal to the proximal border and reaches the middorsal segment
Lateral calcaneocuboid ligament, just above the lateral border
Dorsal cubonavicular ligament, inserting on the medial side of the mid segment
Dorsal $cuneo_3$-cuboid ligament, single or double, inserting in the distal half of the medial dorsal surface
Dorsal $cubometatarsal_4$, $cubometatarsal_5$ ligaments, attached along the distal margin of the bone. The latter has a broader insertion area than the former.

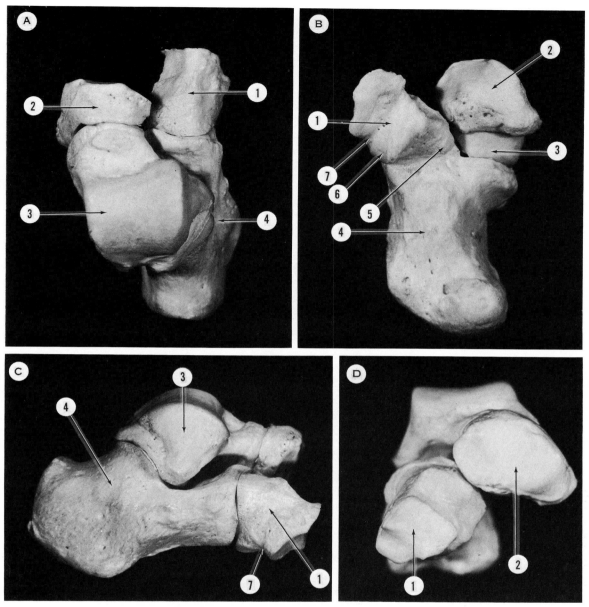

Fig. 2-34.   Subtalar and midtarsal skeleton. (*A*) Dorsal aspect. (*B*) Plantar aspect. (*C*) Lateral aspect. (*D*) Anterior aspect. (1, Cuboid; 2, navicular; 3, talus; 4, calcaneus [elongated ~ contour of Chopart's joint is seen]; 5, beak of cuboid; 6, sesamoid facet of cuboid; 7, canal of peroneus longus.)

PLANTAR SURFACE

The plantar surface faces inferiorly and medially (see Figs. 2-34 and 2-35). It is wider medially and narrower laterally. The medial border is oblique and is directed more posteriorly and slightly medially, while the posterior border is directed more medially and slightly posteriorly. At the junction of these two borders is the beak or coronoid process of the cuboid.

The short lateral border is slightly concave. The anterior border is directed laterally and posteriorly and is divided into a short medial segment and a long lateral segment, which is more inclined posteriorly.

A strong ridge, the tuberositas ossis cuboidei, oriented obliquely anteromedially, divides the plantar surface into a small anterior and a large posterior area. A line extending in the direction of this tuberosity will reach the base of the first metatarsal.

As demonstrated by Stieda and Poirier, there is no cuboidal groove or peroneal groove on the anterior aspect of

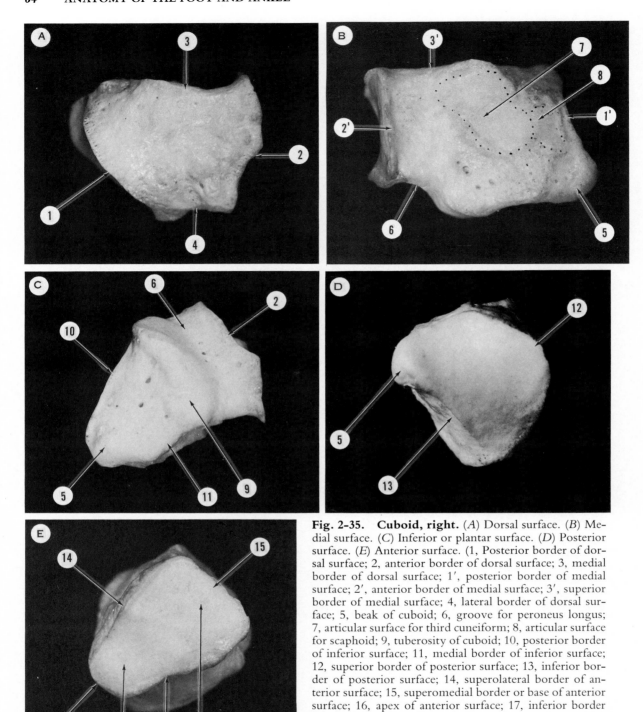

Fig. 2-35.   Cuboid, right. (*A*) Dorsal surface. (*B*) Medial surface. (*C*) Inferior or plantar surface. (*D*) Posterior surface. (*E*) Anterior surface. (1, Posterior border of dorsal surface; 2, anterior border of dorsal surface; 3, medial border of dorsal surface; 1′, posterior border of medial surface; 2′, anterior border of medial surface; 3′, superior border of medial surface; 4, lateral border of dorsal surface; 5, beak of cuboid; 6, groove for peroneus longus; 7, articular surface for third cuneiform; 8, articular surface for scaphoid; 9, tuberosity of cuboid; 10, posterior border of inferior surface; 11, medial border of inferior surface; 12, superior border of posterior surface; 13, inferior border of posterior surface; 14, superolateral border of anterior surface; 15, superomedial border or base of anterior surface; 16, apex of anterior surface; 17, inferior border of anterior surface; 18, articular surfaces corresponding to metatarsals 4 and 5.)

the plantar surface.[18, 22] The tendon of the peroneus longus glides and is reflected over the anterior slope of the cuboidal tuberosity. Furthermore, a gliding facet corresponding to the sesamoid of the peroneus longus tendon is present on the anterolateral aspect of this tuberosity. The sesamoid facet or cuboid facet is present in 93%.[1] It is oval (77%), irregularly quadrilateral (18%) or triangular (5%) and is slightly convex.[1]

The anterior segment of the plantar surface is long and narrow. It is limited anteriorly by the anterior border corresponding to the base of the fourth and fifth metatarsals and posteriorly by the tuberosity of the cuboid. The surface is flat and may appear as a groove due to the elevation of the tuberosity and "to the presence of a slight ledge of bone which is thrown up along its anterior margin."[1]

The posterior segment, located posterior to the ridge, is larger and triangular. The base corresponds to the tuberosity of the cuboid and the apex to the beak. It is a depressed surface and may form a deep concavity.

The plantar surface of the cuboid provides attachment to the following:

Plantar cubometatarsal$_5$, cubometatarsal$_4$ ligaments, which are inserted along the margin of the anterior border

Peroneus longus fibrous tendon sheath, which attaches to the anterior segment behind the cubometatarsal ligaments and over the crest of the cuboidal ridge

Deep fibers of the longitudinal plantar ligament, inserting over the cuboidal tuberosity

Short plantar calcaneocuboid ligament, which inserts on the entire triangular posterior aspect of the surface. A strong band inserts transversely on the beak of the cuboid

Plantar cubonavicular ligament, which attaches to the medial border of the posterior segment and the beak of the cuboid

Plantar cuneo$_3$-cuboid ligament, which inserts on the medial aspect of the cuboid crest and the segment of the medial border immediately behind it

An expansion from the tibialis posterior tendon may insert on the posteromedial corner in conjunction with the plantar cuboscaphoid ligament.

On the posterior aspect of the tuberosity of the cuboid are also attached, in a lateral to medial direction, the opponens and short flexor of the fifth toe, the oblique head of the adductor hallucis, and the flexor hallucis brevis. Some of these attachments are through their connection with the fibrous tunnel of the peroneus longus tendon.

ANTERIOR SURFACE

The anterior surface (see Figs. 2-33–2-35) articulates with the base of the fourth and fifth metatarsals. The long axis is directed downward and laterally. The surface is more or less triangular, with a medial base and a lateral apex. It is divided into two segments by a vertical smooth ridge. The lateral surface, triangular, has a long transverse axis and is larger than the medial; it is slightly concave in the center and corresponds to the base of the fifth metatarsal. The medial surface, rectangular, is smaller than the lateral and slightly concave, and its long axis is vertical; it corresponds to the base of the fourth metatarsal. The two segments of the surface join at an obtuse angle, forming an anterior angular convexity.

POSTERIOR SURFACE

The posterior surface articulates with the calcaneum. It is saddle shaped, concave transversely and convex vertically. The medial end of the surface bears the beak of the cuboid.

This process (the pyramidal apophysis or coronoid of the cuboid) augments the concavity of the articular surface.[23] It lodges in a corresponding fossa of the calcaneum in flexion and adduction of the forefoot.[8] "The process 'undershoots' the os calcis, supporting it in a bracketlike way, in fact in a very similar manner to that in which the plantar point, on the navicular, supports the head of the astralagus."[24]

MEDIAL SURFACE

The medial surface faces medially and upward. It is quadrilateral and is narrower anteriorly. In the middle third, the articular surface for the third cuneiform is present. This articular surface is flat, round, oval, or triangular with a superior base. It is in touch with the superior margin and is separated from the inferior margin by a band of rugosities. The segment posterior to the cuneiform articular surface bears a small articular surface for the scaphoid. The contour of this segment is variable. The facet for the scaphoid occurs with the following frequency: in Gruber's series of 200 feet, it was present in 45.5%; in Pfitzner's series of 437 feet, it was present in 54.5%.[19, 25] This surface extends posteriorly up the posterior articular surface, but occasionally a depression separates the two. The rough surface below the scaphoid surface gives insertion to the plantar cuboscaphoid ligament. The anterior third of the medial surface is a rough area for the attachment of the interosseous cuneo$_3$-cuboid ligament.

LATERAL BORDER

The lateral border is the apex of the cuboid, formed by the junction of the dorsal and plantar surfaces. This border bears a concavity that corresponds to the beginning of the peroneal tunnel.

Scaphoid

The scaphoid (os naviculare) is interposed between the head of the talus and the three cuneiforms (Figs. 2-36 and 2-37). It establishes minimal articular contact with the cuboid and is firmly bound with ligaments to the os calcis. It is an integral part of the talotarsal joint. The scaphoid is pyriform, with the long axis oblique, directed downward and medially. The round base is superolateral and the enlarged apex, inferomedial. The bone is flattened anteroposteriorly and is thicker dorsomedially.

It presents four surfaces—posterior, anterior, dorsal, plantar—and two extremities—lateral, medial.

POSTERIOR SURFACE

The posterior surface is oriented posteriorly and faces the talar head. It does not cover completely the navicular articular surface of the talus. It is biconcave and tear shaped and has the same obliquity as the bone. The concavity of the surface is variable, and in a few cases the surface is nearly flat.[26] Frequently an inferior extension of the articular sur-

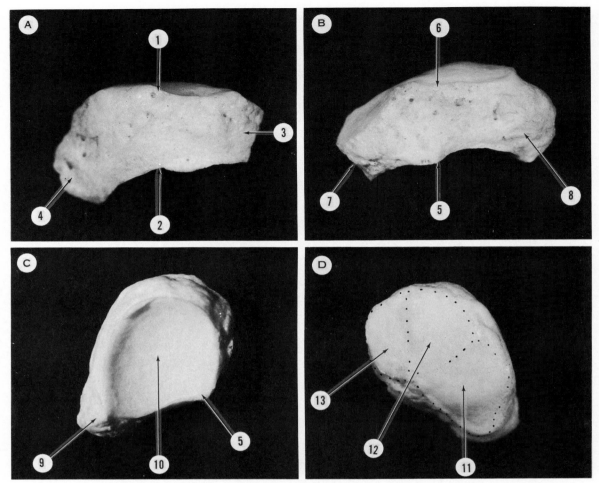

Fig. 2-36. Navicular. (*A*) Dorsal surface. (*B*) Plantar surface. (*C*) Posterior surface. (*D*) Anterior surface. (1, Anterior border of dorsal surface; 2, posterior border of dorsal surface; 3, lateral border of dorsal surface; 4, medial border of dorsal surface; 5, beak of navicular; 6, anterior border of inferior surface; 7, lateral border of inferior surface; 8, medial segment of inferior surface; 9, tuberosity of navicular; 10, talar articular surface; 11, articular surface for first cuneiform; 12, articular surface for second cuneiform; 13, articular surface for third cuneiform.)

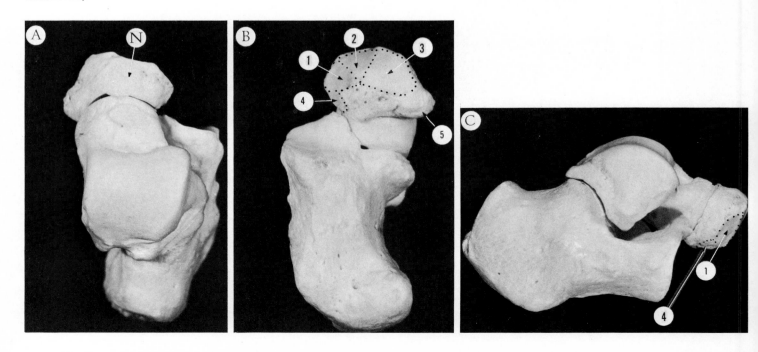

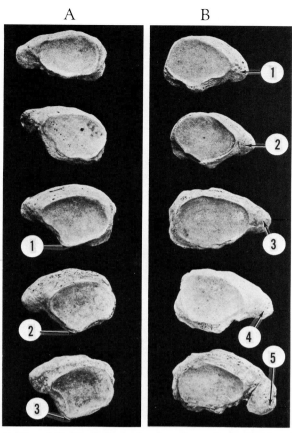

face is present, corresponding to the beak of the navicular (Fig. 2-38). This projection gives a triangular or quadrangular outline to the scaphoid. Dwight considers this extension as a fused secondary cuboid.[27]

ANTERIOR SURFACE

The anterior surface is reniform with inferior concavity. It is entirely articular and corresponds to the three cuneiforms. This surface is angular and faceted but yet is convex in its general contour. It is divided into three facets by two soft crests converging inferiorly, extending from the superior to the inferior border. The medial facet is the largest and corresponds to the first cuneiform. It is convex and triangular with a superolateral convex base and is oriented anteroinferiorly. The middle facet corresponds to the second cuneiform. It is triangular, with a superior base and an inferior apex. The surface is flat or slightly convex. It is oriented anteriorly with a minimal inferior tilt. The lateral facet is the smallest of the three. It is quadrilateral with rounded corners. This surface is flat or minimally concave and is oriented anterolaterally with a minimal inferior inclination.

When the general contour and the orientation of the anterior and posterior surfaces of the navicular are analyzed, it becomes evident that this bone induces a change of direction in the medial bony column. The talar head and neck initiate a medial deviation, whereas the navicular orients the column laterally and inferiorly. This zig-zag arrangement maintains the overall axial alignment of the foot, overcoming the initial divergence (Fig. 2-39).

The inferior convergence of the articular facets on the anterior articular surface determines the formation of the transverse tarsal arch (see Fig. 2-37).

Fig. 2-38. (*A*) Variations in the size of the beak of the navicular, more pronounced in 1, 2, and 3. (*B*) Variations in the size of the tuberosity of the navicular. (From Dwight T: Variations in the Bones of the Hands and Feet: A Clinical Atlas, pp 14–23. Philadelphia, J B Lippincott, 1907)

Fig. 2-37. **Navicular bone (*N*) in relation to hindfoot skeleton.** (*A*) Dorsal view. (*B*) Plantar view. (*C*) Lateral view. (*D*) Medial view. (*E*) Anterior view. (1, Articular surface with third cuneiform; 2, articular surface with second cuneiform; 3, articular surface with first cuneiform; 4, articular surface with cuboid; 5, tuberosity of navicular.)

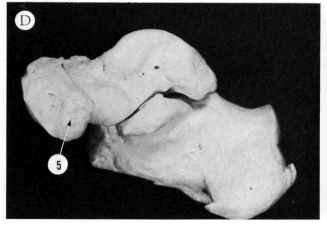
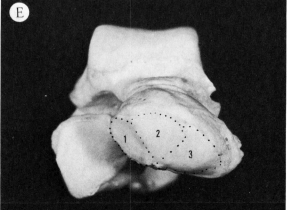

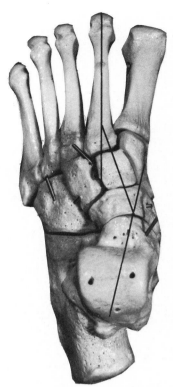

Fig. 2-39. Zig-zag pattern formed by the medial bony column—talus, navicular, cuneiform block, and metatarsals 2 and 3. The talar neck is deflected medially. The distal articular surface of the navicular deflects the cuneiforms laterally, neutralizing the medial deviation.

DORSAL SURFACE

The dorsal surface is strongly convex, narrower laterally and larger medially. The apex of the convexity corresponds to the level of the middle articular facet of the anterior surface. The lateral one fourth of the surface faces superolaterally, and the medial three fourths is oriented superomedially. The posterior border of the surface is concave. The anterior border is angular, formed by three segments united at an obtuse angle. The lateral segment is the shortest, oriented posterolaterally. The middle segment, nearly transverse, is longer. The medial segment is the largest, slightly convex, and oriented downward posteriorly. This segment is inferior to the other two.

The taloscaphoid capsule inserts at the periphery of the posterior articular surface.

The dorsal surface gives attachment to the following:

Superomedial calcaneonavicular ligament, attaching along the superomedial aspect of the surface[28]
Superficial and deep components of the dorsal talonavicular ligament
Tibionavicular component of the superficial deltoid ligament, interlacing fibers with the superomedial calcaneonavicular ligament
Dorsal cuneo$_{1,2,3}$-navicular ligament, originating from the distal segment of the dorsal surface
Dorsal cubonavicular ligament inserting on the lateral segment of the surface.

PLANTAR SURFACE

The plantar surface is irregular and covered with rugosities and is in continuity medially with the tuberosity of the navicular. Frequently, an inferior bony projection—the beak of the navicular—is present in its mid segment.

The segment of the tibialis posterior tendon destined for the cuneiforms passes in a groove lateral to the tuberosity of the navicular and is oriented anterolaterally. The inferior calcaneonavicular ligament inserts on the inferior surface and posterior border, extending from the tuberosity of the navicular to the beak, where the insertion is most powerful.

The mid segment of the inferior surface gives attachment to the plantar cubonavicular ligament, and farther anteriorly, the second and third plantar cuneonavicular ligaments are inserted along the articular margin.

Manners-Smith mentions the rare occurrence (in 13 of 600) on the plantar surface of an articular facet for the os calcis close to the posterior surface, located between the beak of the navicular and the facet for the cuboid.[26]

MEDIAL END

The medial end of the navicular is formed by a bony prominence, the navicular tuberosity. The size of this structure is variable (see Fig. 2-38). When separated from the main bone mass, it is called the *naviculare secundarium*. The tibialis posterior tendon inserts on the tuberosity.

The first plantar cuneonavicular ligament arises from the anterior aspect of the tubercle and the medial cuneonavicular ligament, from the medial aspect.

LATERAL END

The lateral end of the navicular is convex and presents two segments: inferior and superior. A small articular facet for the cuboid occupies most of the inferior surface. This surface is in continuity with the articular facet for the third cuneiform. As indicated by Manners-Smith, the cuboid facet is present in 70% of 600 naviculars and is variable in contour and size.[26] In some instances, it extends from the articular facet of the third cuneiform to the posterior articular surface. This cuboid surface not infrequently extends onto the beak of the navicular.

The superior segment of the lateral end gives insertion to the powerful lateral calcaneonavicular ligament, a component of the bifurcate ligament.

Cuneiforms

The cuneiforms are three in number and are interposed between the scaphoid proximally, the first three metatarsals distally, and the cuboid laterally. The three cuneiforms, in association with the cuboid, form an arcade or transverse arch that acts as a niche for the plantar musculotendinous and neurovascular structures. The cuneiforms are wedge shaped. The first or medial cuneiform has a dorsal crest and plantar base, the second or middle cuneiform and the third or lateral cuneiform have a dorsal base and a plantar crest (see Fig. 2-33).

Proximally, on the dorsum of the foot, the bases of the cuneiforms form a polygonal line with two obtuse angles. The angle between the second and third cuneiforms is oriented posteromedially, and the angle between the bases of the first and second cuneiforms is directed posteriorly. Distally, the second cuneiform is in proximal recess, approximately 8 mm relative to the first cuneiform and 4 mm relative to the third cuneiform. This disposition creates the necessary space to receive and lock the base of the second metatarsal.

FIRST CUNEIFORM

The first cuneiform has five surfaces—anterior, posterior, medial, lateral, inferior—and a crest (Fig. 2-40).

The posterior surface articulates with the scaphoid. It is triangular or pear shaped, with an inferior base and a superior apex. The surface is concave in all directions.

The anterior surface articulates with the base of the first metatarsal. It is reniform, with a convex medial border and a concave lateral border. The surface is elongated in the vertical direction and is oriented anteriorly, with some inferior and medial inclination. The surface is minimally convex in the transverse direction and more or less flat in the vertical dimension. As mentioned by Jones, this facet for the hallux is usually a single surface or (often) notched with a distinct constriction in its mid segment; not uncommonly, it is subdivided into two separate surfaces.[9]

The medial surface is pentagonal, higher distally and lower proximally. The anteroinferior angle is occupied by an oval, smooth surface. The tibialis anterior takes insertion along the inferior and posterior margin of this oval surface. A bursa covers the smooth surface;[29] it corresponds to the cartilaginous sesamoid of the tibialis anterior tendon. The medial surface also provides attachment to the following:

Dorsal cuneo$_1$-navicular ligament
Dorsal intercuneiform$_{1,2}$ ligament, which occupies the lateral aspect of the surface
Dorsal cuneo$_1$-metatarsal$_2$ ligament, arising from the anterolateral corner
Dorsal cuneo$_1$-metatarsal$_1$ broad ligament, arising from the mid segment of the anterior margin
Medial cuneo$_1$-navicular ligament, inserting on the lower and posterior aspect of the surface

The lateral surface, more or less rectangular, is limited along the posterior and superior borders by two articular surfaces. The articular surface corresponding to the second cuneiform is in the shape of an inferiorly reflected L, the vertical arm running along the posterior border and the larger horizontal arm running along the posterior two thirds of the superior border. The horizontal segment is concave anteroposteriorly, and the vertical is concave vertically. The anterior third of the surface along the superior border is occupied by an oval articulating surface, corresponding to the base of the second metatarsal. This surface reaches the anterior articulating surface but is separated from the superior border and the horizontal arm of the cuneiform surface by a small bony band. The angle formed by the two arms of the articulating surfaces is occupied by the insertion

of the intercuneiform$_{1,2}$ ligament, and anterior to it is located a bony eminence that gives attachment to the powerful cuneo$_1$-metatarsal$_2$ ligament (Lisfranc's ligament).

The inferior or plantar surface is rectangular, large, and strongly convex transversely. It provides insertion to the following:

Plantar cuneo$_1$-navicular ligament, attached to the tubercle located on the posterior aspect of the surface
Plantar intercuneiform$_{1,2}$ ligament from the mid segment of the lateral border
Cuneo$_1$-metatarsal$_1$ broad ligament, arising from the distal border of the surface
Cuneo$_1$-metatarsals$_{2,3}$ ligament very strong, which originates from the posterolateral corner
Peroneus longus tendon, inserting anterior to the tubercle and occupying the lateral half of the distal segment

The crest or superior border is round and smooth. The anterior one fourth corresponds to the base of the second metatarsal and is directed posteriorly. The posterior three fourths is directed downward, posteromedially, and corresponds to the second cuneiform.

SECOND CUNEIFORM

The second cuneiform is the smallest of the three and is in recess relative to the other two. The bone presents five surfaces—anterior, posterior, medial, lateral, superior or dorsal—and a crest (Fig. 2-41).

The anterior surface articulates with the base of the second metatarsal. It is triangular, with a dorsal convex base and an inferior apex. The lateral border is slightly concave laterally. The surface is gently convex in its vertical dimension.

The posterior surface is also triangular, with a similar orientation. The lateral border is concave and the medial border, convex. This surface articulates with the scaphoid and presents vertical concavity.

The medial surface articulates with the first cuneiform, with a similar inferiorly reversed L-shaped articular surface. The vertical segment of this articular surface is narrower than the horizontal arm, which may overflow inferiorly. The surface of the bone located at the angle of the two articular arms gives insertion to the interosseous cuneiform$_{1,2}$ ligament. Jones describes a variant to the medial surface with an interosseous groove dividing the horizontal segment into two.[9]

The lateral surface, rectangular, bears also a reversed L-shaped articular surface occupying the superior and posterior borders. It articulates with the third cuneiform. A small tubercle located in the interarticular angle gives insertion to the interosseous cuneiform$_{2,3}$ ligament. From the anteroinferior segment of the surface originates the cuneo$_2$-metatarsal$_2$ or cuneo$_2$-metatarsal$_{2,3}$ ligament.

The dorsal surface is rectangular, minimally convex, and larger posteriorly. A small depression is often present near the posteromedial corner along its medial border. With a corresponding depression on the first cuneiform, a small pit is formed (the intercuneiform fossa).[9] The borders of the dorsal surface give insertion to the dorsal scaphocuneiform$_2$

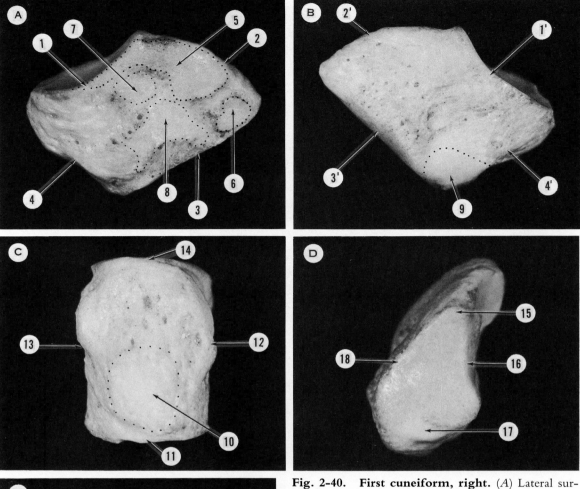

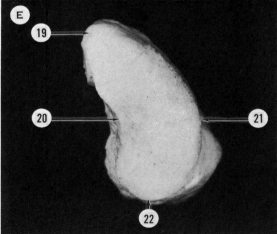

Fig. 2-40. First cuneiform, right. (*A*) Lateral surface. (*B*) Medial surface. (*C*) Plantar surface. (*D*) Posterior surface. (*E*) Anterior surface. (1, 1′, Posterior borders of lateral and medial surfaces; 2, 2′, superior borders of lateral and medial surfaces; 3, 3′, anterior borders of lateral and medial surfaces; 4, 4′, inferior borders of lateral and medial surfaces; 5, articular surface for second cuneiform; 6, articular surface for base of second metatarsal; 7, insertional zone of intercuneiform C_1–C_2 ligament; 8, insertional zone of Lisfranc's ligament C_1–M_2; 9, oval smooth surface for tibialis anterior tendon, where a gliding bursa may be found; 10, tubercle of inferior surface; 11, posterior border of inferior surface; 12, medial border of inferior surface; 13, lateral border of inferior surface; 14, anterior border of inferior surface; 15, apex of navicular articular surface; 16, lateral border of navicular articular surface; 17, round base of navicular articular surface; 18, medial border of navicular articular surface; 19, apex of first metatarsal articular surface; 20, concave lateral border of first metatarsal articular surface; 21, convex medial border of first metatarsal articular surface; 22, inferior border of first metatarsal articular surface.)

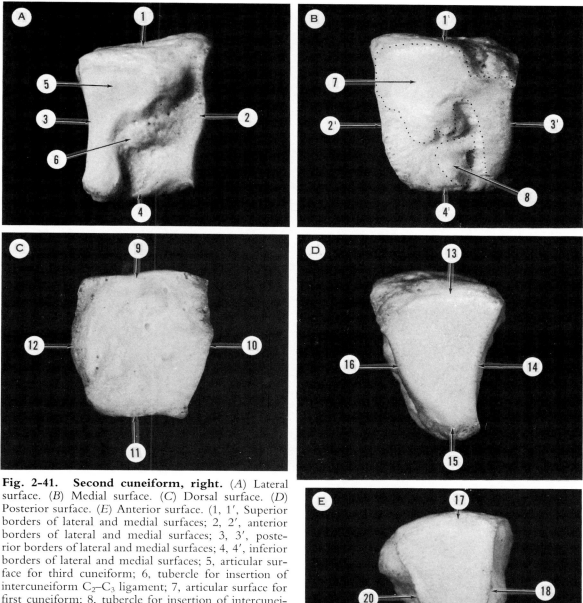

Fig. 2-41. Second cuneiform, right. (*A*) Lateral surface. (*B*) Medial surface. (*C*) Dorsal surface. (*D*) Posterior surface. (*E*) Anterior surface. (1, 1′, Superior borders of lateral and medial surfaces; 2, 2′, anterior borders of lateral and medial surfaces; 3, 3′, posterior borders of lateral and medial surfaces; 4, 4′, inferior borders of lateral and medial surfaces; 5, articular surface for third cuneiform; 6, tubercle for insertion of intercuneiform C_2–C_3 ligament; 7, articular surface for first cuneiform; 8, tubercle for insertion of intercuneiform C_1–C_2 ligament; 9, posterior border of dorsal surface; 10, medial border of dorsal surface; 11, anterior border of dorsal surface; 12, lateral border of dorsal surface; 13, superior border of navicular articular surface; 14, concave lateral border of navicular articular surface; 15, apex of navicular articular surface; 16, medial border of navicular articular surface; 17, superior border of second metatarsal articular surface; 18, medial border of second metatarsal articular surface; 19, apex of second metatarsal articular surface; 20, lateral border of second metatarsal articular surface.)

ligament posteriorly, the dorsal cuneo$_2$-metatarsal$_2$ ligament anteriorly, the dorsal cuneiform$_{1,2}$ ligament medially, and the dorsal cuneiform$_{2,3}$ ligament laterally.

The crest or inferior border is thin and engulfed by the two other cuneiforms. It provides insertion to the plantar cuneo$_2$-navicular ligament and the plantar cuneiform$_{1,2}$ ligament, both masked by the insertion of the tibialis posterior tendon. The crest also gives attachment to the lateral fibrous arm of the Y origin of the flexor hallucis brevis muscle.

THIRD CUNEIFORM

The third cuneiform articulates with the scaphoid proximally, the cuboid laterally, the base of the third metatarsal distally, and the second cuneiform medially. The bone presents five surfaces—anterior, posterior, medial, lateral, dorsal—and a plantar crest (Fig. 2-42).

The anterior surface articulates with the base of the third metatarsal. It is triangular, with the base dorsal and apex

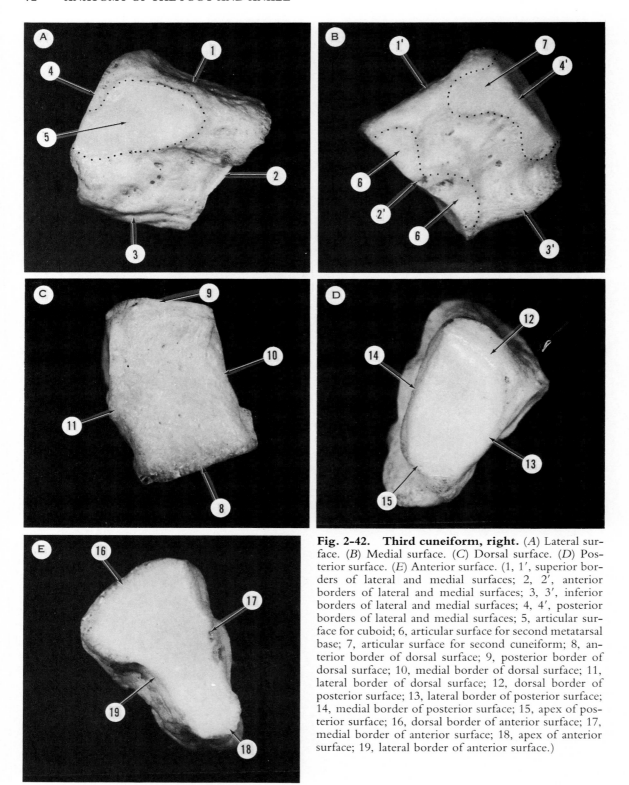

Fig. 2-42.   Third cuneiform, right. (*A*) Lateral surface. (*B*) Medial surface. (*C*) Dorsal surface. (*D*) Posterior surface. (*E*) Anterior surface. (1, 1′, superior borders of lateral and medial surfaces; 2, 2′, anterior borders of lateral and medial surfaces; 3, 3′, inferior borders of lateral and medial surfaces; 4, 4′, posterior borders of lateral and medial surfaces; 5, articular surface for cuboid; 6, articular surface for second metatarsal base; 7, articular surface for second cuneiform; 8, anterior border of dorsal surface; 9, posterior border of dorsal surface; 10, medial border of dorsal surface; 11, lateral border of dorsal surface; 12, dorsal border of posterior surface; 13, lateral border of posterior surface; 14, medial border of posterior surface; 15, apex of posterior surface; 16, dorsal border of anterior surface; 17, medial border of anterior surface; 18, apex of anterior surface; 19, lateral border of anterior surface.)

plantar. The surface is flat or has a minimal transverse concavity.

The posterior surface articulates with the scaphoid, with an oval surface occupying the upper three fourths of the aspect, leaving the inferior one fourth as a blunt pointed area. This surface is oriented posteriorly and medially and is flat.

The medial surface is rectangular. Articulating surfaces occupy vertically the anterior and posterior aspects, leaving the central segment for the insertion of the ligaments. The anterior articulating surface is a narrow band, corresponds to the base of the second metatarsal, and is divided into two segments by the interosseous ligament extending from the third cuneiform to the base of the third metatarsal or possibly to the third and second metatarsals. The intercuneiform$_{2,3}$ ligament inserts posterior to this ligament. The posterior articulating surface is also a vertical facet occupying most of the posterior aspect and leaving only a small, inferior, nonarticulating band. It is in continuity with the surface of the scaphoid and articulates with the second cuneiform. The anterior border of this surface is concave, with a forward extension of the upper segment.

The lateral surface is quadrilateral. A large ovoid facet articulating with the cuboid occupies the posterosuperior corner extending just beyond the midlevels of the posterior and superior borders of the surface. Occasionally a small articulating surface is present in the anterosuperior angle for the base of the fourth metatarsal. The remaining segment of the surface gives insertion to the cuneo$_3$-metatarsal$_3$, or cuneo$_3$-metatarsals$_{3,4}$, or cuneo$_3$-metatarsal$_4$ ligaments. The interosseous cuneo$_3$-cuboid ligament originates posterior to the previous ligament.

The dorsal surface is rectangular. The posterior border is oblique, directed laterally and slightly posteriorly. The medial border is bevelled in the anterior segment in correspondence to the base of the second metatarsal and is followed proximally by a notch occupying the mid segment. The lateral border is oriented posteriorly and medially in the posterior half, whereas the anterior segment makes a gentle change in direction toward the medial aspect of the foot, thus announcing the direction of the third metatarsal. This surface gives insertion posteriorly to the scaphocuneiform$_3$ ligament, medially to the dorsal intercuneiform$_{2,3}$ ligament, and laterally to the cuneo$_3$-metatarsal$_3$ ligament and the cuneo$_3$-metatarsal$_2$ ligament.

The crest or inferior border is round and smooth and posteriorly bears a small tubercle. It provides insertion to the plantar cuneo$_3$-cuboid ligament, plantar cuneo$_3$-navicular ligament, plantar cuneo$_3$-metatarsals$_{3,4}$ ligament (one or both ligaments may be missing), tibialis posterior tendon, oblique head of the adductor hallucis, lateral arm of the Y stem of origin of the flexor hallucis brevis. The last three insertions cover the ligamentous attachments.

Metatarsals

The five metatarsals articulate proximally with the three cuneiforms and the cuboid and form the tarsometatarsal or Lisfranc's joint.

Proximally the bases of the metatarsals are disposed in an arcuate fashion, forming a transverse arch high medially and low laterally (Fig. 2-43). The apex of this arch corresponds to the base of the second metatarsal. The metatarsals are also flexed, thus contributing to the formation of longitudinal arches that are more pronounced medially and barely present laterally. Distally, the five metatarsal heads are located in the same plane horizontally, and no transverse arch is present at this level.

The first metatarsal diverges slightly from the second metatarsal. The intermetatarsal angle formed by the long

axis of these two metatarsals is 2° to 8° in the adolescent and 3° to 9° in the adult.[30] Kelikian mentions that "any measurement in excess of 10 degrees is indicative of varus deformity of the first metatarsal."[31]

In relationship to the axial alignment of the talar neck and the cuneiform block, the metatarsals contribute to the formation of an elongated Z arrangement (see Fig. 2-39).

The first metatarsal is shorter than the second metatarsal. Leboucq measured anatomically the length of these two metatarsals in the adult and the newborn–adolescent group.[32] In the adult, the average shortening of the first metatarsal is 10.5 mm (maximum 14 mm, minimum 7 mm), and in the newborn–adolescent group, the average shortening is 7.45 mm (maximum 10 mm, minimum 5.5 mm). Straus gives the following data concerning the length measurements of the first and second metatarsals: the average ratio of the greatest length of the metatarsal 1 × 100 to the greatest length of the metatarsal 2 is 83 in the adult, 85 in the juvenile, and 86 in the newborn.[30] The metatarsal formula has been expressed in terms of the distal projections of the metatarsal heads relative to each other in mounted skeletons or on radiographs. Morton introduced the formula of $1 = 2>3>4>5$ and stated that "one of the requirements for ideal foot function is an equidistance of the heads of the first and second metatarsal bones from the heel."[33] The metatarsal formula $2>3>1>4>5$ is the one accepted by most anatomists; there are variations such as $2>1>3>4>5$, $2>1 = 3>4>5$, or other combinations, but "no anatomist appears to record a dominant first metatarsal."[9] The general alignment of the metatarsal baseline is oblique, oriented backward and laterally from the base of the first metatarsal. This line and the corresponding tarsal line interlock in two locations: the base of the second metatarsal penetrates the tarsal line proximally at the level of the second cuneiform. The third cuneiform penetrates distally, to a much lesser degree, the metatarsal line at the level of the third metatarsal base. This arrangement secures the second and third metatarsals.

Each metatarsal is formed by a base, a head, and a shaft (Figs. 2-44–2-48).

BASE

First Metatarsal

The base of the first metatarsal is more or less triangular, with lateral, medial, and inferior surfaces supporting the articular surface for the first cuneiform (see Figs. 2-43 and 2-44). This articular surface has its long axis oriented downward and laterally. It is reniform, with the hilum on the lateral side, and presents a slight concavity transversely. It is flat in the direction of the long axis. This articular surface may be subdivided into partially united upper and lower parts.[34]

At the junction of the medial and inferior surfaces is a tubercle for the insertion of the tibialis anterior tendon; a more prominent tuberosity is present at the junction of the inferior and lateral surfaces for the insertion of the peroneus longus tendon. The medial surface provides attachment to the dorsal cuneo$_1$-metatarsal$_1$ ligament. The plantar cuneo$_1$-metatarsal$_1$ ligament inserts on the lateral half of the inferior

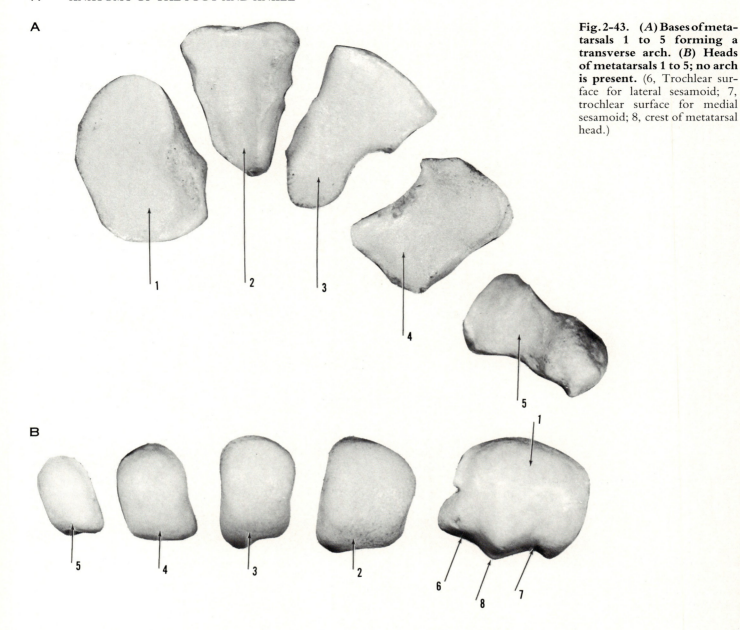

A

B

surface. There is no intermetatarsal ligament between the first and second metatarsal bases.

The lateral surface of the base establishes variable contact with the second metatarsal. Singh gives the following distribution of areas of contact with the second metatarsal in 100 first metatarsals: smooth facet, 21; smooth area with indefinite margins, 40; no area of contact, 39.[34]

Second Metatarsal

The base of the second metatarsal is cuneiform (see Figs. 2-43 and 2-45). The superior surface is flat. The lateral and medial surfaces converge on the plantar aspect to form a crest. These three surfaces support the triangular concave articular surface (base dorsal, apex plantar) for the second cuneiform. The base of the second metatarsal establishes contact with five bones: medially with the first cuneiform

and possibly the base of the first metatarsal, laterally with the third metatarsal and the lateral cuneiform, and proximally with the middle cuneiform.

The dorsal surface provides insertion to the dorsal cuneometatarsal ligaments (C_1-M_2), (C_2-M_2), (C_3-M_2) and to the dorsal intermetatarsal ligament (M_2-M_3). The medial surface bears in the posterosuperior corner a small articulating oval surface that corresponds to a similar surface on the first cuneiform. The remaining segment of the surface provides attachment to the powerful $cuneo_1-metatarsal_2$ ligament (Lisfranc's ligament). Two tonguelike articular surfaces, upper and lower, are present on the lateral surface of the base. They are both oriented longitudinally. The upper surface is longer than the lower and separated from it by a small interval. These articular surfaces correspond anteriorly to the third metatarsal base and posteriorly to the third cuneiform. As reported by Singh, the configuration and

Fig. 2-44.   First metatarsal, right. (*A*) Dorsal surface. (*B*) Plantar surface. (*C*) Lateral surface. (*D*) Medial surface. (1, Head; 2, lateral border of dorsal surface; 2′, superior border of lateral surface; 3, medial border of dorsal surface and plantar surface; 4, proximal border of dorsal surface; 5, lateral border of plantar surface; 5′, inferior border of lateral surface; 6, proximal border of plantar surface; 7, lateral trochlear surface; 8, crest of metatarsal head; 9, medial trochlear surface; 10, tubercle for origin of lateral metatarsophalangeal ligament; 11, tubercle for insertion of peroneus longus tendon; 12, tubercle for origin of medial metatarsophalangeal ligament; 13, insertion site of tibialis anterior tendon.)

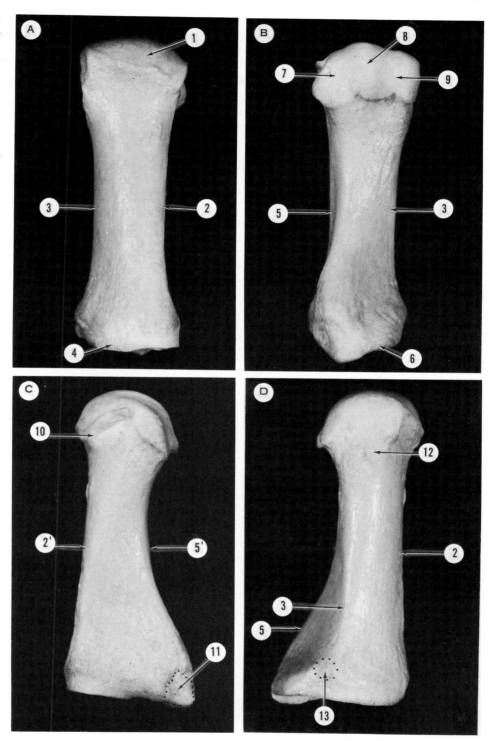

distribution of the articular surface are very variable (Fig. 2-49).[34] The nonarticular segment of the lateral surface provides attachment proximally to the cuneo$_2$-metatarsal$_2$ ligament and distally to the interosseous metatarsal ligament (M$_2$–M$_3$). On the crest are inserted the plantar cuneo$_1$-metatarsal$_2$ ligament, the plantar metatarsal$_{2,3}$ ligament, a slip from the tibialis posterior tendon, a slip from the long plantar ligament, and the adductor hallucis obliquis muscle.

Third Metatarsal

The base of the third metatarsal is also cuneiform, supporting a triangular flat articular surface (base dorsal, apex plantar) for the third cuneiform (see Figs. 2-43 and 2-46). The medial surface presents two articular surfaces for the base of the second metatarsal. These surfaces are plantar and dorsal, flat, and separated by an anteroposterior surface of ru-

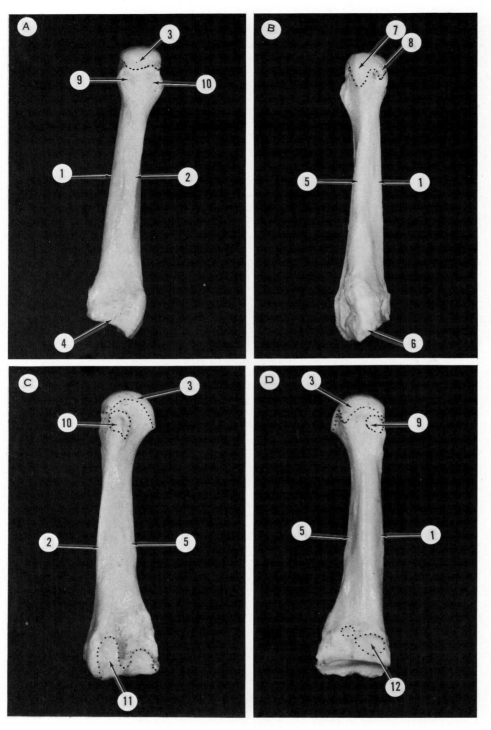

Fig. 2-45. Second metatarsal, right. (*A*) Dorsal surface. (*B*) Plantar surface. (*C*) Lateral surface. (*D*) Medial surface. (1, Medial border of dorsal surface; 2, lateral border of dorsal surface; 3, head; 4, proximal border of dorsal surface; 5, inferior border; 6, crest at base, on plantar aspect; 7, articular surface of head, proximal extension, laterally; 8, articular surface of head, proximal extension, medially; 9, medial tubercle for origin of metatarsophalangeal and metatarsoglenoid ligaments; 10, lateral tubercle for origin of metatarsophalangeal and metatarsoglenoid ligaments; 11, articular surfaces for third cuneiform and third metatarsal; 12, articular surface for first cuneiform.)

gosities giving insertion to the interosseous cuneometatarsal ligament (C_3-M_3).

On the distal segment of the medial surface inserts the interosseous metatarsal ligament (M_2-M_3). The distribution of these surfaces is also variable.[34] The lateral surface bears a large, oval, concave or flat surface corresponding to the base of the fourth metatarsal. A deep groove limits this surface inferiorly and gives insertion to the interosseous cuneo$_3$-metatarsal$_3$ ligament. The interosseous metatarsal ligament$_{3,4}$ inserts anteriorly on a large segment of the lateral surface, which is covered by rugosities. The dorsal surface provides insertion to the dorsal intermetatarsal ligaments (M_2-M_3, M_3-M_4) and to the dorsal cuneo$_3$-metatarsal$_3$ ligament. On the crest are attached the plantar cuneo$_1$-metatarsal$_3$ ligament, the plantar intermetatarsal ligaments (M_2-M_3, M_3-M_4), a slip from the long plantar ligament, a slip from the tibialis posterior tendon, and the adductor hallucis obliquis.

Fig. 2-46.   Third metatarsal, right.
(*A*) Dorsal surface. (*B*) Plantar surface.
(*C*) Lateral surface. (*D*) Medial surface.
(1, Medial border of dorsal surface; 2,
lateral border of dorsal surface; 3, head;
4, medial tubercle for origin of metatarsophalangeal and metatarsoglenoid ligaments; 5, lateral tubercle for origin of
metatarsophalangeal and metatarsoglenoid ligaments; 6, proximal border of
dorsal surface; 7, proximal extension of
articular surface, laterally; 8, proximal
extension of articular surface, medially;
9, inferior border; 10, articular surface
with fourth metatarsal; 11, articular surface with base of second metatarsal.)

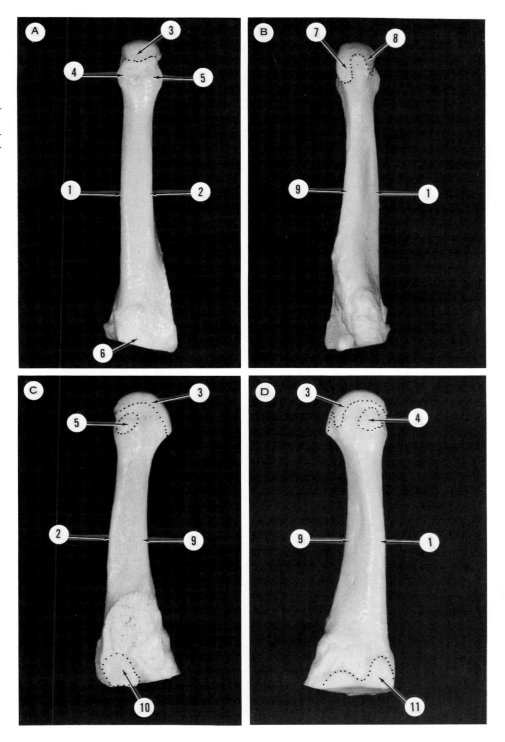

Fourth Metatarsal

The base of the fourth metatarsal is quadrilateral (see Figs.
2-43 and 2-47). The proximal surface, slightly concave,
articulates with the cuboid. On the medial surface, there is
a large dorsal oval facet, corresponding to the base of the
third metatarsal. The very posterior aspect of this surface
corresponds to the third cuneiform. Variations are indicated
in Figure 2-49. The nonarticulating segment provides insertion to the interosseous cuboideometatarsal$_4$ ligament or
the cuneo$_3$-metatarsal$_4$ ligament and, farther distally, to the
interosseous metatarsal (M$_3$-M$_4$) ligament. The lateral surface gives support to a triangular articular surface (base
dorsal, apex plantar), occupying the posterosuperior segment of the surface and articulating with the fifth metatarsal.
A deep vertical groove limits this surface anteriorly. The
interosseous metatarsal ligament M$_4$-M$_5$ inserts on the anterior aspect of the surface. The dorsal aspect of the meta-

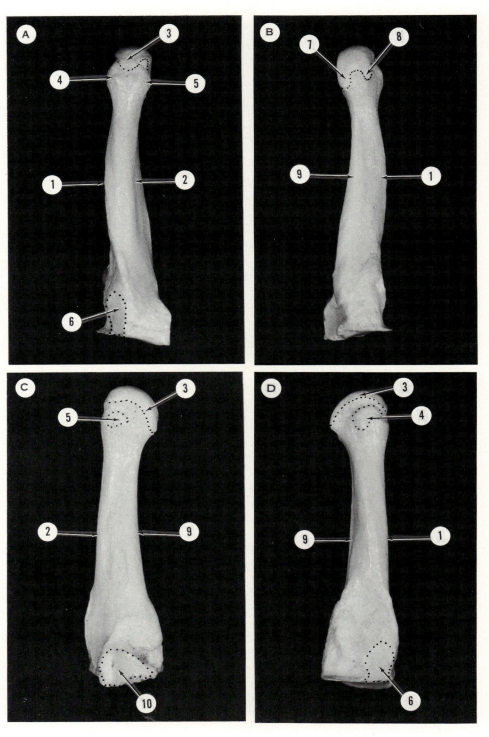

Fig. 2-47. Fourth metatarsal, right. (*A*) Dorsal surface. (*B*) Plantar surface. (*C*) Lateral surface. (*D*) Medial surface. (1, Medial border of dorsal surface; 2, lateral border of dorsal surface; 3, head; 4, medial tubercle for origin of metatarsophalangeal and metatarsoglenoid legaments; 5, lateral tubercle for origin of metatarsophalangeal and metatarsoglenoid ligaments; 6, articular surface with third metatarsal; 7, proximal extension of articular surface, laterally; 8, proximal extension of articular surface, medially; 9, inferior border; 10, articular surface with fifth metatarsal.)

tarsal base provides insertion to the dorsal cuboideometatarsal$_4$ ligament and the dorsal intermetatarsal ligaments (M$_3$-M$_4$, M$_4$-M$_5$). The inferior surface is rectangular and may bear a tubercle. It gives attachment to the plantar intermetatarsal ligaments (M$_3$-M$_4$, M$_4$-M$_5$), the plantar cuboideometatarsal$_4$ ligament, the plantar cuneo$_3$-metatarsal$_4$ ligament, a slip from the longitudinal plantar ligament, a slip from the tibialis posterior tendon, and the adductor hallucis obliquis.

Fifth Metatarsal

The base of the fifth metatarsal is flat in a dorsoplantar direction and is projected laterally and posteriorly as the tubercle of the fifth metatarsal or styloid apophysis (see Figs. 2-43 and 2-48). The latter gives insertion to the peroneus brevis tendon.

The posterior surface presents an inner articulating field that is triangular (medial base, lateral apex), corresponding

Fig. 2-48.   Fifth metatarsal, right. (*A*) Dorsal surface. (*B*) Inferior surface. (*C*) Lateral border. (*D*) Medial surface. (1, Medial border of dorsal surface; 1′, superior border of medial surface; 2, lateral border of dorsal and inferior surfaces; 3, medial border of inferior surface; 3′, inferior border of medial surface; 4, head; 5, base; 6, tuberosity of base; 7, articular surface with fourth metatarsal; 8, lateral tubercle for insertion of lateral metatarsophalangeal and metatarsoglenoid ligaments; 9, medial tubercle for insertion of medial metatarsophalangeal and metatarsoglenoid ligaments; 10, articular surface with cuboid.)

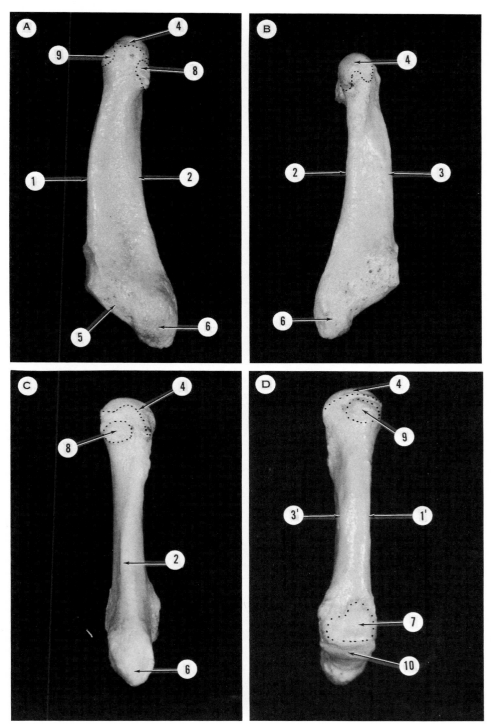

to the cuboid. A smaller lateral field, irregular and nonarticular, contributes with the cuboid to the formation of the cubostyloid groove, which will lead to the cuboid canal for the peroneus longus tendon.

The medial surface bears an oval or triangular surface articulating with the base of the fourth metatarsal. The remaining segment provides insertion to the interosseous metatarsal M_4-M_5 ligament.

The superior surface is flat and gives insertion to the peroneus tertius tendon, the dorsal cuboideometatarsal$_5$ ligament, and the dorsal intermetatarsal (M_4-M_5) ligament.

The inferior surface is broad and bears a medial bony prominence that gives insertion to the plantar intermetatarsal (M_4-M_5) ligament. The proximal segment provides attachment to the plantar short cuboideometatarsal$_5$ ligament and, farther distally, to the broad slip from the long plantar ligament. In the central excavation of the surface inserts the short flexor of the fifth toe. The plantar aspect of the styloid

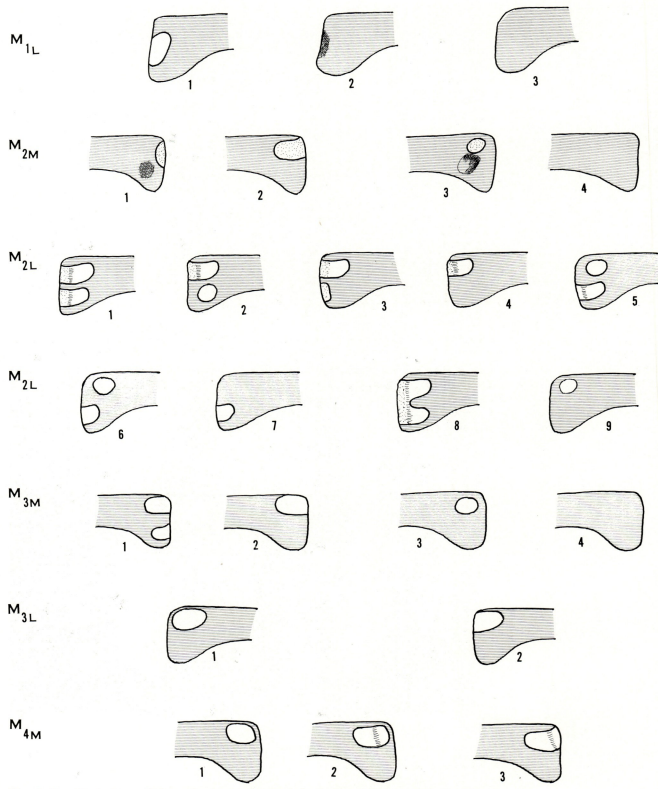

Fig. 2-49.   Variations of the articular surfaces of the bases of the metatarsals. M_{1L}, Base of metatarsal 1, lateral aspect; M_{2M}, base of metatarsal 2, medial aspect; M_{2L}, base of metatarsal 2, lateral aspect; M_{3M}, base of metatarsal 3, medial aspect; M_{3L}, base of metatarsal 3, lateral aspect; M_{4M}, base of metatarsal 4, medial aspect.) (After Singh I: Variations in the metatarsal bones. J Anat 94:345, 1960)

apophysis occasionally gives insertion to the abductor of the fifth toe.

SHAFT

First Metatarsal

The shaft of the first metatarsal is the shortest and the strongest of the metatarsals (see Fig. 2-44). It has a prismatic contour, mainly in the proximal two thirds, and presents three surfaces: dorsomedial, lateral, and inferior. The three borders are superolateral, inferolateral, and inferomedial. The dorsomedial surface is convex and oriented dorsally in the distal third. The lateral surface is flat and smooth and provides insertion to the first dorsal interosseous muscle from its posterior third. The inferior surface has a longitudinally concave contour; this concavity is exaggerated by the plantar tubercles of the base.

Second, Third, and Fourth Metatarsal

The second, third, and fourth metatarsal shafts have a variable plantar concavity to their contour (see Figs. 2-45, 2-46, and 2-47). They are prismatic and present three surfaces: dorsal, medial, and lateral. They have three borders: inferior, dorsolateral, and dorsomedial. The inferior border forms a smooth crest. The dorsal surface is flat and large posteriorly and convex and narrow distally. The medial and lateral surfaces converge toward the plantar crest; the medial surface is slightly convex and becomes more plantar in orientation distally. The fourth metatarsal has a recognizable twist to its shaft along the longitudinal axis, which orients the dorsal surface medially and brings the central plantar crest to a lateral position. The lateral surface then has a dorsolateral orientation.

Fifth Metatarsal

The fifth metatarsal shaft has the same longitudinal axial rotation, to a much greater degree, and this changes the general pattern of orientation of the three surfaces (see Fig.

2-48). The central plantar crest is now in a definite lateral position. The three surfaces of the general pattern—dorsal, lateral, medial—are now converted to dorsal, medial, *inferior* surfaces. The shaft is flat and prismatic, with a medial base and a lateral crest.

The dorsal and plantar interossei muscles originate from the metatarsal shafts as follows (Fig. 2-50): first dorsal interosseous—posterior third lateral surface M_1, medial surface M_2; second dorsal interosseous—lateral surface M_2, upper segment medial surface M_3; third dorsal interosseous—lateral surface M_3, upper segment medial surface M_4; fourth dorsal interosseous—lateral surface M_4, medial surface M_5; first plantar interosseous—lower segment medial surface M_3, plantar crest M_3; second plantar interosseous—lower segment medial surface M_4, plantar crest M_4; third plantar interosseous—inferior surface M_5. The fifth metatarsal also provides origin to the opponens of the fifth from its lateral border.

HEAD

First Metatarsal

The head of the first metatarsal is large and quadrilateral in general contour, with the transverse diameter exceeding the vertical dimension (see Figs. 2-43 and 2-44). This apparent superoinferior flattening is in contradistinction to the heads of the lesser metatarsal heads, which are flattened side to side, transversely.

The articular surface covering the head presents two fields in continuity: superior phalangeal and inferior sesamoidal. The superior articular field is smooth and convex (more in the vertical direction than the transverse). This surface is larger than the corresponding articular surface of the proximal phalanx. Dorsally, this field is limited by a posteriorly convex border that is smooth and overhangs the dorsal surface of the shaft. The inferior articular surface is larger than the superior and is separated into two sloped surfaces by a rounded ridge or crest oriented anteroposteriorly. This crest is not central in location but passes at the junction of the outer third and inner two thirds of the

Fig. 2-50. Cross section through metatarsal shafts M_1 to M_5—origin of interossei muscles. (D_1 to D_4, dorsal interossei 1 to 4; P_1 to P_3, plantar interossei 1 to 3.)

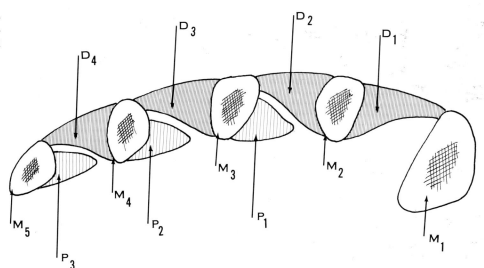

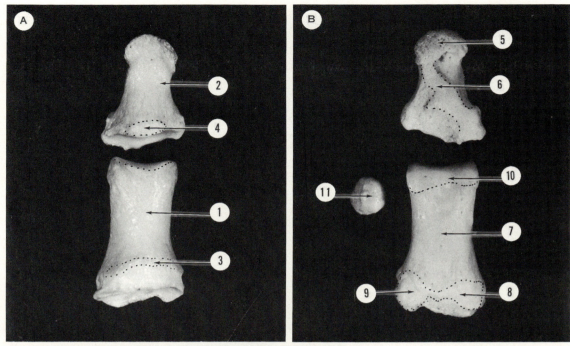

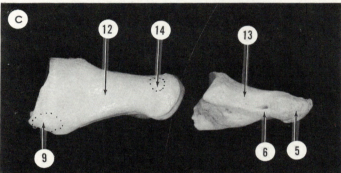

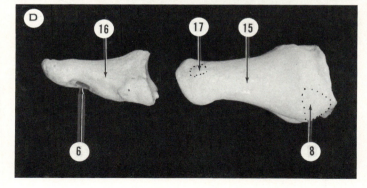

Fig. 2-51.   Phalanges of the big toe, right. (*A*) Dorsal aspect. (*B*) Plantar aspect. (*C*) Lateral aspect. (*D*) Medial aspect. (1, Dorsal aspect of proximal phalanx; 2, dorsal aspect of distal phalanx; 3, insertion zone for capsule and extensor hallucis brevis; 4, insertion zone for extensor hallucis longus; 5, tuft of distal phalanx; 6, bony ridge forming a "flying buttress" extending obliquely from the tibial side at the base to the fibular side at the level of the tuft; this is an insertion site for the flexor hallucis longus tendon; 7, plantar aspect of proximal phalanx; 8, medial tubercle for insertion of tendons of medial head of flexor hallucis brevis and abductor hallucis; 9, lateral tubercle for insertion of tendons of lateral head of flexor hallucis brevis and adductor hallucis; 10, head of proximal phalanx; 11, sesamoid; 12, lateral aspect of proximal phalanx; 13, lateral aspect of distal phalanx; 14, tubercle for insertion of lateral interphalangeal and phalangeoglenoid ligaments; 15, medial aspect of proximal phalanx; 16, medial aspect of distal phalanx; 17, tubercle for insertion of medial interphalangeal and phalangeoglenoid ligaments.)

articular surface. The sloped surfaces are grooved, and each corresponds to a sesamoid. The inner groove is more pronounced than the outer groove. When the sesamoids are small, an intermediate groove is present over the ridge, due to the pressure of the flexor hallucis longus tendon.[35]

Well-developed bony tubercles or epicondyles are located on the sides of the metatarsal head. They are in contact with or very close to the articular surface. The inner tubercle is more developed than the outer. These tubercles provide insertion to the metatarsophalangeal collateral ligaments and to the suspensory metatarsoglenosesamoid ligaments.

Lesser Metatarsals

The heads of the lesser metatarsals are quadrilateral and flattened transversely (see Figs. 2-43–2-48). The articular surface is condylar, extending more on the plantar aspect than on the dorsal. The plantar articular segment has a proximal central concave border and two marginal articular proximal extensions. Usually the lateral extension is more pronounced than the medial. On the sides of the metatarsal heads, a groove separates the articular surface from the pronounced tubercle for the origin of the metatarsophalangeal ligaments and for the metatarsoglenoid ligaments. When observed in the lateral profile, the metatarsal head has an elliptic articular contour and the lateral tubercle is superior. When viewed from the dorsum, the narrow neck is seen to flare up into the lateral tubercles.

Phalanges

LARGE TOE

The large toe has two phalanges; proximal and distal (Fig. 2-51).

Proximal Phalanx

The proximal phalanx has a large base directed transversely and bears an oval, concave articular surface, the glenoid cavity, smaller than the corresponding articular surface of the metatarsal head. A transverse crest or bony prominence is present on the dorsum of the base at a small distance from the articular surface. The extensor hallucis brevis inserts on this tubercle. On the plantar aspect, two tubercles, lateral and medial, give insertion to the intrinsic muscles of the big toe. The larger medial plantar tubercle gives insertion to the medial head of the short flexor and to the abductor hallucis. The less prominent lateral plantar tubercle gives insertion to the lateral head of the short flexor and to the adductor hallucis. The plantar plate inserts firmly on the plantar border of the surface.

The shaft of the proximal phalanx is convex dorsally and flat on the plantar aspect, with slight grooving at each end for the flexor hallucis longus tendon. The head is flat vertically. The articular surface is trochlear and is larger and more concave on the plantar aspect. The surface is strongly convex in the dorsoplantar direction. A small fossa is present on the plantar aspect, just proximal to the articular surface. The collateral ligaments insert on small tubercles located on the head in a superolateral position behind the articular cartilage.

Distal Phalanx

The distal phalanx has a large, transversely oriented base bearing the articular surface corresponding to the trochlear surface of the proximal phalangeal head. This surface is convex centrally and concave laterally. The transverse tubercle on the dorsum of the base, close to the articular surface, gives insertion to the extensor hallucis longus tendon. This proximal position of the extensor tendon allows a large insertion of the ungual matrix on the dorsum of the phalanx. On the plantar aspect of the shaft, the flexor hallucis longus tendon inserts on a tuberosity, directed toward the fibular side and strongly marked on the tibial side. This obliquely directed ridge may reach the distal tuberositas unguicularis in a bridge fashion on the fibular side, forming a "flying buttress."[36] Occasionally a bony projection is present at the base, giving origin to side ligaments inserting on the base of the tuberositas unguicularis. The flexor hallucis longus thus makes a broad attachment over the oblique tuberosity, the side ligaments reaching the distal tuberosity.[36]

The shaft of the distal phalanx is not at right angles to the articular surface but deviates to the fibular side, and

Wilkinson gives the deflection measurements as mean, 14.7° (S.D. 4.1°)—male 8° to 23°, female 10° to 22°.[36] A comparable figure was present in the big toes in 10 fetuses.

LESSER TOES

The lesser toes (Fig. 2-52) have three phalanges: proximal, middle, and distal.

Proximal Phalanx

The proximal phalanx is the longest of the three, being slightly longer than the other two phalanges combined. The base is large and transverse, with an oval articular surface for the metatarsal head. Two plantar tubercles give insertion to the interossei muscles: The medial tubercles of the third, fourth, and fifth toes give insertion to the first, second, and third plantar interossei. The medial tubercle of the second toe gives insertion to the first dorsal interosseous. The lateral tubercles of the second, third, and fourth toes give insertion to the second, third, and fourth dorsal interossei. The lateral tubercle of the fifth toe gives insertion to its abductor and short flexor.

The shaft is convex dorsally and flat inferiorly, with slight concavity at both distal and proximal ends.

The head is flat and supports a trochlear type of articular surface that extends more on the plantar aspect. A small tubercle is present on each side of the head in a superolateral position for the origin of the collateral ligaments.

Middle Phalanx

The middle phalanx is very short. The base bears a transverse articular surface corresponding to the trochlear contour of the proximal phalangeal head. The middle slip of the long extensor tendon inserts on the dorsum of the base. The shaft is convex dorsally. The flat plantar surface gives insertion to the two slips of the flexor brevis. The distal articular head is also transversely oriented; it is rather flat transversely but presents a strong convexity in the dorsoplantar direction. The middle phalanx of the fifth toe is fused to the distal phalanx in 37% (Fig. 2-53).[19]

Distal Phalanx

The distal phalanx is rudimentary. It is more or less triangular, with a crescent-shaped contour of the distal tuberositas unguicularis. The base supports an articular surface, transverse, corresponding to the head of the middle phalanx. The extensor terminal tendon inserts on the dorsum of the base and the long flexor of the toe on the plantar aspect of the base and shaft. The dorsum of the shaft and the crescent-shaped distal tuberosity support the ungual matrix.

Sesamoids

The sesamoids are small, round bones deriving their names from the sesame seed. Their anatomic location is always the same even though certain sesamoids are not always present or occur infrequently.

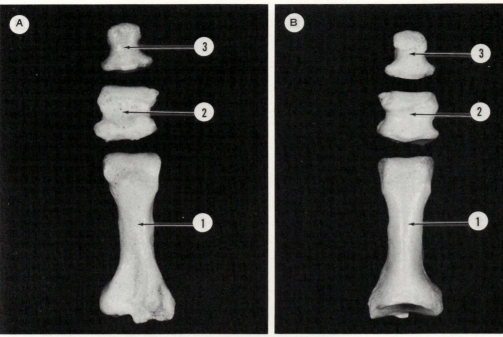

Fig. 2-52.   Second toe, right. (*A*) Plantar view. (*B*) Dorsal view. (*C*) Medial view. (1, Proximal phalanx; 2, middle phalanx; 3, distal phalanx; 4, tubercle for attachment of first dorsal interosseous tendon and metatarsophalangeal ligament; 5, attachment site of medial collateral ligament of interphalangeal joint; 6, tubercle of origin of medial collateral ligament of interphalangeal joint.)

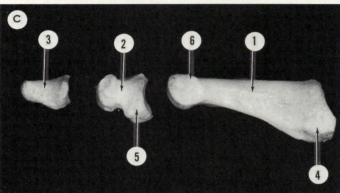

The sesamoids are embedded, partially or totally, in the substance of a corresponding tendon. Structurally, some sesamoids always ossify, whereas others remain cartilaginous or fibrocartilaginous for life; this accounts for the discrepancies encountered in the studies reporting the frequency of occurrence of a given sesamoid. Anatomically the sesamoids are part of a gliding or pressure-absorbing mechanism and are located within the flexor hallucis brevis tendons, the plantar plates of the metatarsophalangeal and interphalangeal joints, the intrinsic tendons of the lesser toes, the peroneus longus tendon, the tibialis posterior tendon, and the tibialis anterior tendon (Fig. 2-54).

THE BIG TOE

The sesamoids of the big toe (Fig. 2-55) are three in number: two constant at the level of the plantar aspect of the metatarsophalangeal joint, and one inconstant at the level of the plantar aspect of the interphalangeal joint.

The Metatarsophalangeal Joint

The two sesamoids of the metatarsophalangeal joint (Figs. 2-56 and 2-57), lateral and medial, are plantar in location. They are embedded in the thick plantar plate and present two surfaces: inferior, convex, nonarticular, insertional, and superior, articular with the metatarsal head.

The overall configuration of the sesamoids is variable, as they may be semiovoid, circular, or bean shaped. The variations of contour are well depicted by Kewenter (Fig. 2-58).[37] The two sesamoids are not of the same size and configuration: the medial sesamoid is usually larger than the lateral and is ovoid and elongated, whereas the latter is smaller and more circular. Kewenter provides the following

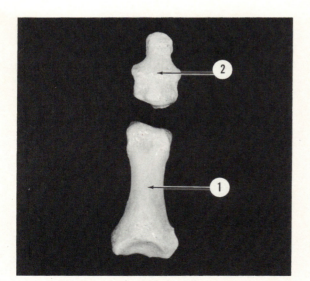

Fig. 2-53.   Little toe, dorsal aspect. (1, Proximal phalanx; 2, fused middle and distal phalanges.)

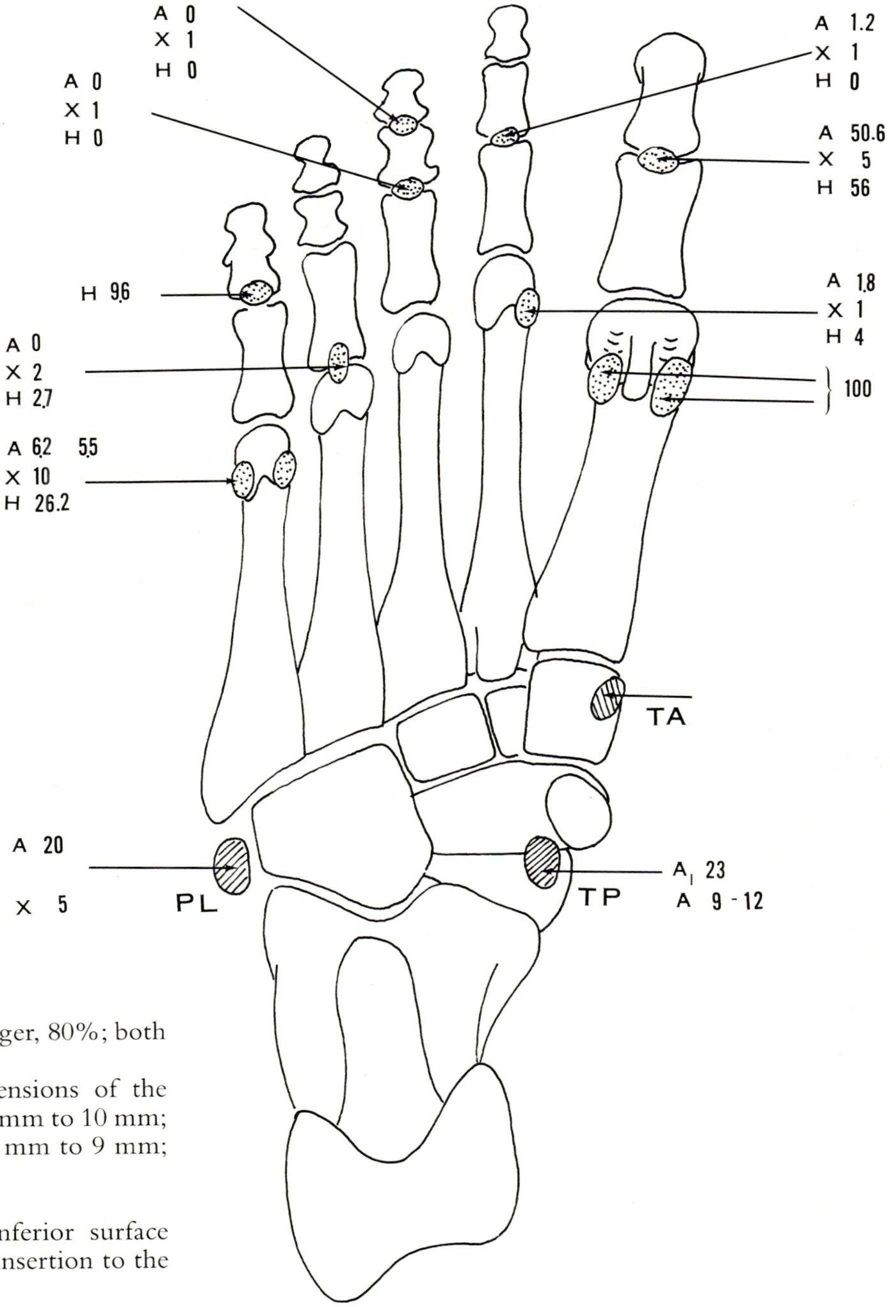

Fig. 2-54. Sesamoids of the foot. Percentage of occurrence based on: *A,* anatomic investigation; *X,* roentgenographic investigation; *H,* histoembryologic investigation. For the toes: *A,* from Pfitzner W: Die Sesambeine des Menschen. In Schwalbe (ed): Morphologische Arbeiten, Vol I, pp 517–762. Jena, Gustav Fischer, 1892; *X,* from Bizarro AH: On sesamoids and supernumerary bones of the limbs. J Anat 55:258, 1921; *H,* from Trolle D: Accessory Bones of the Human Foot: A Radiological, Histoembryological, Comparative Anatomical and Genetic Study, pp 20–21. Copenhagen, Munksgaard, 1948. PL—Os peroneum in peroneus longus tendon in ossified form: *A,* from Anatomical Society, Collective Investigations: Sesamoids in the gastrocnemius and peroneus longus. J Anat Physiol 32:182, 1897; *X,* from Jones FW: Structure and Function as Seen in the Foot, 2nd ed, p 97. London, Baillière, Tindall & Cox, 1949. TP—Sesamoid in tibialis posterior tendon: *A₁,* from, Storton CE: In Grant JCB (ed): Grant's Atlas of Anatomy, 5th ed. Baltimore, Williams & Wilkins, 1962; *A,* from Pfitzner W: Beiträge zur Kenntniss des Menschlichen Extremitätenskelets: VI. Die Variationen in Aufbau des Fussskelets. In Schwalbe (ed): Morphologische Arbeiten, pp 245–527. Jena, Gustav Fischer, 1896. TA—Sesamoid in tibialis anterior tendon.

information on their size: medial sesamoid larger, 80%; both equal, 15%; lateral sesamoid larger, 5%.[37]

Gillette reports the most common dimensions of the nondeformed sesamoids as length—lateral, 9 mm to 10 mm; medial, 12 mm to 15 mm; width—lateral, 7 mm to 9 mm; medial, 9 mm to 11 mm.[38]

Nonarticular Surface. The convex inferior surface and borders of the lateral sesamoid provide insertion to the following:

Lateral head of the flexor hallucis brevis
Three components of the oblique head of the adductor hallucis
Transverse component of the adductor hallucis
Deep transverse metatarsal ligament
Suspensory lateral metatarsosesamoid ligament
Lateral border of the flexor hallucis longus fibrous tunnel
Lateral longitudinal septum of the plantar aponeurosis to the big toe
Vertical and arciform fibrous fibers contributing to the formation of the pre-flexor tendon space

The convex inferior surface and borders of the medial sesamoid provide insertion to the following:

Medial head of the flexor hallucis brevis
Abductor hallucis tendon
Suspensory medial metatarsosesamoid ligament
Medial border of the flexor hallucis longus fibrous tunnel
Medial longitudinal septum of the plantar aponeurosis of the big toe
Vertical and arciform fibers contributing to the formation of the pre-flexor tendon space

The medial slope of the lateral sesamoid and the lateral slope of the medial sesamoid contribute to the formation of the proximal segment of the flexor hallucis longus tunnel. The pre-flexor tendon space retains an adipose cushion over-

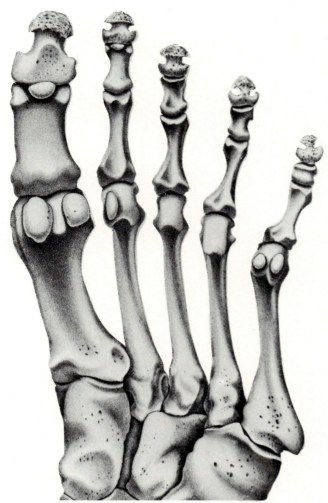

Fig. 2-55.   Sesamoids of toes. (From Pfitzner W: Die Sesambeine des Menschen. In Schwalbe [ed]: Morphologische Arbeiten, Vol I, pp 517–762. Jena, Gustav Fischer, 1892)

lying both sesamoids and the flexor hallucis longus tendon.

Articular Surface.   The lower two thirds of the large metatarsal head has a double trochlear contour—large medial and small lateral. The trochlear surfaces are separated by a central crest oriented anteroposteriorly. The articular surface of each sesamoid fits against the corresponding trochlear surface. In the well-developed sesamoid the articular surface is concave longitudinally and bears a soft longitudinal crest corresponding to the trochlear groove. On each side, the surface is slightly convex in the transverse direction, adapting to the trochlear surface. This arrangement has brought forth the comparison of the sesamotrochlear joint to the patellofemoral joint or to the cubitohumeral joint.[38,39] In their anatomic position, the two sesamoids are not transverse but incline obliquely toward the central metatarsal ridge. They are firmly connected to each other and to the base of the proximal phalanx through the powerful plantar plate and form an anatomic and functional unit that moves relative to the metatarsal head; this

unit is called the *phalangeosesamoid apparatus*.[38] It is suspended from the head of the metatarsal by the metatarsosesamoid and metatarsophalangeal ligaments. Normally the sesamoids move with the proximal phalanx and follow the latter in the metatarsophalangeal dislocations.

The sesamoids are connected to each other mainly by their incorporation in the substance of the plantar plate. From within the joint, the following intrinsic connecting ligaments are recognized (see Figs. 2-56 and 2-57):

An intersesamoid, thin fibrous transverse band

Lateral and medial sesamophalangeal short ligaments inserting on the plantar tubercles of the proximal phalanx. These ligaments are also attached to a transverse band extending from one side of the phalanx to the other.

The metatarsosesamoid ligaments, which originate from the posteromedial and posterolateral aspects of the metatarsal head and insert on the corresponding sesamoid. The medial ligament is stronger and sends

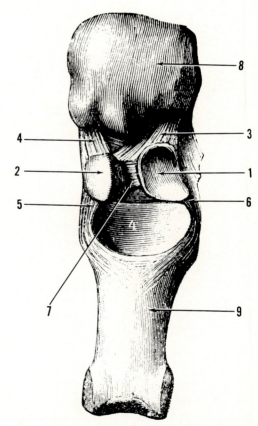

Fig. 2-56.   Phalangeosesamoid apparatus of the big toe. The dorsal capsule of the metatarsophalangeal joint has been excised and the first metatarsal head reflected backward. (1, Medial sesamoid; 2, lateral sesamoid; 3, medial metatarsosesamoid ligament sending direct fibers to medial sesamoid and oblique fibers to lateral sesamoid; 4, lateral metatarsosesamoid ligament; 5, lateral short sesamophalangeal ligament; 6, medial short sesamophalangeal ligament; 7, intersesamoid transverse ligament; 8, head of first metatarsal; 9, proximal phalanx of big toe.) (From Gillette: Des os sésamoides chez l'homme. Anat Physiol, pp 506–538, 1872)

oblique fibers to the lateral sesamoid from the posterior aspect of the plate.[38]

The sesamoids of the metatarsophalangeal joint may be partite; the frequency of occurrence is reported by Kewenter as male, 36.6% ± 2.3%; female, 30.1% ± 2.3%.[37] The patterns of partition are shown in Figure 2-58.[37]

The Interphalangeal Joint

This sesamoid is single and transversely oriented and has two surfaces: nonarticular and articular. The nonarticular surface is embedded in the plantar plate and attached to the flexor hallucis longus tendon. The articular surface is divided by a transverse crest into two facets: anterior and posterior. The anterior surface is smaller and articulates with the distal phalanx; the posterior surface is larger and articulates with the trochlear surface of the proximal phalangeal head. The sesamoid is attached to the proximal phalanx with short plantar sesamoid ligaments and forms a distal phalangeal-sesamoid apparatus. The solitary sesamoid moves with the distal phalanx. Its occurrence is not constant

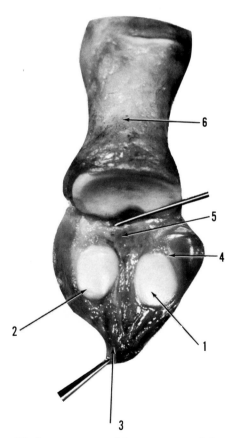

Fig. 2-57. **Phalangeosesamoid apparatus of the metatarsophalangeal joint of the big toe, left.** (1, Medial sesamoid; 2, lateral sesamoid; 3, capsule-synovial attachment to metatarsal neck inferiorly; 4, metatarsoglenoid ligament; 5, transverse ligament, lifted by probe, uniting lateral and medial sesamophalangeal ligaments; synovial pouch is present distal to this ligament; 6, proximal phalanx of big toe.)

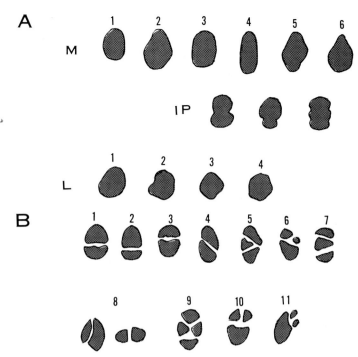

Fig. 2-58. **Variations in contour and partition of the sesamoids of the metatarsophalangeal joint of the big toe.** (A) M, medial sesamoid; L, lateral sesamoid. IP, intermediary partite; (B) Partite sesamoids. (Redrawn from Kewenter U: Die Sesambiene des I Metatarso-phalangeal-gelenks des Menschen. Acta Orthop Scand [Suppl] 2: 43, 1936)

and is reported as follows: Bizarro[40] (roentgenographic study), 5%; Pfitzner[41] (anatomic investigation), 50.6%; Trolle[42] (histoembryologic study), 56%.

THE LESSER TOES

The sesamoids of the lesser toes, when present, are connected to the long flexor tendons or the intrinsic muscles. Their occurrence is less frequent or rare. Pfitzner, in an anatomic study of 384 feet, provides the following frequencies of occurrence: second toe—metatarsophalangeal joint, tibial side, 1.8%, fibular side, 0; distal interphalangeal, 0.8%; fifth toe—metatarsophalangeal joint, tibial side, 5.5%, fibular side, 6.2%.[41]

The roentgenographic investigations and the histoembryologic studies yield a different distribution, presented in Figure 2-58.[40,42]

THE PERONEUS LONGUS TENDON

This sesamoid (os peroneum, sesamum peroneum; Fig. 2-59) is located in the substance of the peroneus longus tendon at the level of the cuboid tunnel where it angulates to enter the sole of the foot. The articular surface glides along the anterior slope of the plantar oblique tuberosity of the cuboid. The sesamoid is always present in an ossified, cartilaginous, or fibrocartilaginous stage.[43] It may remain a fibrocartilaginous nucleus for life. The os peroneum occurs

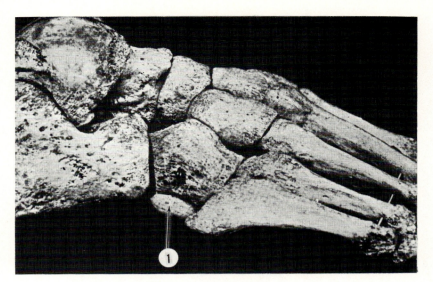

Fig. 2-59. Os peroneum (1). (From Dwight T: Variations of the Bones of the Hands and Feet: A Clinical Atlas, pp 14–23. Philadelphia, J B Lippincott, 1907)

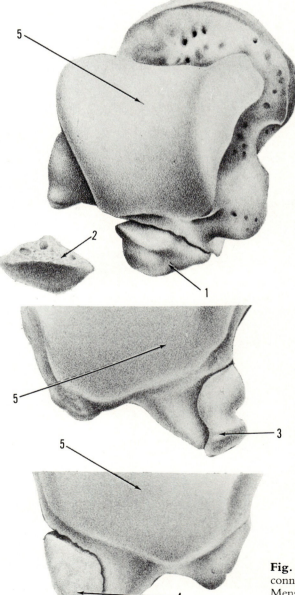

with the following frequency: anatomic study[43]—fully ossified, 20%, not fully ossified, 75%; radiographic investigation,[9] 5%. The os peroneum is frequently round but may be elongated or divided into several portions.[44]

THE TIBIALIS POSTERIOR TENDON

This sesamoid is located in the tibialis posterior tendon as it crosses the inferior calcaneonavicular ligament on the plantar aspect of the navicular tuberosity, and its occurrence is reported with the following frequency: Pfitzner[19] (729 feet), before age 50, 9.2%, after age 50, 11.9%; Storton[45] (348 feet), 23% (paired, 52.5%, unpaired, 47.5%).

THE TIBIALIS ANTERIOR TENDON

This sesamoid is located in the substance of the tibialis anterior tendon near its insertion at the level of the antero-inferior corner of the medial surface of the first cuneiform. An articular surface is found in this location on the cuneiform.

Accessory Bones

The accessory bones are developmental anomalies.[46] They are "either normal parts or prominences of the ordinary tarsal bones that are abnormally separated from the main elements or they are subdivisions of the main elements."[9] They may, on the other hand, not only complete the canonical element in contour but also represent "a free element which appears to be additional to the adjacent portion of its canonical element."[46]

Multiple accessoria may be present in a single foot, and they are unilateral in about half or even more than half of the cases.[46] They may be multipartite. For a comprehensive

Fig. 2-60.   Os trigonum. (1, 3, 4, Variations in contour; 2, anterior talar connecting surface; 5, talus.) (From Pfitzner W: Beitrage zur Kenntnis des Menschlichen Extremitätenskelets: VI. Die Variationen in Aufbau des Fussskelets. In Schwalbes [ed]: Morphologische Arbeiten, pp 245–527. Jena, Gustav Fischer, 1896)

account of the accessory bones of the foot, we refer to the classic work of Pfitzner and the studies of Dwight, Marti, Trolle, O'Rahilly, and Kohler and Zimmer.[19,27,42,44,46,47]

The more commonly occurring accessory bones are the os trigonum, the os tibiale, and the os intermetatarseum, 1–2. The following accessory bones occur less frequently: os sustentaculi, os calcaneus secundarius, os cuboides secundarium, os talonaviculare dorsale, os intercuneiforme, os cuneometatarsale 1 plantare, os vesalianum, os subtiale, os subfibulare.

OS TRIGONUM

The os trigonum[49] (Fig. 2-60) has already been described in the study of the talus. It is located at the level of the posterolateral tubercle of the talus. Its reported occurrence ranges from 1.7% to 7.7%. It is to be differentiated from the trigonal process and its fracture (Shepherd's fracture).

OS TIBIALE

The os tibiale (os tibiale externum, accessory navicular, naviculare secundarium; Figs 2-61 and 2-62) is an accessory

bone located on the posteromedial aspect of the tuberosity of the navicular. It is incorporated by the insertional fibers of the tibialis posterior tendon on the tuberosity of the navicular. It is to be differentiated from the sesamoid of the tibialis posterior tendon, which is located in the plantar portion of the tendon at the level of the inferior calcaneonavicular ligament. The sesamoid is located in the lateral aspect of the navicular tuberosity on the roentgenographic anteroposterior projection of the foot. A typical accessory navicular bone is pyramidal (see Fig. 2-60). The base is anterior and corresponds to the posteromedial aspect of the navicular tuberosity. The connection is fibrous or fibrocartilaginous. The apex is posterior. The contour of the os tabiale is very variable, and the roentgenographic morphological variations are described by Mouchet and Moutier (Fig. 2-63).[50] The bone is at times semilunate, round, or ovoid and is rudimentary, not articulating with the tuberosity of the navicular. At times it is partially or completely incorporated in the navicular tuberosity, which may then acquire the form of a bent hook.

The frequency of occurrence is as follows: Harris and Beath[51] (roentgenographic), 4.1%; Hoerr and co-workers[52] (501 adolescents, roentgenographic), girls, 3% to 8%, boys,

Fig. 2-61. Accessory navicular (1, 2). (From Dwight T: Variations of the Bones of the Hands and Feet: A Clinical Atlas, pp 14–23. Philadelphia, J B Lippincott, 1907)

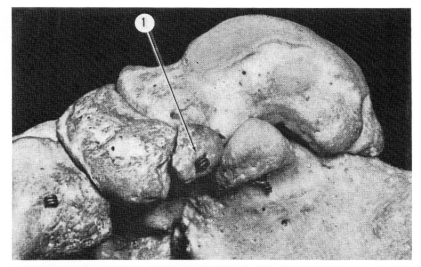
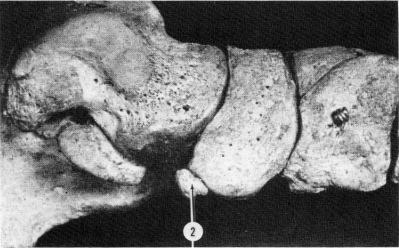

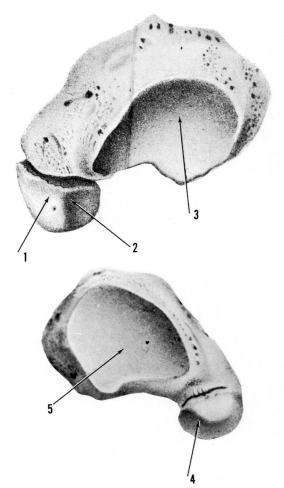

Fig. 2-62.   Accessory navicular. (Top) 1, 2, Accessory navicular with two facets; 3, navicular. (Bottom) 4, Accessory navicular attached to navicular [5].) (From Pfitzner W: Beiträge zur Kenntniss des Menschlichen Extremitätenskelets: VI. Die Variationen in Aufbau des Fussskelets. In Schwalbe [ed]: Morphologische Arbeiten, pp 245–527. Jena, Gustav Fischer, 1896)

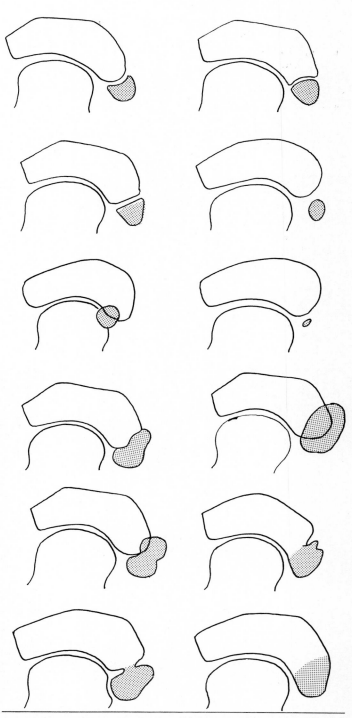

Fig. 2-63.   Variations in the roentgenographic forms of the accessory navicular. (From Mouchet A, Moutier G: Osselets surnuméraires du tarse [ossa tarsalia]. Presse Médicale, 23: 370, 1925)

4% to 9%; Bizarro[40] (roentgenographic), 2%; Holland[53] (roentgenographic), 10% to 12%; Pfitzner[19] (425 feet, anatomic), 11.5%; Trolle[42] (histoembryologic), 6.4%; Dwight[27] (anatomic), about 10%.

Zadek and Gold studied roentgenographically the fate of 14 accessory naviculars in children and adolescents.[54] Of 14 accessory naviculars, 5 fused totally to the navicular, 3 fused partially to the navicular, and 6 remained as independent accessory bones.

The terminology of os tibiale *externum* is confusing, as it relates to the phylogenetic concept of this accessory bone relative to the old representation of the primitive tetrapod foot. In the present concept of the primitive tetrapod foot and the development of the mammalian foot elements (Fig. 2-64), the head of the talus is formed by the two centrale proximale (fibulare and tibiale), the navicular is formed by the two centrale distale (fibulare and tibiale), and the tibiale, now medial to the talar head in this concept, forms the accessory navicular or os tibiale.[42] The tibiale is the third

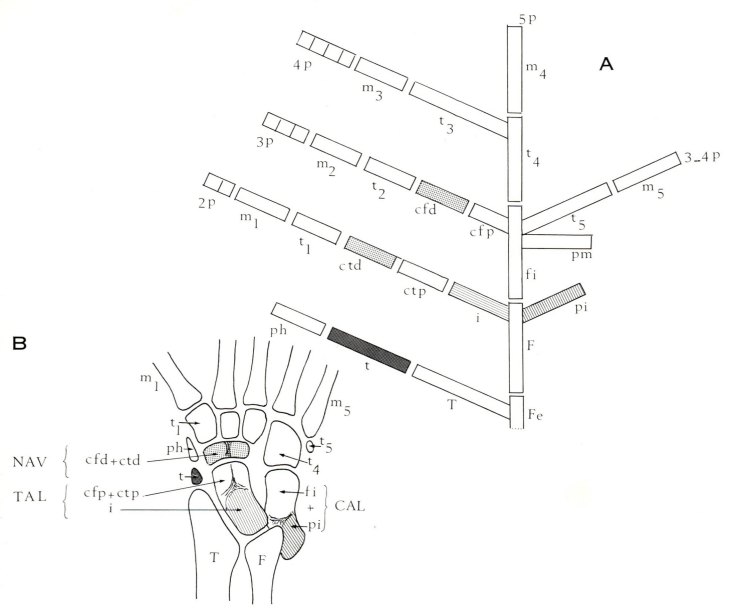

Fig. 2-64. **(A) Development of the primitive tetrapod foot.** The basal cord is formed by the femur (*Fe*), the fibula (*F*), the fibulare (*Fi*), the tarsale₄ (*T₄*), the metatarsale₄ (*M₄*), and five phalanges (*5p*). From the tibial side of the basal cord, 4 rays lead off. The first ray arises from the femur and is formed by the tibia (*T*), the tibiale (*t*), and the prehallux (*ph*). The second ray arises from the distal end of the fibula and is formed by the intermedium (*i*), the centrale tibiale proximale (*ctp*), the centrale tibiale distale (*ctd*), the tarsale₁ (*t₁*), the metatarsale₁ (*m₁*), and two phalanges (*2p*). The third ray takes off from the distal end of the fibulare and is formed by the centrale fibulare proximale (*cfp*), the centrale fibulare distale (*cfd*), the tarsale₂ (*t₂*), the metatarsale₂ (*m₂*), and three phalantes (*3p*). The fourth ray takes off from the tarsale₄ and is formed by the tarsale₃ (*t₃*), the metatarsale₃ (*m₃*), and four phalanges (*4p*). From the fibular side of the basal cord the following take off: the pisiform, arising from the distal end of the fibula (*pi*), and a distal ray, arising from the distal end of the fibulare and formed by the tarsale₅ (*t₅*), the metatarsale₅ (*m₅*), and three or four phalanges (*3-4p*). The postminimus (*pm*) has a similar origin. **(B) The foot of the living mammal has developed in the following manner from the elements of the primitive tetrapod foot:** The tibiale (*t*) of the first ray forms the accessory navicular. The talus is formed by the intermedium (*i*) of the second tibial ray and the proximal tibial and fibular centrales (*ctp* + *cfp*) of the second and third tibial rays. The navicular is formed by the distal tibial and fibular centrale (*ctd* + *cfd*) of the second and third tibial rays. The cuneiform₁ is formed by the tarsale₁, the cuneiform₂ is formed by the tarsale₂, and the cuneiform₃ is formed by the tarsale₃. The calcaneus is formed by the fibulare (*fi*) of the basal cord and the pisiform (*pi*). The cuboid is formed by the tarsale₄ (*t₄*) of the basal cord. (Diagrams redrawn after and data from Trolle D: Accessory Bones of the Human Foot: A Radiological, Histoembryological, Comparative Anatomical and Genetic Study, pp 150–151. Copenhagen, Munksgaard, 1948)

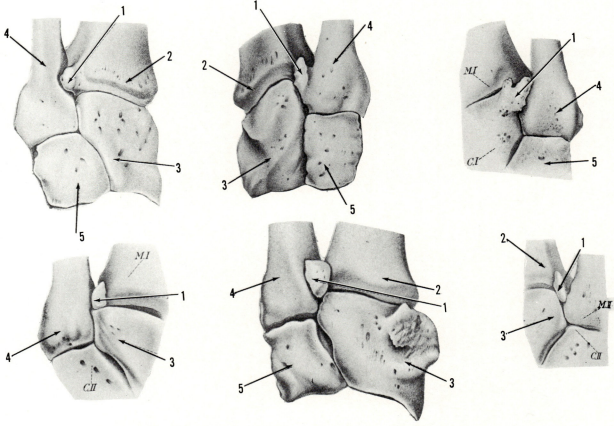

Fig. 2-65.   Os intermetatarseum. The os intermetatarseum is seen arising from the first or second metatarsal or from the first cuneiform. It may also present as an independent ossicle. (1, Os intermetatarseum; 2, first metatarsal; 3, first cuneiform; 4, second metatarsal; 5, second cuneiform.) (From Pfitzner W: Beiträge zur Kenntniss des Menschlichen Extremitäten skelets: VI. Die Variationen in Aufbau des Fussskelets. In Schwalbe [ed]; Morphologische Arbeiten, pp 245–527. Jena, Gustav Fischer, 1896)

element participating in the formation of the navicular. The term *externum* is "only misleading and ought to be dropped."[42]

OS INTERMETATARSEUM 1, 2

The os intermetatarseum is found between the medial cuneiform and the base of the first and second metatarsals.[55] The bone has variable size and contour, and it may be free or fused. A comprehensive description of the variations is given by Pfitzner (Fig. 2-65), Dwight (Fig. 2-66), and Schinz.[19,27,56] The os intermetatarseum is usually spindle shaped, fused to the distal dorsolateral corner of the medial cuneiform, and tapers distally while projecting between the first and second metatarsal bones. This accessory bone may fuse with the second metatarsal bone and project then anteriorly and medially. It may also fuse to the first metatarsal. When fused with one bone, the os intermetatarseum is in contact with the two others, and Dwight describes a case in which an articular surface is present with the three surrounding bones.[27] Friedl describes this bone as a sesamoid of the first dorsal interosseous muscle.[57] Henderson reports the association of hallux valgus and os intermetatarseum in

both feet of a brother and sister;[58] a tendinous structure is described extending from the tip of the accessory bone through the belly of the first dorsal interosseous and attaching to the lateral aspect of the proximal phalanx of the big toe.

The frequency of occurrence of the os intermetatarseum is as follows: Pfitzner[19] (anatomic), 8.2%; Dwight[27] (anatomic), 10%; Gruber[55] (anatomic), 8%; Bizarro[40] (roentgenographic), 0; Faber[59] (roentgenographic), 1.2%; Trolle[42] (histoembryologic), 6.8%.

OS SUSTENTACULI

The os sustentaculi is an accessory bone located at the posterior aspect of the sustentaculum tali (Fig. 2-67).[19] It occurs rarely as a distinct bone (0.47%)[19] and is connected with fibrous tissue or fibrocartilage to the sustentaculum. Dwight has "never seen it separate."[27] Kohler and Zimmer have observed this bone on four occasions.[44] Hoerr and co-workers give a frequency of roentgenographic occurrence of 2% to 3% in boys and none in girls in a total adolescent population of 501.[52]

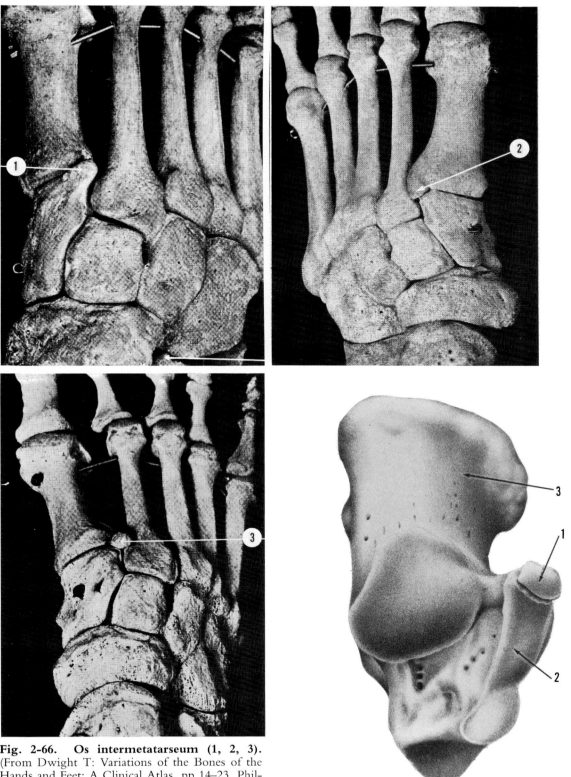

Fig. 2-66.   Os intermetatarseum (1, 2, 3).
(From Dwight T: Variations of the Bones of the
Hands and Feet: A Clinical Atlas, pp 14–23. Phil-
adelphia, J B Lippincott, 1907)

Fig. 2-67.   Os sustentaculi. (1, Os sustentaculi; 2, sustentaculum
tali; 3, calcaneus.) (From Pfitzner W: Beiträge zur Kenntniss des
Menschlichen Extremeitätenskelets: VI. Die Variationen in Aufbau
des Fussskelets. In Schwalbe [ed]: Morphologische Arbeiten, pp
245–527. Jena, Gustav Fischer, 1896)

OS CALCANEUS SECUNDARIUS

The os calcaneus secundarius is located dorsally in the interval between the anteromedial angle of the os calcis, the cuboid, the navicular, and the head of the talus (Fig. 2-68).[60] The configuration is variable, being round or angular. According to Kohler and Zimmer, "a rounded form is an expression of underdevelopment; a triangular form is seen much more frequently."[44]

The reported frequencies of occurrence are as follows: Pfitzner[19] (840 feet, anatomic), 2%; Stieda[60] (120 feet, anatomic), 2.5%; Gruber[61] (719 feet, anatomic), one case; Laidlaw[21] (750 feet, anatomic), three cases; Hoerr and co-workers[52] (510 adolescents, roentgenographic), boys, 7% to 11%, girls, 6% to 7%.

OS CUBOIDES SECUNDARIUM

The os cuboides secundarium, an accessory bone is of rare occurrence.[61] It is located on the plantar aspect of the foot between the cuboid, navicular, talus, and os calcis. Dwight gives the description of a free cuboides secundarium.[62] Holland mentions having seen it once roentgenographically as a "small circular shadow."[53]

This bone is recognized as a process connected to the cuboid (Fig. 2-69) or "more frequently fused with the scaphoid" (Fig. 2-70).[27] Hoerr and associates give a roentgenologic occurrence of 1% to 3% in 501 adolescent feet.[52]

OS TALONAVICULARE DORSALE

This accessory bone (os supranavicular, talonavicular ossicle, Pirie's bone) is located dorsally at the talonavicular joint near the midpoint.[63] Pfitzner considers it an avulsed exostosis and calls it *supranavicular spurium*(?).[19] Pirie describes this "normal ossicle" and reports subsequently on 14 cases, of which 4 were bilateral.[64, 65] Kohler and Zimmer observed it in "20 instances in the course of approximately two years."[44] Hoerr and co-workers report a roentgenographic rate of occurrence of 15% in boys and 11% in girls in a group of 134 adolescents.[52]

OS INTERCUNEIFORME

This ossicle is located on the dorsum of the foot between the proximal segments of the internal and middle cuneiforms and in front of the navicular (Fig. 2-71).[66] It is wedge shaped. Dwight mentions having seen this bone twice. Hoerr and co-workers report the frequency of occurrence of this accessory bone at 1% in boys and 1% in girls in a population of 367 adolescents.[52] Jones mentions the presence of "a little pit at the junction of the two tibial cuneiforms with the navicular that suggests that a very small free ossicle may have been present in the recent state."[9]

OS CUNEO$_1$ METATARSALE$_1$ PLANTARE

This accessory bone (pars peronea metatarsalis primi) is located on the plantar aspect of the foot between the base of the first metatarsal and the medial cuneiform (Fig. 2-72).[19] Its occurrence is rare.

OS VESALIANUM

The os vesalianum "has been the subject of much controversy and a good deal of confusion."[53] Holland reproduced

Fig. 2-68. Os calcaneus secundarius. ([*A*] 1, Os calcaneus secundarius; [*B*] 2, os calcaneus secundarius; 3, os intercuneiform.) (From Dwight T: Variations of the Bones of the Hands and Feet: A Clinical Atlas, pp 12–23. Philadelphia, J B Lippincott, 1907)

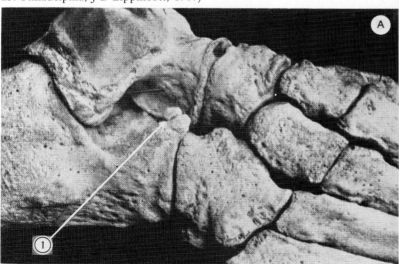

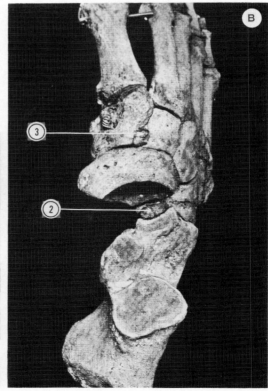

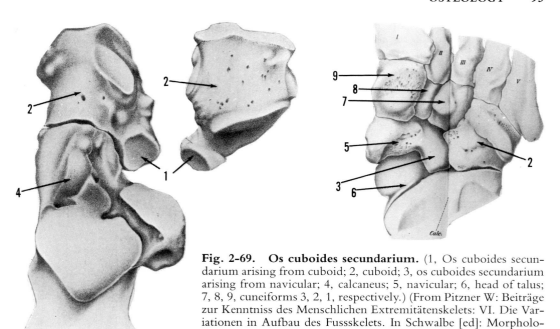

Fig. 2-69.   Os cuboides secundarium. (1, Os cuboides secundarium arising from cuboid; 2, cuboid; 3, os cuboides secundarium arising from navicular; 4, calcaneus; 5, navicular; 6, head of talus; 7, 8, 9, cuneiforms 3, 2, 1, respectively.) (From Pitzner W: Beiträge zur Kenntniss des Menschlichen Extremitätenskelets: VI. Die Variationen in Aufbau des Fussskelets. In Schwalbe [ed]: Morphologische Arbeiten, pp 245–527. Jena, Gustav Fischer, 1896)

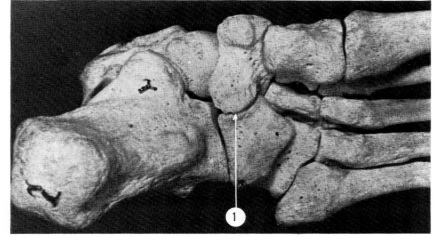

Fig. 2-70.   Os cuboides secundarium (1) arising from navicular. (From Dwight T: Variations of the Bones of the Hands and Feet: A Clinical Atlas, pp 14–23. Philadelphia, J B Lippincott, 1907)

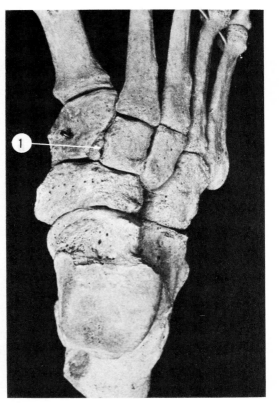

Fig. 2-71.   Os intercuneiform (1). (From Dwight T: Variations of the Bones of the Hands and Feet: A Clinical Atlas, pp 14–23. Philadelphia, J B Lippincott, 1907)

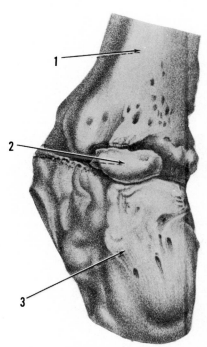

Fig. 2-72.   Os cuneo I-metatarsal I plantare. (1, First metatarsal; 2, os cuneo I–metatarsal I plantare; 3, first cuneiform.) (From Pfitzner W: Beiträge zur Kenntniss des Menschlichen Extremitätenskelets: VI. Die Variationen in Aufbau des Fussskelets. In Schwalbe [ed]: Morphologische Arbeiten, pp 245–527. Jena, Gustav Fischer, 1896)

Fig. 2-73.   Fifth metatarsal base. (1, Ossification within apophysis of base; 2, ossification within apophysis of base with fragmentation; 3, ununited apophysis of fifth metatarsal base; 4, position of os vesalianum.)

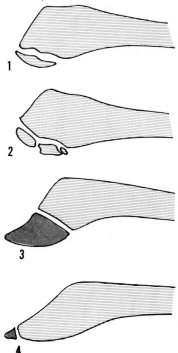

two illustrations from the 1725 edition of *The Works of Vesalius* (edited by Boerhave) depicting a plantar and a dorsal view of the lateral tarsus and the fifth metatarsal.[53] The dorsal view shows a small bone located between the well-formed tuberosity of the fifth metatarsal and the cuboid. The plantar view shows a small bone at the tip of the same tuberosity. The original description of the os vesalianum, translated by Holland, is as follows: "a small bone, opposite to the outer side of the joint, and placed proximately to the little toe, and probably articulating with the cuboid."[53]

This accessory bone is of rare occurrence. Dameron, in a roentgenographic study of 1000 feet, mentions its detection in one case.[67] Sporadic cases have been reported by Lequerrière and Drevon, Holland, and others.[53,68]

The os vesalianum is to be differentiated from the following (Fig. 2-73): the ossifying apophysis of the fifth metatarsal base, a fracture of the base of the fifth metatarsal bone or a nonunion of the same, an ununited apophysis of the fifth metatarsal base, and the sesamoid within the peroneus longus tendon. The following may help to differentiate the entities:[67]

The os vesalianum is located just proximal to the tip of the well-developed tuberosity of the fifth metatarsal. The opposing surfaces may be sclerotic.

The ossification center of the apophysis is linear initially and longitudinally oriented, parallel to the metatarsal shaft.

The fracture of the apophysis or base of the fifth metatarsal is transverse in direction and may pass through the cubometatarsal joint or metatarsal M_4-M_5 joint.

OS SUBTIBIALE, OS SUBFIBULARE

The os subtibiale is an accessory bone located under the medial malleolus. It may present as a round or angular ossicle. It is to be differentiated from a secondary ossification center of the medial malleolus or from a sequela of trauma. Powell, in a roentgenographic study of 100 healthy children aged 6 to 12 years, found an accessory ossification center to the medial malleolus in 20%.[69] Both ankles in 50 adults without history of injury were studied by the same author, and separate submalleolar ossicles were found in 4% of the ankles.

The *os subfibulare* is an accessory bone located under the tip of the lateral malleolus in a posterior position. Kohler and Zimmer mention having seen several cases in adults.[44] The ossicle may be round or comma shaped or present an articular facet facing the lateral malleolus. It is to be differentiated from a secondary ossification center of the lateral malleolus (which occurs in 1%) and from the sequela of trauma.

Coalition and Bipartition

COALITION

Coalition is the union of two or more bony elements. It may be fibrous (syndesmosis), cartilaginous (synchondrosis), or osseous (synostosis) and may involve the tarsus, the tarsometatarsal elements, or the phalanges. Pfitzner, in an anatomic study of 750 feet, reported an overall occurrence of coalition in 2% with the following distribution:[19] talocalcaneal, 1; talonavicular, 1; calcaneonavicular, 15; cubonavicular, 3; intercuneiform$_{2-3}$, 1; cuneo$_3$-metatarsal$_3$, 15.

Harris reports the following anatomic sites involved in 102 patients with tarsal coalition:[70] talocalcaneal, 66 (medial 62, posterior 4); calcaneonavicular, 29; cubonavicular, 1; talonavicular, 1; calcaneocuboid, 1; multiple intertarsal, 4.

Talocalcaneal Coalition

The talocalcaneal coalition occurs mainly on the medial side. Prior to the advent of roentgenographic investigation, the condition was recognized and reported by the anatomists.[71-74] Pfitzner described and gave a clear illustration of his only coalition occurring between the posterior end of the sustentaculum tali and the talus (Fig. 2-74).[19]

Few clinical reports[75-79] were present prior to the comprehensive study of the talocalcaneal coalition by Harris and Beath,[80] who correlated this anatomic variation with the etiology of peroneal spastic flatfoot. Harris described four anatomic types of medial talocalcaneal coalition:[70]

Complete (synostosis): a bony bridge unites the talus and the calcaneus at the level of the sustentaculum tali.
Incomplete (synchondrosis, syndesmosis): a cartilaginous or fibrous bridge unites the talar and calcaneal projections on the posterior aspect of the sustentaculum tali.
Rudimentary: a calcaneal sustentacular element extends from the posterior aspect of the sustentaculum tali and impinges on the medial aspect of the talus.
Rudimentary: a talar element extends from the posteromedial talar tubercle toward the os calcis just posterior to the sustentaculum tali.

The talocalcaneal coalition occurs more frequently at the level of the middle calcaneal facet or the posterior part of the sustentaculum tali; it sometimes occurs (but rarely) at the level of the posterior talocalcaneal joint.[75,81-83] It may involve the anterior calcaneal facet, as reported by Conway and Cowell in their comprehensive study related to the roentgenographic demonstration of the tarsal coalitions.[84]

Calcaneonavicular Coalition

Cruveilhier described and illustrated the first anatomic specimen of calcaneonavicular coalition (Fig. 2-75).[85] He mentioned that "this anatomic variety, which is certainly not a pathologic ossification, has already been seen many times." This specimen was provided by M. Fischer, who encountered an unusual resistance while doing a Chopart disarticulation of the foot: "This resistance was an abnormal ossification but by no means pathologic, uniting the anterior facet of the os calcis to the scaphoid."[85]

Subsequently, many anatomists reported on this union.[19,86-97] Pfitzner described 15 cases of calcaneaonavicular coalition (Fig. 2-76, A), and Dwight presented the photograph and roentgenogram of a calcaneonavicular synchondrosis (Fig. 2-76, B).[19,27] The clinical recognition of this coalition and its correlation with flatfeet is attributed to Slomann, who described three forms:[98,99] abnormal projections between the two bones (amphiarthrosis); fibrous union between the bony projections (syndesmosis) and often containing one or more osseous nuclei (ossa calcanea secundaria) embedded in the fibrous tissues; osseous union between the two bones (synostosis). Many clinical reports pertaining to the recognition and treatment of the condition confirmed the frequent occurrence of this coalition.[100-110]

When a synostosis is present, it is at least 1 cm wide, whereas in the amphiarthrosis, the width of the coalition is less than 0.5 cm.[110]

The reports in the literature indicate the inheritance of this coalition.[111-113] Leonard reported a study of 31 patients with spastic flatfoot in association with tarsal coalition.[114] Ninety-eight first-degree relatives of these patients were studied; 39% of the relatives presented a tarsal coalition

Fig. 2-74. Talocalcaneal coalition. (1, Coalition site, posteromedial; 2, posterior talocalcaneal segmental interline; 3, posteromedial talar tubercle; 4, medial aspect of talus.) (From Pfitzner W: Beiträge zur Kenntniss des Menschlichen Extremitätenskelets: VI. Die Variationen in Aufbau des Fussskelets. In Schwalbe [ed]: Morphologische Arbeiten, pp 245–527. Jena, Gustav Fischer, 1896)

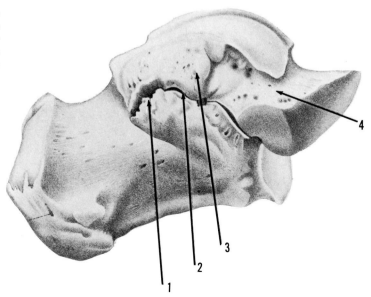

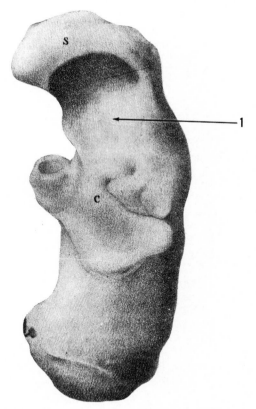

Fig. 2-75. Calcaneonavicular coalition. (1, Calcaneonavicular coalition; *S*, scaphoid; *C*, calcaneus.) (From Cruveilhier J: Anatomie Pathologique du Corps Humain ou Descriptions avec Figures Lithographieés et Colorées des Diverses Altérations Morbides dont le Corps Humain est Susceptible, Vol. 1. Paris, Baillière, 1829–1835. Courtesy of Northwestern University Medical Library)

(25%, calcaneonavicular; 14%, talocalcaneal and other coalitions). In 80% of these patients and in 84% of their relatives, the coalition was bilateral. Leonard concluded that "tarsal coalitions are inherited, most probably as a unifactorial disorder of autosomal dominant inheritance, very nearly of full penetrance."[114] Interestingly, none of the relatives with tarsal coalition had any evidence of peroneal spastic flatfoot.

Talonavicular Coalition

The first anatomic description of the talonavicular coalition was given by Anderson.[115] He described the synostosis in two anatomic specimens of a male subject, age 34, with "small and well shaped" feet. The fusion was so complete that the skeletal element was called *an astragaloscaphoid bone*. The head of this coalesced bone articulates laterally and on the external segment of the inferior surface with the cuboid. The inner surface is nonarticular, and the anterior surface articulates with the cuneiforms. A small elevated articular surface on the inferior aspect of the head, located in the middle of a depression, articulates with the sustentaculum tali.

Chaput described a talonavicular synostosis in an adult, involving the right foot, and both feet were flat.[72] Pfitzner had only one specimen of such coalition in 750 feet (Fig. 2-77).[19] Only sporadic cases are described in the literature.[84, 116–133]

Schreiber reported on five cases of talonavicular synostosis, three having the fusion bilaterally and two unilaterally.[134] Two patients had accompanying ball-and-socket ankle joint.

Calcaneocuboid Coalition

Robert mentioned a bilateral calcaneocuboid synostosis attributed to Auzias.[135] Wagoner reported on a 9-year-old boy with bilateral and complete calcaneocuboid synostosis.[136] Both feet were flat and symptomatic. Few cases are reported in the literature.[137–143] A bilateral case of calcaneocuboid synostosis reported by Brobeck also featured a very prominent base of the fifth metatarsal bone articulating with the calcaneus;[143] this coalition seems to be in frequent association with other anomalies. Stern and co-workers, Poznanski and co-workers, and Kelikian mentioned the presence of the calcaneocuboid coalition in the hand-foot-uterus syndrome.[143–146]

Kozlowski described a bilateral calcaneocuboid synostosis in a 14-year-old girl with bilateral hypoplasia of the distal ulna.[147] Schauerte and St. Aubin documented the occurrence of a sequential fusion of the tarsal joints in type I acrocephalosyndactyly (Apert's syndrome), the calcaneocuboid coalition being stage one, followed by the fusion of the lateral cuneiform and third metatarsal, and finally involving the navicular and the medial cuneiform.[148]

Craig and Goldberg reported on an 8-year-old girl with craniofacial dysostosis (Crouzon's syndrome) and bilateral isolated calcaneocuboid coalition, with one foot symptomatic.[149]

Cubonavicular Coalition

Cruveilhier illustrated a foot (Fig. 2-78) with cubonavicular coalition in association with synostosis between cuneiform 2-metatarsal 2 and cuneiform 3-metatarsal 3.[85] The text, however, does not carry a description of the cubonavicular union. Gruber presented four cases of cubonavicular coalition through the presence of a cuboides secundarium.[150] Pfitzner reported on three cases with a cuboides secundarius fused to the cuboid on the plantar side; in two specimens, they coalesced with the navicular, and the third specimen had a cuboides secundarius fused to the navicular and coalesced with the cuboid (Fig. 2-79).[19]

A true joint between the navicular and the cuboid is found frequently, as reported by the following anatomists: Gruber,[150] in 200 feet, 45.5%; Pfitzner,[19] in 437 feet, 50.4%; Dwight,[27] in 200 feet, about 60%.

When the joint is absent, normally the two bones are connected by ligaments. Dwight mentioned having "seen bony connection once and cartilaginous once or twice."[27]

The literature is very scarce in regard to the cubonavicular coalition.[151,152]

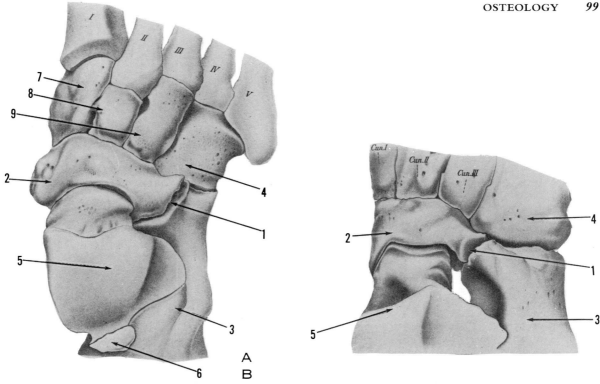

A
B

Fig. 2-76.   (A) Calcaneonavicular coalition. (1, Calcaneonavicular coalition; 2, navicular; 3, os calcis; 4, cuboid; 5, talus; 6, os trigonum; 7,8,9, cuneiforms 1,2,3, respectively.) (From Pfitzner W: Beiträge zur Kenntniss des Fussskelets. In Schwalbe [ed]: Morphologische Arbeiten, pp, 245–527. Jena, Gustav Fischer, 1896) **(B) Calcaneonavicular coalition.** (1, Calcaneonavicular coalition; 2, peroneal trochlear process, prominant.) (From Dwight T: Variations of the Bones of the Hand and Feet: A Clinical Atlas, pp 14–23. Philadelphia, J B Lippincott, 1970)

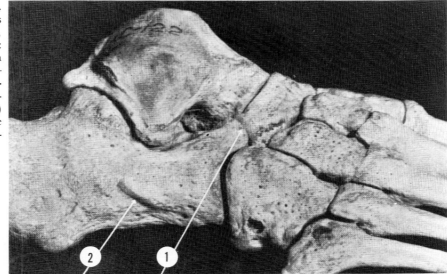

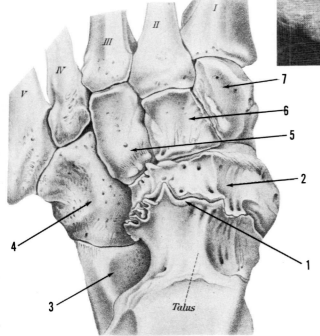

Fig. 2-77.   Talonavicular coalition. (1, Talonavicular coalition; 2, navicular; 3, calcaneus; 4, cuboid; 5, 6, 7, cuneiforms 3, 2, 1, respectively.) (From Pfitzner W: Beiträge zur Kenntniss des Menschlichen Extremitätenskelets: VI. Die Variationen in Aufbau des Fussskelets. In Schwalbe [ed]: Morphologische Arbeiten, pp 245–527. Jena, Gustav Fischer, 1896)

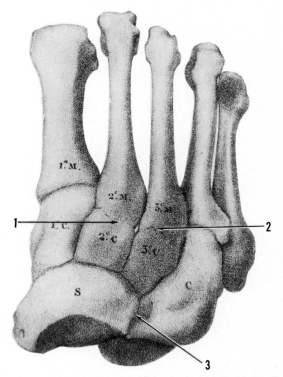

Fig. 2-78.   Cubonavicular coalition. (*S*, Scaphoid; *C*, Cuboid; 1, cuneiform₂ - metatarsal₂ coalition; 2, cuneiform₃ - metatarsal₃ coalition; 3, cubonavicular coalition.) (From Cruveilhier J: Anatomie Pathologique du Corps Humain ou Descriptions avec Figures Lithographiées des Diverses Altérations Morbides dont le Corps Humain est Susceptible, Vol 1. Paris Baillière, 1829–1835)

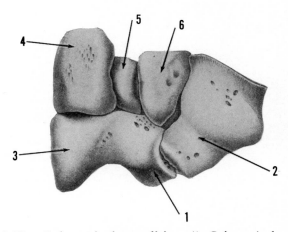

Fig. 2-79.   Cubonavicular coalition. (1, Cubonavicular coalition; 2, cuboid; 3, navicular; 4, 5, 6, cuneiforms 1, 2, 3, respectively.) (From Pfitzner W: Beiträge zur Kenntniss des Menschlichen Extremitätenskelets: VI. Die Variationen in Aufbau des Fussskelets. In Schwalbe [ed]: Morphologische Arbeiten, pp 245–527. Jena, Gustav Fischer, 1896)

Cuneonavicular Coalition

Lagrange described the foot of a 46-year-old woman with a bony fusion between the navicular and the three cuneiforms.[153] The coalition is, however, not limited to these

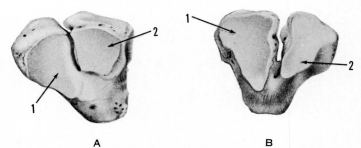

Fig. 2-80.   Intercuneiform II–III coalition. (*A*) (1, Cuneiform₂; 2, cuneiform₃.) (*B*) (1, Cuneiform₃; 2, cuneiform₂.) Coalesced from plantar aspect. (From Pfitzner W: Beiträge zur Kenntniss des Menschlichen Extremitätenskelets: VI. Die Variationen in Aufbau des Fussskelets. In Schwalbe [ed]: Morphologische Arbeiten, pp 245–527. Jena, Gustav Fischer, 1896)

skeletal elements, as the second and third metatarsals are fused to the cuniforms. Furthermore, the cuboid and metatarsals 4, 5 are also synostosed.

Lusby reported on the first isolated case of a cuneonavicular coalition.[154] The synostosis was present between the lateral cuneiform and the navicular; the patient was asymptomatic.

Gregersen reported on a bilateral cuneonavicular coalition in association with a bipartite navicular.[155] The medial half of the navicular was synostosed to the first cuneiform and the lateral half fused to the third cuneiform. The patient was 42 years old and presented bilateral symptomatic flatfeet.

Intercuneiform 2, 3 Coalition

One case of synostosis between the second and third cuneiforms was described by Pfitzner.[19] The two cuneiforms were synostosed on the plantar aspect, and the joint between them was undisturbed (Fig. 2-80). The union occurred through the enlarged plantar aspect of the third cuneiform, corresponding to the processus uncinatus cuneiformis 3. Pfitzner also mentioned that he had never seen a coalition between the first and second cuneiforms.[19]

Cuneo₂-Metatarsal₂ and Cuneo₃-Metatarsal₃ Coalitions

Cruveilhier described and illustrated one specimen with the second cuneiform fused to the second metatarsal bone and the third cuneiform to the third metatarsal (Fig. 2-81).[85] The synostosis was complete, and Cruveilhier stated also "it is obvious that this union is not the result of a disease." He furthermore advises that such a synostosis may create a surgical handicap and "this inconvenience could also be encountered during the partial amputation of the foot at the tarso-metatarso articulations, after the ingenious method of Lisfranc."[85]

Pfitzner found the coalition between the third cuneiform and the third metatarsal in 15 cases in 750 feet.[19] The synostosis was usually on the plantar aspect (Fig. 2-82) and included, in 14 cases, one third to one fourth of the joint

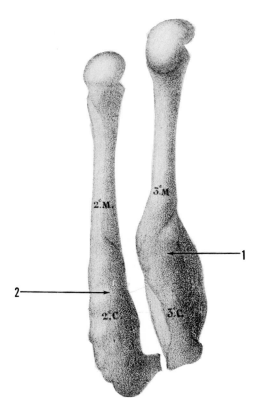

Fig. 2-81. Cuneo₃-metatarso₃ coalition (1) and cuneo₂-metatarso₂ coalition (2). (From Cruveilhier J: Anatomie Pathologique du Corps Humain ou Descriptions avec Figures Lithographiées et Colorées des Diverses Altérations Morbides Dont Le Corps Humain est Susceptible, Vol 1. Paris Baillière, 1829–1835)

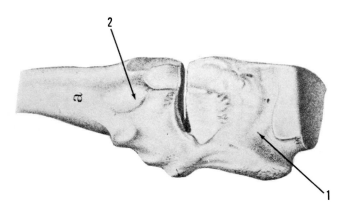

Fig. 2- 82.   Cuneo₃- metatarso₃ coalition. (1, Third cuneiform; 2, third metatarsal.) (From Pfitzner W: Beiträge zur Kenntniss des Menschlichen Extremitätenskelets: VI. Die Variationen in Arbeiten, pp 245-527. Jena, Gustav Fischer, 1896)

surfaces. A complete synostosis was present in one case and a partial central synostosis in two others.

Interphalangeal Coalition

The interphalangeal coalition involves mainly the middle and distal phalanges of the little toe (Fig. 2-83).[19] The monumental investigation of Pfitzner yielded the following re-

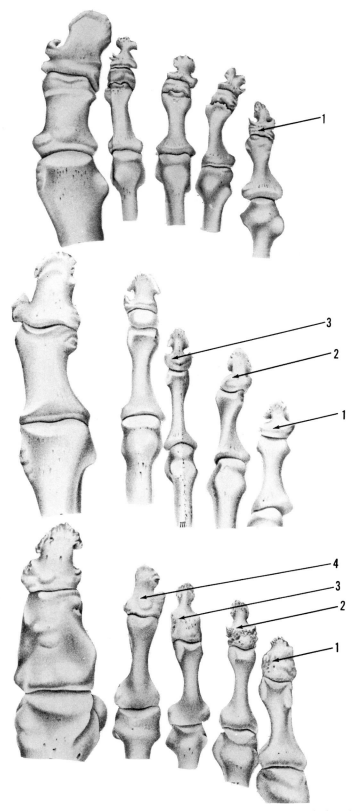

Fig. 2-83.   Interphalangeal coalition of middle and distal phalanges of (1) toe 5, (2) toe 4, (3) toe 3, (4) toe 2. (From Pitzner W: Beiträge zur Kenntniss des Menschlichen Extremitätenskelets: VI. Die Variationen in Aufbau des Fussskelets. In Schwalbe [ed]: Morphologische Arbeiten, pp 245–527. Jena, Gustav Fischer, 1896)

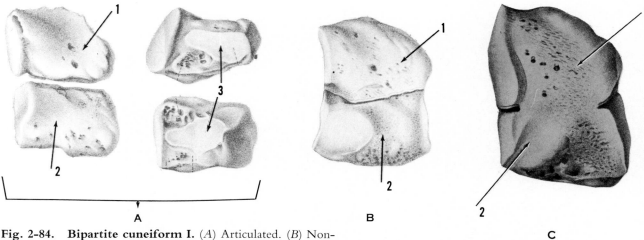

Fig. 2-84. Bipartite cuneiform I. (*A*) Articulated. (*B*) Non-osseous union. (*C*) Fused. (1, Dorsal; 2, plantar; 3, articular surface.) (From Pfitzner W: Beiträge zur Kenntniss des Menschlichen. Extremitätenskelets: VI. Die Variationen in Aufbau des Fussskelets. In Schwalbe [ed]: Morphologische Arbeiten, pp 245–527. Jena, Gustav Fischer, 1896)

sults: in 91 feet in embryos 5 months or older and children up to 7 years, 37 coalitions (40.7%); in 838 adult feet, 310 coalitions (37%).[19] The coalition seems more frequent in females:[53] males, 35.5%; females, 40.2%.

Coalition of the middle and terminal phalanges may involve toes other than the fifth, but this is relatively rare. According to Pfitzner, when the other toes are involved, the progression is from lateral to medial and in an orderly fashion.[19] The fourth never shows a coalition when a coalition is not present in the fifth, nor the third if not present in the fourth and fifth, nor the second if not present already in the lesser three toes.

Multiple, Massive, and Associated Coalitions

Cruveilhier, Lagrange, and Morestin have described multiple coalitions in the same foot.[74,85,153] Massive or multiple tarsal coalitions are recorded in the literature.[156–165]

Tarsal coalitions may also occur in association with other malformations: carpal fusions, carpal synostosis with radial head subluxation, symphalangism, and partial adactylia.[163–169] This may also occur in the following clinical entities: type I acrocephalosyndactyly (Apert's syndrome),[148] hand-foot-uterus syndrome,[170] craniofacial dysostosis (Crouzon's syndrome),[170] acropectorovertebral dysplasia (F syndrome),[170] arthrogryposis (occasionally),[170] and otopalatodigital syndrome (OPD syndrome).[170]

The occurrence of massive or multiple tarsal synostosis in Nievergelt–Pearlman syndrome is well established. Murakami, reporting 3 cases and reviewing the total of 13 cases in the literature, found tarsal fusions in 12.[171]

BIPARTITION

Bipartite First Cuneiform

The bipartite first cuneiform was first described by Morel.[172] Four cuneiforms were present in the left foot, and a

trace of partition was observed in the first cuneiform of the right foot.

The presence of this skeletal variation has been recorded by anatomists.[173–178] Gruber observed 10 complete and 5 incomplete bipartitions, and in a study of 2500 feet, the frequency of occurrence of a perfect bipartition was reported as 1 in 320.[179,180] Pfitzner, examining 750 feet, found and illustrated two bipartite first cuneiforms (Fig. 2-84).[19] Hartman and Mordret observed two such variations in 200 feet.[181] Roentgenographic recognition of the bipartition of this bone was reported early by many authors.[182–186] Barclay, after describing the roentgenographic recognition of this anatomic variation bilaterally in a jockey aged 34, mentioned that "cases of partial division seem to be fairly common, and several examples were found in the osteological collection here," and she produced diagrams of two such specimens.[184]

Barlow gave the following anatomic description of a bilateral bipartite first cuneiform in a male of age 82.[187]

The bone is divided by a horizontal cleft into a dorsal small and a plantar larger segment. A diarthrodial joint is present between these two segments on the medial half of the cleft. The *dorsal segment* articulates anteriorly with the dorsal part of the first metatarsal base. Its posterior surface articulates with the navicular. The supero-medial surface gives attachment to ligaments connecting to the bones with which it articulates. The lateral surface is articular in the posterior half with the middle cuneiform. The anterior half of this lateral surface articulates with the second metatarsal base dorsally and gives insertion in its plantar half to the interosseous ligament. The inferior surface gives insertion laterally to a strong interosseous ligament uniting the dorsal plantar segments and the middle cuneiform. The *plantar segment* articulates anteriorly with the base of the first metatarsal and posteriorly with the navicular. The medial surface gives insertion to the tibialis anterior at the antero-inferior angle. The inferior surface has a prominent tubercle at its proximal end for the attachment of a portion of the tibialis posterior. A tubercle at the antero-inferior angle of the lateral surface gives insertion to the peroneus longus tendon. The two segments of the bipartite 1 cuneiform are together slightly larger than an undivided medial cuneiform.

Bipartite Navicular

The bipartite navicular was not recognized prior to the roentgenographic era. In 1937 Volk reported on two cases of bipartite navicular.[188] Zimmer in 1938 described roentgenographically and histologically a case of bipartite navicular in a 19-year-old patient.[189] Roentgenographically, on the dorsoplantar view, the smaller fragment is a comma-shaped structure measuring 12 mm by 21 mm, superimposed on the first and second cuneiforms and the main navicular segment. On the lateral view, the smaller fragment is dorsal in location, triangular in contour, separated from the main navicular fragment by a cleft directed upward and anteriorly. No disease could be found histologically.

In 1941, Fine Licht reported on four cases, two of which were bilateral.[190] Typically, on the dorsoplantar projection of the roentgenogram, the smaller fragment is wedge shaped, with the base directed medially and the apex laterally. On the lateral view, the same fragment is again wedge shaped, the apex directed in a plantar direction.

Sporadic reporting of individual cases of bipartite navicular is further found in the literature.[191,192]

REFERENCES

1. Edwards, ME: The relations of the peroneal tendons to the fibula, calcaneus and cuboideum. Amer J Anat 42, No. 1: 213, 1928
2. Inman VT: The Joints of the Ankle, pp 2, 12, 13, 19, 23, 26, 38–39, 94–97. Baltimore, Williams & Wilkins, 1976
3. Lang J, and Wachsmuth W: Praktische Anatomie Bein und Statik, pp 353, 361. Berlin, Springer-Verlag, 1972
4. Singh I: Squatting facets on the talus and tibia in Indians. J Anat 93:540, 1959
5. Barnett, CH, Napier JR: The axis of rotation at the ankle joint in man: Its influence upon the form of the talus and the mobility of the fibula. J Anat 86:1, 1952
6. Sewell, RBS: A study of the astragalus, Part II. J Anat Physiol 38:423, 1904
7. Rouvière H, Canela Lazaro M: Le ligament péroneo-astragalo-calcanéen. Ann Anat Pathol 9, No. 7:745, 1932
8. Farabeuf LH: Précis de Manuel Opératoire, Nouvelle ed, p 840. Paris, Masson, 1889
9. Jones FW: Structure and Function as Seen in the Foot, 2nd ed, pp 39–40, 76–77, 83, 87, 97, 117–120. London, Baillière, Tindall & Cox, 1949
10. Sewell RBS: A study of the astragalus. Part IV. J Anat Physiol 40:152, 1906
11. Gamble FO, Yale I: Clinical Foot Roentgenology, p 153. Baltimore, Williams & Wilkins, 1966
12. Steindler A: Kinesiology of the Human Body, 3rd ed, p. 405. Springfield, Charles C Thomas, 1970
13. Laidlaw PP: The varieties of the os calcis. J Anat Physiol 38:133, 1904
14. Boehler L: Diagnosis, pathology and treatment of fractures of the os calcis. J Bone Joint Surg 13:77, 1931
15. Manter JT: Movements of the subtalar and transverse tarsal joints. Anat Rec 80:397, 1941
16. Bunning PSC, Barnett CH: A comparison of adult and foetal talocalcaneal articulations. J Anat 99:71, 1965
17. Gruber W: Ueber den eine Thierbildung Reprasentirenden Normalen, und uber den Exostotisch Gewordenen Processus Trochlearis Calcanei. Virchows Arch [Pathol Anat] 70:128, 1877
18. Stieda L: Der M. Peroneus Longus und die Fussknochen. Anat Anz 4:606–607, 624–640, 652–661, 1889
19. Pfitzner W: Beiträge zur Kenntniss des Menschlichen Extremitätenskelets: VI. Die Variationen in Aufbau des Fussskelets. In Schwalbe (ed): Morphologische Arbeiten, pp 245–527. Jena, Gustav Fischer, 1896
20. Morestin H: Note pour servir à l'étude de l'anatomie du calcaneum. Bull Soc Anat Paris, 69:737, 1894
21. Laidlaw PP: The os calcis, Part II. J Anat Physiol 39:168, 1905
22. Poirier P, Charpy A: Traité d'Anatomie Humaine, Vol 1, pp 263–264, 758. Paris, Masson, 1899
23. Paturet G: Traité d'Anatomie Humaine, Vol 2, p 573. Paris, Masson, 1951
24. Manners-Smith T: A study of the cuboid and os peroneum in the primate foot. J Anat Physiol 42:399, 1908
25. Gruber, W: Ueber den Fortsatz des Hockers des Kahnbeins der Fusswurzel—Processus Tuberositatis Navicularis—und dessen Auftreten als Epiphyse oder als Besonderes Arti-kulirendes Knochelchen. Arch Anat Physiol Wiss Med: 281, 1871
26. Manners-Smith T: A study of the navicular in the human and anthropoid foot. J Anat Physiol 41:261, 1907
27. Dwight T: Variations of the Bones of the Hands and Feet: A Clinical Atlas, pp. 14–23. Philadelphia, JB Lippincott, 1907
28. Barclay-Smith E: The astragalo-calcaneo-navicular joint. J Anat Physiol 30:399, 1896
29. Breathnack, AS (ed): Frazer's Anatomy of the Human Skeleton, 6th ed, p 149. Boston, Little Brown, 1965
30. Straus WL Jr: Growth of the human foot and its evolutionary significance. Contrib Embryol 19, No. 101:116, 119, 1927
31. Kelikian H: Hallux Valgus Allied Deformities of the Forefoot and Metatarsalgia, pp 102, 112. Philadelphia, WB Saunders, 1965
32. Lebaucq H: Le développement du premier métatarsien et de son articulation tarsienne chez l'homme. Arch Biol 3:343, 1882
33. Morton DJ: The Human Foot: Its Evolution, Physiology & Functional Disorders, p 179, Columbia University Press, 1935
34. Singh I: Variations in the metatarsal bones. J Anat 94:345, 1960
35. Haines RW, McDougall A: The anatomy of hallux valgus. J Bone Joint Surg [Br] 36:272, 1954
36. Wilkinson JL: The terminal phalanx of the great toe. J Anat 88:537, 1954
37. Kewenter U: Die Sesambeine des I Metatarso-phalangeal-gelenks des Menschen. Acta Orthop Scand [Suppl] 2:43, 1936
38. Gillette: Des os sesamoides chez l'homme. J Anat Physiol, pp 506–538, 1872
39. Sabatier M: Traité Complet d'Anatomie ou Description de toutes les Parties du Corps Humain, Vol 1, p 231. Paris, Didot, 1775
40. Bizarro AH: On sesamoids and supernumerary bones of the limbs. J Anat 55:258, 1921
41. Pfitzner W: Die Sesambeine des Menschen. In Schwalbe: Morphologische Arbeiten, Vol I, pp 517–762, Jena, Gustav Fischer, 1892
42. Trolle, D: Accessory Bones of the Human Foot: A Radiological, Histoembryological, Comparative Anatomical and Genetic Study, pp 20–53, 150–151, 165. Copenhagen, Munksgaard, 1948
43. Anatomical Society, Collective Investigation: Sesamoids in the gastrocnemius and peroneus longus. J Anat Physiol 32:182, 1897
44. Kohler A, Zimmer EA: Borderlands of the Normal and Early Pathologic in Skeletal Roentgenology, 3rd ed, pp. 460, 464–468, 489, 502, 507. New York, Grune & Stratton, 1968
45. Storton CE: In Grant JCB (ed): Grant's Atlas of Anatomy, 5th ed. Baltimore: Williams & Wilkins, 1962
46. O'Rahilly R: Developmental deviations in the carpus and the tarsus. Clin Orthop 10:9, 15, 1957
47. Marti T: Die Skelettvarietaten des Fusses ihre Klinische und Unfallmedizinische Bedentug, pp 27–111. Berne, Hans Huber, 1947
48. O'Rahilly R: A survey of carpal and tarsal anomalies. J Bone Joint Surg [Am] 35:635, 1953
49. Rosenmuller JC: De Nonnullis Musculorum Corporis Humani Varietatibus, p 8. Leipzig, 1804
50. Mouchet A, Moutier G: Osselets surnuméraires du tarse (ossa tarsalia). Presse Médicale 23:370, 1925
51. Harris RI, Beath T: Army Foot Survey, Vol 1, p 52. Ottawa, National Research Council of Canada, 1947
52. Hoerr NL, Pyle DI, Francis CC: Radiographic Atlas of Skeletal Development of the Foot and Ankle, A Standard of Reference, pp 41–44. Springfield, Charles C Thomas, 1962
53. Holland CT: The Accessory Bones of the Foot With Notes on a Few Other Conditions, the Robert Jones Birthday Volume, pp 160, 162–167, 170, London, Oxford University Press, 1928
54. Zadek I, Gold AM: The accessory tarsal scaphoid. J Bone Joint Surg [Am] 30:957, 1948
55. Gruber W: Abhandlungen aus er Menschlichen und Vergleichenden Anatomie, pp 111–113. Leipzig, St. Petersburg University, 1852

56. Schinz HR: Roentgen-Diagnostics, 1st American ed (Case JT, ed), p 124. New York, Grune & Stratton, 1951
57. Friedl E: Das Os Intermetatarseum und die Epiphysenbildung am Processus Trochlearis Calcanei. Dtsch Z Chir 188:150, 1924
58. Henderson, RS: Os intermetatarseum and possible relationship to hallux valgus. J Bone Joint Surg [Br] 45:117, 1963
59. Faber A: Ueber das Os Intermetatarseum. Orthop Chir 61:186, 1934
60. Stieda L: Ueber Sekundare Fusswurzelknochen. Arch Anat Physiol Wiss Med: 108, 1869
61. Gruber W: Uber einen Neven Secundaren Tarsalknochen-Calcaneus Secundarius-mit Bemerkungen uber den Tarsus uber haupt. Mém Acad Impériale Sci Saint-Petersbourg 7:1, 1871
62. Dwight T: Description of a free cuboides secundarium, with remarks on that element and on the calcaneus secundarius. Anat Anz 37:218, 1910
63. Hyrtl J: Ueber die Trochlearfortsatze der Menschlichen Knochen. Denkschrift Wiener Akad Math Naturaw 18:141, 1860
64. Pirie AH: A normal ossicle in the foot frequently diagnosed as a fracture. Arch Radiol Electrother 24:93, 1920
65. Pirie, AH: Extra bones in the wrist and ankle found by roentgen rays. Am J Roentgenol: 573, 1921
66. Dwight, R: Os intercuneiforme tarsi, os paracuneiforme tarsi, calcaneus secundarius. Anat Anz 20:465, 1902
67. Dameron, TB Jr: Fractures and anatomical variations of the proximal portion of the fifth metatarsal. J Bone Joint Surg [Am] 57, No. 6:788, 1975
68. Lequerrière, Drevon: On the vesalian bone. J Radiol Elec 395, 1916
69. Powell, HDW: Extra centre of ossification for the medial malleolus in children: Incidence and significance. J Bone Joint Surg [Br] 43, No.1:107, 1961
70. Harris, RI: Follow-up notes on articles previously published in the J Retrospect: Peroneal spastic flat foot (rigid valgus foot). J Bone Joint Surg [Am] 47, No. 8:1657, 1965
71. Zuckerkandl E: Ueber einen Fall von synostose zwischen Talus und Calcaneus. Allgem Wiener Med Z 22:292, 1877
72. Chaput: Etude anatomo-pathologique de deux pièces de pied plat valgus (tarsalgie des adolescents) guéris par ankylose, suivie de quelques considérations sur la pathogénie et le mécanisme de ces lésions. Progres Med 14:857, 1886
73. Leboucq H: De la soudure congénitale de certains os du tarse. Bull Acad Med Brux 4:103, 1890
74. Morestin H: De l'ankylose calcaneo-astragalienne. Bull Soc Anat Paris 69:985, 1894
75. Bentzon PGK: Bilateral congenital deformity of the astragalo-calcaneal joint: Bone coalescence between os trigonum and the calcaneus. Acta Orthop Scand 1:359, 1930
76. Burman, MS, Sinberg SE: An anomalous talocalcaneal articulation: Double ankle bones. Radiology 34:239, 1940
77. Gaynor, SS: Congenital astragalocalcaneal fusion. J Bone Joint Surg 18:479, 1936
78. Grashey R: Articulatio talo-calcanea (os sustentaculi). Rontgenpraxis, 14:139, 1942
79. Sutro C: Anomalous talo-calcaneal articulation: Cause for limited subtalar movements. Am J Surg 74:64, 1947
80. Harris, RI, Beath T: Etiology of peroneal spastic flat foot. J Bone Joint Surg [Br] 30:624, 1948
81. Maier K: Beitrage zur Verschmelzung des Os Trigonum mit dem Kalkaneus. Fortschr Geb Rontgenst 98:664, 1963
82. Outland T, Murphy ID: Relation of tarsal anomalies to spastic and rigid flat feet. Clin Orthop 1:217, 1953
83. Shands, AR and Wentz IJ: Congenital anomalies, accessory bones and osteochondritis in the feet of 850 children. Surg Clin North Am 33:1643, 1953
84. Conway JJ, Cowell HR: Tarsal coalition: Clinical significance and roentgenographic demonstration. Radiology 92:799, 1969
85. Cruveilhier J: Anatomie Pathologique du Corps Humain ou Descriptions, avec Figures Lithographiées et Colorées des Diverses Altérations Morbides dont le Corps Humain est Susceptible, Vol. 1. Paris, Baillière, 1829–1835
86. Wedding CF: Quaedam de Ancylosibus, p 24. Berlin, 1832
87. Smith RW: Congenital malformation of the tarsus. Dublin Q J Med Sci 9:109, 1850
88. Verneuil, in Robert A: Des Vices Congénitaux de Conformation des Articulations. Thesis, Paris, 1851
89. Gurlt E: Beiträge zur vergleichenden pathologischen Anatomie der Gelenkkrankheiten, p 620. Berlin, 1853
90. Humphrey GM: A Treatise on the Human Skeleton, p 80. Cambridge, 1858
91. Gruber W: Ueber den Fortsatz des Höckers des Kahnbeins der Fusswurzel-Processus tuberositatis navicularis-und dessen Auftreten als Epiphyse oder als besonderes artikulirendes Knöchelchen. Arch Anat Physiol Wiss Med: 281, 1871
92. Gruber W: Beobarhtungen aus der Menschlichen und Vergleichenden Anatomie, Vol 1, pp 15–18. Berlin, 1879
93. Zuckerkandl E: Neue Mittheilungen über coalition von Fusswurzelknochen. Wien Med Jahrb:125, 1880
94. Holl M: Beiträge zur chirurgischen Osteologie des Fusses. Langenbecks Arch Klin Chir 25:211, 1880
95. Weber M: Ober coalescentia calcaneo-navicularis. Versl Med Kongl Acad Vmet Afd Naturk: 121, 1882
96. Petrini, P: Articulation anomale entre le calcaneum et le scaphoide. Atti del' XI Cong Med Internaz Roma, Vol 2, Anatomia, pp. 71–79. Roma, 1894
97. Morestin H: Note sur un scaphoide s'articulant par de larges facettes avec le cuboide et le calcaneum. Bull Soc Anat Paris 69:798, 1894
98. Slomann HC: On coalition calcaneo-navicularis. J Orthop Surg 19:586, 1921
99. Slomann, HC: On the demonstration and analysis of calcaneo-navicular coalition by roentgen examination. Acta Radiol 5:304, 1926
100. Badgley CE: Coalition of the calcaneus and the navicular. Arch Surg 15:75, 1927
101. Bentzon, PG: Coalitio calcaneo-navicularis, mit besonderer Bezungnahme auf die operative Behandlung des durch diese Anomalie bedingten Plattfusses. Verh Dtsch Orthop Ges 23:269, 1929
102. Seddon HJ: Calcaneo-scaphoid coalition. Proc R Soc Med 26:419, 1933
103. Herschel H, Von Ronnen JR: The occurrence of calcaneo navicular synostosis in pes valgus contracture. J Bone Joint Surg [Am] 32:280, 1950
104. Hark FW: Congenital anomalies of the tarsal bones. Clin Orthop 16:21, 1960
105. Kendrick JJ: Treatment of calcaneo-navicular bar. JAMA 172:1242, 1960
106. Braddock GTF: A prolonged follow-up of peroneal spastic flat foot. J Bone Joint Surg [Br] 43:734, 1961
107. Rutt A: Zur genese der coalitio calcaneo-naviculare. Z Orthop 96:96, 1962
108. Simmons, EH: Tibialis spastic varus foot with tarsal coalition. J Bone Joint Surg [Br] 47:533, 1965
109. Mitchell, GP, Gibson JMC: Excision of calcaneonavicular bar for painful spasmodic flat foot. J Bone Joint Surg [Br] 49:281, 1967
110. Heikel HUA: Coalitio cancaneo-navicularis and calcaneus secundarius. Acta Orthop Scand 31:78, 1961
111. Webster FS, Roberts WM: Tarsal anomalies and peroneal spastic flat foot. JAMA 146:1099, 1951
112. Wray JB, Herndon CN: Hereditary transmission of congenital coalition of the calcaneus to the navicular. J Bone Joint Surg [Am] 45:365, 1963
113. Glessner JR Jr, Davis GL: Bilateral calcaneonavicular coalition occurring in twin boys. Clin Orthop Rel Res 47:173, 1966
114. Leonard MA: The inheritance of tarsal coalition and its relationship to spastic flat foot. J Bone Joint Surg [Br] 56:520, 1974
115. Anderson RJ: The presence of an astragalo-scaphoid bone in man. J Anat Physiol 14:452, 1879
116. Holland, CT: Two cases of rare deformity of feet and hands. Arch Rad Elect 22:234, 1918
117. Blencke H: Ein seltner Fall von Synostosis talonavicularis. Z Orthop Chir 47:594, 1925–1926
118. Esau: Angeborene Missbildungen der Füsse (Randdefekt). Dtsch Z Cir 194:263, 1925–1926

119. Bullitt, JB: Variations of the bones of the foot: Fusion of the talus and navicular, bilateral and congenital. Am J Radiol 20:548, 1928

120. Illievitz AB: Congenital malformations of the feet: Report of a case of congenital fusion of the scaphoid with the astragalus and complete absence of one toe. Am J Surg 4:550, 1928

121. Haglund P: Ein fall von vollständiger coalitio talo-navicularis. Z Orthop Chir 51:93, 1929

122. Lapidus PR: Congenital fusion of the bones of the foot with a report of a case of congenital astragaloscaphoid fusion. J Bone Joint Surg 14:888, 1932

123. Hayek W: Synostosis talonavicularis. Z Orthop Chir 60:231, 1934

124. Rothberg AS, Feldman FW, Schuster OF: Congenital fusion of astragalus and scaphoid: bilateral: inherited. NY Med 35:29, 1935

125. Lapidus PW: Bilateral congenital talonavicular fusion: Report of a case. J Bone Joint Surg 20:775, 1938

126. Jaubert de Beaujeu A, Benmussa: Synstose, astragaloscaphoidienne congénital bilatérale et isolée. J Radiol Elect 23:348, 1939

127. O'Donoghue DH, Sell, LS: Congenital talonavicular synostosis: A case report of a rare anomaly. J Bone Joint Surg 25:925, 1943

128. Boyd HB: Congenital talonavicular synostosis. J Bone Joint Surg 26:682, 1944

129. Weitzner I: Congenital talonavicular synostosis associated with hereditary multiple ankylosing arthropathies. Am J Roentgenol 56:185, 1946

130. Chambers CH: Congenital anomalies of the tarsal navicular with particular reference to calcaneo-navicular coalition. Br J Radiol 33:584, 1950

131. Austin FG: Symphalangism and related fusions of tarsal bones. Radiology 56:882, 1951

132. Sanghi JK, Roby HR: Bilateral peroneal spastic flat feet associated with congenital fusion of the navicular and talus: A case report. J Bone Joint Surg [Am] 43:1237, 1961

133. Challis J: Hereditary transmission of talonavicular coalition in association with anomaly of the little finger. J Bone Joint Surg [Am] 56:1273, 1974

134. Schreiber RR: Talonavicular synostosis. J Bone Joint Surg [Am] 45, No. 1:170, 1963

135. Auzias, in Robert A: Des vices congénitaux de conformation des articulations, p 22. Thesis, Paris, 1851

136. Wagoner GW: A case of bilateral congenital fusion of the calcanei and cuboids. J Bone Joint Surg 10:220, 1928

137. Bargellini D: Fusione calcaneo-cuboidea e piede piatto. Arch Ital Chir 21:386, 1928

138. Esau: Angeborene Synostose im Bereich des Carpus und Tarsus. Rontgenprazis 5:235, 1933

139. Rey: Angeborne Verschmelzung von Calcaneus und Kuboid. Zentralbl Chir 59:1666, 1932

140. Mestern J: Erbliche Synostosen den Hand-und Fusswurzelknochen. Rontgenpraxis 6:594, 1934

141. Veneruso L: Unilateral congenital calcaneo-cuboid synostosis with complete absence of a metatarsal and toe. J Bone Joint Surg 27:718, 1945

142. Mahaffey HW: Bilateral congenital calcaneo cuboid synostosis. J Bone Joint Surg 27:164, 1945

143. Brobeck O: Congenital bilateral synosteosis of the calcaneus and cuboid and of the triquetral and hamate bones. Acta Orthop Scand 25:217, 1956

144. Stern AM, Gall, JC Jr, Perry BL et al: The hand-foot-uterus syndrome. J Pediatr 77:109, 1970

145. Poznanski AK, Stern AM, Gall JC Jr: Radiographic findings in hand-foot-uterus syndrome (HFUS). Radiology 96:129, 1970

146. Kelikian H: Congenital Deformities of the Hand and Forearm, p 131. Philadelphia, WB Saunders, 1974

147. Kozlowski K: Hypoplasie bilatérale congénitale du cubitus et Synostose bilatérale calcanéo-cuboide chez une fillette. Ann Radiol 1–2:389, 1965

148. Schauerte EW, St. Aubin PM: Progressive synosteosis in Apert's syndrome (acrocephalosyndactyly): With a description of roentgenographic changes in the feet. Am J Roentgenol 97:67, 1966

149. Craig CL, Goldberg MJ: Calcaneo-cuboid coalition in Crouzon's syndrome. J Bone Joint Surg [Am] 59:826, 1977

150. Gruber W: Ueber einen neuen sekundären tarsalknochen-Calcaneus secundarius-mit Bemerkungen über den Tarsus überhaupt. Mem Acad Sci St. Petersbourg. 17:1871

151. Waugh W: Partial cubo-navicular coalition as a case of peroneal spastic flat foot. J Bone Joint Surg [Br] 39:520, 1957

152. Del Sel JM, Grand NE: Cubo-navicular synostosis. J Bone Joint Surg [Br] 41:149, 1959

153. Lagrange: Anomalie du pied, soudure des os du tarse et du métatarse. Bull Soc Anat Paris: 577, 1881

154. Lusby JLJ: Naviculo-cuneiform synostosis. J Bone Joint Surg [Br] 41:149, 1959

155. Gregersen HN: Naviculocuneiform coalition. J Bone Joint Surg [Am] 59:128, 1977

156. Bersani FA, Samilson RL: Massive familial tarsal synostosis. J Bone Joint Surg [Am] 39:1187, 1957

157. Basu SS: Naviculo-cuneo-metatarso phalangeal synostosis. Indian J Surg 25:750, 1963

158. Kadelbach G: Ein Beiträg zu den Fusswurzelsynostosen. Arch Orthop Unfallchir 40:363, 1940

159. Sloane MWM: A case of anomalous skeletal development in the foot. Anat Rec 96:23, 1946

160. Zock E: Ein Beiträg zu den synostosen der Fusswurzel. Zentralb Chir 78:845, 1953

161. Vizkelety T: Eine seltene Form der Synostose der Fusswurzelknochen. Z Orthop 97:245, 1963

162. Rompe G: Ankylosen der Unteren Sprunggelenkes nach offenem Unterschenkelbruch. Arch Orthop Unfallchir 54:339, 1962

163. Pearlman HS, Edkin RE, Warren RF: Familial tarsal and carpal synostosis with radial head subluxation. J Bone Joint Surg [Am] 46:585, 1964

164. Miller EM: Congenital ankylosis of joints of hands and feet. J Bone Joint Surg 4:560, 1922

165. Lissoos I, Soussi J: Tarsal synostosis with partial adactylia. Med Proc 11:224, 1965

166. Devoldere J: A case of familial congenital synostosis in the carpal and tarsal bones. Arch Chir Neerland 12:185, 1960

167. Austin FH: Symphalangism and related fusions of tarsal bones. Radiology 56:882, 1951

168. Slater P, Rubinstein H: Aplasia of interphalangeal joints associated with synostoses of carpal and tarsal bones. Q Bull Sea View Hosp 7:429, 1942

169. Harle TS, Stevenson JR: Hereditary symphalangism associated with carpal and tarsal fusions. Radiology 89:91, 1967

170. Poznanski AK: The Hand in Radiologic Diagnosis, pp 267, 270, 304, 358. Philadelphia, WB Saunders, 1974

171. Murakami Y: Nievergelt-Pearlman syndrome with impairment of hearing. J Bone Joint Surg [Br] 57, No. 3:367, 1975

172. Morel: Diversités Anatomiques: Recueil Period d'Observ, pp 432–434. Paris, 1757

173. Jones S: A right foot showing two internal cuneiforms. Trans Pathol Soc 15: 189, 1864

174. Smith T: A foot having four cuneiforms. Trans Pathol Soc 17:222, 1866

175. Turner W: Report on the progress of anatomy. J Anat 3:447, 1869

176. Stieda L: Uber sekundare Fusswurzelknochen. Mullers Arch: 109, 1869

177. Ledentu M: Anomalie du Squelette du pied: Cunéiforme supplementaire. Bull Soc Anat Ser 14:13, 1869

178. Friedlowsky A: Uber Vermehrung der Handwurzelknochen durch ein Os Carpale Intermedium und uber sekundare Fusswurzelknochen. Sitzungsber Akad Wissensbh 61:591, 1870

179. Gruber W: Vorläfige Mittheilung über die secundären Fusswurzelknochen des Mensche. Arch Anat Physiol Wiss Med: 286, 1864

180. Gruber W: Monographie über das Zweigetheilte erste Keilbein der Fusswurzel-Os Cuneiforme I bipartitum Tarsi-beim Menschen. Mem Acad Sci St. Petersbourg 24, No. 11, 1877

181. Hartman H, Mordret J: Sur un point de l'anatomie du premier cuneiform. Bull Soc Anat Paris: 71, 1889

182. Hasselwander A: Studies on the ossification of the human foot. Z Morphol:466, 1903
183. Haenisch GF: Die röntgenographie der Knochen und Gelenke und ihr Wert für die Orthopaedische Chirurgie. Dtsch Med Wochenschr 42:1039, 1913
184. Barclay M: A case of duplication of the internal cuneiform bone of the foot. J Anat 67:175, 1932
185. Friedl E: Divided cuneiform I in childhood. Rontgenpraxis 6: 193, 1934
186. Hiedsieck E: Os cuneiform I bipartitum. Rontgenpraxis 8:712, 1936
187. Barlow TE: Os cuneiform I Bipartitum. Am J Phy Anthropol 29:95, 1942
188. Volk C: Zwei Fälle von Os naviculare pedis bipartitum. Z Orthop Grenzgebiete: 396, 1937
189. Zimmer, EA: Krankheiten, Verletzungen und Varietäten des os Naviculare pedis. Arch Orthop Unfal Chir 38:402, 1938
190. Fine Licht E: On bipartite os naviculare pedi. Acta Radiol 22:377, 1941
191. Hatoff A: Bipartite navicular bone as a cause of flat foot. Am J Dis Child 80:991, 1950
192. Mau H: Zur Kenntnis des Naviculare bipartitum pedis. Z Orthop 93:404, 1960

Retaining Systems and Compartments

The tendons and the neurovascular bundles pass from the leg into the foot through a nearly 90° turn. To prevent their bowstringing or subluxation, retaining retinacular systems are necessary.

On the convex dorsal surface of the foot, the thin investing fascial layers provide flat compartments; at the sole of the foot, the thick plantar aponeurosis and its extensions create deep compartments.

The major retaining structures and compartments to be considered are the following: extensor retinaculum, superior and inferior; peroneal retinaculum, superior and inferior; dorsal aponeurosis of the foot and dorsal compartments; tibiotalocalcaneal tunnel and flexor retinaculum; plantar aponeurosis; plantar compartments and fascial spaces. The retaining systems of the extensor and flexor mechanisms of the toes are discussed in subsequent chapters.

Extensor Retinaculum

The extensor tendons of the foot and the toes are retained in the distal leg by the superior extensor retinaculum and at the level of the ankle–foot by the inferior extensor retinaculum (Fig. 3-1).

SUPERIOR EXTENSOR RETINACULUM

The superior extensor retinaculum (ligamentum transversum cruris) is a transverse aponeurotic band formed by the reinforcement of the distal segment of the superficial aponeurosis of the leg. The proximal and distal borders are difficult to delineate and are more or less surgically created. This transverse ligament is attached laterally on the lateral crest of the lower fibula and the lateral surface of the lateral malleolus and medially on the anterior crest of the tibia and the medial malleolus. Laterally the superior extensor retinaculum is in continuity with the superior peroneal retinaculum and medially with the apical fibers of the flexor retinaculum.

The digital extensors, the peroneus tertius tendon and the tibialis anterior tendon, pass under the ligament. In 25% of the cases, there is a separate tunnel for the tibialis anterior tendon, formed by the dissociation of the fibers into a superficial and a deep layer.[1] The apical fibers of the flexor retinaculum contribute to the formation of this tunnel by passing superficially and deep to the tibialis anterior tendon before inserting on the deep surface of the transverse ligament. The superomedial band of the inferior extensor retinaculum also provides fibers to the deep layer of the same tunnel.

INFERIOR EXTENSOR RETINACULUM

The inferior extensor retinaculum (anterior annular ligament of the tarsus, ligamentum cruciatum of Weitbrecht, frondiform ligament of Retzius, ligamentum lamboideum) is a Y- or X-shaped retaining structure located on the anterior aspect of the tarsus and the ankle (Figs. 3-1–3-5).[1–6] It is a complex structure and has four components: the stem or frondiform ligament, the oblique superomedial band, the oblique inferomedial band, the oblique superolateral band.

Stem or Frondiform Ligament

The stem or frondiform ligament is a sling ligament retaining the tendons of the extensor digitorum longus and peroneus tertius against the talus and the calcaneus. This ligament has three roots: lateral, intermediary, and medial.

The lateral root is superficial, originates in the sinus tarsi lateral to the origin of the extensor digitorum brevis muscle, and blends with the deep fascia and the inferior peroneal retinaculum. The boundaries of this superficial root are difficult to delineate by dissection; tensing of the extensor tendons or inversion of the foot facilitates recognition of its borders.

The intermediary root arises from the sinus tarsi medial to the origin of the extensor digitorum brevis muscle and

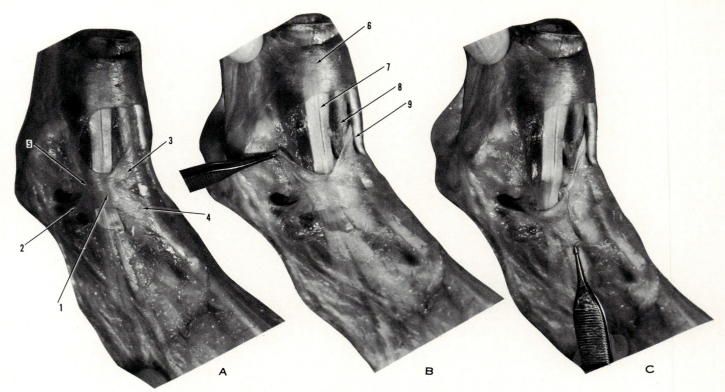

Fig. 3-1. (*A*) **Inferior extensor retinaculum** *in situ*. (*B*) **Superolateral band of** (*A*) **detached.** (*C*) **Superolateral band of** (*A*) **reflected, demonstrating the frondiform or sling arrangement around the extensor digitorum longus tendons.** (1, Inferior extensor retinaculum, cruciate form; 2, stem of inferior extensor retinaculum; 3, oblique superomedial band of inferior extensor retinaculum; 4, oblique inferomedial band of inferior extensor retinaculum; 5, oblique superolateral band of inferior extensor retinaculum; 6, superior extensor retinaculum; 7, extensor digitorum longus tendons; 8, extensor hallucis longus tendon; 9, tibialis anterior tendon.)

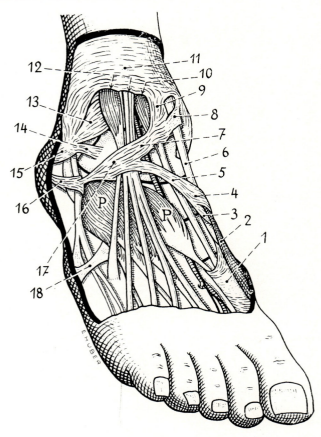

Fig. 3-2. **Inferior extensor retinaculum.** (1, Medial transverse retinacular band of dorsum of foot; 2, abductor hallucis muscle; 3, 4, superficial and deep laminae of oblique inferomedial band of inferior extensor retinaculum; 5, oblique inferomedial band of inferior extensor retinaculum; 6, tibialis anterior tendon; 7, oblique superomedial band of inferior extensor retinaculum; 8, 9, superficial and deep components of oblique superomedial retinaculum forming tunnel of tibialis anterior tendon; 10, extensor hallucis longus tendon; 11, aponeurosis of leg; 12, extensor digitorum longus and peroneus tertius tendons; 13, anteroinferior tibiofibular ligament; 14, anterior talofibular ligament; 15, superior peroneal retinaculum; 16, inferior peroneal retinaculum; 17, stem of inferior extensor retinaculum or frondiform ligament; P, extensor digitorum brevis muscle.) (From Meyer P: La morphologie du ligament annulaire antérieur du cou-de-pied chez l'homme. Comptes-Rendus Assoc Anat 84:286, 1955)

Fig. 3-3.   Diagram after dissection under magnification. The talus has been ostectomized obliquely in the direction of the canalis tarsi. The posterior half of the talus has been removed. Further exposure of the sinus tarsi and canal was obtained by removing bone from the talus with a rongeur. (1, Lateral root of inferior extensor retinaculum; 2, intermediary root of inferior extensor retinaculum; 3, medial root of inferior extensor retinaculum; 4, lateral calcaneal component of medial root; 5, medial calcaneal component of medial root; 6, talar component of medial root attached into canalis tarsi; 7, oblique talocalcaneal band of medial root; 8, talar body attachment of medial root; 9, loop formed by medial root of inferior extensor retinaculum turning around extensor digitorum longus tendon; 10, reflected component of oblique superomedial band of inferior extensor retinaculum forming a sling for extensor hallucis longus tendon; 11, tunnel for tibialis anterior tendon; 12, interosseous ligament of canalis tarsi, oblique in direction, forming an X with medial calcaneal component of the medial root of inferior extensor retinaculum; 13, tendons of peronei; 14, peroneus tertius tendon; 15, extensor digitorum longus tendons; 16, extensor hallucis longus tendon; 17, tibialis anterior tendon; 18, talus; 19, os calcis.)

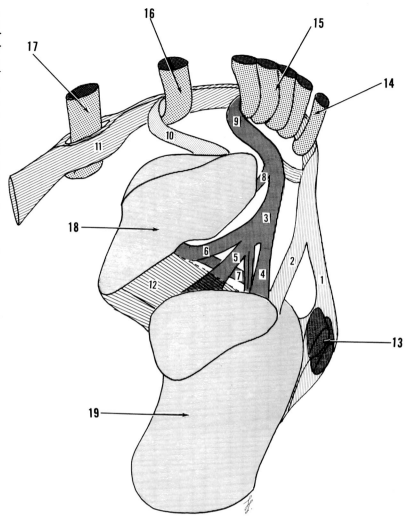

just posterior to the origin of the cervical ligament. At times this root is fasciculated, and one large fascile may divide the origin of the extensor hallucis brevis from that of the lesser toes.

The intermediary root extends upward and unites with the lateral root, forming the superficial component of the stem of the inferior extensor retinaculum. Once formed, the stem courses obliquely upward and inward across the neck of the talus. It passes over the peroneus tertius and extensor digitorum longus tendons and bifurcates into the oblique superomedial and inferomedial bands.

The medial root completes the formation of the retinacular sling for the extensor digitorum longus tendons and the peroneus tertius and forms the deep part of the stem. It has three components: two calcaneal (lateral and medial) and one talar.

The lateral calcaneal component is formed by vertical fibers and inserts in the sinus tarsi just posterior to the intermediary root and establishes connection at this level. The major medial calcaneal component enters the tarsal canal very obliquely and inserts on the floor of the canal along its longitudinal axis, usually anterior to the ligament

of the tarsal canal. The fibers of the ligament are oriented downward and laterally, whereas those of the medial calcaneal root are oriented downward and medially, forming an X.

The talar component of the medial root attaches to the talus on the roof of the tarsal canal, joining the insertion fibers of the ligament of the tarsal canal. Arcuate fibers with inferior concavity unite the two calcaneal components of the medial root. An oblique band of the medial root originates at the calcaneal attachment of the intermediate root, extends medially upward, and joins the talar insertion of the ligament of the tarsal canal. This ligament has been described by Barclay Smith and, more recently, by Cahill who named it the *oblique talocalcaneal band*.[3,4]

The medial root, ascending upward and medially, is applied against the lateral aspect of the talar neck. It passes anterior to the insertion of the anterior talofibular ligament. A bursa may be interposed between the two structures in 50% to 80% of the cases. Occasionally, instead of the bursa, one finds adipose tissue or even a fibrous band of attachment.

(Text continues on p. 113.)

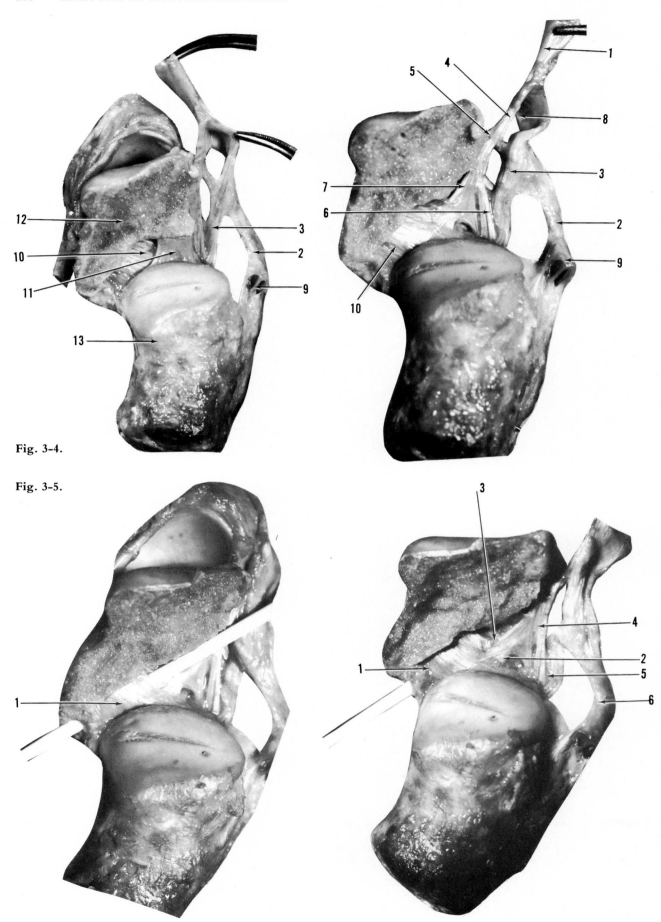

Fig. 3-4.

Fig. 3-5.

Fig. 3-4. Anatomic preparation of the roots of the inferior extensor retinaculum.
(1, Stem of inferior extensor retinaculum; 2, lateral root inserting on the inferior retinaculum of peronei [9]; 3, intermediary root of inferior extensor retinaculum; 4, medial root of inferior extensor retinaculum; 5, talar body attachment of medial root; 6, lateral calcaneal attachment of medial root; 7, oblique calcaneal component of medial root; 8, sling or pulley for extensor digitorum longus and peroneus tertius tendons; 9, inferior retinaculum of peronei tendons; 10, interosseous ligament of tarsal canal; 11, anterior capsule-ligament of posterior talocalcaneal joint; 12, ostectomized talus, posterior half removed; 13, calcaneus.)

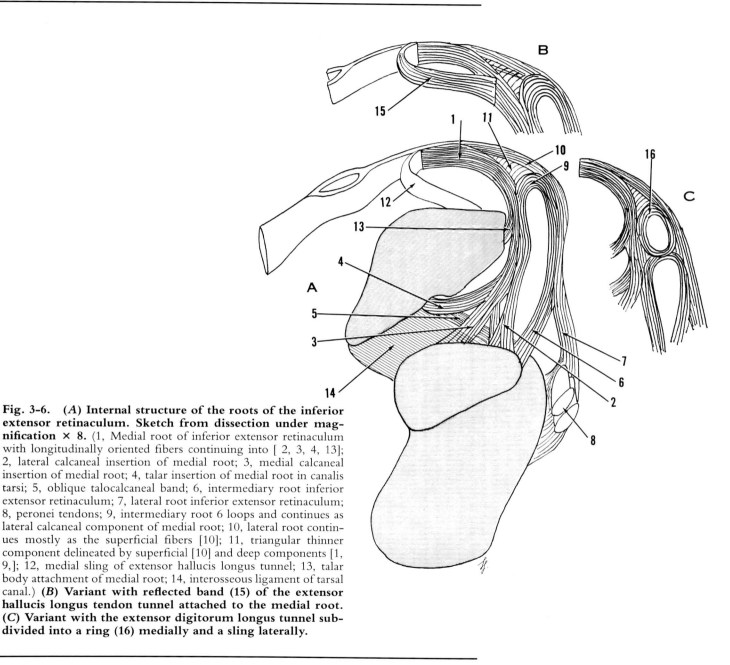

Fig. 3-6. **(A) Internal structure of the roots of the inferior extensor retinaculum. Sketch from dissection under magnification × 8.** (1, Medial root of inferior extensor retinaculum with longitudinally oriented fibers continuing into [2, 3, 4, 13]; 2, lateral calcaneal insertion of medial root; 3, medial calcaneal insertion of medial root; 4, talar insertion of medial root in canalis tarsi; 5, oblique talocalcaneal band; 6, intermediary root inferior extensor retinaculum; 7, lateral root inferior extensor retinaculum; 8, peronei tendons; 9, intermediary root 6 loops and continues as lateral calcaneal component of medial root; 10, lateral root continues mostly as the superficial fibers [10]; 11, triangular thinner component delineated by superficial [10] and deep components [1, 9,]; 12, medial sling of extensor hallucis longus tunnel; 13, talar body attachment of medial root; 14, interosseous ligament of tarsal canal.) **(B) Variant with reflected band (15) of the extensor hallucis longus tendon tunnel attached to the medial root. (C) Variant with the extensor digitorum longus tunnel subdivided into a ring (16) medially and a sling laterally.**

Fig. 3-5. Anatomic preparation of the roots of the inferior extensor retinaculum.
(1, Interosseous ligament of canalis tarsi [white rod passing anterior to the ligament]; 2, medial calcaneal component of medial root of inferior extensor retinaculum crosses anteriorly [1]; 3, talar insertion of medial root; 4, lateral calcaneal component of medial root; 5, intermediary root of inferior extensor retinaculum; 6, lateral root of inferior extensor retinaculum.)

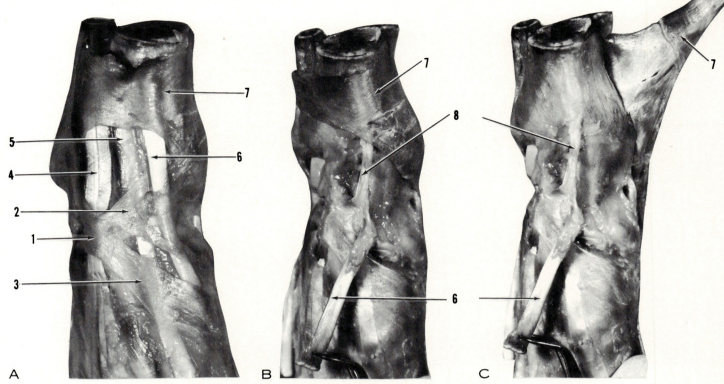

Fig. 3-7. Anatomy of the oblique superomedial band of the inferior extensor retinaculum forming the pulleys for the tibialis anterior tendon. (*A*) The deep fibers of the oblique superomedial band of the inferior extensor retinaculum pass under the tibialis anterior tendon proximally, whereas the superficial fibers pass more distally. (*B*) Tibialis anterior tendon reflected downward exposing (8). (*C*) Superior extensor retinaculum reflected medially with the flexor retinaculum, which is in continuity and covers the medial aspect of the ankle. (1, Stem of inferior extensor retinaculum; 2, oblique superomedial band of inferior extensor retinaculum. The deep component [8] of this band passes proximally under the tendon of the tibialis anterior, penetrates under the superior extensor retinaculum, and attaches to the tibia. The former is in continuity with the flexor retinaculum; 3, oblique inferomedial band of inferior extensor retinaculum; 4, extensor digitorum longus tendon; 5, extensor hallucis longus tendon; 6, tibialis anterior tendon; 7, superior extensor retinaculum; 8, deep tibial attachment of oblique superomedial band of the inferior extensor retinaculum.)

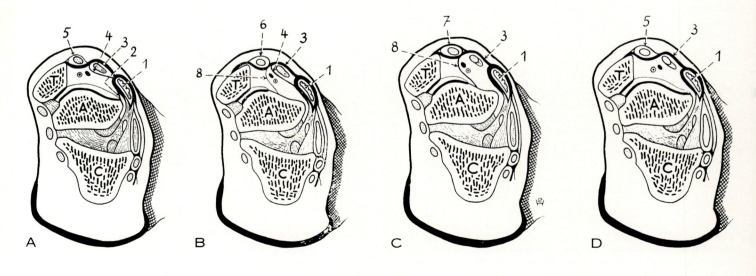

After crossing the superior surface of the talar neck, the medial root forms a loop, joins the deep surface of the stem, and completes the sling for the extensor digitorum longus and peroneus tertius tendons. The internal architecture of the frondiform ligament and some of its variations are depicted in Figure 3-6.

Oblique Superomedial Band

The oblique superomedial band continues the direction of the stem, passes over the tendon of the extensor hallucis longus and under the tendon of the tibialis anterior, and inserts on the anterior aspect of the medial malleolus. Occasionally the insertion fans out and reaches the anterior tibial crest and the medial surface of the medial malleolus, interchanging fibers with the superior extensor retinaculum and the flexor retinaculum (Fig. 3-7).

On the medial border of the extensor hallucis longus tendon, the deep fibers of the superomedial band loop around the tendon in a recurrent manner and have a variable insertion (Fig. 3-8), *viz.,* on the apex of the lateral sling or on the deep surface of the medial root in 50% of the cases, on the anterior aspect of the talar neck in 25% of the cases (Fig. 3-9), or on the lateral sling and the anterior aspect of the talar neck in 25%.[1] In the latter cases, the tendon of the extensor hallucis longus and the anterior neurovascular bundle are in the same compartment. Exceptionally, the deep layer of this segment of the retinaculum is absent.

Farther medially, at the level of the tibialis anterior tendon, there is a bifurcation of the superomedial band, forming superior and inferior retention systems. The superior tunnel has a thick deep wall and a very thin or even absent superficial wall. The inferior tunnel is well formed, with insertional fibers reaching the medial malleolus or occasionally blending with the fibers of the inferior arm of the extensor retinaculum.

Oblique Inferomedial Band

The oblique inferomedial band arises from the apex of the lateral sling, advances inferomedially, and reaches the medial border of the foot at the level of the cuneo$_1$-navicular joint.

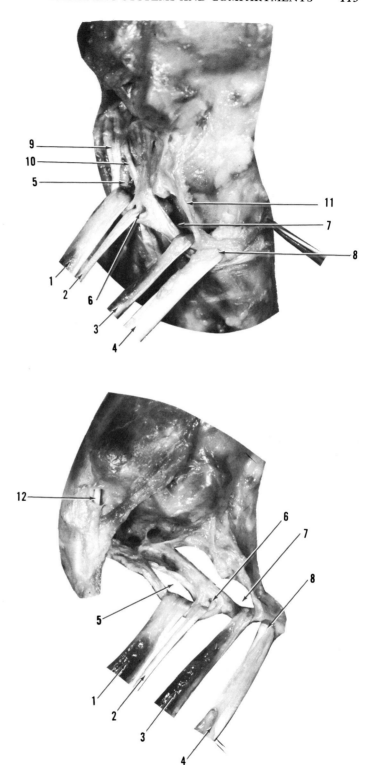

Fig. 3-8.   Cross sections through the sinus tarsi and canal; variations of the insertion made of the deep lamina or sling or reflected fibers of the extensor hallucis longus tunnel. (A) Deep fibers attached to the apex of the lateral sling of the extensor digitorum communis (50% occurrence). (B) Deep fibers attached to the deep surface of the lateral sling and to the anterior surface of the talus, forming a separate compartment to the neurovascular bundle (25% occurrence). (C) Deep fibers attached to the anterior aspect of the talus. The extensor hallucis longus tendon and the neurovascular bundle are in the same compartment (25% occurrence). (D) Absence of deep fibers and sling around the extensor hallucis longus tendon (rare). (1, Frondiform ligament; 2, talar attachment of [1]; 3, oblique superomedial band of inferior extensor retinaculum; 4, deep lamina of the extensor hallucis longus sling; 5, 6, 7, superficial lamina of tibialis anterior tunnel; 8, talar attachment of extensor hallucis longus sling.) Meyer P: La morphologie du ligament annulaire antérieur du cou-de-pied chez l'homme. Comptes-Rendus Assoc Anat 84:286, 1955)

Fig. 3-9.   Inferior extensor retinaculum. (1, extensor digitorum longus tendons, toes 5, 4, 3; 2, extensor digitorum longus tendon to second toe; 3, extensor hallucis longus tendon; 4, tibialis anterior tendon; 5, tunnel for extensor digitorum longus, toes 5, 4, 3; 6, tunnel extensor digitorum longus, toe 2; 7, tunnel for extensor hallucis longus; 8, tunnel for tibialis anterior; 9, stem of lateral and intermediary roots of inferior extensor retinaculum; 10, medial root of inferior extensor retinaculum; 11, talar attachment of extensor hallucis longus sling; 12, peronei tendons.)

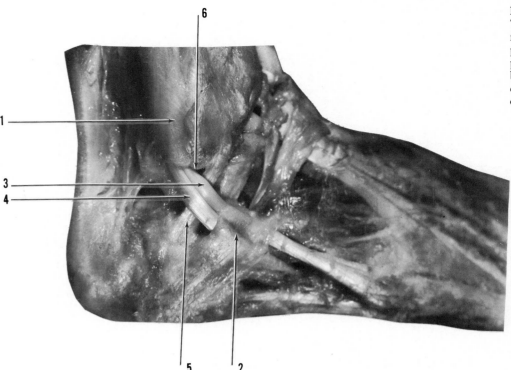

During its course, the 1-cm to 2-cm–wide band passes over the dorsalis pedis vessels, the deep peroneal nerve, and the extensor hallucis longus tendon. At the level of the tibialis anterior tendon, most of the fibers pass superficial to the tendon and the remaining fibers slide under te tendon, forming a tunnel. The terminal segment splits to envelop the abductor hallucis muscle; deep fibers insert on the navicular and the medial cuneiform.

The level of division of the inferior extensor retinaculum into the oblique superomedial and inferomedial band is variable; it may be lateral to the extensor hallucis longus tendon, medial to the extensor hallucis longus tendon, or medial to the tibialis anterior tendon. The last is the least frequent, and when it occurs, the two division bands are in continuity except for a short distance on the medial aspect of the tibialis anterior tendon.[1]

Oblique Superolateral Band

The oblique superolateral band, when present, gives a cruciate configuration to the inferior extensor retinaculum, as described by Weitbrecht.[2] This band is present in 25% of the cases, but the size varies considerably, from 2 mm to 25 mm.[1] It originates from the lateral sling, from the superomedial band, or from both. The band is directed upward and laterally, crosses the anterior tibiofibular ligament, and inserts on the lateral surface of the lateral malleolus and the lateral crest of the lower segment of the fibula. The fibers blend with those of the superior extensor and the superior peroneal retinacula.

Peroneal Retinaculum

The peroneal retinaculum (external annular ligament of the tarsus) is formed laterally by the thickening of the superficial aponeurosis at the level of the hindfoot and is divided into a superior and an inferior component.

SUPERIOR PERONEAL RETINACULUM

The superior peroneal retinaculum is an obliquely oriented quadrilateral lamina. It originates from the lateral border of the retromalleolar groove and the tip of the lateral malleolus. The fibrous band passes over the peronei tendons and inserts on the Achilles tendon and the posterior aspect of the lateral surface of the calcaneus.

INFERIOR PERONEAL RETINACULUM

The inferior peroneal retinaculum is in continuity with the lateral root of the inferior extensor retinaculum (Fig. 3-10). It originates from the posterior segment of the lateral rim of the sinus tarsi. The superficial fibers are oriented downward and posteriorly, cross the trochlear process, and insert on the lateral surface of the os calcis just above the posterolateral tubercle. The deep layer attaches on the apex of the trochlear process. It provides superior and inferior arciform fibers and forms two fibrous tunnels over the superior and inferior surfaces of the trochlear process (Fig. 3-11). The upper tunnel lodges the peroneus brevis tendon and the lower tunnel the peroneus longus tendon. Distal to the bony eminence, the inferior peroneal retinaculum forms two nearly circular separate fibrous tunnels for the peronei tendons.

Dorsal Aponeurosis and Dorsal Compartments of the Foot

A comprehensive study of the dorsal aponeurosis of the foot and the dorsal compartment (Fig. 3-12) is presented by Bellocq and Meyer.[7]

As one dissects the dorsum of the foot and removes the skin, a very thin layer of connective tissue is encountered—fascia superficialis—covering the superficial sensory nerves and veins. Next is a semitransparent, relatively thin fascia located under the superficial nerves and veins, investing all the musculotendinous units of the dorsum of the foot. This layer is the superficial lamina or superficial dorsal aponeurosis. A true osteofascial space (the spatium dorsalis pedis) is created as this aponeurosis inserts on the foot skeleton at the lateral and medial margins. More precisely, the lateral

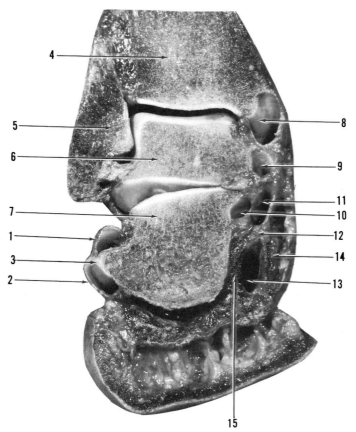

Fig. 3-11. Frontal cross section of the ankle-hindfoot. (1, Tunnel of peroneus brevis tendon; 2, tunnel of peroneus longus tendon; 3, peroneal trochlear process, well developed in this specimen; 4, tibia; 5, lateral malleolus; 6, talus; 7, calcaneus, 8, tunnel of tibialis posterior tendon; 9, tunnel of flexor digitorum longus tendon; 10, tunnel of flexor hallucis longus tendon; 11, upper chamber of tarsal tunnel for the medial plantar neurovascular bundle; 12, interfascicular ligament; 13, lower chamber of tarsal tunnel for the lateral plantar neurovascular bundle; 14, abductor hallucis muscle covered by the split layers of the flexor retinaculum; 15, quadratus plantae muscle.)

Fig. 3-12. Frontal cross section of right foot passing through the anterior tarsus—view of anterior segment. (*S*, scaphoid; *C*, cuboid.) *Layers* (1, Skin; 2, fascia superficialis covering the superficial veins and nerves; 3, superficial dorsal aponeurosis; 4, *first layer,* superficial tendinoconnective, formed by the tendons of the tibialis anterior [14], extensor hallucis longus [15], extensor digitorum longus [4'], peroneus tertius [17], and their fibrosynovial sheath connected with a layer of connective tissue. This layer attaches to the superficial dorsal aponeurosis on the medial border of the tibialis anterior tendon sheath and to the lateral border of the peroneus tertius tendon sheath; 5, *second layer,* formed by the extensor digitorum brevis and its investing facia, attaches to the superficial layer at the level of the deep surface of the extensor hallucis longus sheath, covering the underlying doralis pedis vessels. The lateral wing of this layer is attached to the cuboid and to the superficial aponeurosis medial to the peroneus brevis tendon [18]; 6, *third layer,* adipoconnective, carries the dorsalis pedis vessels and the deep peroneal nerve and its branches.) *Spaces:* (7, Subcutaneous space; 8, first fascial space between superficial dorsal aponeurosis and the superficial tendinoconnective layer; 9, second fascial space between the superficial tendinoconnective layer and the extensor digitorum brevis and its investing fascia; 10, third fascial space between the extensor digitorum brevis with its investing deep fascia and the neurovascular adipoconnective layer; 11, fourth fascial space between the neurovascular adipoconnective layer and the tarsal osteoarticular layer proximally and the dorsal interosseous aponeurosis distally; 12, connection of the superficial dorsal aponeurosis with the first layer, medially; 13, connection of the superficial dorsal aponeurosis with the first layer, laterally; 14, tibialis anterior tendon; 15, extensor hallucis longus tendon; 16, dorsalis pedis artery, veins, and deep peroneal nerve; 17, peroneus tertius tendon; 18, peroneus brevis tendon; 19, peroneus longus tendon; 20, sural nerve and short saphenous vein.) (Redrawn from Bellocq P, Meyer P: Contribution a l'étude de l'aponevrose dorsale du pied [fascia dorsalis pedis, P.N.A.] Acta Anat 30:67, 1957.)

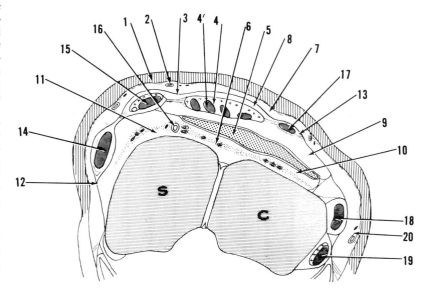

insertion is on the os calcis, the cuboid, and the tuberosity and lateral border of the fifth metatarsal, and the medial insertion extends from the sustentaculum tali to the tuberosity of the scaphoid and the medial border of the first metatarsal.

This superficial dorsal aponeurosis extends fibers to the chorion of the skin, thus forming the retinacula cutis, and closes the subcutaneous space of the foot at its margins. Other connective fibers reach the sheath of the abductor of the big toe medially and the abductor of the little toe laterally.

The dorsal osteoaponeurotic space is subdivided into four gliding subspaces by three layers of tissue.

The *first layer,* located under the superficial dorsal aponeurosis, is formed by the tendons of the tibialis anterior, extensor hallucis longus, extensor digitorum longus, and peroneus tertius, surrounded by synovial sheaths or loose connective tissue united to each other. This superficial tendinoconnective layer unites with the superficial dorsal aponeurosis near the tibialis anterior medially and the outer aspect of the peroneus tertius laterally.

The *second layer* is formed by the extensor digitorum brevis and its investing fascia, the deep lamina of the dorsal aponeurosis. This aponeurosis attaches medially to the synovial sheath of the extensor hallucis longus. It courses laterally, passes over the dorsalis pedis vessels, and at the medial border of the extensor digitorum brevis, splits into two layers. The thick superficial layer and the thin deep layer merge on the lateral border of the muscle and attach laterally on the superficial dorsal aponeurosis and the tarsus.

The *third layer* is adipoconnective carrying the dorsalis pedis artery and the accompanying veins and the deep peroneal nerve and its branches. The dorsal interosseous aponeurosis is the last investing layer covering the metatarsals and the interossei muscles.

The four fascial spaces of the dorsal fibro-osseous compartment of the foot located between the above-described three soft-tissue layers and the dorsal aponeurosis are as follows:

Space 1: Located between the superficial dorsal aponeurosis and the superficial tendinoconnective layer

Space 2: Located between the superficial tendinoconnective layer and the extensor digitorum brevis

Space 3: Located between the deep surface of the extensor digitorum brevis with its investing fascia and the neurovascular adipoconnective layer

Space 4: Located between the neurovascular adipoconnective layer and the tarsal osteoarticular layer proximally and the dorsal interosseous aponeurosis distally

Space 2 has been investigated by Latarjet and Etienne-Martin with injection studies.[8] When distended, this space is well delineated, located under the layer formed by the long extensor tendons of the second, third, fourth, and fifth toes and the extensor digitorum brevis. This space is in the form of a trapezoid, with the small base proximal and the large base distal (Fig. 3-13). The proximal border does not reach the inferior extensor retinaculum, but variations are possible. The distal border is located in the middle of the

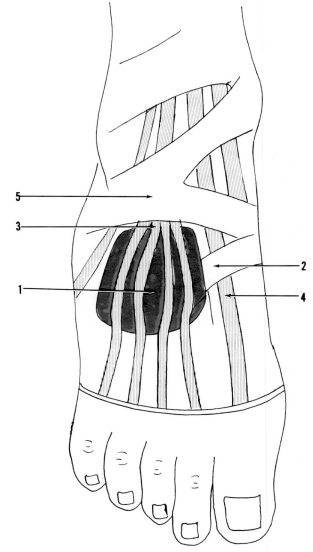

Fig. 3-13.   Gliding mechanism or cellular bursa or space located on the dorsum of the foot behind the extensor digitorum longus tendons. (1, Cellular space; 2, medial transverse retinacular band of dorsum of foot; 3, extensor digitorum longus tendons; 4, extensor hallucis longus tendon; 5, inferior extensor retinaculum.) (Redrawn from Latarjet A, Etienne-Martin M: L'appareil de glissement des tendons extenseurs des doigts et des orteils sur le dos de la main et sur le dos du pied. Ann Anat Pathol Anat Normal 9:605, 1932)

dorsum of the foot and may send extentions under the tendons; this border has a variable location. Medially the distended bursa reaches the tendon of the extensor hallucis longus but does not lift the latter.

In the distal segment at the level of the base of the metatarsals, the tendons are located in a fibrous sheath, with surrounding loose connective tissue or synovial sheaths. As the tendinoconnective superficial and deep layers are converted into fibrous sheaths, they adhere to the dorsal interosseous aponeurosis or remain separate from it, delineating fibroadipose small spaces (Fig. 3-14).

Fig. 3-14. Coronal cross section of right foot at the level of the distal segment of the metatarsal shafts: view of anterior segment. The extensor tendons and their sheaths adhere to the dorsal interosseous aponeurosis in certain locations and delineate with the latter fibroadipose small spaces. (1, Point or area of adhesion of the extensor tendon sheaths to the dorsal interosseous aponeurosis; 2, small spaces limited above by the extensor tendon sheaths and laterally and medially by their adhesion to the dorsal interosseous aponeurosis, which with the metatarsals forms the floor of the space; 3, extensor hallucis longus and brevis of the big toe with their sheaths, including an accessory tendinous band on the medial side; 4, premetatarsal$_1$ space; 5, dorsalis pedis artery and veins; M_1 to M_5, metatarsal shafts; D_1 to D_4, dorsal interossei muscles; P_1 to P_3, plantar interossei muscles.) (Redrawn from Bellocq P, Meyer P: Contribution a l'étude de l'aponevrose dorsale du pied [fascia dorsalis pedis, P.N.A.]. Acta Anat 30: 67, 1957)

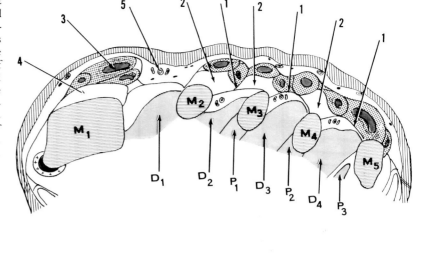

Fig. 3-15. Cross section of left ankle 2 cm, proximal to the tip of the medial malleolus, seen from lower surface of section. (1, Superficial aponeurosis of leg; 2, deep aponeurosis of leg; 3, tendon of tibialis posterior in its tunnel; 4, tendon of flexor digitorum longus in its tunnel; 5, posterior tibial artery and veins, posterior tibial nerve laterally in their compartment; 6, flexor hallucis longus with tendon medially and low muscle fibers laterally in its compartment; 7, posterior peroneal vessels in the same compartment as [6]; 8, achilles tendon covered by the split superficial aponeurosis [1]; the pre-Achilles space between the superficial and deep aponeuroses is filled with adipose tissue; 9, sural nerve; 10, lesser saphenous vein; Both [9] and [10] are in separate compartments; 11, peroneus longus tendon; 12, peroneus brevis tendon, U shape; both peronei are located in a compartment; 13, extensor digitorum longus tendon and tunnel; 14, dorsalis pedis, artery and veins; 15, extensor hallucis longus tendon and tunnel in common with [14]; 16, tibialis anterior tendon and tunnel; 17, synovial fringe of tibiofibular syndesmosis; 18, anteroinferior tibiofibular ligament; 19, anterolateral tubercle of distal tibia; 20, distal tibia; 21, lateral malleolus.)

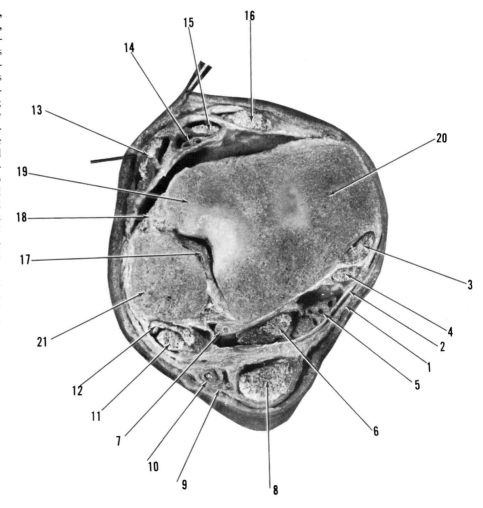

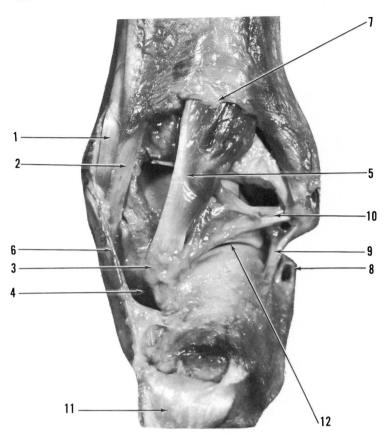

Fig. 3-16. Posterior aspect of ankle and inferior talocalcaneal joint. (1, Tibialis posterior tendon with fibrous sheath excised; 2, flexor digitorum longus tendon with fibrous sheath excised; 3, flexor hallucis longus tendon in its tunnel on posterior border of talus; 4, compartment for posterior tibial neurovascular bundle; 5, flexor hallucis longus, which still has low descending muscle fibers at the level of the ankle on the lateral side; 6, flexor retinaculum; 7, intermediary aponeurosis of the leg; 8, tunnel of peronei; 9, calcaneofibular ligament; 10, posterior talofibular ligament; 11, reflected Achilles tendon; 12, posterior talocalcaneal joint interline.)

The superficial dorsal aponeurosis is reinforced along the medial and lateral borders of the foot by two aponeurotic transverse bands, medial and lateral (see Fig. 3-2).[1] The medial transverse band originates from the medial cuneiform and metatarsal 1 bones and may form a terminal fibrous tunnel for the tibialis anterior tendon. Directed laterally, the fibers pass under the inferior arm of the extensor aponeurosis but over the tendon of the extensor hallucis longus and occasionally over the tendon of the extensor hallucis brevis. The transverse fibers terminate on the cuneiforms and the first metatarsal. Occasionally the metatarsal insertion may extend up to the level of the metatarsophalangeal joint and forms an osteofibrous tunnel for the two extensor tendons.[1]

The lateral transverse band is inconstant and located at the level of the base of the fifth metatarsal bone. It originates from the latter, bridges over the metatarsal or digital extensions of the peroneus tertius or the peroneus brevis tendon, and inserts on the fifth or the fourth metatarsal.

Tibiotalocalcaneal Tunnel

The tibiotalocalcaneal tunnel (Richet's tunnel, tarsal tunnel, calcaneal tunnel), a major passageway, extends from the distal end of the tibia to the level of the plantar aspect of the navicular.[9–12] It is posteromedial in location and is concave anteriorly. The tunnel may be divided into two components: upper, tibiotalar and lower, talocalcaneal.

UPPER, TIBIOTALAR TUNNEL

The upper, tibiotalar tunnel (Figs. 3-15–3-17) corresponds to the posterior aspect of the distal tibia, the retromedial malleolar surface, the posterior border of the talus with its central sulcus flanked by the posterior tubercles, and the posterior segment of the medial talar surface. The osseous canal is converted into a large tunnel or deep compartment by the covering deep aponeurosis of the leg. The latter is attached medially to the posteromedial border of the tibia and the posterior border of the medial malleolus and laterally to the fibrous sheath of the peronei tendons. Farther distally, the deep aponeurosis attaches to the superomedial surface of the os calcis and continues anteriorly with the flexor retinaculum. Anteriorly, at the level of the tibiotalar tunnel, the deep aponeurosis is adherent to the covering superficial aponeurosis; in the posterior segment, the two aponeuroses part: the superficial aponeurosis courses toward the medial border of the Achilles tendon and the deep aponeurosis courses laterally toward the sheath of the peronei tendons.

In the proximal tibial segment of the tunnel (see Fig. 3-15) are located, medially to laterally, the following structures: the fibrous tunnel of the tibialis posterior tendon; the fibrous tunnel of the flexor digitorum longus, adherent to the former; the superficial compartment for the posterior tibial neurovascular bundle; and the large loose compartment for the flexor hallucis longus muscle–tendon unit and the peroneal vessels laterally.

Fig. 3-17. Anatomic preparation of the posteromedial aspect of the ankle and upper segment of the tibiotalar tunnel. The crossing tendons have been reflected downward after excision of their fibrous tendon sheaths; the implantations of the latter have been preserved. The joint levels are indicated by transverse partial incisions. The tendinous fibrous sheath as indicated in this preparation contributes to the reinforcement of the posterior capsuloligamentous complex. (1, Incisions indicating level of tibiotalar joint; 2, incisions indicating level of posterior talocalcaneal joint; 3, retromedial malleolar canal of tibialis posterior tendon; 4, canal of flexor digitorum longus tendon; 5, oblique canal of flexor hallucis longus tendon; 6, tibialis posterior tendon, reflected; 7, flexor digitorum longus tendon, reflected; 8, flexor hallucis longus tendon, reflected. In the upper segment the tunnels of the two flexors are separated by an intertendinous space.)

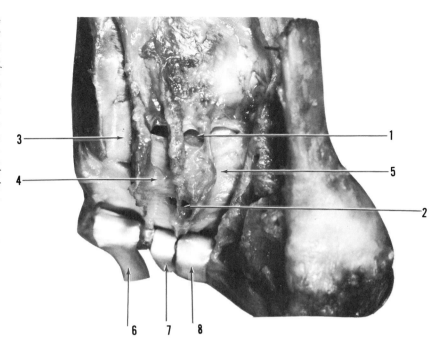

In the distal malleolar–talar segment of the tunnel, the same relationship is present, with some modifications. The flexor hallucis longus is all tendinous and passes through a strong fibrous tunnel on the posterior border of the talus. The peronei vessels have parted. The posterior tibial neurovascular compartment is superficial and overlies the tunnel of the flexor hallucis longus and the intertendinous interval between the flexor hallucis longus and flexor digitorum longus tunnels. The adherent segment of the superficial and deep aponeuroses is attached to the tibialis posterior and the flexor digitorum longus fibrous tunnel and forms the cover of the neurovascular compartment (Fig. 3-18).

LOWER, TALOCALCANEAL TUNNEL

The lower, talocalcaneal tunnel or tarsal tunnel corresponds from above downward to the medial surface of the talus, the sustentaculum tali, and the large excavated medial surface of the os calcis (Fig. 3-19). The osseous floor and canal is converted into a tunnel by the flexor retinaculum above and the abductor hallucis muscle below.

The **flexor retinaculum** (laciniate ligament, medial annular ligament; Fig. 3-20) is formed by the juxtaposition of the superficial and deep aponeuroses. It is triangular, with a proximal malleolar apex, an inferior base along the superior border of the abductor hallucis muscle, and an anterior and a posterior border.

The apex of the flexor retinaculum inserts on the anterior and medial surfaces of the medial malleolus and extends farther laterally toward the tibialis anterior tendon. It divides into two bands, upper and lower (Figs. 3-21 and 3-22). The upper fibers pass over the tibialis anterior tendon and terminate on the deep surface of the superior extensor retinaculum. The lower fibers pass under the tibialis anterior

Fig. 3-18. Posterior aspect of the ankle and hindfoot. Compartment of the posterior tibial neurovascular bundle (1) is covered by the adherent superficial and deep aponeuroses of the leg (2). This compartment is superficial to the tunnel of the flexor hallucis longus (5), and the intertendinous space (6) and posterior to the tunnel of the flexor digitorum longus (3) and the tibialis posterior tendon (4).

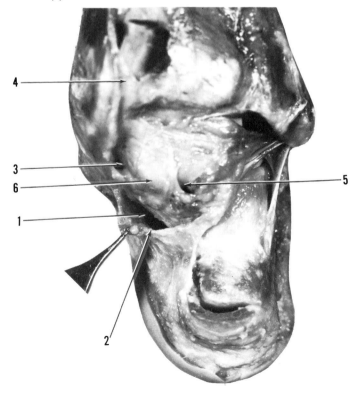

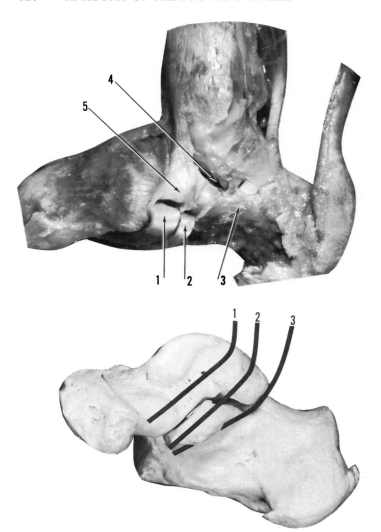

Fig. 3-19.   Anatomic preparation demonstrating the talo-calcaneal canal, the crossing tendons and their relationship to the tibiotalar joint, the talus, and the calcaneus. The tibialis posterior tendon passes above the sustentaculum tali. The flexor digitorum longus tendon crosses the medial opening of the canalis tarsi and passes over the medial border of the sustentaculum tali. A longitudinal incision through the anterior border of its sheath leads to the sustentaculotalar interline, but this relationship varies. The flexor hallucis longus tendon passes under the sustentaculum tali. (1, Tibialis posterior tendon; 2, flexor digitorum longus tendon; 3, flexor hallucis longus tendon; 4, medial opening of tarsal canal; 5, medial calcaneonavicular ligament.)

tendon, cross over the tibial insertion of the inferior extensor retinaculum, and terminate on the anterior tibia. With this arrangement, the apical fibers contribute to the formation of the proximal fibrous tunnel of the tibialis anterior tendon.

The base of the flexor retinaculum corresponds to the superior border of the abductor hallucis muscle. It extends its insertion to the medial tuberosity of the os calcis and reaches the lowest segment of insertion of the Achilles tendon. At the superior border of the abductor hallucis muscle,

the vertical descending fibers of the flexor retinaculum split and incorporate the muscle. The superficial fibers correspond to the superficial aponeurosis and the deep fibers to the deep aponeurosis. Both layers unite at the inferior border of the muscle and are in continuity with the plantar fascia.

The anterior and posterior borders are difficult to delineate, as the former is in continuity with the dorsal aponeurosis of the foot and the latter with the superficial aponeurosis of the leg. The anterior border corresponds approximately to a vertical line drawn from the anterior border of the medial malleolus to the medial border of the foot. The posterior border corresponds more or less to an oblique line extended from the anterior aspect of the medial malleolus to the posterosuperior corner of the os calcis.

The lower segment of the calcaneal canal is divided into two chambers—upper and lower—by the *transverse interfascicular lamina*.[12] The transverse interfascicular lamina is triangular and has a proximal free concave border (Figs. 3-23–3-25). The lateral border of the lamina inserts on the medial surface of the os calcis between the upper border of the quadratus plantae muscle and the tunnel of the flexor hallucis longus. The medial border inserts proximally on the deep covering aponeurosis of the abductor hallucis muscle

Fig. 3-20.   Medial aspect of the ankle and the flexor retinaculum. (1, Plantar fat; 2, anterior border of flexor retinaculum; 3, deep layer of sheath of abductor hallucis; 4, superficial layer of sheath of abductor hallucis; 5, superficial fibers of flexor retinaculum continued by retinaculum cutis; 7, posterior border of retinaculum; 8, sheath of Achilles tendon; 9, superficial aponeurosis cruris; 10, adherent superficial and deep aponeurosis cruris; 12, apex of flexor retinaculum; 13, projection of tibialis anterior tendon; 14, 16, superficial aponeuroses of foot; 15, oblique inferomedial band of inferior extensor retinaculum; 17, 18, superior and inferior borders of abductor hallucis muscle.) (From Bellocq P, Meyer P: Le ligament annulaire interne du cou-de-pied. Arch Anat Hist Embryol 37: 23, 1954)

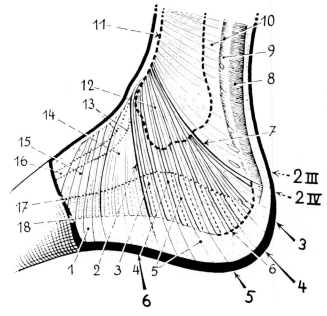

Fig. 3-21.   Diagram of the apical insertion of the flexor retinaculum, based on dissection under magnification. (1, Flexor retinaculum; 2, segment of flexor retinaculum covering abductor hallucis muscle; 3, 4, apical insertion of flexor retinaculum. One band passes over the tibialis anterior tendon and a deeper band passes under the same tendon. Both bands cross over the tibial insertion of the oblique superomedial band of the inferior extensor retinaculum and insert on the deep surface of the superior extensor retinaculum, creating continuity of the two; 5, superior extensor retinaculum; 6, oblique deep component of superomedial band of inferior extensor retinaculum; 7, distal superficial component of the oblique superomedial band of inferior extensor retinaculum; 8, oblique inferomedial band of inferior extensor retinaculum; 9, superficial aponeurosis cruris; 10, deep aponeurosis cruris; 11, tibialis anterior tendon with its 3 retaining systems; 12, Achilles tendon incorporated within split layers of superficial aponeurosis cruris.)

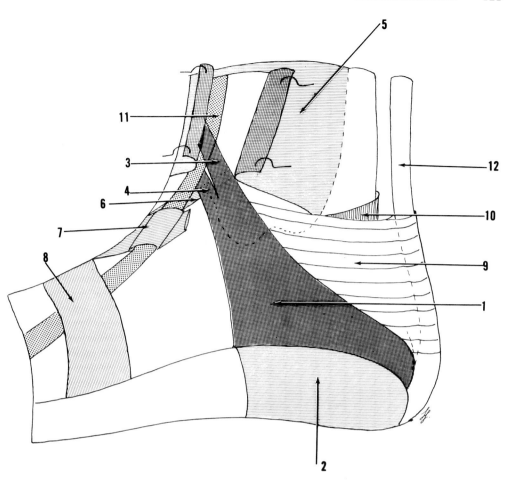

at the level of the proximal border of the muscle; farther distally the insertion shifts to the mid segment and finally to the lower border of the same.

In its terminal portion, the interfascicular lamina is narrow and corresponds to the interval between the abductor hallucis muscle and the medial border of the flexor digitorum brevis. It is in continuity with the medial intermuscular septum of the sole of the foot.

In the talocalcaneal tunnel, the tibialis posterior tendon with its fibrous sheath crosses the medial surface of the talus and passes over the posterior talotibial segment of the deltoid ligament, the tibiocalcaneal segment of the deltoid ligament, the superomedial calcaneonavicular ligament, and the inferior calcaneonavicular ligament (Fig. 3-26). Subsequently, the tibialis posterior tendon divides into three parts: navicular, plantar, and recurrent. The navicular segment terminates on the tuberosity of the navicular, the plantar segment continues under the inferior calcaneonavicular ligament and enters the planta pedis, and the recurrent portion inserts on the sustentaculum tali.

The tunnel of the flexor digitorum longus crosses the posteromedial talar tubercle and the posterior fibers of the deltoid ligament, passes over the medial border of the sustentaculum tali, and farther distally, shares a common tunnel with the flexor hallucis longus tendon.

The canal on the lower segment of the sustentaculum tali

is in direct continuity with the canal of the posterior border of the talus (Fig. 3-27). The tunnel of the flexor hallucis longus attaches to the inferior surface of the sustentaculum tali, and farther distally, the tendon shares a common sheath with the flexor digitorum longus.

The neurovascular tunnel is initially superficial and corresponds to the interval between the tunnel of the flexor digitorum longus and the flexor hallucis longus (Fig. 3-28). Gradually, as the latter approaches the former, the intertendinous space disappears and the neurovascular tunnel is located on the medial surface of the os calcis, posterior to the flexor hallucis longus tunnel.

In the lower segment of the calcaneal canal, the neurovascular tunnel is divided into upper and lower chambers by the interfascicular septum (Figs. 3-29 and 3-30). The lower chamber is limited laterally by the quadratus plantae muscle covering the medial calcaneal surface, medially by the abductor hallucis muscle covered by the deep aponeurosis, above by the interfascicular septum, and below by the space between the inferior borders of the abductor hallucis and the quadratus plantae. The upper chamber is limited medially by the flexor retinaculum, laterally by the tunnel of the flexor hallucis longus, above by the tunnel of the flexor digitorum longus, and below by the interfascicular septum.

(Text continues on p. 127.)

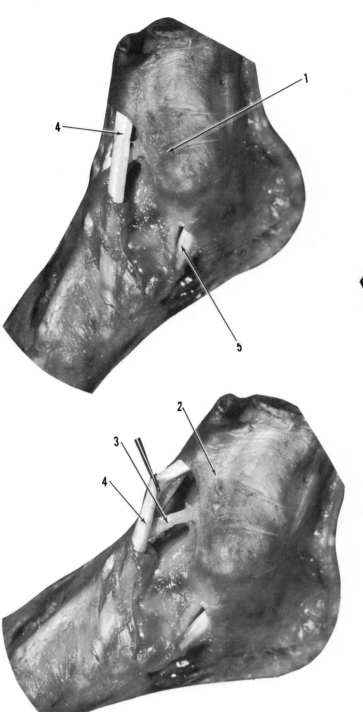

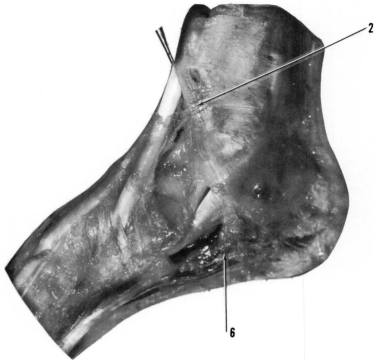

Fig. 3-22.   Apical insertion of flexor retinaculum. (1, Flexor retinaculum; 2, direction of apical fibers of flexor retinaculum demonstrated by traction with forceps; superficial fibers are passing over tibialis anterior tendon; 3, deep component of oblique superomedial band of inferior extensor retinaculum passing under flexor retinaculum; 4, tibialis anterior tendon; 5, tibialis posterior tendon and anterior border of flexor retinaculum; 6, abductor hallucis muscle covered by flexor retinaculum.)

Fig. 3-23. The lower calcaneal segment of the tarsal tunnel leading to the porta pedis. (1, Interfascicular ligament transversely oriented and inserting under flexor hallucis longus tendon and on the calcaneus, above the superior border, of the quadratus plantae [which has been removed in this specimen]; 2, upper chamber of calcaneal canal for medial plantar neurovascular bundle; 3, lower chamber of calcaneal canal for lateral plantar neurovascular bundle; this chamber leads to middle plantar space of sole of foot; 4, medial calcaneal origin of quadratus plantae muscle; 5, abductor hallucis muscle; 6, medial investing fascia of abductor hallucis muscle reflected after detachment of its calcaneal insertion; 7, flexor digitorum brevis muscle; 8, medial intermuscular membrane; 9, flexor hallucis longus tendon covered by its tenosynovial sheath; 10, tip of hemostat emerging through lower chamber of calcaneal canal; 11, flexor hallucis longus tendon; 12, flexor digitorum longus tendon; 13, tibialis posterior tendon; 14, Achilles tendon.)

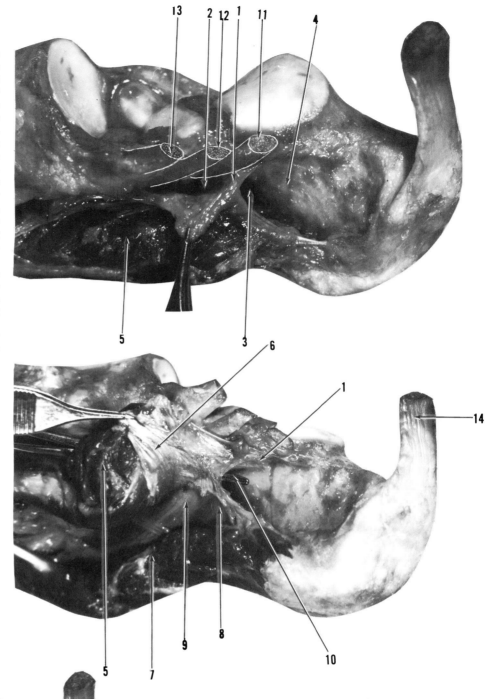

Fig. 3-24. Lower chamber of the lower segment of the calcaneal canal. (1, Interfascicular ligament with hemostat underneath; 2, second attachment site of investing sheath of abductor hallucis muscle; 3, abductor hallucis muscle; 4, flexor hallucis longus tendon; 5, flexor digitorum longus tendon; 6, tibialis posterior tendon.)

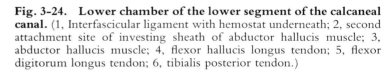

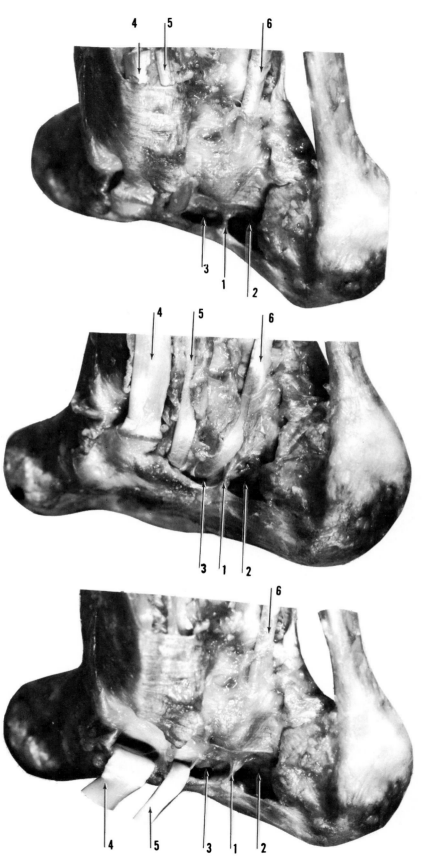

Fig. 3-25.   Compartments of the lower segment of the tarsal tunnel. In the top figure the tendons are maintained in their fibrous tunnels. In the middle figure a segment of the fibrous tunnels has been excised. (1, Interfascicular septum; 2, lower chamber of tarsal tunnel for lateral plantar neurovascular bundle; 3, upper chamber of tarsal tunnel for medial plantar neurovascular bundle; 4, tibialis posterior tendon; 5, flexor digitorum longus tendon; 6, flexor hallucis longus tendon.)

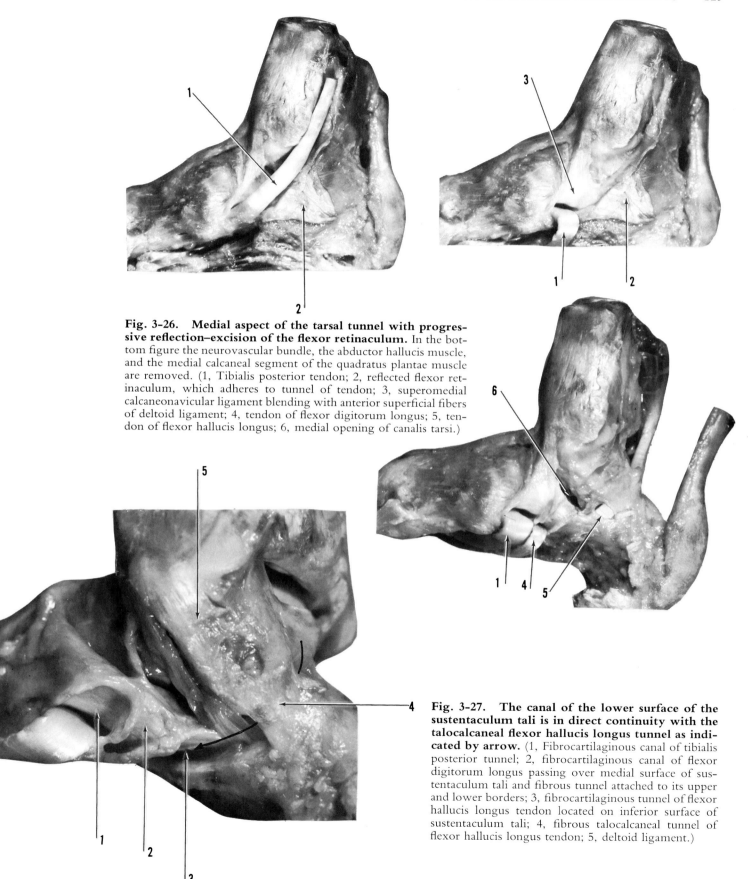

Fig. 3-26.   Medial aspect of the tarsal tunnel with progressive reflection–excision of the flexor retinaculum. In the bottom figure the neurovascular bundle, the abductor hallucis muscle, and the medial calcaneal segment of the quadratus plantae muscle are removed. (1, Tibialis posterior tendon; 2, reflected flexor retinaculum, which adheres to tunnel of tendon; 3, superomedial calcaneonavicular ligament blending with anterior superficial fibers of deltoid ligament; 4, tendon of flexor digitorum longus; 5, tendon of flexor hallucis longus; 6, medial opening of canalis tarsi.)

Fig. 3-27.   The canal of the lower surface of the sustentaculum tali is in direct continuity with the talocalcaneal flexor hallucis longus tunnel as indicated by arrow. (1, Fibrocartilaginous canal of tibialis posterior tunnel; 2, fibrocartilaginous canal of flexor digitorum longus passing over medial surface of sustentaculum tali and fibrous tunnel attached to its upper and lower borders; 3, fibrocartilaginous tunnel of flexor hallucis longus tendon located on inferior surface of sustentaculum tali; 4, fibrous talocalcaneal tunnel of flexor hallucis longus tendon; 5, deltoid ligament.)

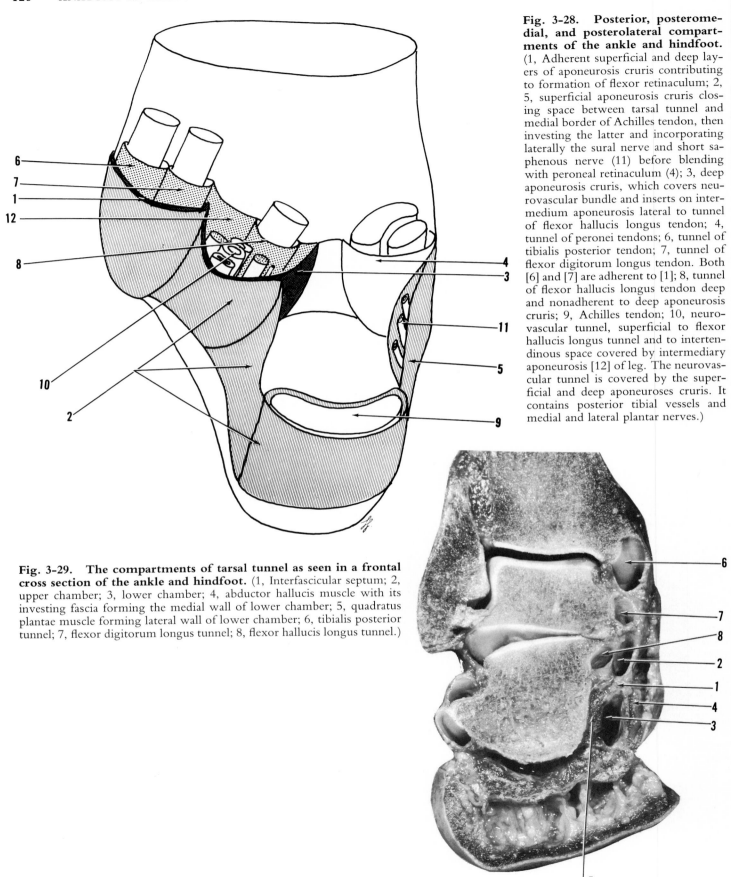

Fig. 3-28. Posterior, posterome-dial, and posterolateral compart-ments of the ankle and hindfoot. (1, Adherent superficial and deep layers of aponeurosis cruris contributing to formation of flexor retinaculum; 2, 5, superficial aponeurosis cruris closing space between tarsal tunnel and medial border of Achilles tendon, then investing the latter and incorporating laterally the sural nerve and short saphenous nerve (11) before blending with peroneal retinaculum (4); 3, deep aponeurosis cruris, which covers neurovascular bundle and inserts on intermedium aponeurosis lateral to tunnel of flexor hallucis longus tendon; 4, tunnel of peronei tendons; 6, tunnel of tibialis posterior tendon; 7, tunnel of flexor digitorum longus tendon. Both [6] and [7] are adherent to [1]; 8, tunnel of flexor hallucis longus tendon deep and nonadherent to deep aponeurosis cruris; 9, Achilles tendon; 10, neurovascular tunnel, superficial to flexor hallucis longus tunnel and to intertendinous space covered by intermediary aponeurosis [12] of leg. The neurovascular tunnel is covered by the superficial and deep aponeuroses cruris. It contains posterior tibial vessels and medial and lateral plantar nerves.)

Fig. 3-29. The compartments of tarsal tunnel as seen in a frontal cross section of the ankle and hindfoot. (1, Interfascicular septum; 2, upper chamber; 3, lower chamber; 4, abductor hallucis muscle with its investing fascia forming the medial wall of lower chamber; 5, quadratus plantae muscle forming lateral wall of lower chamber; 6, tibialis posterior tunnel; 7, flexor digitorum longus tunnel; 8, flexor hallucis longus tunnel.)

Within the upper segment of the neurovascular compartment, the posterior tibial nerve has already divided into the medial and lateral plantar nerves just proximal to the tip of the medial malleolus. The posterior tibial artery divides into the medial and lateral plantar arteries proximal to the free concave border of the interfascicular septum (Fig. 3-31). The medial plantar neurovascular bundle penetrates the upper chamber of the calcaneal canal above the interfascicular septum, and the lateral plantar neurovascular bundle penetrates the lower chamber and reaches the middle plantar compartment of the planta pedis. In both chambers the nerve is anterior to the corresponding artery.

Plantar Aponeurosis

The plantar aponeurosis is the strong, fibrous, investing layer of the sole of the foot (Figs. 3-32 and 3-33). It is subcutaneous and extends from the heel to the ball of the foot. It is connected to the skin with retinacular vertical fibers proximally and transverse septae distally. Two longitudinally oriented intermuscular septae connect the plantar aponeurosis to the deep planta pedis. Smaller deep sagittal extensions bind the distal segment of the plantar aponeurosis to the depth of the ball of the foot.

In 1840, Maslieurat-Lagémard gave the first detailed description of the insertion of the plantar aponeurosis.[13] Henkel, in 1913, provided the most comprehensive study of the plantar aponeurosis.[14] The recent work of Bojsen-Møller and Flagstad confirmed and revived Henkel's work and brought further understanding of the insertions of the plantar aponeurosis and the anatomy of the ball of the foot.[15]

The plantar aponeurosis has three components, central, lateral, and medial.

CENTRAL COMPONENT

The central or major component of the plantar aponeurosis is triangular, with a posterior apex and an anterior base. It originates from the plantar aspect of the posteromedial calcaneal tuberosity. It conforms to the convexity of the tuberosity and may receive contributions from the Achilles tendon and especially from the plantaris tendon.

The origin of the central component of the aponeurosis is approximately 1.5 cm to 2 cm in width. The fibers group into a longitudinally oriented, thick, shiny, gently twisted band that gradually enlarges.

At the mid metatarsal level, the aponeurosis divides into five longitudinally oriented segments that gradually diverge. Proximal to the metatarsal heads, each longitudinally oriented band divides into a superficial and a deep tract (lacertus aponeuroticus superficialis and profundus; Fig. 3-34).[14] The diversion of the deep tracts is completed as they reach the corresponding metatarsophalangeal complex.

(Text continues on p. 130.)

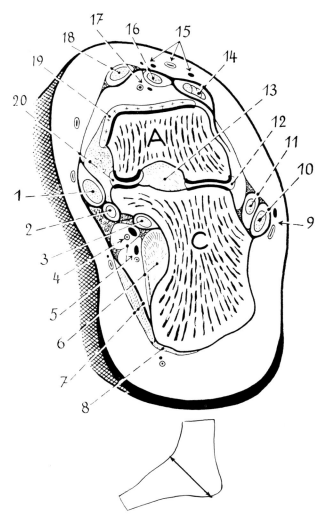

Fig. 3-30. Oblique cross section in direction of arrow; terminal section of calcaneal tunnel. (1, Tibialis posterior tendon and tunnel; 2, flexor digitorum longus tendon and tunnel; 3, flexor hallucis longus tendon and tunnel; 4, upper chamber with medial neurovascular bundle; 5, interfascicular lamina, lower chamber, and lateral plantar neurovascular bundle; 6, quadratus plantae muscle and covering fascia; 7, abductor hallucis muscle and investing fascia; 8, middle segment of superficial plantar aponeurosis; 9, sural nerve and short saphenous vein; 10, tunnel and tendon of peroneus longus; 11, tunnel and tendon of peroneus brevis; 12, talocalcaneal posterolateral articulation; 13, interosseous talocalcaneal ligament; 14, frondiform ligament and extensor digitorum communis tendons; 15, superficial peroneal nerve and superficial vein; 16, sling and tendon of extensor hallucis longus; 17, anterior tibial neurovascular bundle; 18, fibrous tunnel of tibialis anterior tendon; 19, tibiotalar joint cavity; 20, superficial dorsal aponeurosis of foot and deltoid ligament.) (From Bellocq P, Meyer P: Contribution a l'étude du canal calcanéen. Comptes-Rendus Assoc Anat 89: 292, 1956)

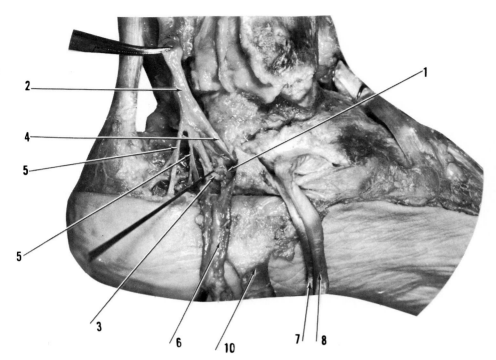

Fig. 3-31.   Medial aspect of tarsal tunnel. (1, Interfascicular ligament; 2, posterior tibial nerve; 3, lateral plantar nerve entering lower chamber; 4, medial plantar nerve entering upper chamber; 5, medial calcaneal nerves; 6, posterior tibial vessels reflected downward; 7, flexor digitorum longus tendon reflected downward; 8, tibialis posterior tendon reflected downward; 9, flexor hallucis longus tendon, deep to neurovascular bundle; 10, reflected flexor retinaculum.)

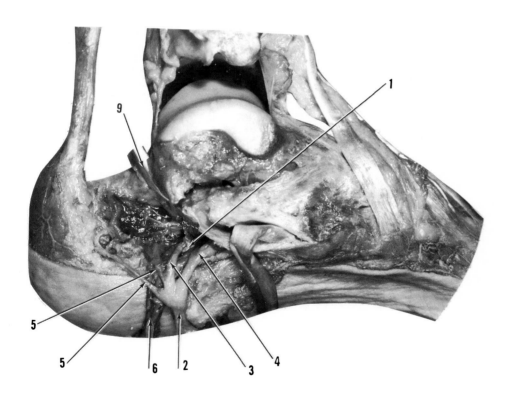

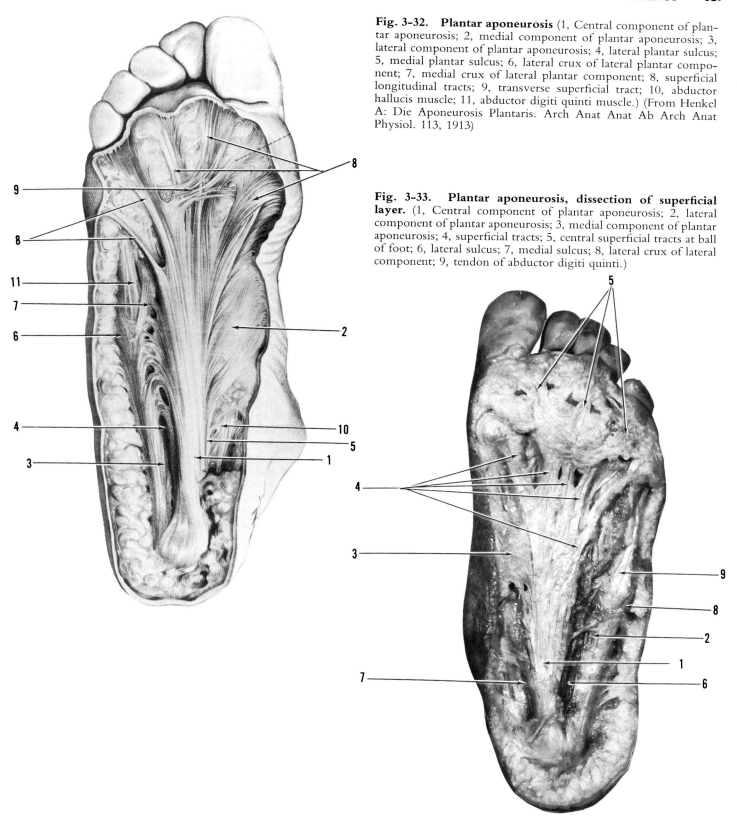

Fig. 3-32. Plantar aponeurosis (1, Central component of plantar aponeurosis; 2, medial component of plantar aponeurosis; 3, lateral component of plantar aponeurosis; 4, lateral plantar sulcus; 5, medial plantar sulcus; 6, lateral crux of lateral plantar component; 7, medial crux of lateral plantar component; 8, superficial longitudinal tracts; 9, transverse superficial tract; 10, abductor hallucis muscle; 11, abductor digiti quinti muscle.) (From Henkel A: Die Aponeurosis Plantaris. Arch Anat Anat Ab Arch Anat Physiol. 113, 1913)

Fig. 3-33. Plantar aponeurosis, dissection of superficial layer. (1, Central component of plantar aponeurosis; 2, lateral component of plantar aponeurosis; 3, medial component of plantar aponeurosis; 4, superficial tracts; 5, central superficial tracts at ball of foot; 6, lateral sulcus; 7, medial sulcus; 8, lateral crux of lateral component; 9, tendon of abductor digiti quinti.)

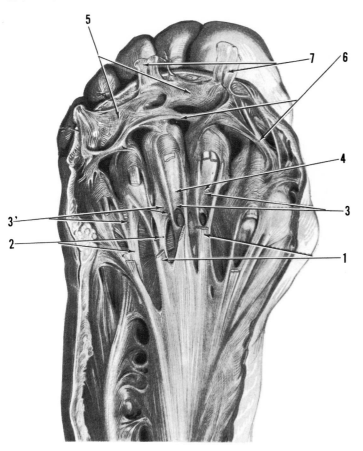

Fig. 3-34.   Deep components of plantar aponeurosis. (1, Superficial longitudinal tracts, transected and reflected distally [7]; 2, sagittal septae of plantar aponeurosis; 3, crossing fibers of the sagittal septae of the same ray at the level of the plantar plates [4]; 3′, crossing fibers between sagittal septae of adjacent rays; 5, natatory ligament; 6, mooring ligament or deep transverse aponeurotic tract.) (From Henkel A: Die Aponeurosis Plantaris. Arch Anat Anat Ab Arch Anat Physiol, 113, 1913)

Proximal to the metatarsal heads, sagittal septae extend from the deep surface of the longitudinal superficial aponeurotic bands (Fig. 3-37). These 10 septae arise in pairs from each of the five longitudinal bands (see Fig. 3-34).

The sagittal septae are oriented toward the corresponding metatarsophalangeal joint and pass on each side of the long flexor tendon, forming an arch of entrance for this tendon (Fig. 3-38). They insert sequentially on the interosseous fascia, the fascia of the transverse head of the adductor hallucis, the deep transverse metatarsal ligament, and the plantar plate and its junction with the accessory collateral ligament of the metatarsophalangeal joint.

The sagittal septae may cross fibers and form with the longitudinal band a true foramina of entrance for the flexor tendons. Crossing fibers may also extend into the insertional fibers of the adjacent septum. Such a thick crossing band is seen in Figure 3-38, extending from the longitudinal septum of the big toe to the second toe, the plantar plate, and the deep transverse metatarsal ligament.

The medial septum of the aponeurotic band of the big toe inserts on the plantar plate and the medial sesamoid and connects with the fascia of the medial head of the flexor hallucis brevis.

The lateral band of the same aponeurotic band inserts on the transverse metatarsal ligament, the plantar plate, and the lateral sesamoid and connects with the fascia of the lateral head of the flexor hallucis brevis muscle.

The proximal extension of the sagittal septae is limited by the origin of the lumbrical muscles.

At the level of the metatarsal heads, the sagittal septae are in continuity with vertical connective tissue fibers that arise from the sides of the fibrous flexor tendon sheath and the deep transverse metatarsal ligaments (see Fig. 3-35). The vertical fibers pass through the superficial aponeurosis and insert into the skin. Some of the vertical fibers cross over the flexor tendon sheath and form a pretendinous compartment retaining an adipose cushion (Fig. 3-39).[15]

At the level of the metatarsophalangeal joint, from the tibial side, a thin septum is extended, which forms a lumbrical compartment. In the intermetatarsal capitular space and over the plantar aspect of the deep transverse metatarsal ligament, an encapsulated fat body covers the common digital neurovascular bundle (Figs. 3-39 and 3-40).[15]

Distal to the metatarsal heads, a transverse retinacular system attaches to the fibrous flexor tendon sheaths and arches over the intertendinous spaces, forming the mooring ligament.

At the level of the web space, the distal segment of the ball of the foot is crossed by six to eight transverse bands

The central three superficial tracts continue more or less in the direction of the toes. One tract reaches the interval between the first and second toes. The next tract is located at the base of the third toe or in the interval between the third and fourth toes. The third central superficial tract reaches the base of the fifth toe or the interval between the fourth and fifth toes. Anterior to the metatarsal heads, the three central superficial components insert into the skin and from their deep surfaces send transversely oriented fibers, contributing to the formation of the natatory ligament (Fig. 3-35).

The two marginal superficial tracts run to the margins of the foot. The medial tract continues the direction of the big toe and the lateral tract that of the fifth toe, thus differing by their orientation from the central band. They contribute minimally to the formation of the transversely oriented natatory ligament.

Proximal to the metatarsal heads, the plantar aponeurosis is crossed superficially by transversely oriented retinacular bands separated by adipose tissue and forms the fasciculus aponeuroticum transversum (Fig. 3-36). Transversely oriented in the middle, the retinacular bands curve longitudinally at the margins and help form the ligamentum natatorum. At the level of the big toe, these fibers contribute to the medial longitudinal band. The subcutaneous transverse bands connect with the skin, and from their transverse segment, oblique fibers extend into the depth and connect with the longitudinal septae of the plantar aponeurosis and the bases of the proximal phalanges.[15]

or a weblike retinacular system forming the natatory ligament (Fig. 3-41).[14–16*]

The fibers of the natatory ligament are deep to the longitudinally oriented terminal fibers of the superficial aponeurotic bands and originate from the fibrous flexor tendon sheaths and the mooring ligament. The proximal lamellae receive a contribution from the superficial longitudinal tracts of the plantar aponeurosis. The distal lamellae insert on the deep surface of the skin, but there is no insertion on the skin at the level of the plantodigital crease, where a transverse band of adipose tissue is interposed between the skin and the most frontal part of the natatory ligament. The digital neurovascular bundle passes under the bridging segment of the natatory ligaments.

On the superficial plantar aspect of the ball of the foot, the adjoining longitudinal superficial aponeurotic bands, crossed proximally by the transverse aponeurotic fibers and

* Poirier and Charpy use the term *ligament palmant interdigital,* which should translate as *palmant = natatory; palmaire* would translate as *palmar* and *plantaire* as *plantar.*[16]

distally by the natatory ligaments, delineate a quadrilateral or oval space through which protrudes the fat body, forming the plantar monticuli. These adipose windows correspond to the common digital neurovascular bundles.

The medial border of the central component of the plantar aponeurosis is in continuity in the mid segment and distally, with longitudinal thin fibers covering the abductor hallucis muscle, and it blends with the dorsal aponeurosis. Proximally, a sulcus is present between the medial border of the plantar aponeurosis and the abductor hallucis. Superficially, this sulcus is bridged sparsely by oblique aponeurotic fibers (Fig. 3-42). The depth corresponds to the proximal segment of the medial intermuscular septum.

The lateral border of the central component of the plantar aponeurosis corresponds to the lateral sulcus. A fine network of aponeurotic fibers fills in the sulcus superficially, and fatty lobules are trapped in the intervals (Fig. 3-42). The depth of sulcus corresponds to the lateral intermuscular septum. The central segment of the plantar aponeurosis is

(Text continues on p. 136.)

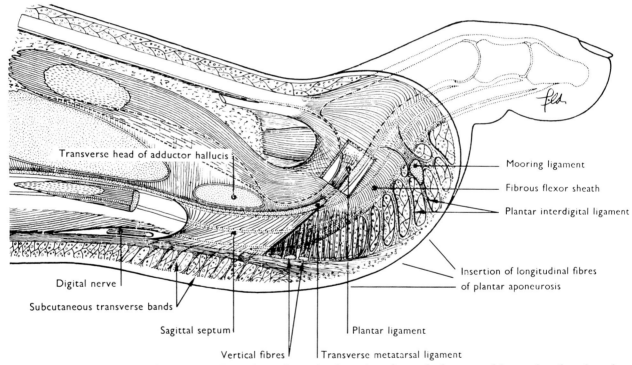

Fig. 3-35. "Drawing of a sagittal section through the second interstice showing the internal architecture of the three areas of the ball of the foot. The sagittal septum is attached to the proximal phalanx through the transverse metatarsal ligament and the plantar ligament of the joint. The vertical fibers and the lamellae of the plantar interdigital ligament are attached to the proximal phalanx through the fibrous flexor sheath." (From Bojsen-Møller F, Flagstad KE: Plantar aponeurosis and internal architecture of the ball of the foot. Anat 121: 599, 1976. By permission of Cambridge University Press)

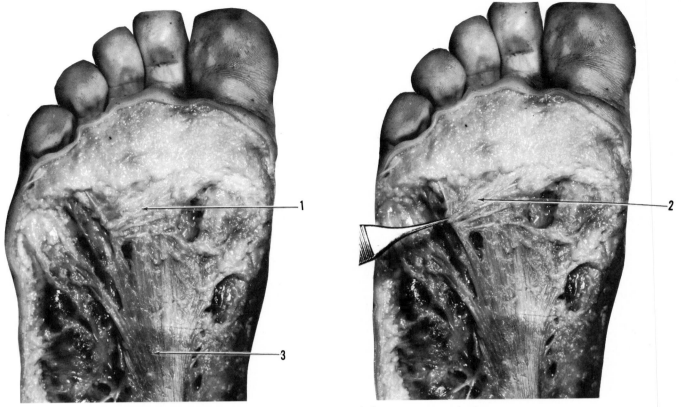

Fig. 3-36. Plantar aponeurosis. (1, Superficial transverse tract of plantar aponeurosis; 2, superficial transverse tract with side traction applied to emphasize direction of fibers; 3, superficial central component of plantar aponeurosis.)

Fig. 3-37. Plantar aponeurosis. (1, Superficial longitudinal tract continuing as [3]; 2, lateral sagittal septum arising from superficial tract of second toe; 4, medial sagittal septum to the second toe.)

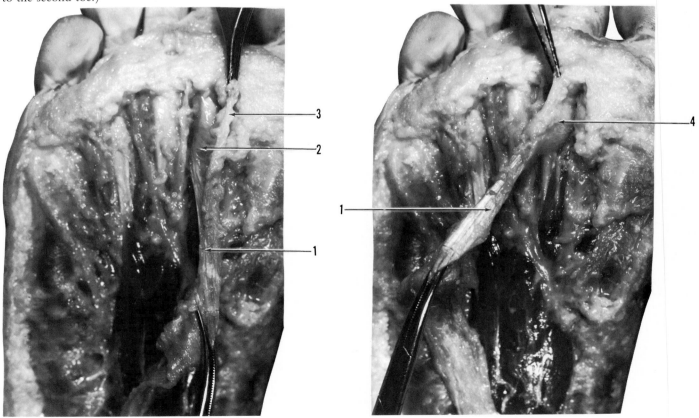

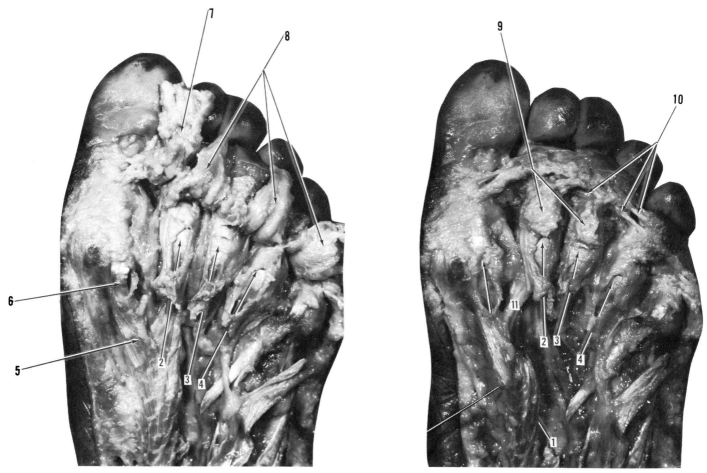

Fig. 3-38. Plantar aponeurosis. (1, Arrow indicates direction of flexor hallucis longus [6] passing distally between the two sagittal septae arising from the longitudinal tract [5]; 2, 3, 4, arrows indicating direction of long flexors tendons of toes 2, 3, 4, passing through foraminae formed by septae of corresponding longitudinal aponeurotic tracts; 7, reflected distal end of longitudinal aponeurotic tract; 8, reflected intermetatarsal head fat bodies; 9, pre-flexor tendon adipose cushions; 10, transverse mooring ligament; 11, connecting band between septae of first and second toes.)

Fig. 3-39. Diagram of deep insertion of plantar aponeurosis. (1, Superficial longitudinal tract; 2, sagittal septae arising proximal to metatarsal heads; 3, foramina for long flexor tendons formed by two septae of the ray; 4, crossing fibers of two septae under long flexor tendons; 5, oblique insertional fibers of sagittal septae on deep transverse metatarsal ligament; 6, vertical fibers arising at level of metatarsal head from sides of fibrous tunnel (9) of long flexor tendons (10) and deep transverse metatarsal ligament. Some of these vertical fibers arch over the flexor tunnel and form a pre-tendinous space retaining an adipose cushion [7]; 8, fat body that lies over plantar aspect of deep transverse metatarsal ligament; 11, transverse component of adductor hallucis muscle.)

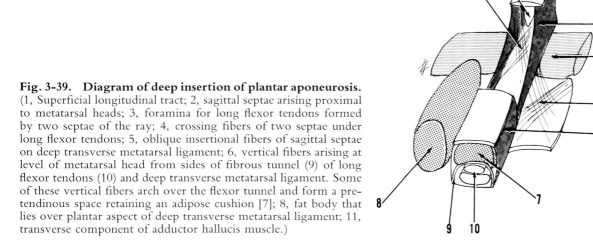

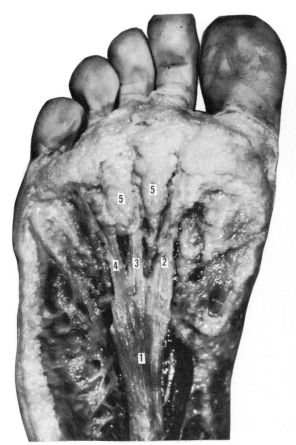

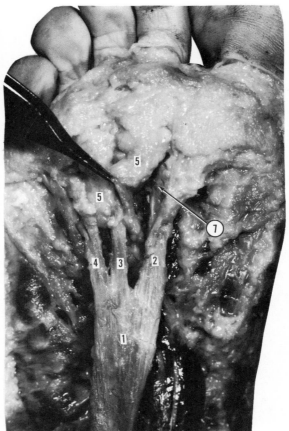

Fig. 3-40. Plantar aponeurosis and ball of the foot. (1, Central component of plantar aponeurosis; 2, 3, 4, superficial longitudinal tracts; 5, fat bodies; 6, reflected fat bodies exposing underlying neurovascular bundle; 7, sagittal septum or deep insertion of plantar aponeurosis. The insertion of the septum is proximal to the metatarsal head.)

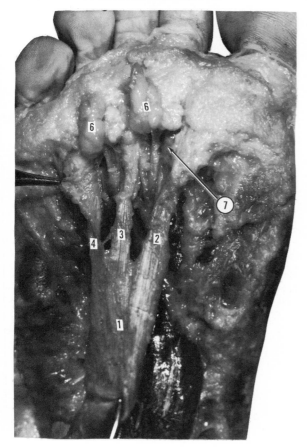

Fig. 3-42. Anatomy of the lateral and medial sulci located between the components of the plantar aponeurosis. Specimen dissected under magnification × 8. (1, Lateral sulcus bridged by retinacular meshlike connective retaining network for subcutaneous adipose tissue [5], which is reflected off interstices; 2, medial sulcus bridged by less-complex connective system; 3, central component of plantar aponeurosis; 4, medial component of plantar aponeurosis; 6, adipose tissue reflected off central component.)

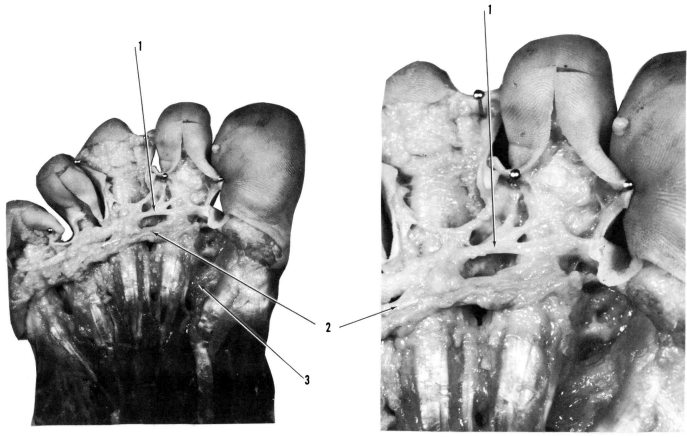

Fig. 3-41. Natatory ligament. The fibers of the natatory ligament are deep to the longitudinally oriented terminal fibers of the superficial aponeurotic bands, which insert on the dermis of the ball of the foot. (1, Natatory ligament, crossing web space, with retinacular arrangement and general transverse orientation; 2, transverse mooring ligament; 3, deep transverse metatarsal ligament between first and second toes.)

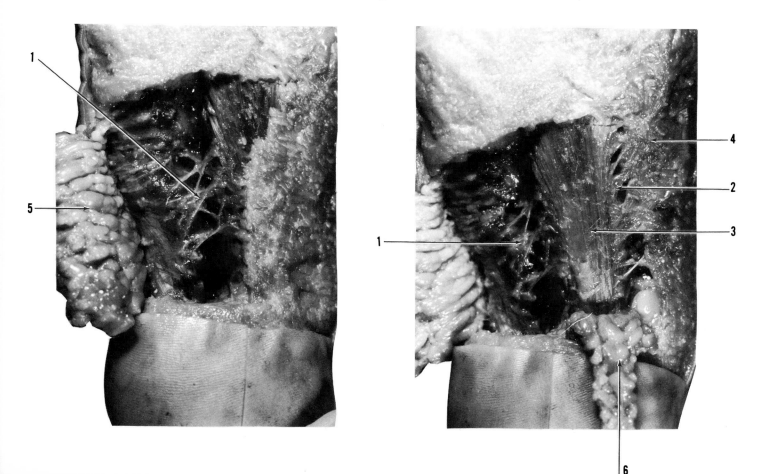

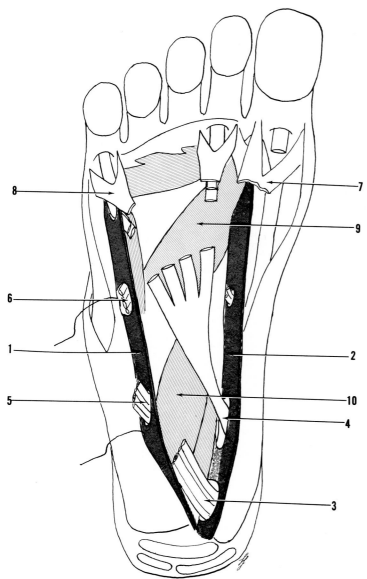

Fig. 3-43. **Intermuscular longitudinal septae.** (1, Lateral intermuscular septum perforated twice by lateral plantar neurovascular bundle [5, 6] and by long flexor of fifth toe; 2, medial intermuscular septum perforated by lateral plantar neurovascular bundle [3] and flexor digitorum longus tendon [4]; 7, 8, longitudinal septae of plantar aponeurosis; 9, oblique head of adductor hallucis muscle; 10, quadratus plantae muscle.)

connected laterally and medially to the intermuscular longitudinal septae of the planta pedis.[17]

The lateral intermuscular septum (Fig. 3-43) is attached to the medial calcaneal tubercle, the calcaneocuboid ligament, and the sheath of the peroneus longus. Distally, the septum splits, encloses the third plantar interosseous muscle, and inserts on the medial border of the fifth metatarsal shaft and on the base of the proximal phalanx at the insertion site of the tendon. At this level, it blends with the medial sagittal septum of the fifth deep aponeurotic tract of the plantar aponeurosis.

The medial intermuscular septum (Fig. 3-43) is less well defined and is formed by a set of vertical fascicles arranged like a comb, leaving passages for the tendons and neurovascular structures. Posteriorly, the medial intermuscular septum is formed by the interfascicular lamina of the calcaneal tunnel. This lamina is attached to the medial surface of the os calcis, above the proximal border of the quadratus plantae. Distally, the medial longitudinal speptum is attached to the navicular, the medial cuneiform, and the lateral aspect of the first metatarsal shaft after passing between the adductor hallucis and the flexor hallucis brevis, and it contributes to the formation of their sheaths.

PERONEAL OR LATERAL COMPONENT

The peroneal component of the plantar aponeurosis was extensively analyzed by Loth and Henkel[14, 18, 19] This component is variable. It was present in 92% and absent in 7% in a study of 410 plantar aponeuroses.[18] This peroneal component may be of four types (Fig. 3-44): complete and well developed, complete and thin, incomplete with only partial distal extension, or absent distal segment.[18]

The well-developed peroneal component originates from the lateral margin of the medial calcaneal tubercle in close connection with the origin of the abductor digiti minimi muscle. The aponeurosis is 1 cm to 1.5 cm wide at the origin. It extends in the direction of the cuboid and bifurcates into a medial and a lateral component (Fig. 3-45). The lateral band or crux is the stronger component and inserts on the base of the fifth metatarsal and forms the calcaneometatarsal ligament. A longitudinal extension band may be present in close connection with the tendon of the abductor digiti minimi. Some fibers take a dorsal course and unite with the dorsal aponeurosis. The medial band or crux turns around the abductor digiti minimi muscle, passes into the depth under the neurovascular bundle to the fifth toe, and blends with the plantar plate of the fourth and, occasionally, of the third metatarsophalangeal joints. This band gives origin to the transverse component of the adductor hallucis muscle.[19]

TIBIAL OR MEDIAL COMPONENT

The medial component of the plantar aponeurosis is thin posteriorly and thicker anteriorly. It forms the covering fascia of the abductor hallucis muscle. The fibers are oriented distally and medially and are in continuity with the dorsal aponeurosis of the foot, the inferomedial arm of the inferior extensor retinaculum, and the flexor retinaculum.

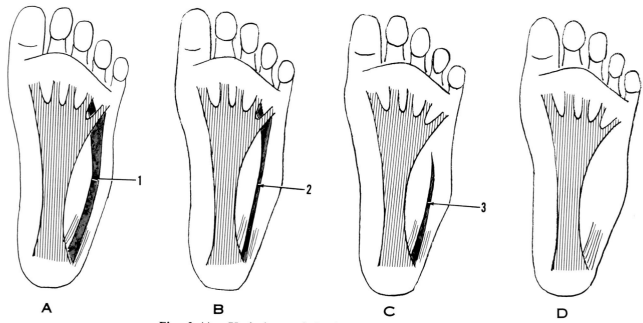

Fig. 3-44.   Variations of the lateral component of the plantar aponeurosis. *(A,1)* Complete and well developed. *(B,2)* Complete and thin. *(C,3)* Incomplete with partial distal extension. *(D)* Incomplete with no distal extension. (Redrawn from Loth EM: Etude anthropologique sur l'aponévrose plantaire. Bull Mem Soc Anthro Paris 4: 601, 1913)

Fig. 3-45.   Plantar aponeurosis. (1, Lateral component; 2, lateral crux of [1]; 3, medial crux of [1]; 4, tendon of abductor digiti quinti.)

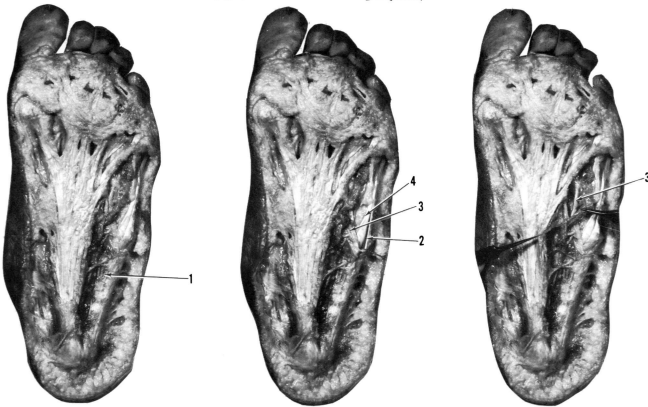

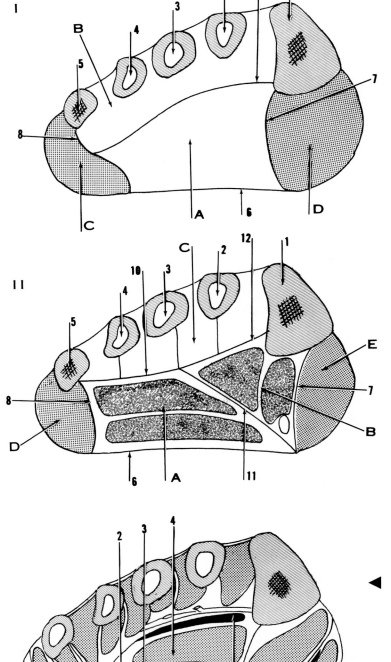

Fig. 3-46. Plantar compartments of the sole of the foot. (*I*) Classical interpretation. (*A*, central compartment; *B*, interosseous compartment; *C*, lateral or peroneal compartment; *D*, medial or tibial compartment; 1–5, metatarsals 1 to 5; 6, central segment of plantar aponeurosis; 7, medial intermuscular septum; 8, lateral intermuscular septum; 9, interosseous fascia.) (*II*) Modified interpretation. (*A*, Superficial part of central or intermediary compartment; *B*, middle part of central or intermediary compartment; *C*, deep part of central or intermediary compartment; *D*, lateral compartment; *E*, medial compartment; 10, horizontal stem of Y septum; 11, inferomedial limb of Y septum; 12, superomedial limb of Y septum.) (Concept *II* and diagram of *II* adapted from Kamel R, Sakla BF: Anatomical compartments of the sole of the human foot. Anat Rec 140: 57, 1961)

Fig. 3-47. Fascial spaces of the sole of the foot: cross section of foot at the level of the middle of the fifth metatarsal bone (proximal surface). *Central compartment:* F_1, Fascial space between central plantar aponeurosis (1) and flexor digitorum brevis (2); F_2, fascial space between flexor digitorum brevis (2) and quadratus plantae (3); F_3, fascial space between quadratus plantae (3) and oblique head of adductor hallucis (4); F_4, fascial space between adductor hallucis (4) and interosseous fascia. *Medial compartment:* F_5, fascial space located between investing fascia of abductor hallucis and deep surface of muscle. *Lateral compartment:* F_6, fascial space located between investing fascia of abductor digiti quinti and deep surface of muscle. (Redrawn after Grodinsky M: A study of the fascial spaces of the foot and their bearing on infections. Surg Gynecol Obstet 49: 737, 1929)

Plantar Compartments and Fascial Spaces

COMPARTMENTS

The sole of the foot is divided into four compartments (Fig. 3-46): central, medial or tibial, lateral or peroneal, and interosseous.

The central compartment is limited superficially by the central segment of the plantar aponeurosis, laterally and medially by the lateral and medial intermuscular septae, and dorsally by the tarsometatarsal skeleton covered distally by the interosseous fascia. The space contains the flexor digitorum brevis muscle, the flexor digitorum longus tendons with four lumbricals, the quadratus plantae muscle, the adductor hallucis muscle, the peroneus longus tendon, and the plantar segment of the tibialis posterior tendon.

The medial compartment is limited superficially and medially by the medial segment of the plantar aponeurosis, laterally by the medial intermuscular septum, and dorsally by the inferior surface of the first metatarsal shaft. The space contains the abductor hallucis and flexor hallucis muscles and the flexor hallucis longus tendon. The terminal portions of the peroneus longus and tibialis posterior tendons are also in this compartment.

The lateral compartment is limited superficially and laterally by the lateral segment of the plantar aponeurosis and medially by the lateral intermuscular septum. The space contains the abductor, short flexor, and opponens muscles of the little toe.

The interosseous compartment is limited below by the interossei fascia and above by the central metatarsals 2, 3, 4 and contains the interossei muscles.

Wood-Jones locates in the central compartment not only the muscles mentioned above but also the lateral head of the flexor hallucis brevis.[20]

FASCIAL SPACES

Potential fascial spaces are present in the central, medial, and lateral compartments, as described by Grodinsky.[17]

Central Compartment

There are four fascial spaces of the central compartment (Fig. 3-47).

Fascial Space 1. Fascial space 1 or median plantar space M_1 is located between the deep surface of the central part of the plantar aponeurosis and the flexor digitorum brevis muscle. In the posterior third the space is completely obliterated as the muscle takes origin from the aponeurosis. Only a sharp dissection separates the two structures. Anteriorly, this short space ends at the level of or proximal to the middle of the metatarsal bones where the fascial floor and the muscular roof come together. A careful dissection reveals three very thin connective tissue septae dividing the space into four compartments of unequal length. Posteriorly, the first

and fourth compartments terminate at the level of the base of the fifth metatarsal. The second compartment, which is the longest, extends posteriorly to within 2 cm to 3 cm of the medial calcaneal tubercle. The third compartment is the shortest and terminates into the second 2.5 cm distal to the base of the fifth metatarsal.[17] Each longitudinal compartment lies proximal to the subcutaneous spaces between the five longitudinal bands of the plantar aponeurosis.

Fascial Space 2. Fascial space 2 or median plantar space M_2 is located between the deep surface of the flexor digitorum brevis and the quadratus plantae muscle, joined by the flexor digitorum longus tendon. The space is triangular, with the apex located along a line joining the navicular tubercle to the medial calcaneal tubercle, 1 cm distal to the latter. Anteriorly, the space terminates at the origin of the fibrous flexor tendon tunnel.[21] On the tibial aspect of the flexor tunnel, there is an extension along the four lumbrical tunnels. In the posterior aspect of the fascial space 2, a transverse septum is present between the flexor digitorum brevis and the quadratus plantae muscle and unites the medial and lateral intermuscular septae (Fig. 3-48).

Fascial Space 3. Fascial space 3 or median plantar space M_3 is the interval located dorsal to the quadratus plantae muscle and the flexor digitorum longus. The deep surface is formed posteriorly by the tarsal bones and ligaments, the fibrous tunnel of the peroneus longus, the superficial surface of the adductor hallucis muscle, and the segment of the interossei uncovered by the adductor hallucis muscle. The floor is covered by a fascia. A septum formed of loose areolar connective tissue fibers limits the space anteriorly and extends along a line drawn from the middle of the fifth metatarsal to the head of the first metatarsal.[17] Four anterior extensions may lead to the spaces under the lumbrical muscles.

Fascial Space 4. This potential space (fascial space 4 or median plantar space M_4) is located on the dorsal aspect of the adductor hallucis obliquis muscle. The first intermetatarsal space, the proximal half of the second intermetatarsal space, and a small portion of the proximal part of the third interspace, with their corresponding interossei, from the dorsal limit of the space. The lateral boundary is along a line extending from the base of the fourth metatarsal bone to the lateral aspect of the base of the proximal phalanx of the big toe (Fig. 3-49).

Medial Compartment

The fascial space of the medial compartment is a potential closed space located between the investing fascia and the deep surface of the abductor hallucis. It extends from the medial calcaneal tubercle to the point where the tendon blends with the medial head of the flexor hallucis brevis muscle.

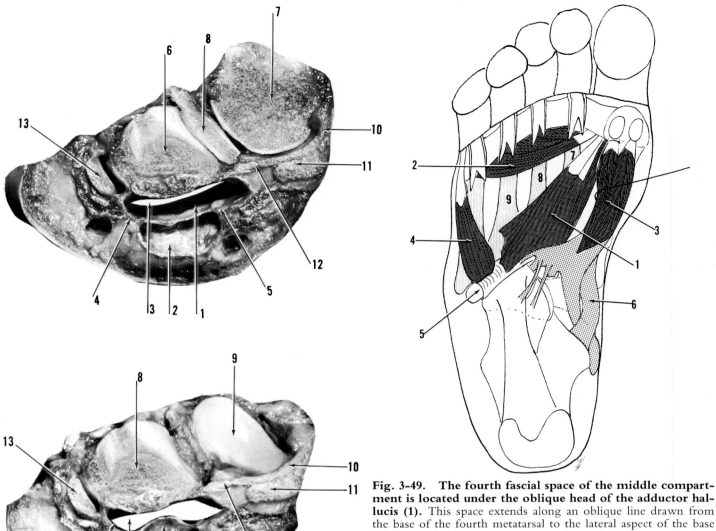

Fig. 3-48.   Distal view of transverse cross section of the
left foot, passing through the proximal segment of the
cuboid, the beak of the os calcis, and the distal segment
of the talar head. (1, Transverse septum dividing central
compartment into compartment for flexor digitorum brevis
[2] and compartment for quadratus plantae [3]. This septum
extends from the lateral intermuscular septum [4] to the medial intermuscular septum [5]; 6, cuboid; 7, talar head supported by os calcis [8], inferior calcaneonavicular ligament
[12], superomedial calcaneonavicular ligament (10), tibialis
posterior tendon [11], and navicular [9]; 13, peroneus longus
tendon and tunnel.)

Fig. 3-49.   The fourth fascial space of the middle compartment is located under the oblique head of the adductor hallucis (1). This space extends along an oblique line drawn from
the base of the fourth metatarsal to the lateral aspect of the base
of the proximal phalanx of the big toe. (2, Transverse head of
adductor hallucis muscle; 3, flexor hallucis brevis, retracted; 4,
flexor digiti quinti; 5, peroneus longus tendon and sheath; 6, deep
component of tibialis posterior tendon; 7, 8, 9, metatarsal shafts
2, 3, 4.)

Lateral Compartment

The fascial space of the lateral compartment is a potential space located between the deep surface of the abductor digiti quinti and its investing fascia. It extends from the os calcis to about the level of the head of the fifth metatarsal.

COMMUNICATIONS BETWEEN COMPARTMENTS AND FASCIAL SPACES

The compartments of the sole of the foot are normally closed spaces. The sites of perforation of the septae by the tendons arriving from the calcaneal canal and the entrance points of the plantar neurovascular bundles are sealed off by connective areolar tissue that would yield to increased compartmental or interfascial pressure.

Injection studies have established patterns of communications.[17, 21–23] Grodinsky, in his study of 58 injections of feet with colored paraffin or colored gelatin, provided the following data:[17]

Injection of the median plantar space M_1 spreads plantarly through the plantar aponeurosis into the subcutaneous area or dorsally into the median space M_2.

Injection of the median plantar space M_2 spreads within the middle compartment into the fascial spaces M_3 (100%) or M_1 (75%) or anteriorly in the lumbrical spaces (100%). If the local pressure increases, the spread may extend into the surrounding compartments. Proximally, the spread may reach the calcaneal canal through the flexor digitorum longus and flexor hallucis longus tendons (50%), the lateral plantar neurovascular bundle (50%), or the medial plantar neurovascular bundle (25%). An extension into the lateral compartment may also occur (25%).

Injection of the median plantar space M_3 located dorsal to the quadratus plantae and flexor digitorum longus spreads within the fascial compartments M_2 (75%), M_4 (40%), or M_1 (50%), the latter either directly or indirectly after reaching the fascial space M_2 or the lumbrical grooves. An anterior extension may also occur into the lumbrical spaces (75%). With increased pressure, the connective tissue seal around the piercing long flexors yields (90%), resulting in local accumulation of injected mass or proximal extension along the flexor tendons to or beyond the flexor retinaculum and distal along the flexor hallucis longus up to its insertion. Pooling of injected material may take place on the medial aspect of the os calcis, deep to the lateral plantar and posterior tibial neurovascular bundles. Anterior extension may occur through the third and fourth interosseous spaces and the distal half of the second interosseous space into the dorsal subaponeurotic space (40%). Occasionally the injected mass flows along the long flexor tendon sheaths to almost the level of the metatarsophalangeal joint. Rarely, it may break into the long flexor synovial sheath of the third toe. Infrequently, an extension may be seen into the lateral compartment or on the deep side of the flexor hallucis brevis muscle.

Injection of the median plantar space M_4 extends into the fascial space M_3 (100%), the dorsal subaponeurotic spaces through the first and second interosseous spaces (50%), or the deep side of the flexor hallucis brevis muscle.

Injection of the medial or tibial plantar space remains localized to the space or the subcutaneous interval.

Injection of the lateral plantar space extends into the subcutaneous area (100%) or the fascial space M_2 (66%) or penetrates the peroneus longus tunnel (66%).

Kamel and Sakla describe three compartments—lateral, medial, intermediate—in the sole of the foot, with a partition pattern in variance with the common description as presented above (see Fig 3-46).[22]

The lateral compartment is limited by the lateral plantar aponeurosis and the lateral intermuscular septum. The space retains the abductor digiti minimi brevis and flexor digiti minimi brevis muscles. The injection of colored celloidin solution into this compartment showed this to be a closed space not communicating with the other compartments.

The medial compartment is limited by the medial plantar aponeurosis and the medial intermuscular septum. The space contains the abductor hallucis muscle. It also is a closed, noncommunicating space.

The intermediate or central space is divided by horizontally laid Y septum into three parts: *superficial, middle, deep*. The Y-shaped septum extends horizontally from the medial side of the fifth metatarsal shaft and bifurcates at the level of the third metatarsal into an upper and a lower limb. The upper limb is directed upward and medially and attaches to the lateral side of the first metatarsal bone. The lower limb is directed downward and medially and blends with the medial border of the central segment of the plantar aponeurosis.

The *superficial compartment* is limited below by the central segment of the plantar aponeurosis, laterally by the lateral intermuscular septum, dorsally by the stem of the Y septum, and medially by the inferomedial bifurcation arm of the Y septum. This space contains the flexor digitorum brevis, the quadratus plantae, and the flexor digitorum longus with its four lumbricals. The dye injected between the flexor digitorum brevis and the flexor digitorum longus follows the latter through the calcaneal canal into the deep compartment of the leg.

The *middle compartment* is limited by the bifurcation arms of the Y-shaped septum laterally and by the medial intermuscular septum medially. The space contains the flexor hallucis longus, flexor hallucis brevis, and adductor hallucis muscles. The injection of the space extends into the calcaneal canal and the deep compartment of the leg.

The *deep compartment* of the intermediate space is limited below by the stem and the superomedial arm of the Y septum and above by the central metatarsals 2, 3, 4. The space contains the interossei muscles and is subdivided by three vertical septae attached to the corresponding metatarsals. This compartment is a non-communicating, closed space.

A subcutaneous space is described located superficial to the posterior and plantar aspect of the os calcis.[23] In this location, a large calcaneal bursa is present.[24]

REFERENCES

1. Meyer P: La morphologie du ligament annulaire anterieur du cou-de-pied chez l'homme. Comptes-Rendus Assoc Anat 84:286, 1955
2. Weitbrecht J: Syndesmology or a Description of the Ligaments of the Human Body: Arranged in Accordance With Anatomical Dissections and Illustrated With Figures Drawn From Fresh Subjects, p 191, 1742. Translated by E. Kaplan. Philadelphia, WB Saunders, 1969
3. Smith BE: The astragalo-calcaneo-navicular joint. J Anat Physiol 30:390, 1896
4. Cahill DR: The anatomy and function of the contents of the human tarsal sinus and canal. Anat Rec 153:1, 1965
5. Retzius A: Bemerkungen über ein schleuderformiges Band in dem Sinus Tarsi des Menschen und Mehrerer Thiere. Arch Anat Physiol 497, 1841
6. Smith JW: The ligamentous structures in the canalis and sinus tarsi. J Anat 92:616, 1958
7. Bellocq P, Meyer P: Contribution a l'étude de l'aponevrose dorsale du pied (fascia dorsalis pedis, P.N.A.). Acta Anat 30:67, 1957
8. Latarjet A, Etienne-Martin M: L'appareil de glissement des tendons extenseurs des doigts et des orteils sur le dos de la main et sur le dos du pied. Ann Anat Pathol Anat Normal 9:605, 1932
9. Bellocq P, Meyer P: Contribution a l'étude du canal calcaneén. Comptes-Rendus Assoc Anat 89:292, 1956
10. Richet A: Traité Pratique d'Anatomie Médico-Chirurgicale, 5th ed, pp 1311–1312. Paris, Lauwereyns, 1877
11. Baumann J: La région de passage de la loge posterieure de la jambe à la plante du pied. Ann Anat Pathol Anat Normal Medico-chir 7:201, 1930
12. Raiga, A: Le canal calcaneen. La Presse Méd 31:808, 1923
13. Maslieurat-Lagémard: De l'anatomie descriptive et chirurgicale des aponevroses et des synoviales du pied: De leur appliction à la thérapeutique et à la médecine operatoire. Gaz Med Paris, 274, 1840
14. Henkel A: Die Aponeurosis Plantaris. Arch Anat Anat Ab Arch Anat Physiol, 113, 1913.
15. Bojsen-Møller F, Flagstad KE: Plantar aponeurosis and internal architecture of the ball of the foot. J Anat 121: 599, 1976
16. Poirier P, Charpy A: Traité de'Anatomie Humaine, Vol 2, p 300. Paris, Masson et Cie, 1901
17. Grodinsky M: A study of the fascial spaces of the foot and their bearing on infections. Surg Gynecol Obstet 49:737, 1929
18. Loth EM: Etude anthropologique sur l'aponévrose plantaire. Bull Mem Soc Anthro Paris 4:601, 1913
19. Loth EM: Die Plantar aponeurose beim Menschen und den übrigen primaten. Korr Bl Deutsch Anthrop Ges, 1907
20. Wood Jones F: Structure and Function as Seen in the Foot, 2nd ed, p 63. London, Baillière, Tindall & Cox, 1949
21. Liaras H: Tissu cellulaire et topographic plantaire: Connexions de la plante et du mollet. Ann Anat Pathol Anat Normal 12:537, 1935
22. Kamel R, Sakla BF: Anatomical compartments of the sole of the human foot. Anat Rec 140:57, 1961
23. Loeffler RD, Ballard A: Plantar fascial spaces of the foot and a proposed surgical approach. Foot and Ankle 1:11, 1980
24. Testut L, Jacob O: Traité d'Anatomie Topographique avec Applications Médico-chirurgicales, 2nd ed, Vol 2, p 1075. Paris, Doin, 1909

4

The human frame is to a large extent but clay in the dissector's hands—clay from which many an artificially isolated product can be modeled; and of all structures in the body, the ligaments are the most plastic in this respect.

Barclay-Smith, 1896

Syndesmology

The distal segment of the fibular shaft and the lateral malleolus are firmly attached to the distal tibia and form a movable articulating system embracing the talar body. The inferior tibiofibular articulation is an integral part of the ankle joint. The subdivision of the ankle joint, as presented in the German literature, into an upper ankle joint (talocrural) and lower ankle joint (subtalar, talocalcaneonavicular) has merit from the anatomic and functional points of view, because these two joints are closely integrated and determine the major field of motion of the ankle–foot complex.

Ligaments of the Inferior Tibiofibular Joint

The three ligaments uniting the distal fibular shaft and the lateral malleolus to the distal tibia are the anterior tibiofibular ligament, the posterior tibiofibular ligament, and the interosseous ligament. The lower segment of the interosseous membrane also participates in the stabilization of the distal fibular shaft.

ANTERIOR TIBIOFIBULAR LIGAMENT

The anterior tibiofibular ligament (Figs. 4-1 and 4-2) is a flat, fibrous lamina. It originates from the longitudinal tubercle located on the anterior border of the lateral malleolus in front of the upper segment of the articulating surface for the talus and from the lower segment of the anterior border of the fibular shaft. The fibers are directed upward and medially and insert on the anterolateral tubercle of the tibia; some fibers reach the anterior surface of the distal tibia. The fibers increase in length from above downward, the lower fibers being the longest—close to 25 mm.

The anterior tibiofibular ligament is divided into two or three bands or may be multifascicular. Vessels from the anterior peroneal artery penetrate through the interlaminar spaces. During their oblique course, the most inferior fibers cover the tibiofibular corner of the joint and pass over the corresponding segment of the talus. The lowest fibers at their fibular site reach the origin of the anterior talofibular ligament.

POSTERIOR TIBIOFIBULAR LIGAMENT

The posterior tibiofibular ligament (Figs. 4-1 and 4-3) has two components: superficial and deep.

The superficial component originates from the posterior border of the tubercle located above the digital fossa of the lateral malleolus. The origin extends distally to the upper part of the posterior border of the digital fossa and proximally to the ridge separating the lateral and medial fibular surfaces posteriorly. The fibers are directed upward and medially, and the major insertion is on the posterolateral tibial tubercle. The remaining fibers continue their course and insert on the distal tibia, and they may reach the lateral border of the groove for the tibialis posterior tendon.

The deep component is the *transverse ligament*. This ligament is thick, strong, and conoid with a twist to its fibers; it originates from the round posterior fibular tubercle located above the digital fossa and from the upper segment of the digital fossa. The fibers are directed upward, medially, and posteriorly. At the posterior border of the tibial articular surface, the fibers change direction and become horizontal or transverse. This ligament inserts on the lower part of the posterior border of the tibial articular surface and reaches the medial border of the medial malleolus. The insertion is the strongest on the outer half. The transverse ligament descends below the posterior tibial margin and constitutes a true posterior labrum deepening the tibial articular surface (Figs. 4-1 and 4-4). The posterior half of the medial surface of the lateral malleolus is deficient in articular surface but is filled by the transverse ligament, which establishes contact with the talar surface and leaves its imprint as a bevelled triangular facet on the posterior half of the lateral border of the superior talar surface.

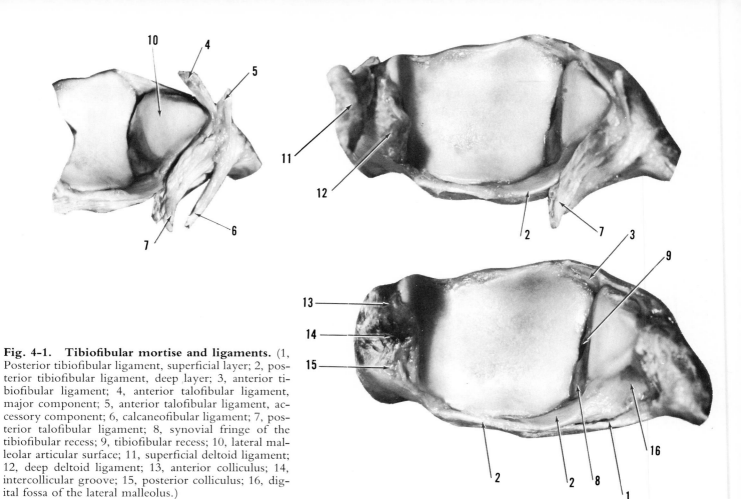

Fig. 4-1. Tibiofibular mortise and ligaments. (1, Posterior tibiofibular ligament, superficial layer; 2, posterior tibiofibular ligament, deep layer; 3, anterior tibiofibular ligament; 4, anterior talofibular ligament, major component; 5, anterior talofibular ligament, accessory component; 6, calcaneofibular ligament; 7, posterior talofibular ligament; 8, synovial fringe of the tibiofibular recess; 9, tibiofibular recess; 10, lateral malleolar articular surface; 11, superficial deltoid ligament; 12, deep deltoid ligament; 13, anterior colliculus; 14, intercollicular groove; 15, posterior colliculus; 16, digital fossa of the lateral malleolus.)

Fig. 4-2. Anterior tibiofibular ligament. (1, Anterior tibiofibular ligament with three fascicles; 2, anterior tibiofibular ligament with multiple fascicles; 3, anterior talofibular ligament, major component; 4, anterior talofibular ligament, accessory component; 5, lateral malleolus; 6, tibia.)

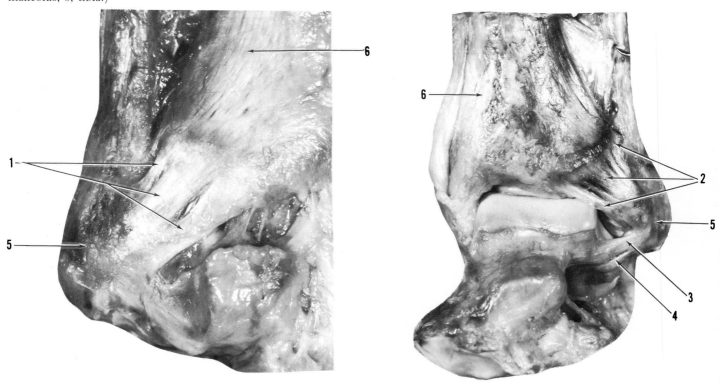

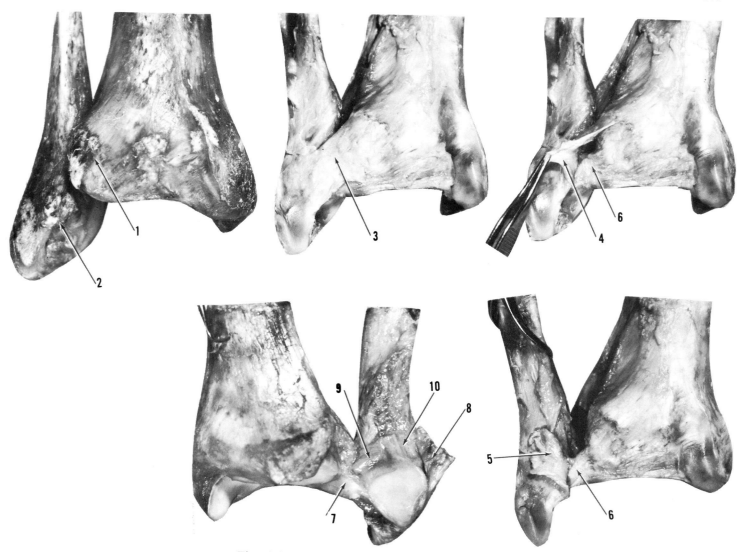

Fig. 4-3. Posterior tibiofibular ligament. (1, Posterolateral tibial tubercle; 2, lateral malleolus; 3, posterior tibiofibular ligament, superficial layer; 4, partially detached posterior tibiofibular ligament, superficial layer; 5, completely detached posterior tibiofibular ligament, superficial layer; 6, posterior tibiofibular ligament, deep layer, posterior aspect; 7, posterior tibiofibular ligament, deep layer, anterior aspect; 8, anterior tibiofibular ligament; 9, synovial fringe of tibiofibular recess; 10, tibiofibular synovial recess.)

INTEROSSEOUS LIGAMENT

The interosseous ligament (Fig. 4-5) is a reddish ligament formed by a dense mass of short fibers intermingled with adipose tissue and vessels. These fibers form a vault over the underlying synovial recess and may be perforated in some specimens. The ligament originates from the antero-inferior triangular segment of the medial aspect of the distal fibular shaft. This area of origin is higher anteriorly and lower posteriorly, and the fibers insert on a similar corresponding area on the lateral surface of the distal tibia.

The fibula is in contact with the tibia only through a minute, crescent-shaped, cartilage-coated articular surface in continuity with the articular surface of the lateral malleo-lus.[1] A semilunar cavity is present above this tibiofibular interline and is limited proximally by the concave base of the interosseous ligament. The anterior segment of the cavity corresponds to a synovial recess communicating with the ankle joint through the linear opening. This synovial recess is about 1 cm in height. The posterior part of the semilunar cavity is smaller and occupied by a reddish synovial fringe that originates only from the peroneal surface and descends into the ankle joint between the fibula and the lateral talar surface (Figs. 4-1 and 4-6). In dorsiflexion of the ankle, the synovial fringe retreats toward the upper chamber, and in plantar flexion, it descends into the ankle joint.[2, 3]

(Text continues on p. 148.)

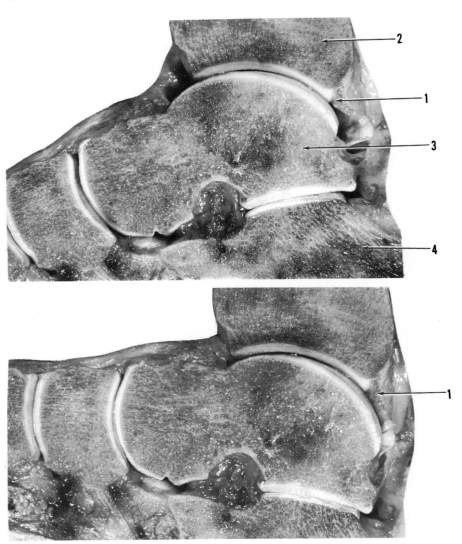

Fig. 4-4.   Sagittal cross section of the ankle. (1, Tibial attachment of the deep component of the posterior tibiofibular ligament forming a labrum; 2, tibia; 3, talus; 4, os calcis.)

Fig. 4-5.   Interosseous ligament. (1, Anterolateral tibial tubercle; 2, lateral malleolus; 3, anterior tibiofibular ligament; 4, transected anterior tibiofibular ligament; 5, interosseous membrane; 6, interosseous ligament; 7, tibiofibular synovial recess.)

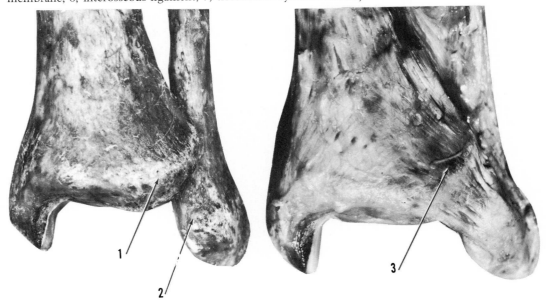

(continued)

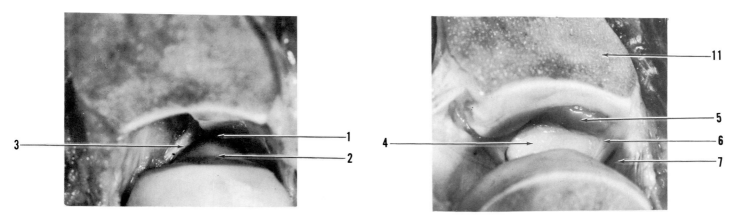

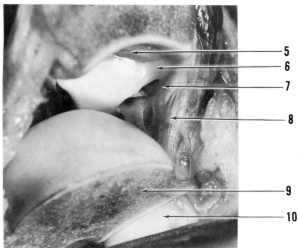

Fig. 4-6.   Sagittal section of the tibia and talus. (1, Talofibular joint; 2, lateral talar articulating surface; 3, anterior talofibular ligament; 4, lateral malleolar articulating surface; 5, tibiofibular synovial fringe; 6, 7, posterior tibiofibular ligament; 8, posterior talofibular ligament; 9, talus; 10, posterior articular surface of calcaneus.)

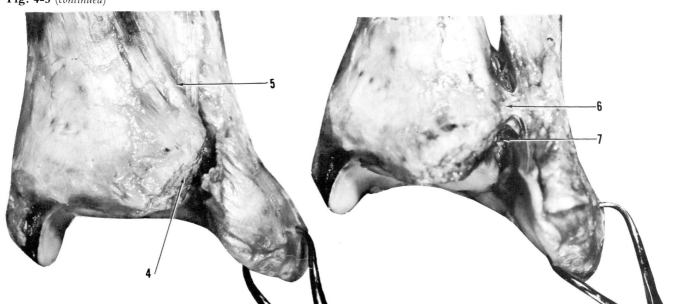

Fig. 4-5 (*continued*)

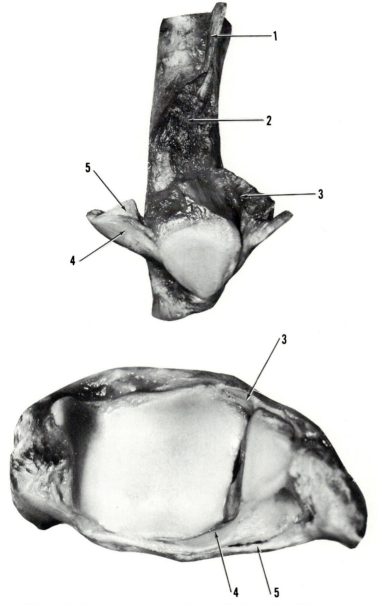

Fig. 4-7. Interosseous membrane. (1, Insertion of interosseous membrane; 2, insertion zone of tibiofibular interosseous ligament; 3, anterior tibiofibular ligament; 4, posterior tibiofibular ligament, deep component; 5, posterior tibiofibular ligament, superficial component.)

INTEROSSEOUS MEMBRANE

The interosseous membrane is in continuity with the apex of the interosseous ligament (Fig. 4-7). The anterior fibers are oblique, directed downward and laterally, whereas the posterior fibers are nearly vertical.

Ligaments Uniting the Distal Tibiofibular Complex to the Talus, Calcaneus, and Navicular

The distal tibiofibular complex is firmly connected to the talus and the os calcis. The talus is anchored to the fibula anteriorly and posteriorly and to the tibia medially. The calcaneus is anchored to the fibula laterally and to the tibia medially. The anterior connection of the tibia to the talus and to the navicular is of lesser magnitude.

LATERAL LIGAMENT OF THE ANKLE

Anterior Talofibular Ligament

The anterior talofibular ligament (Figs. 4-8 and 4-9) is a flat, quadrilateral, relatively strong ligament measuring approximately 15 mm × 8 mm × 2 mm, 20 mm × 6 mm × 2 mm,[4] or 12 mm × 5 mm.[5] This ligament is formed by two distinct bands separated by an interval that allows the penetration of vascular branches. The upper band is larger than the lower. A third band occasionally may be present. The ligament originates from the inferior oblique segment of the anterior border of the lateral malleolus. The upper band reaches the origin of the anterior tibiofibular ligament and the lower band that of the calcaneofibular ligament; in many specimens, these two ligaments are united with arciform fibers at their malleolar origin. The anterior talofibular ligament courses anteromedially and inserts, not on the talar neck, but on the talar body just anterior to the lateral malleolar articular surface. Two flat tubercles are occasionally seen, corresponding to the insertion of the two bands. The anterior talofibular ligament is in close connection to the capsule of the talofibular joint. In the neutral position of the talus, the ligament is horizontal. In dorsiflexion, the ligament is directed slightly upward. In plantar flexion, the ligament firmly braces the talar body as it stretches over the nearly right angle formed by the union of the anterior and lateral surfaces of the talar body (Fig. 4-10); in this position, the ligament is directed downward, medially, and anteriorly.

Calcaneofibular Ligament

The calcaneofibular ligament (Figs. 4-8 and 4-11) is a strong cordlike or flat oval ligament and measures approximately 30 mm × 5 mm × 3 mm, 20 mm × 4 mm to 8 mm in diameter,[4] 30 mm to 40 mm × 5 mm,[2] or 30 mm to 40 mm × 4 mm to 5 mm.[3] It originates from the lower segment of the anterior border of the lateral malleolus just

(Text continues on p. 153.)

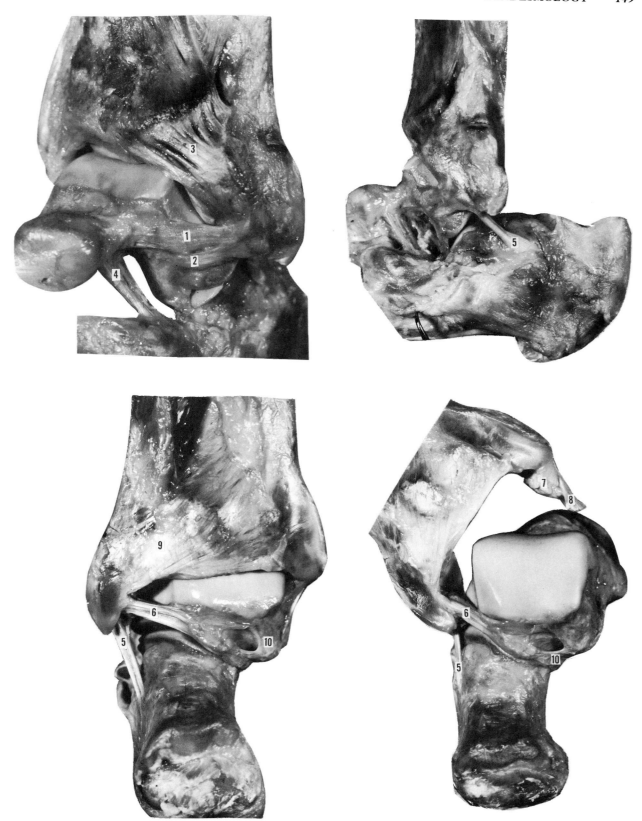

Fig. 4-8. Anterior talofibular ligament. (1, Anterior talofibular ligament, main component; 2, anterior talofibular ligament, accessory component; 3, anterior tibiofibular ligament, fasciculated; 4, cervical ligament; 5, calcaneofibular ligament; 6, posterior talofibular ligament; 7, deltoid ligament, deep layer; 8, deltoid ligament, superficial layer; 9, posterior tibiofibular ligament; 10, fibrous tunnel of flexor hallucis longus tendon.)

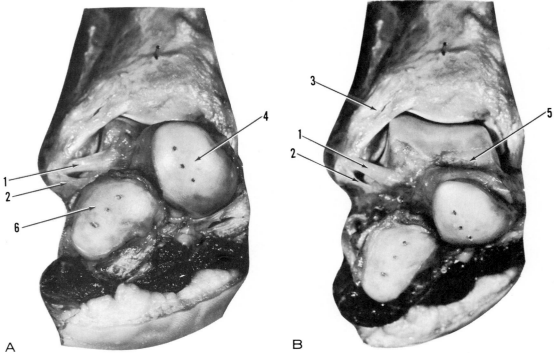

A   B

Fig. 4-9.   Anterior talofibular ligament. (*A*) Dorisiflexion. (*B*) Plantar flexion. (1, Anterior talofibular ligament, major component. The ligament is oriented upward, medially in dorsiflexion [*A*], and downward, medially in plantar flexion [*B*]; 2, Anterior talofibular ligament, accessory component; 3, anterior tibiofibular ligament; 4, navicular articular surface of the talus; 5, talus; 6, cuboidal articular surface of the os calcis.)

Fig. 4-10.   Anterior talofibular ligament in plantar fexion. (1, Anterior talofibular ligament inserting on the anterior surface of the talar body and under tension in plantar flexion; 2, anterior tibiofibular ligament.)

Fig. 4-11.   Calcaneofibular ligament. (1, Calcaneofibular ligament; 2, superior peroneal retinaculum; 3, peronei tendons, brevis anteriorly and longus posteriorly; 4, inferior peroneal retinaculum; 5, stem of inferior extensor retinaculum; 6, tip of lateral malleolus, *free of insertion;* 7, anterior talofibular ligament, major component; 8, anterior talofibular ligament, accessory component.) (*continued*)

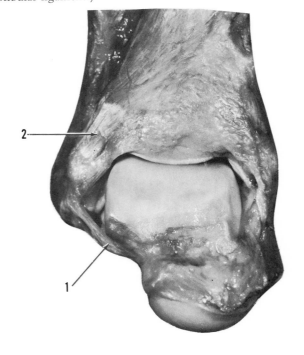

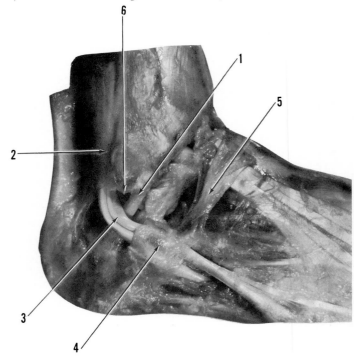

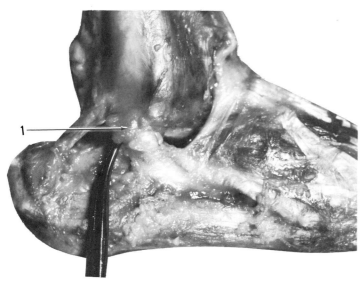

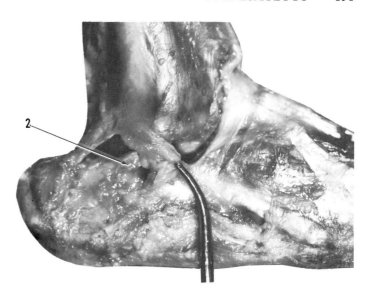

Fig. 4-12.   Calcaneofibular ligament. (1, Adipose tissue covering the posterior segment of the calcaneofibular ligament; 2, exposure of the posterior segment of the calcaneofibular ligament by reflection of the adipose tissue; 3, calcaneofibular ligament exposed after resection of the peronei tendons.)

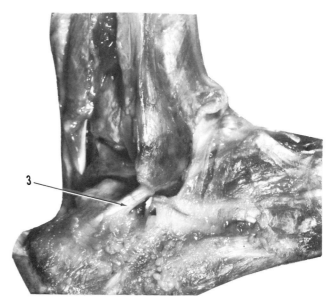

Fig. 4-11 (*continued*)

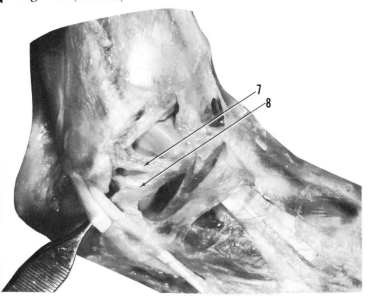

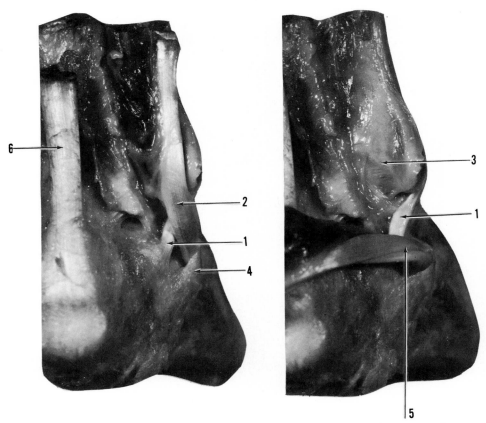

Fig. 4-13. Posterolateral aspect of the ankle. (1, Calcaneofibular ligament and peronei tendons (2) crossing in ✕; 3, sulcus of peronei tendons on posterior surface of lateral malleolus; 4, inferior, peroneal retinaculum; 5, reflected peronei tendons; 6, Achilles tendon.)

Fig. 4-14. Anatomical variations of the calcaneofibular ligament in seventy-five ankles. (*Left* to *Right*) Vertical, horizontal, fan shaped, oblique. (Redrawn after Ruth CJ: The surgical treatment of injuries of the fibular collateral ligaments of the ankle. J Bone Joint Surg [A] 43: 233, 1961)

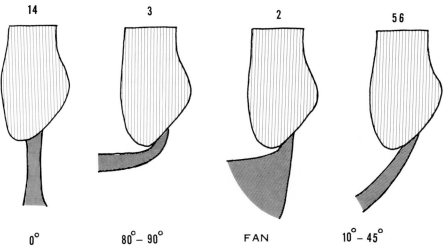

below the origin of the inferior band of the anterior talofibular ligament. The origin does not extend to the tip of the lateral malleolus, which is left free. Near the origin, arciform fibers may unite the calcaneofibular ligament and the inferior band of the anterior talofibular ligament. With the foot in neutral position, the ligament courses posteriorly, inferiorly, and medially and is crossed superficially by the peronei tendons and their sheaths, which may leave an imprint on the ligament (Figs 4-12 and 4-13). Only approximately 1 cm of the ligament remains uncovered by the crossing peronei.

The calcaneofibular ligament inserts on a small tubercle (tuberculum ligamenti calcaneo fibularis) located on the posterior aspect of the lateral calcaneal surface, posterosuperior to the peronei processus trochlearis. The insertion of the ligament is variable. Laidlaw, in a study of 750 calcanei, gives the following location of the calcaneal insertion of the ligament: typical location, 64.5%; anterior location, 25.5%; posterior location, 5.5%; downward location, 4.5%.[6] The variable insertions result in variable obliquity of the ligament relative to the long axis of the fibula.

Ruth, in a study based on 30 dissected specimens and observations of 55 ankles during surgery, provides the following data with regards to the angle formed by the long axis of the calcaneofibular ligament and the long axis of the fibula (Fig. 4-14): 10° to 45°, 74.66%; 0°, 18.66%; 80° to 90°, 4%; fan shaped, 2.66%.[5] The valgus or varus position considerably affects the direction of and the angle formed by the calcaneofibular ligament. The obliquity of the ligament is increased with valgus of the heel and decreased with varus (Fig. 4-15). The obliquity of the ligament is also variable with the position of the ankle joint (Fig. 4-16). The calcaneofibular ligament crosses the talocalcaneal joint and is separated from it by the lateral talocalcaneal ligament. The interval between the two ligaments is filled with adipose tissue.

Posterior Talofibular Ligament

The posterior talofibular ligament (Figs. 4-8 and 4-17) is a very strong ligament situated in a nearly horizontal plane. Trapezoidal in contour, the ligament measures approximately 30 mm in posterior length, 5 mm in width at the fibular origin, and 5 mm to 8 mm in thickness. The ligament originates on the medial surface of the lateral malleolus from the lower segment of the digital fossa (Fig. 4-18). Thick and fasciculated, it courses horizontally toward the lateral and posterior aspects of the talus. The short transverse and intermediary fibers insert along the lateral surface of the talus in a groove along the posteroinferior border of the lateral malleolar articular surface up to its mid segment. The long fibers are directed posteromedially and insert on the posterior surface of the talus. The medial end expands and attaches on the posterolateral tubercle, the trigonal process, or the os trigonum (when present) and contributes to the formation of the floor of the flexor hallucis longus tunnel. When viewed posteriorly, the ligament is triangular, with a lateral apex and a medial base. The upper fibers of

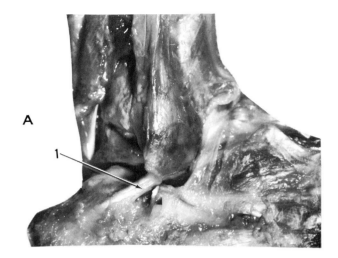

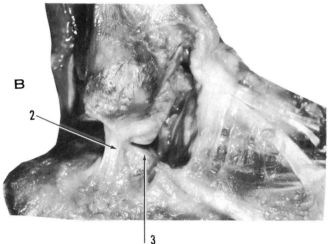

Fig. 4-15. The heel in valgus and varus. (*A*) Heel in valgus; obliquity of calcaneofibular ligament (1) is increased. (*B*) Heel in varus, obliquity of calcaneofibular ligament (2) is decreased. In this specimen the ligament is vertical. (3, Posterior calcaneal surface seen in varus.)

the posterior segment are in continuity medially with the superficial talotibial ligament, forming a posterior ligamentous sling.

Occasionally a band originates from the superior border of the posterior talofibular ligament near its origin, courses upward and medially, and inserts on the posterior tibial margin, blending with the fibers of the transverse component of the posterior tibiofibular ligament (Fig. 4-19); this insertion may reach the posterior surface of the medial malleolus. Paturet designates this ligament the *posterior intermalleolar ligament*.[7] The posterior talofibular ligament is intracapsular but extrasynovial. The fibular origin is covered by the peronei retinaculum (Fig. 4-20). The superomedial segment is crossed by the tendon of the flexor hallucis longus (Fig. 4-21).

(Text continues on p. 157.)

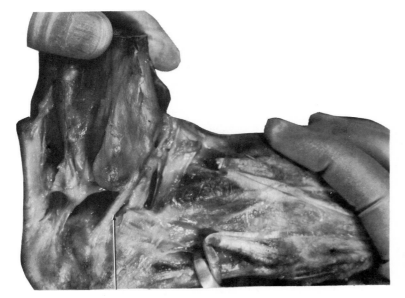

Fig. 4-16.   Obliquity of the calcaneofibular ligament (arrows). (*A*) In neutral position of the ankle. (*B*) In plantar flexion. (*C*) In dorsiflexion.

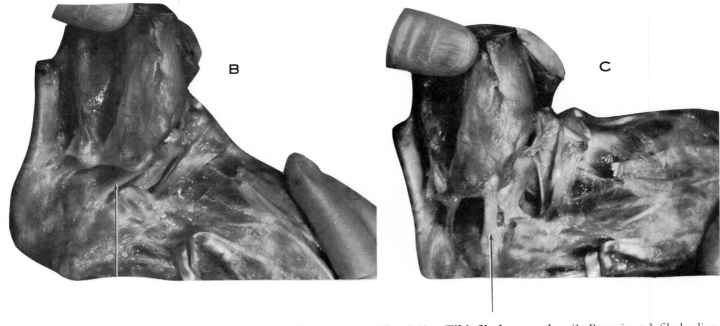

Fig. 4-18.   Tibiofibular mortise. (1, Posterior talofibular ligament; 2 calcaneofibular ligament; 3, anterior talofibular ligament, major component; 4, anterior talofibular ligament, accessory component.)

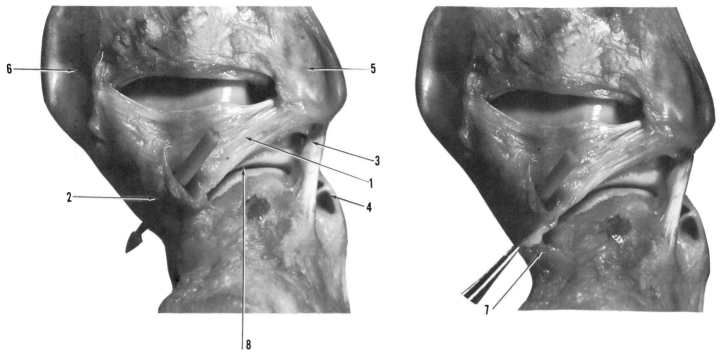

Fig. 4-17.   Posterior aspect of the ankle. (1, Posterior talofibular ligament; 2, fibrous tunnel of the flexor hallucis longus tendon; 3, calcaneofibular ligament; 4, inferior peroneal retinaculum; 5, sulcus of the peronei tendons on posterior surface of the lateral malleolus; 6, sulcus of tibialis posterior tendon on posterior aspect of the medial malleolus; 7, posterior talocalcaneal ligament; 8, posterior calcaneal articular interline.)

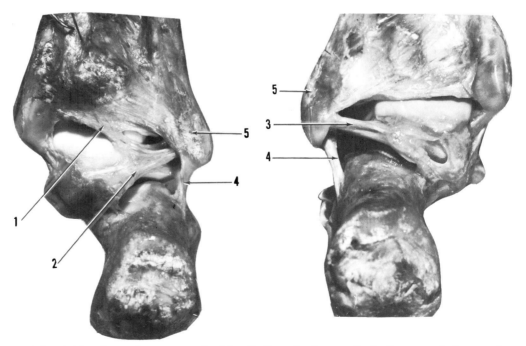

Fig. 4-19.   Posterior aspect of ankle. (1, Posterior intermalleolar ligament; 2, 3, posterior talofibular ligament; 4, calcaneofibular ligament; 5, lateral malleolus.)

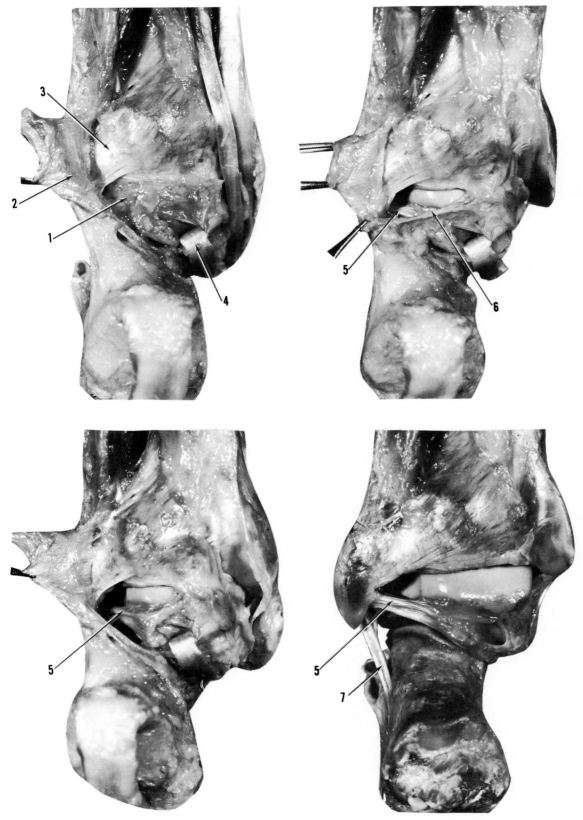

Fig. 4–20.   Posterior aspect of ankle. (1, Adipose tissue and capsule covering the posterior talofibular ligament; 2, ligament of Rouvière Canela Lazaro; 3, posterior tibiofibular ligament; 4, reflected tendon of flexor hallucis longus; 5, posterior talofibular ligament; 6, reflected posterior capsule; 7, calcaneofibular ligament.)

Fibulotalocalcaneal Ligament

The fibulotalocalcaneal ligament of Rouvière and Canela Lazaro (Figs. 4-22–4-24) is an extrinsic ligament that occupies the posterolateral corner of the ankle and posterior subtalar joints. In 1924, Dujarier described briefly and produced a clear illustration of a posterior fibulocalcaneal ligament arising from the posterior aspect of the lateral malleolus and inserting on the posterosuperior aspect of the calcaneus laterally.[8] He qualified this ligament as being abnormal and mentioned that in certain clubfeet, this ligament is considerably developed, forming the posterior fibulocalcaneal ligament of Bessel-Hagen (Fig. 4-25).

In 1932, Rouvière and Canela Lazaro, in a comprehensive study, described the peroneotalocalcaneal ligament.[9] This ligament is independent of the capsules and ligaments of the neighboring joints. It originates from the medial border of the peroneal groove located on the posterior border of the lateral malleolus, in common with the origin of the posterior tibiofibular ligament. Inferiorly, the origin may descend to the tip of the lateral malleolus and quite frequently may reach the origin of the calcaneofibular ligament.

At the origin, the peroneotalocalcaneal ligament is in close connection with the fibrous sheath of the peronei but soon separates from it and is directed downward, medially and posteriorly. This flat structure then divides into two fibrous laminae; superomedial and inferolateral. The superomedial lamina or talar component inserts on the posterolateral tubercle of the talus and contributes to the formation of the flexor hallucis longus fibrous tunnel. The inferolateral or peroneocalcaneal lamina is the major component of the ligament. It is directed downward and posteriorly, enlarges, and inserts nearly transversely on the entire width of the superior surface of the calcaneus. At times the calcaneal insertion is oblique, directed forward and medially. In approximately two thirds of the cases, the insertion remains localized to the superior surface of the calcaneus or reaches the lateral surface of the os calcis; the lateral border of the ligament is then separated by a small interval from the insertion of the calcaneofibular ligament. In the remaining one third, the calcaneal insertion clearly extends to the lateral calcaneal surface and blends with the insertion of the calcaneofibular ligament.

The frequency of occurrence of this ligament is 60% present as a well-defined ligament, 20% present as a thin, weak structure but with ligamentous texture, 20% absent and replaced by a thin fascia.[9] Occasionally both components of the ligament are united, forming a continuous lamina.

On close analysis and as described by Rouvière and Canela Lazaro, the fibulotalocalcaneal ligament is the very thick inferior and suscalcaneal portion of the deep aponeurosis of the leg between the tunnel of the flexor hallucis longus and the tunnel of the peronei.[9] This ligament limits the dorsiflexion of the foot.

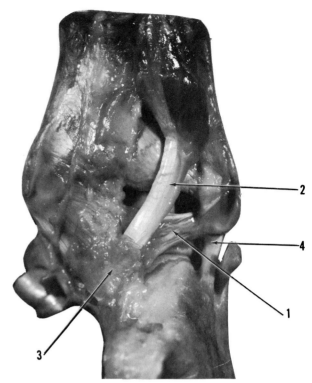

Fig. 4-21. Posterior aspect of ankle. (1, Posterior talofibular ligament crossed by the flexor hallucis longus tendon [2]; 3, tunnel of flexor hallucis longus; 4, calcaneofibular ligament.)

MEDIAL LIGAMENT OR DELTOID LIGAMENT

The medial malleolus provides attachment to the ligaments necessary to stabilize the talus and the naviculocalcaneal complex medially (Fig. 4-26, A). The insertion of the talotibial fibers are concentrated on the posteromedial aspect of the talus, whereas the peritalar fibers insert mainly on the sustentaculum tali.

The remaining fibers of the ligament have received variable acceptance as ligaments, due to the relative strength to qualify them; this applies particularly to the superficial anterior talotibial ligament.

The interpretation of the disposition of the fibers of the medial ligament as being one or two layers (superficial and deep) has brought forth a plethora of descriptions (Fig. 4-26, B–E). On close examination, if one accepts the element of variability with regards to the lesser components of this ligament, the descriptions then fall into a harmonious pattern.

(Text continues on p. 164.)

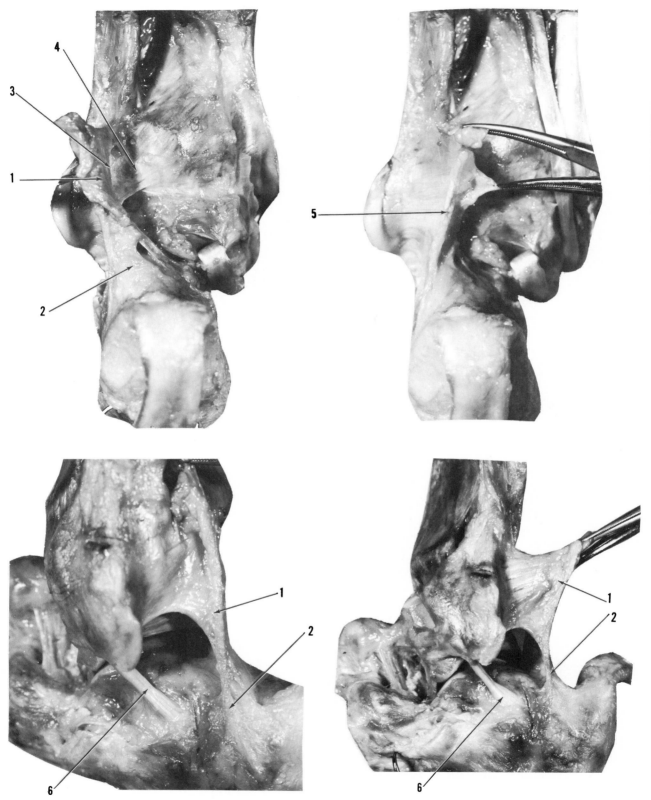

Fig. 4-22. Fibulotalocalcaneal ligament. (1, Fibulotalocalcaneal ligament of Rouvière Canela Lazaro; 2, calcaneal insertion of [1]; 3, common origin of [1] with the posterior tibiofibular ligaments [4]; 5, connection of [1] with superior peroneal retinaculum; 6, calcaneofibular ligament.)

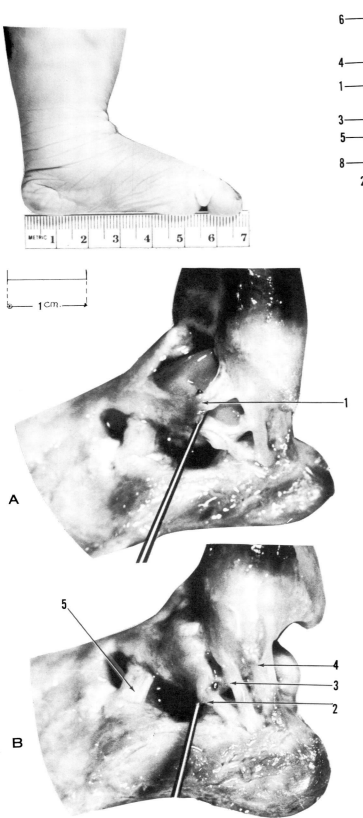

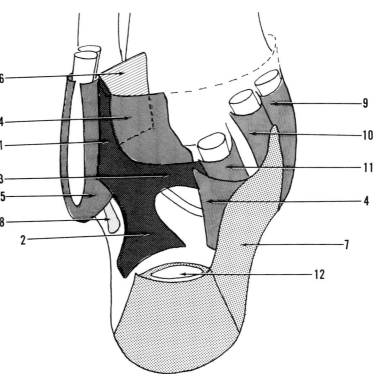

Fig. 4-23. Fibulotalocalcaneal ligament. (1, Stem of fibulo-talocalcaneal ligament of Rouvière Canela Lazaro; 2, calcaneal component, inferolateral, of [1]; 3, talar component, superomedial, of [1]; 4, deep crural aponeurosis; 5, retinaculum of peronei tendons; 6, posterior tibiofibular ligament; 7, superficial crural aponeurosis; 8, calcaneal insertion of calcaneofibular ligament; 9, tunnel of tibialis posterior tendon; 10, tunnel of flexor digitorum longus; 11, tunnel of flexor hallucis longus; 12, Achilles tendon.)

Fig. 4-24. Foot of a fetus. (A, B, C,) Ligaments of lateral aspect of the ankle. (1, Anterior talofibular ligament lifted by probe in (A); 2 lateral talocalcaneal ligament lifted by probe in (B); 3, calcaneofibular ligament; 4, ligament of Rouvière Canela Lazaro [posterior calcaneofibular] lifted by probe in (C); 5, cervical ligament.)

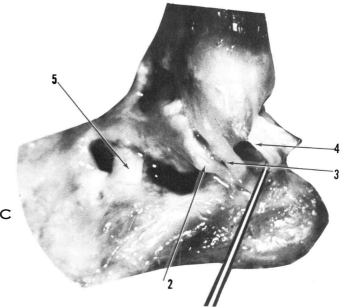

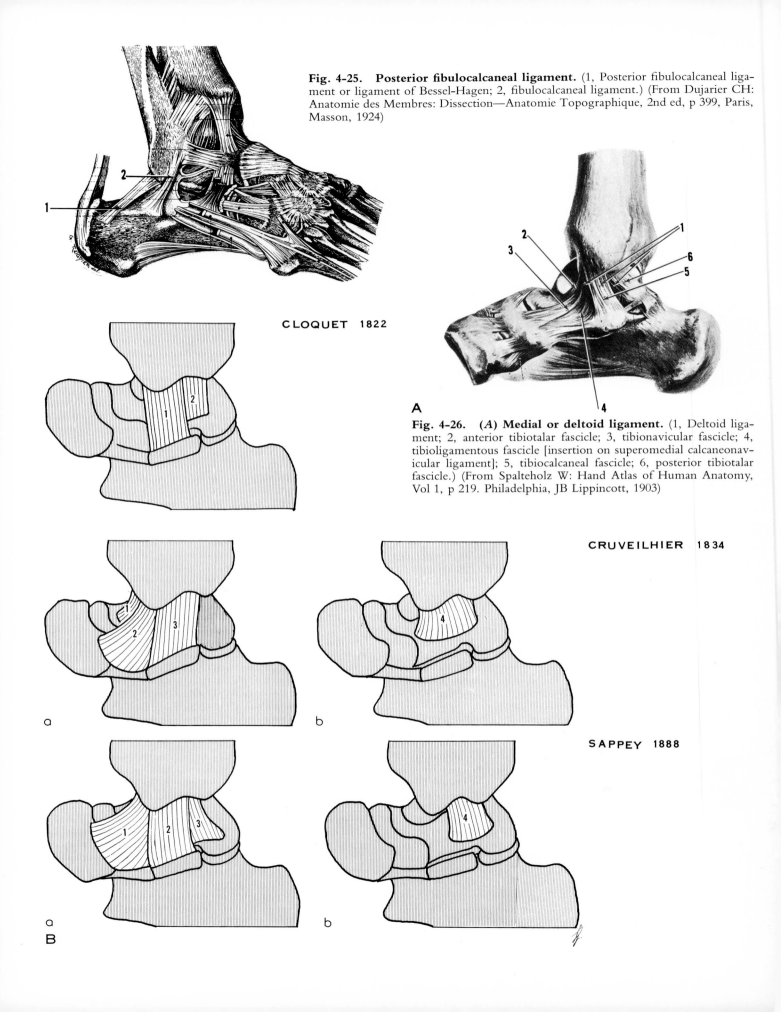

Fig. 4-25. Posterior fibulocalcaneal ligament. (1, Posterior fibulocalcaneal ligament or ligament of Bessel-Hagen; 2, fibulocalcaneal ligament.) (From Dujarier CH: Anatomie des Membres: Dissection—Anatomie Topographique, 2nd ed, p 399, Paris, Masson, 1924)

CLOQUET 1822

A

Fig. 4-26. (A) Medial or deltoid ligament. (1, Deltoid ligament; 2, anterior tibiotalar fascicle; 3, tibionavicular fascicle; 4, tibioligamentous fascicle [insertion on superomedial calcaneonavicular ligament]; 5, tibiocalcaneal fascicle; 6, posterior tibiotalar fascicle.) (From Spalteholz W: Hand Atlas of Human Anatomy, Vol 1, p 219. Philadelphia, JB Lippincott, 1903)

CRUVEILHIER 1834

SAPPEY 1888

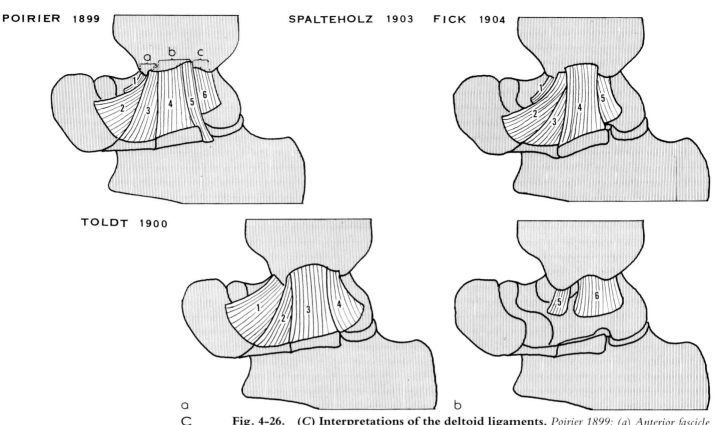

POIRIER 1899

SPALTEHOLZ 1903 FICK 1904

TOLDT 1900

a

b

C

Fig. 4-26. **(C) Interpretations of the deltoid ligaments.** *Poirier 1899: (a) Anterior fascicle* or anterior tibiotalar. Origin, anterior border of medial malleolus; insertion, superficial fibers to superior surface of scaphoid (2), deep fibers to medial surface of talar neck (1) and on inferior calcaneonavicular ligament (3). *(b) Middle fascicle* or tibiocalcaneal. Origin, cutaneous surface of medial malleolus near its apex; insertion, middle fibers to sustentaculum tali (4), anterior fibers on inferior calcaneonavicular ligament (3), posterior fibers on calcaneal canal behind sustentaculum tali (5). *(c) Posterior fascicle* or posterior tibiotalar. Origin, at bifurcation of apex of medial malleolus; insertion, medial surface talus under tibial facet (6). *Toldt 1900:(a) Superficial: Tibionavicular ligament:* origin, anterior border of medial malleolus; insertion, navicular and dorsal calcaneonavicular ligament (1); *Calcaneotibial ligament:* origin, medial subcutaneous surface of medial malleolus; insertion, inferior calcaneonavicular ligament (2), sustentaculum tali (3), medial tubercle of talus (4). *(b) Deep: Anterior talotibial ligament;* origin, apex of medial malleolus; insertion, medial aspect of neck of talus under large segment of articular surface (5); *Posterior talotibial ligament:* origin, posterior border and fossa of medial malleolus; insertion, medial surface of talus, mid and posterior segment (6). *Spalteholz 1903-Fick 1904:* Several layers, divisible according to the lower attachment. *Anterior talotibial ligament:* origin, tip of medial malleolus; insertion, below anterior portion of medial articular surface of talus (1). Most of ligament is hidden under tibionavicular and calcaneotibial ligaments. *Tibionavicular ligament:* origin, medial surface of medial malleolus just above origin of anterior talotibial ligament; insertion, dorsal and medial aspect of navicular (2) and medial margin of plantar calcaneonavicular ligament (3). At origin, ligament is partially hidden beneath calcaneotibial ligament. *Calcaneo-tibial ligament:* (most superficial component): origin, medial surface of medial malleolus; insertion, sustentaculum tali (4). *Posterior talotibial ligament:* origin, behind tip of medial malleolus; insertion, on medial aspect of talus, mid and posterior segment reaching the posteromedial tubercle of talus (5).

◀ **Fig. 4-26.** **(B) Interpretations of the deltoid ligament.** *Cloquet 1822:* Origin, apex of medial malleolus and its depression; insertion, medial aspect of talus (2), calcaneus (1); few fibers to fibrous tunnel of flexor digitorum longus. *Cruveilhier 1834:(a) Superficial.* Origin, apex and borders of medial malleolus; insertion, talus neck (1), scaphoid (2), inferior calcaneoscaphoid ligament (2), calcaneus (3). *(b) Deep.* Origin: Apex and borders of medial malleolus. Insertion: Entire medial aspect talus under articular cartilage. *Sappey 1888:(a) Superficial.* Anterior: origin, anterior border of medial malleolus; insertion, scaphoid (1), inferior calcaneoscaphoid ligament (1). Posterior: origin, apex of medial malleolus; insertion, sustentaculum tali (2), tubercle of posterior aspect of talus (3) medial to tunnel of flexor hallucis longus. *(b) Deep.*(4) Origin, fossa occupying apex of medial malleolus; insertion, imprint on posterior extremity of medial talar surface.

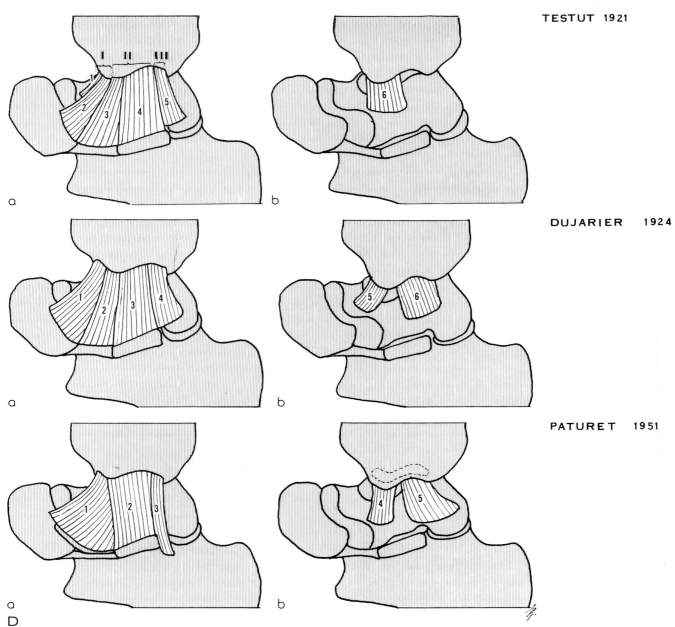

TESTUT 1921

DUJARIER   1924

PATURET   1951

Fig. 4-26.   (D) Interpretations of the deltoid ligament. *Testut 1921:* (*a*) *Superficial:* Origin, from inferior border and fossa of medial malleolus; insertion, I, *Anterior fibers:* talar neck (1), superior surface of scaphoid (2). II,*Middle fibers:* inferior calcaneonavicular ligament (3), sustentaculum tali (4). III, *Posterior fibers:* posteromedial talar tubercle (5). (*b*) *Deep:* Origin, apex of medial malleolus; insertion, medial surface of talus below articular surface. *Dujarier 1924:* (*a*) *Superficial:* Origin, anterior and medial surface of medial malleolus; *Insertion, anterior fibers,* navicular (1); *middle fibers,* inferior calcaneonavicular ligament (2), sustentaculum tali (3); *posterior fibers,* occasionally present and inserting on posteromedial tubercle of talus (4); (*b*) *Deep: Anterior tibiotalar ligament* (Very thin, capsular): origin, anterior border and apex of medial malleolus; insertion, talar neck (5). *Posterior tibiotalar ligament:* origin, apex and sulcus of medial malleolus; insertion, round facet below and posterior to medial articular surface of talus (6). *Paturet 1951:* (*a*) *Superficial:* Origin, anterior border and medial surface of medial malleolus; insertion, *anterior fibers,* Superior and medial surface navicular (1), medial surface of neck of talus, superior talonavicular ligament (1); *middle fibers,* inferior calcaneonavicular ligament, sustentaculum tali (2); *posterior fibers* (less numerous), medial surface of calcaneus, posterior to sustencalum tali, reaching upper part of calcaneal canal (3). (*b*) *Deep:* Origin, apex and posterior part of medial malleolus; insertion, *anterior fibers,* medial surface of talus below comma-shaped articular surface (4); *Posterior fibers,* on posteromedial tubercle, reaching tunnel of flexor hallucis longus (5).

GRAY 1954 – 1973

YASHAR 1961

PANKOVICH & SHIVARAM 1979

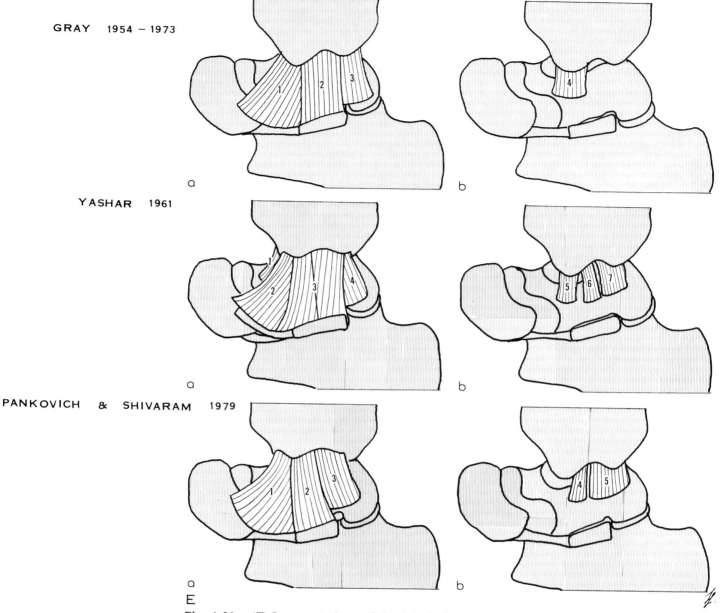

E

Fig. 4-26. (E) Interpretations of the deltoid ligament. *Gray 1954–1973: (a) Superficial:* Origin, apex, anterior and posterior borders of medial malleolus; insertion, *tibionavicular,* on navicular and plantar calcaneonavicular ligament (1); *calcaneotibial,* on sustentaculum (2); *posterior talotibial,* medial surface of talus and posterior medial tubercle (3). *(b) Deep* (anterior talotibial): Origin, tip of medial malleolus; insertion, medial surface of talus (4). *Yashar 1961: (a) Superficial: Anterior and superficial tibiotalar fascicle* (1): origin, anterior border of medial malleolus; insertion, inner surface of talar neck; *Tibioscaphoid fascicle* (2): origin, anterior border of medial malleolus; insertion, scaphoid superior surface and medial calcaneoscaphoid ligament; *Tibioligamentous ligament:* origin, medial malleolus above apex; insetion, medial calcaneoscaphoid ligament and sustenaculum tali (3); *Tibiocalcaneal:* origin, medial surface of medial malleolus; insertion, posterior segment of sustentaculum tali (3); *Posterior and superficial talotibial ligament:* origin, medial surface of medial malleolus; insertion, medial aspect of talus, posteromedial talar tubercle (4). *(b) Deep: Deep anterior tibiotalar ligament:* origin, apex of medial malleolus; insertion, medial surface of talus (5); *Deep posterior tibiotalar ligament:* origin (2 portions): posterior border of anterior colliculus, intercollicular groove, posterior colliculus; insertion, medial surface of talus, posterior segment (6 and 7). *Pankovich and Shivaram 1979: (a) Superficial: Tibionavicular:* origin, anterior colliculus; insertion, dorsomedial aspect of navicular and plantar calcaneonavicular ligament (1); *Tibiocalcaneal ligament:* origin, midportion of medial surface of anterior colliculus; insertion, medial border of sustentaculum tali (2); *Superficial talotibial ligament;* origin, posterior part of medial surface of anterior colliculus and adjacent part of posterior colliculus; insertion, anterior portion of medial talar tubercle (3). *(b) Deep: Deep anterior talotibial ligament:* origin, intercollicular groove and adjoining anterior colliculus; insertion, medial surface of talus near its neck (4); *Deep posterior talotibial ligament:* origin, intercollicular groove and inferior segment of posterior colliculus; insertion, medial surface of talus from medial tubercle to posterior third of articular surface of talar trochlea (5).

A practical understanding of this ligament requires the consideration of a few points:

The entire medial ligamentous complex is invested, expect in the very anterior part, by the deep crural fascia in continuity with the flexor retinaculum (Figs. 4-27 and 4-28).

The anterior border of the ligament is covered by the tibialis anterior tendon with its underlying adipose tissue. This anterior border is in continuity laterally with the thin anterior capsule.

A major segment—mid and posterior—of the ligament is covered by the obliquely crossing tibialis posterior and flexor digitorum longus tendons. The fibrosynovial floors of these tunnels blend with the underlying

ligament (Figs. 4-29 and 4-30); minute dissection usually is necessary to separate the two.

The medial ligament, except for its deep talotibial component, is a continuous fibrous lamina, and any division into components is usually artificial (Figs. 4-31–4-33). It is only by referring to the insertion of the fibers that descriptive differentiation is possible.

Posteriorly, the ligament is in continuity with the posterior capsule and the posterior talofibular ligament.

The medial ligament is divided into two layers, superficial and deep, each being formed by multiple fascicles. The superficial layer or deltoid ligament is broad and triangular. For the purpose of description the following components are considered.

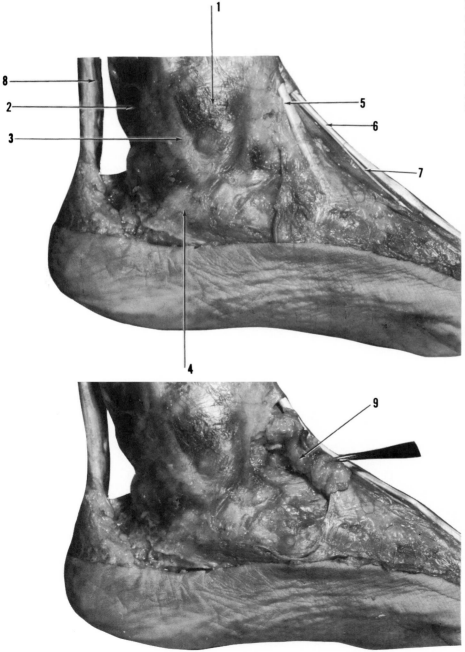

Fig. 4-27. Medial aspect of ankle. (1, Medial malleolus covered by superficial aponeurosis cruris and flexor aponeurosis; 2, deep aponeurosis cruris covering the fibrous tunnel of the tibialis posterior tendon [3]; 4, flexor retinaculum; 5, tibialis anterior tendon; 6, extensor hallucis longus tendon; 7, accessory band of [6]; 8, Achilles tendon; 9, retrotibialis anterior tendon fat pad being reflected.)

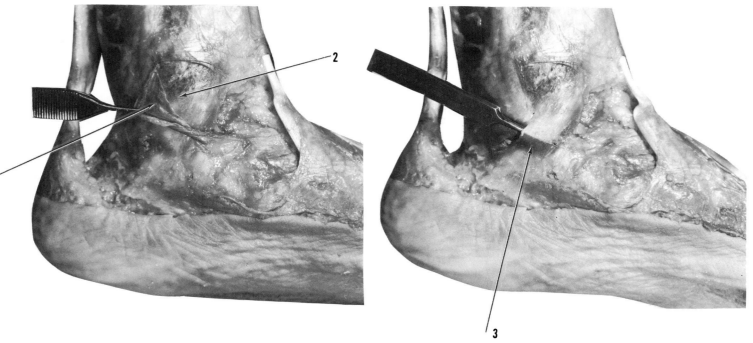

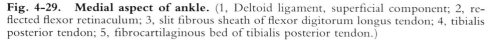

Fig. 4-28. Medial aspect of ankle. (1, Reflected superficial aponeurosis cruris; 2, medial aponeurosis and origin of flexor retinaculum; 3, flexor retinaculum lifted with tissue forceps.)

Fig. 4-29. Medial aspect of ankle. (1, Deltoid ligament, superficial component; 2, reflected flexor retinaculum; 3, slit fibrous sheath of flexor digitorum longus tendon; 4, tibialis posterior tendon; 5, fibrocartilaginous bed of tibialis posterior tendon.)

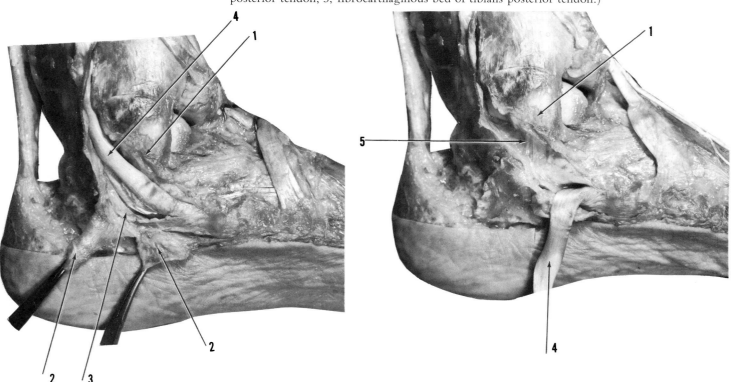

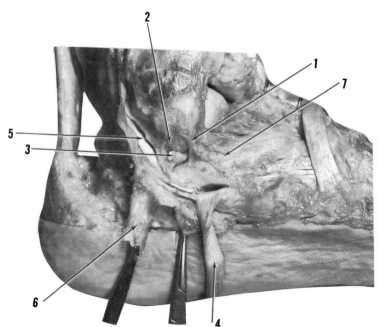

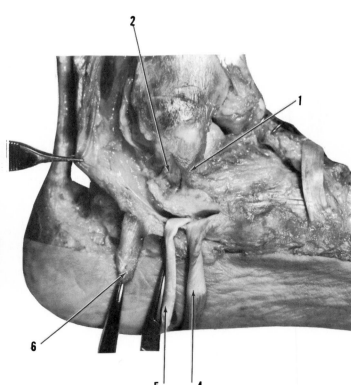

Fig. 4-30.   Medial aspect of ankle. (1, Deltoid ligament, talonavicular and taloligamentous component; 2, deltoid ligament, talocalcaneal ligament separation from [1] with fat pad [3]; 4, tibialis posterior tendon; 5, flexor digitorum longus tendon; 6, reflected flexor retinaculum; 7, superomedial calcaneonavicular ligament.)

Fig. 4-31.   Medial aspect of ankle. (1, Deltoid ligament, tibionavicular component; 2, deltoid ligament, tibioligamentous component, reflected; 3, deltoid ligament, tibiocalcaneal component; 4, interfascicular fat pad; 5, interval occupied by [4].)

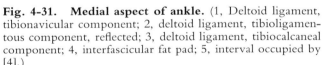

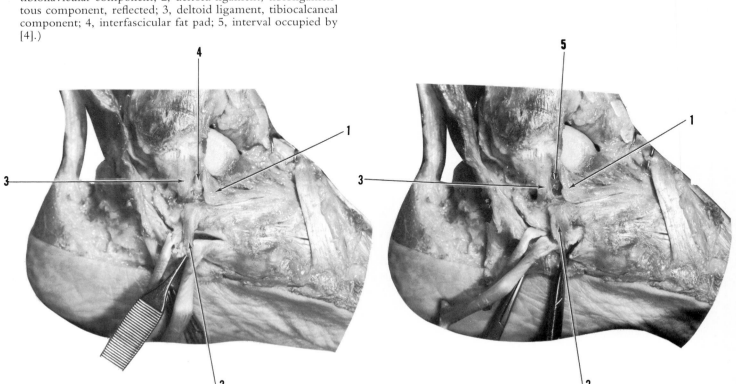

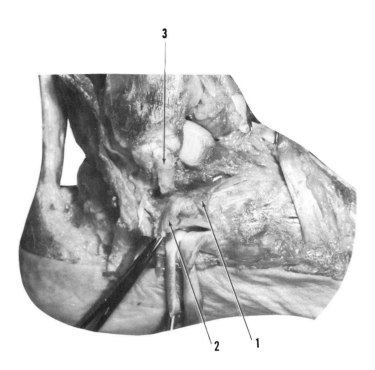

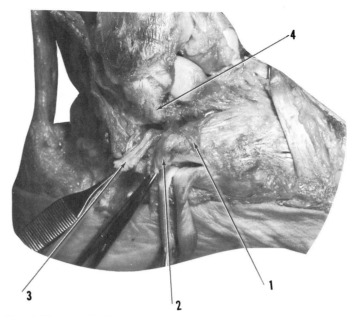

Fig. 4-32.   Medial aspect of ankle. (1, Deltoid ligament, talonavicular component, reflected; 2, deltoid ligament, taloligamentous component reflected; 3, deltoid ligament, talocalcaneal ligament; 4, deltoid ligament, deep talotibial component.)

Anterior Superficial Tibiotalar Fascicle and Tibionavicular Fascicle

These two ligaments (Fig. 4-34) have a common origin on the anterior border of the anterior colliculus. The fibers of origin extend to the medial corner of the anterior margin of the tibial quadrilateral inferior articular surface. As specified by Beau, the fibers delineate an anterolateral concave border and farther distally divide into two layers.[10] The deep fibers insert on the dorsum of the talar neck slightly posterior to the talar head and to the talonavicular capsule; this component is the anterior and superficial tibiotalar ligament. The superficial fibers extend beyond the talonavicular interline and insert on the dorsomedial aspect of the navicular in a curvilinear fashion, extending medially a very short distance from the articular margin; this component is the tibionavicular ligament. The two ligaments overlap except at the most median site, where the talar fibers do not extend onto the navicular.

Tibioligamentous Fascicle

The tibioligamentous fascicle originates from the anterior segment of the anterior colliculus. The fibers present a gentle anterior concavity and insert on the superior border of the superomedial calcaneonavicular ligament. The anterior superficial tibiotalar fascicle, the tibionavicular fascicle, and the tibioligamentous fascicle constitute the broader but weaker component of the medial ligament (Fig. 4-35).

Tibiocalcaneal Ligament

The tibiocalcaneal ligament (Fig. 4-36) is the strongest superficial component. It originates from the medial aspect of the anterior colliculus, descends vertically, and inserts on the medial border of the sustentaculum tali after interlacing its fibers with those of the superomedial calcaneonavicular ligament.[11] This ligament is in continuity with the preceding tibioligamentous.fascicle. In certain specimens, the origin of the latter overlaps the origin of the tibiocalcaneal ligament, and the interval is filled with adipose tissue. The tibiocalcaneal ligament measures approximately 1 cm in width at the origin and 1.5 cm at the insertion. The average length is 2 cm to 3 cm and the thickness 2 mm to 3 mm. It is a substantial structure.

Superficial Posterior Tibiotalar Ligament

The superficial posterior tibiotalar ligament originates from the posterior part of the medial surface of the anterior colliculus and the medial surface of the posterior colliculus (Fig. 4-37). The fibers are directed posteriorly, inferiorly, and laterally and insert on the posteromedial talar tubercle, reaching the flexor hallucis longus tunnel.[3, 12–16] The posterior border of the tibiocalcaneal ligament is distinct from this ligament or the two may be in continuity; if they are in continuity, the superficial layer is represented as a large, fibrous, fan-shaped lamina deserving the "deltoid" denomination. The superficial posterior tibiotalar ligament is separated from the underlying posterior deep tibiotalar ligament with adipose tissue (more so anteriorly) and is in continuity along its superolateral border with the posterior talotibial capsule and the posterior talofibular ligament. The occasional absence of this ligament or its fusion to the deep talotibial ligament accounts for some of the variations in description.

(Text continues on p. 172.)

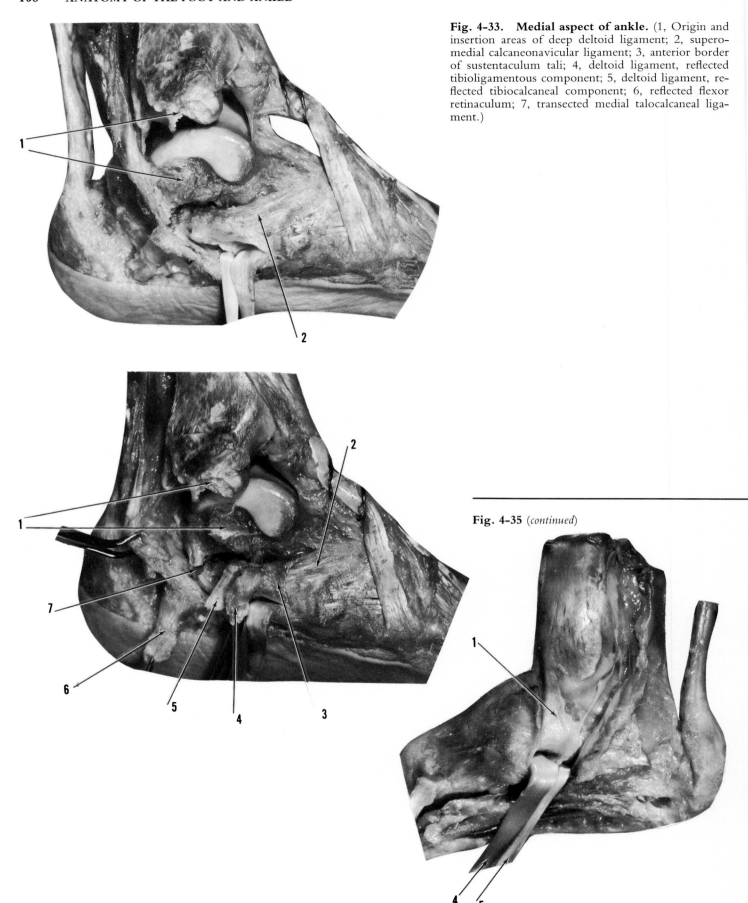

Fig. 4-33.   Medial aspect of ankle. (1, Origin and insertion areas of deep deltoid ligament; 2, superomedial calcaneonavicular ligament; 3, anterior border of sustentaculum tali; 4, deltoid ligament, reflected tibioligamentous component; 5, deltoid ligament, reflected tibiocalcaneal component; 6, reflected flexor retinaculum; 7, transected medial talocalcaneal ligament.)

Fig. 4-35 (continued)

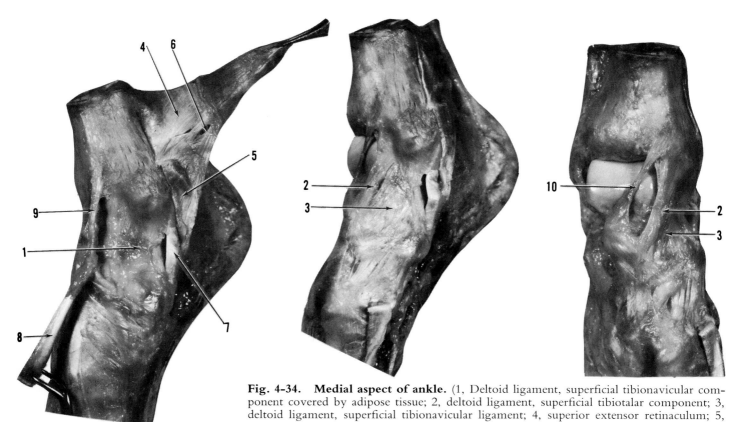

Fig. 4-34.   Medial aspect of ankle. (1, Deltoid ligament, superficial tibionavicular component covered by adipose tissue; 2, deltoid ligament, superficial tibiotalar component; 3, deltoid ligament, superficial tibionavicular ligament; 4, superior extensor retinaculum; 5, flexor retinaculum in continuity with [4]; 6, tunnel of tibialis anterior tendon; 7, tibialis posterior tendon; 8, reflected tibialis anterior tendon; 9, deep attachment of oblique superomedial band of inferior extensor retinaculum; 10, anterior talotibial ligament.)

Fig. 4-35.   Medial aspect of ankle. (1, Deltoid ligament, tibioligamentous component; 2, deltoid ligament, tibionavicular and superficial tibiotalar components; 3, superomedial calcaneonavicular ligament covered by fibrocartilage; 4, reflected tibialis posterior tendon; 5, reflected flexor digitorum longus tendon.)

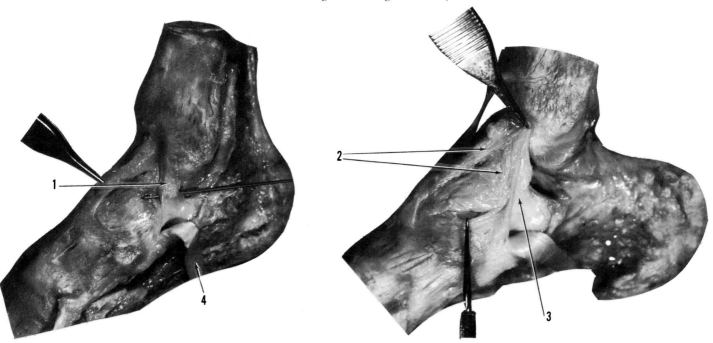

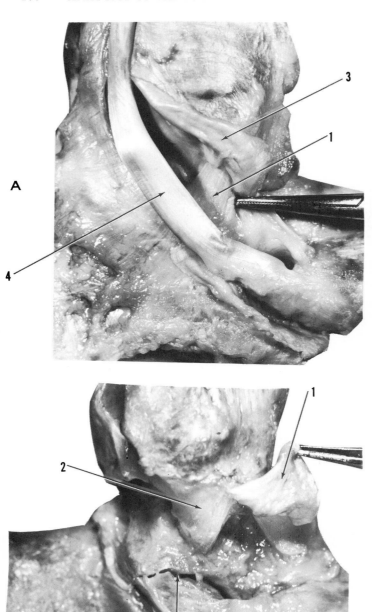

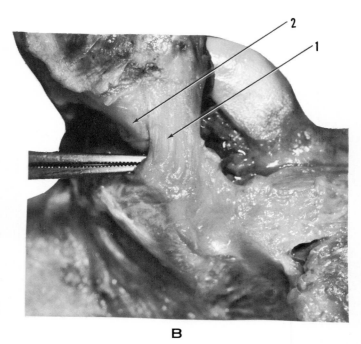

Fig. 4-36.   Medial aspect of ankle. (*A*) Deltoid ligament, tibiocalcaneal component (1), crossed by tibialis posterior tendon (4), exposed by reflecting its sheath and the aponeurosis cruris, superficial and deep, forming the flexor retinaculum (3). (*B*) Deltoid ligament, tibiocalcaneal component (1), covering deep tibiotalar component (2). (*C*) Reflected talocalcaneal component (1) of deltoid ligament exposing deep tibiotalar component (2) of deltoid ligament. (5, Medial and posterior talocalcaneal articular interline.)

Fig. 4-37.   Posteromedial aspect of ankle. (*A*) (1, Superficial and posterior tibiotalar component of deltoid ligament; 2, open tunnel of tibialis posterior tendon formed of fibrocartilage; 3, open tunnel of flexor digitorum longus tendon; 4, open tunnel of flexor hallucis longus tendon; 5, tunnel of flexor hallucis longus on posterior aspect of talus; 6, line indicating direction of flexor hallucis longus tendon.) (*B*) (1, Incised superficial and posterior tibiotalar component of deltoid ligament; 2, inferior calcaneonavicular ligament.) (*C*) (1, Reflected superficial and posterior tibiotalar component of deltoid ligament exposing deep posterior talotibial component [2].) (*D*) Detached superficial (1) and deep (2) fascicles of posterior talotibial component of deltoid ligament.

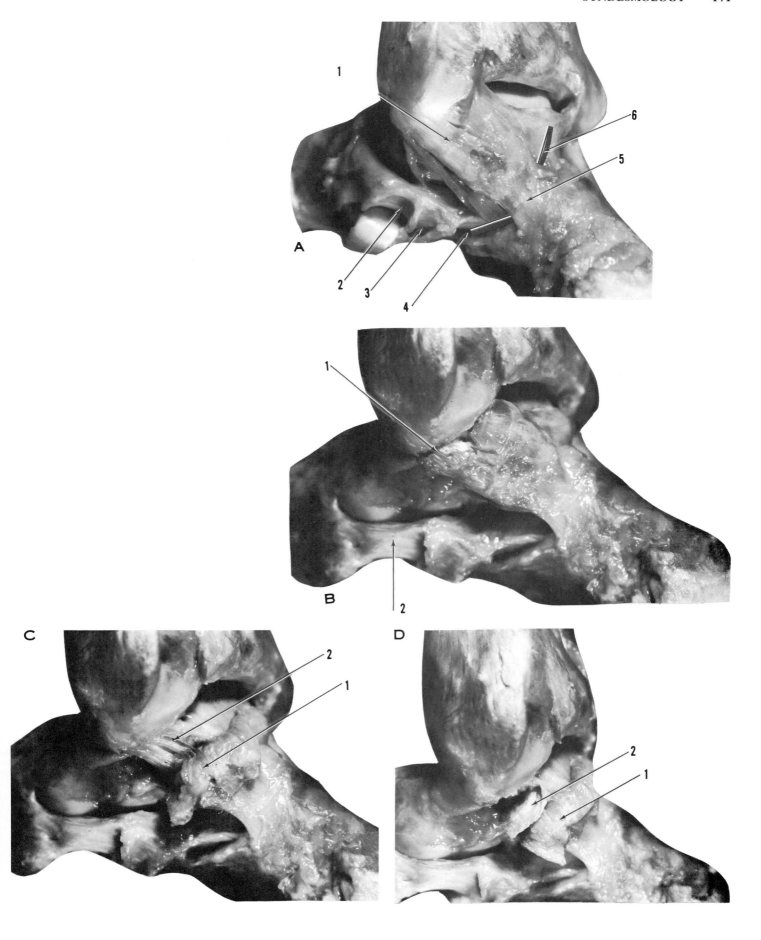

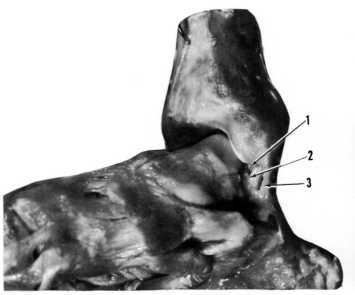

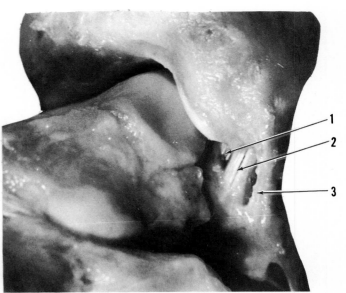

Fig. 4-38.   Deltoid ligament. (1, 2, Fasciculated deep component, talotibial; 3, superficial tibiocalcaneal component.)

Fig. 4-39.   Calcaneonavicularcuboid complex. (1, Lateral calcaneonavicular ligament; 2, medial calcaneocuboid ligament; 3, dorsolateral calcaneocuboid ligament; 4, sinus tarsi; 5, canalis tarsi; 6, navicular articular surface for talar head; 7, inferior calcaneonavicular ligament; 8, medial and anterior articular surfaces of os calcis; 9, posterior articular surface of os calcis; 10, inferior peroneal retinaculum.)

Deep Layer of Deltoid Ligament

The deep layer of the deltoid ligament (Fig. 4-37) is short and strong. It is formed by a small anterior and a very strong posterior component.[7, 13, 15, 16]

Deep Anterior Tibiotalar Ligament.   The deep anterior tibiotalar ligament originates from the tip of the anterior colliculus and the anterior part of the intercollicular groove and inserts on the medial surface of the talus distal to the anterior segment of the comma-shaped talar articular surface. This ligament is "of variable size in different specimens, sometimes hardly discernible, and in some cases completely absent."[16]

Deep Posterior Tibiotalar Ligament.   The deep posterior tibiotalar ligament is the strongest component of the entire medial ligament. In most cases, it is conical, with the base superior and the apex posteroinferior. The approximate measurements are 1.5 cm width at origin, 1 cm width at insertion, 1.5 cm length, and 1 cm thickness at origin. The size of the ligament is variable. The thickness varies from 0.5 cm to 1.5 cm and the width from 1.5 cm to 2 cm.[2, 17]

This ligament originates from the intercollicular fossa (which measures about 1 cm in width), the entire anterior surface of the posterior colliculus, and the upper segment of the posterior surface of the anterior colliculus. The fibers are directed downward, posteriorly, and laterally and insert on the medial surface of the talus on an oval elevation located under the tail of the comma-shaped articular surface. The insertion reaches the posteromedial talar tubercle. This intra-articular but extrasynovial ligament may be fasciculated (Fig. 4-38) or divided into two distinct bands.[15] Beau, in his comprehensive study of the ligaments of the ankle, considers this ligament as the homologue of the posterior talofibular ligament and describes it, not as a medial ligament, but as a posterior ligament of the ankle, bracing the talus posteriorly.[10]

Anterior Tibiotalar Fascicle, Capsule, and Fat Pad.
The anterior capsule of the talotibial joint is thin, reinforced by an oblique fibrous band extending from the medial malleolus to the talar neck. This anterior tibiotalar fascicle (see Fig. 4-34) is narrow in the middle and broader at the origin and the insertion. The tibial attachment of the anterior capsule is 5 mm to 6 mm proximal to the articular margin (see Fig. 4-4). The talar insertion surrounds the cribriform fossa of the neck and is approximately 8 mm from the anterior trochlear margin. Laterally and medially, the anterior capsular insertion is close to the malleolar facets of the talus.

A prearticular fat pad is present anteriorly, extending transversely between the capsule and the tendons. This fat pad is thicker medially (see Fig. 4-26) and reinforces the anterior capsule.

Ligaments of the Calcaneonavicular Joint and Acetabulum Pedis

The head of the talus is received into a deep socket or acetabulum pedis formed by the navicular, the anterior and middle calcaneal articulating surfaces, the calcaneonavicular component of the bifurcate ligament, the superomedial calcaneonavicular ligament, and the plantar calcaneonavicular ligament (Figs. 4-39 and 4-40). The flexibility of the acetabulum pedis permits the adaptability in form and size of the containing socket as necessitated by the relative displacements of the talar head calcaneus and navicular.

SUPEROMEDIAL CALCANEONAVICULAR LIGAMENT

The superomedial calcaneonavicular ligament (ligamentum neglectum; Fig. 4-41) is illustrated by Bourgery and Jacob, analyzed and illustrated as a component of a common tibio-calcaneonavicular ligament by Henle, and described as an individual ligament by Lane.[18-20] A comprehensive study of the superomedial calcaneonavicular ligament was provided by Barclay-Smith, and a recent investigation is reported by Volkmann.[11, 21]

The superomedial calcaneonavicular ligament is quadrilateral, inseparable from the inferior calcaneonavicular ligament. It originates from the medial and anterior borders of the sustentaculum tali. This band is directed upward, anteriorly, and laterally, twists upon itself, winds around the medial segment of the talar head, and inserts on the superomedial aspect of the navicular and, to a lesser degree, on the lateral aspect of the tuberosity of the navicular. The tibionavicular, tibioligamentous, and tibiocalcaneal components of the superficial deltoid ligament interlace with it. The segment of the ligament that does not connect with the deltoid ligament blends with the superior talonavicular ligament. The superficial aspect of the ligament is further hidden by a thick fascial or fibrocartilanginous layer forming the floor of the tunnel of the crossing tibialis posterior tendon. As mentioned by Barclay-Smith, "it requires great care to dissect away this fascial stratum, and to remove the deposited cartilage, in order to expose the proper calcaneonavicular fibers."[11]

Fig. 4-40. Talocalcaneonavicular complex. (1, Talus; 2, navicular; 3, os calcis; 4, articular surface of navicular for talar head; 5, anterior calcaneal surface; 6, middle calcaneal surface; 7, inferior calcaneonavicular ligament; 8, superomedial calcaneonavicular ligament; 9, posterior calcaneal surface; 10, lateral calcaneonavicular ligament; 11, medial root of inferior extensor retinaculum blending with interosseous talocalcaneal ligament [12] of canalis tarsi; 13, cervical ligament.)

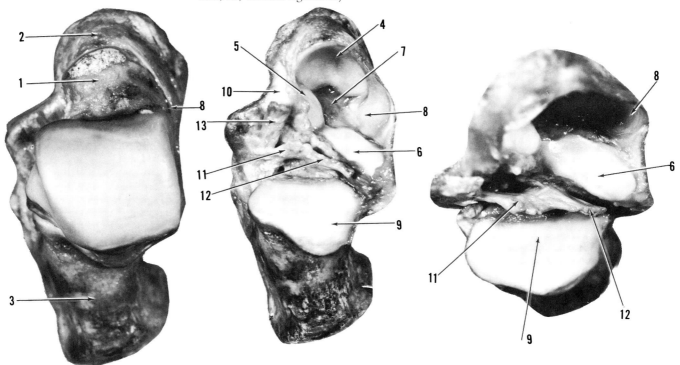

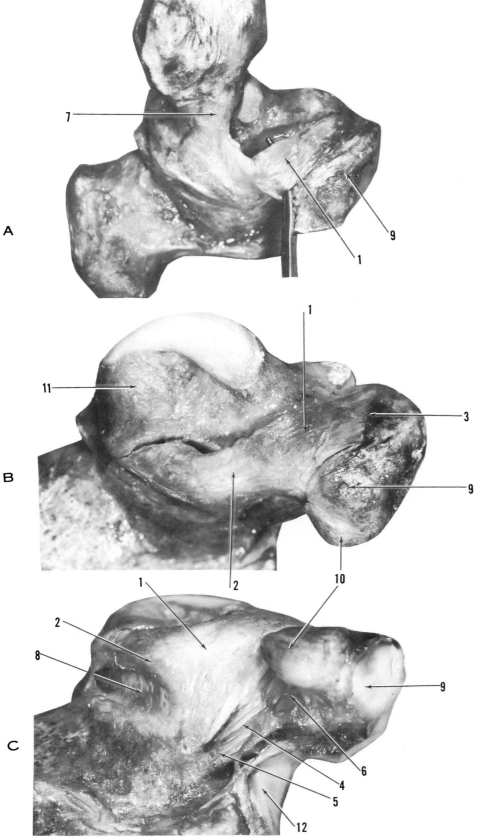

Fig. 4-41.   Superomedial calcaneonavicular ligament. (*A*) Medial view of ankle. (*B*) Medial view of talocalcaneonavicular complex. (*C*) Inferomedial view of talocalcaneonavicular complex. (1, Superomedial calcaneonavicular ligament; 2, origin.of [1] from anterior border of sustentaculum tali; 3, insertion of [1] on superomedial aspect of navicular; 4, inferior calcaneonavicular ligament; 5, origin of [4] from coronoid fossa of os calcis; 6, insertion of [4] on inferior segment of navicular; 7, deltoid ligament, tibiocalcaneal component; 8, canal of flexor hallucis longus tendon on inferior surface of sustentaculum tali; 9, navicular; 10, tuberosity of navicular; 11, talus; 12, cuboidal surface of os calcis.)

The articular surface of this thick ligament is smooth and fibrocartilaginous, giving support to the medial aspect of the talar head, not to the inferior.

INFERIOR CALCANEONAVICULAR LIGAMENT

The inferior calcaneonavicular ligament (spring ligament; Figs. 4-41 and 4-42) is trapezoidal and fasciculated and corresponds to the inferior segment of the talar head unsupported by the articular surfaces. It originates from the upper part of a small excavation, the coronoid cavity, located on the inferior surface of the calcaneus between the anterior border of the sustentaculum tali and the cuboidal articular surface. The thick bundle of fibers extends forward, fans out, and inserts on the inferior surface of the navicular. This ligament is very fasciculated, and the lateral bundle, the strongest inserts on the beak of the navicular. Longitudinal intervals are present between the bundles, and occasionally the ligament clearly has two components. A thick layer of adipose tissue covers the plantar aspect of the ligament, and the fat extends through the longitudinal interligamentous intervals into the joint cavity and is covered by synovial tissue. The medial border of the ligament is in continuity with the superomedial calcaneonavicular ligament.

LATERAL CALCANEONAVICULAR LIGAMENT AND BIFURCATE LIGAMENT

The bifurcate ligament (ligament of Chopart; Fig. 4-43) is formed by the lateral calcaneonavicular ligament and the medial calcaneocuboid ligament. This ligament is disposed in a V, and each component has a distinct origin on the os calcis.

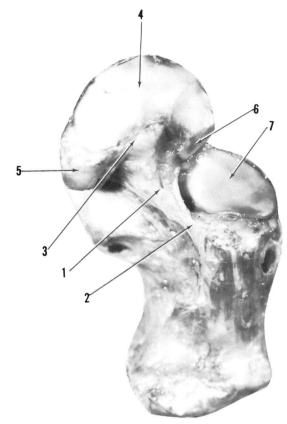

Fig. 4-42. Inferior view of calcaneonavicular complex. (1, Inferior calcaneonavicular ligament; 2, origin of [1] from coronoid fossa of os calcis; 3, insertion of [1] on inferior surface of navicular [4]; 5, tuberosity of navicular; 6, articular surface of navicular for cuboid; 7, articular surface of calcaneus for cuboid.)

Fig. 4-43. Dorsal view of mid tarsus and ankle joint. (1, Lateral calcaneonavicular ligament; 2, medial calcaneocuboid ligament; 3, dorsolateral calcaneocuboid ligament; 4, lateral calcaneocuboid ligament; 5, cervical ligament; 6, dorsal cubonavicular ligament; 7, dorsal cuneo₃cuboid ligament; 8, dorsal navicular-cuneo₃ ligament; 9, 10, intermediate and medial roots of inferior extensor retinaculum; 11, 12, anterior talofibular ligaments; 13, anterior tibiofibular ligament.)

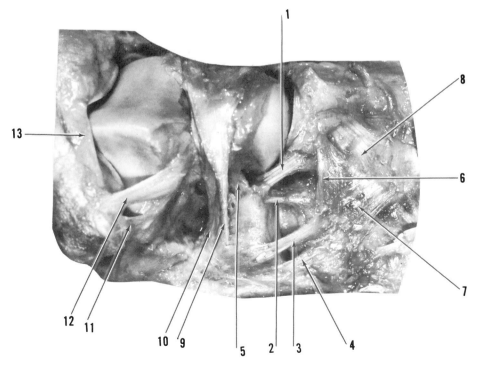

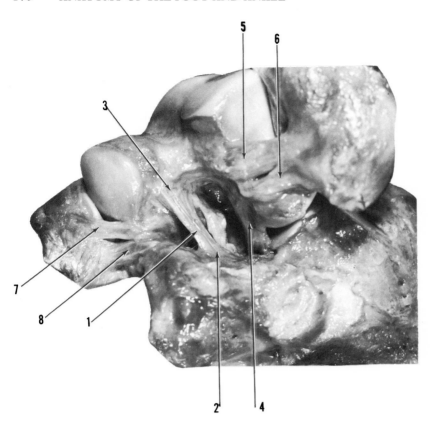

Fig. 4-44. Lateral view of sinus tarsi. (1, Cervical ligament; 2, origin of [1] from sinus tarsi; 3, insertion of [1] on talar neck; 4, capsule of posterior talocalcaneal joint; 5, 6, anterior talofibular ligaments; 7, 8, lateral calcaneonavicular ligaments.)

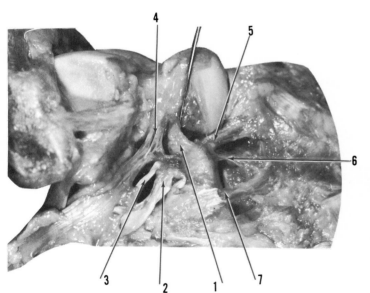

Fig. 4-45. Dorsolateral view of sinus tarsi. (1, Cervical ligament; 2, 3, intermediate and medial roots of inferior extensor retinaculum; 4, cervical attachment of medial root of inferior extensor retinaculum; 5, lateral calcaneonavicular ligament; 6, medial calcaneocuboid ligament; 7, dorsolateral calcaneocuboid ligament.)

The lateral calcaneonavicular ligament originates from the anteromedial corner of the sinus tarsi, immediately lateral to the facies articularis talaris anterior, and reaches the lateral aspect of a small tubercle (the intermediary tubercle).[22] The surface of origin measures approximately 1 cm.[22] The ligament extends anteriorly upward and medially and inserts on the posterosuperior segment of the lateral end of the navicular. The ligament measures an average of 2 cm to 2.5 cm in length and 1 cm in width.[23] Barclay-Smith considers two sets of fibers forming this ligament.[11] The inferior fibers are very short, fasciculated, and separated from the most lateral band of the inferior calcaneonavicular ligament by an interval filled with fat. The upper and the more superficial fibers are longer, stronger, and usually not fasciculated; they represent the main component of the ligament.

The medial calcaneocuboid ligament originates from the anterior aspect of the intermediary tubercle, lateral to the origin of the lateral calcaneonavicular ligament. It is directed anteriorly and slightly inferiorly and inserts on the dorsum of the cuboid 1.5 cm anterior to the posterior border of the cuboid.[23] This ligament measures approximately 1 cm in length and 0.5 cm in width.[23]

The two arms of the bifurcate ligament form an average angle of 30° in the transverse plane and an average angle of 20° in the vertical or sagittal plane.[23]

The lateral calcaneonavicular ligament is usually stronger than the calcaneocuboid component. The latter may be absent, and Köktürk provides the following information based on the dissection of 40 feet: both ligaments present in

57.5%, medial calcaneocuboid ligament absent in 40.0%, lateral calcaneonavicular ligament absent in 2.5%.[22]

Ligaments of the Talocalcaneonavicular Joints

The calcaneonavicular complex is a functional unit moving around the talus. All ligaments connecting the talus to this complex is a functional unit moving around the talus. All ligaments connecting the talus to this complex are considered as ligaments of the talocalcaneonavicular joint. The extracapsular ligaments of the sinus tarsi and tarsal canal are the major elements guiding the motion of the calcaneonavicular complex relative to the talus. Furthermore, any instantaneous motion between the calcaneus and the talus occurs simultaneously at the anterior and posterior talocalcaneal joints and at the talonavicular joint. In clinical and functional terms, the hindfoot carries the forefoot and *vice versa*. The advantage of the functional rather than the conventional anatomic grouping of the ligaments is evident when confronting the understanding and correction of clinical problems.

CERVICAL LIGAMENT

The cervical ligament (external talocalcaneal ligament, anterolateral talocalcaneal ligament, anterior talocalcaneal ligament, a portion of the interosseous ligament; Fig. 4-44) is the strongest ligament connecting the talus and the calcaneus.[11, 24-26] It originates in the anteromedial segment of the sinus tarsi from the cervical tubercle located on the medial aspect of the bony eminence giving origin to the extensor digitorum brevis muscle. The prominence of the cervical tubercle is variable. The origin of the cervical ligament is posterolateral to the origin of the lateral calcaneonavicular ligament and anterior to the intermediate root of the inferior extensor retinaculum (Figs. 4-45 and 4-49). In the neutral position of the os calcis, the cervical ligament takes an oblique course and is directed upward, anteriorly, and medially and inserts on the inferior aspect of the talar neck, where a tubercle may be present. In our series of 100 tali, the tuberculum cervicis tali was recognized in 37%. The long axis of the ligament makes an angle of 45° to 50° with the long axis of the calcaneus in the sagittal plane and nearly parallels the average direction of the calcaneofibular ligament (Fig. 4-46). The position of the os calcis determines the orientation of the ligament. In valgus, the cervical ligament is more horizontal, and in varus, it is more vertical. The angle formed by the long axis of the ligament and the horizontal line in the frontal plane is 16° in valgus and 75° in varus as measured in the specimen shown in Figure 4-47. The cervical ligament is in the form of a rectangular band, and its measurements are as follows: length, 20 mm; width, 10 mm; or length, 19.6 mm; width, 11.6 mm; thickness, 2.8 mm.[25] As mentioned by Smith, the cervical ligament is separate from the ligament of the canalis tarsi in the majority.[26] Of 22 feet, in 1 specimen the two ligaments were continuous, in another specimen, the ligaments were joined by an oblique band.[26]

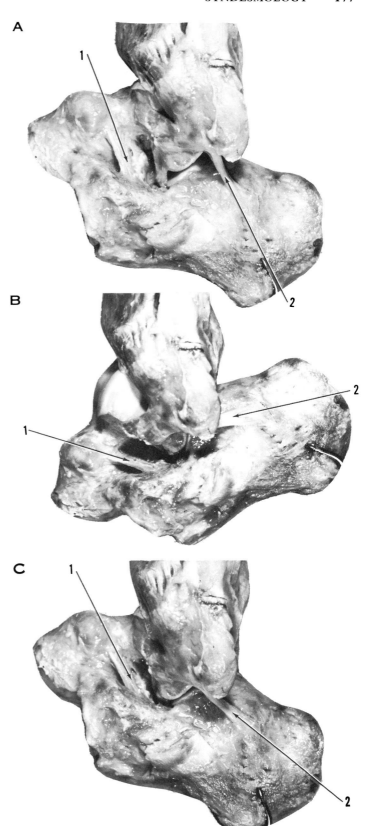

Fig. 4-46. Orientation of cervical ligament (1) and calcaneofibular ligament (2) in neutral (*A*), plantar flexion (*B*), and dorsiflexion (*C*). In (*A*) and (*C*) the ligaments are nearly parallel.

A

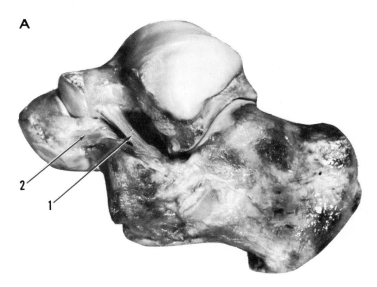

B

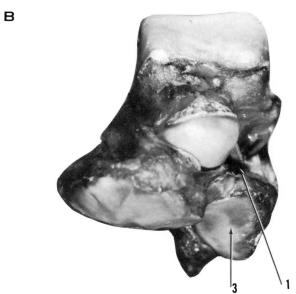

C

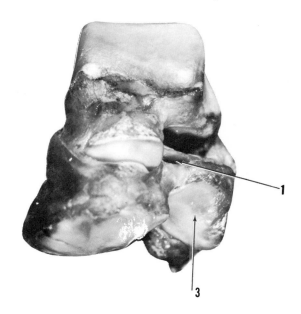

Fig. 4-47. Cervical ligament. (*A*) (1, Cervical ligament; 2, lateral calcaneonavicular ligament.) (*B*) Calcaneus (3) in varus. The cervical ligament (1) is nearly vertical. (*C*) Calcaneus (3) in valgus. The cervical ligament (1) is nearly horizontal.

LIGAMENT OF THE TARSAL CANAL

This ligament (interosseous talocalcaneal ligament; Figs. 4-48 and 4-49) of the tarsal canal is a flat, oblique band that originates from the sulcus calcanei of the tarsal canal close to the anterior capsule of the posterior talocalcaneal joint but independent from it.[11, 25, 26] The fibers are directed obliquely upward and medially, with an angle of inclination of 40° to 45° relative to the horizontal; they insert on the sulcus tali medially. Cahill provides the following average measurements of the ligament: length, 15 mm; width, 5.6 mm; thickness, 1.6 mm.[25] The inner fibers are shorter than the outer fibers.

The ligament of the tarsal canal may be distinguished from the thickened segment of the anterior capsule of the posterior talocalcaneal joint since the fibers of the latter are vertically oriented whereas the former takes an oblique course. The liagment is crossed anteriorly in an X by the canalicular portion of the medial root of the inferior extensor retinaculum. The talar insertion of the ligament is joined by the talar portion of the medial root and by the "oblique talocalcaneal band."[25] The oblique talo-calcaneal band extends from the calcaneal attachment of the intermediate extensor retinacular root to the talar portion of the tarsal canal. These two talar extensions from the medial and intermediate roots of the extensor retinaculum were clearly recognized by Barclay-Smith in 1896.[11] In reference to the latter extension, Barclay-Smith describes "very close associated with and lying on a plane anterior to that of the deep limb is a ligament which at its attachment to the os calcis is often blended with its outer band; passing upwards and inwards, it is attached to the groove on the astragalus, forming the roof of the canalis tarsi."[11]

LATERAL TALOCALCANEAL LIGAMENT

The lateral talocalcaneal ligament (see Fig. 4-12) is a flat, short, rectangular ligament, parallel to the calcaneofibular ligament. It originates from the antero inferior aspect of the lateral talar process, extends downward and posteriorly, and inserts on the os calcis just lateral to the posterior articular surface. This ligament is slightly anterior and medial to the calcaneofibular ligament. Occasionally it is difficult to separate these two ligaments, due to their intimate adherence.

POSTERIOR TALOCALCANEAL LIGAMENT

The posterior talocalcaneal ligament is a short, flat, quadrilateral ligament directed downward and laterally. It originates from the lateral surface and apex of the posterolateral talar tubercle and inserts on the superior and medial aspect of the os calcis. It may also give insertion to the fibrous roof of the flexor hallucis longus tunnel (see Fig. 4-17). At

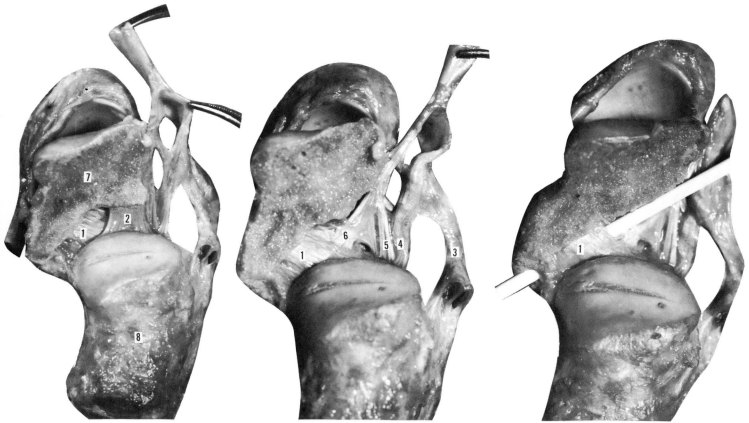

Fig. 4-48.   Anatomic preparation of canalis tarsi. Posterior half of talus is removed through an oblique osteotomy. (1, Talocalcaneal interosseous ligament of canalis tarsi; 2, anterior capsular ligament of posterior talocalcaneal joint; 3, insertion of lateral root of inferior extensor retinaculum on inferior peroneal retinaculum; 4, intermediate root of inferior extensor retinaculum; 5, 6, medial roots of inferior extensor retinaculum; 7, talus; 8, os calcis.)

the talar origin, the posterior talocalcaneal ligament may interchange fibers with the posterior talofibular ligament. Occasionally the posterior talocalcaneal ligament is formed by two fascicles. The lateral band originates from the posterolateral tubercle, extends downward and medially, and inserts on the dorsum of the os calcis. The medial band originates from the posteromedial talar tubercle, extends downward and laterally, and inserts on the superomedial aspect of the os calcis next to the insertion of the lateral band. The two fascicles form a V with a talar base and calcaneal apex.

When an os trigonum is present, the posterior talocalcaneal ligament originates from it and forms a trigonocalcaneal ligament.

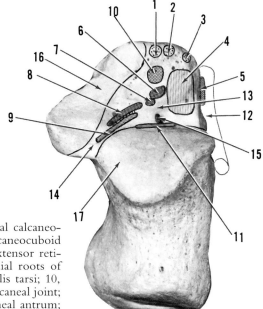

Fig. 4-49.   Insertion sites in the sinus tarsi and canalis tarsi. (1, Lateral calcaneonavicular ligament; 2, medial calcaneocuboid ligament; 3, dorsolateral calcaneocuboid ligament; 4, extensor digitorum brevis muscle; 5, lateral root of inferior extensor retinaculum; 6, intermediate root of inferior extensor retinaculum; 7, 8, medial roots of inferior extensor retinaculum; 9, interosseous talocalcaneal ligament of canalis tarsi; 10, cervical ligament; 11, capsular ligament of anterior aspect of posterior talocalcaneal joint; 12, tunnel of peronei; 13, sinus tarsi; 14, canalis tarsi; 15, foramina of calcaneal antrum; 16, anterior and middle calcaneal articular surfaces; 17, posterior calcaneal articular surface.)

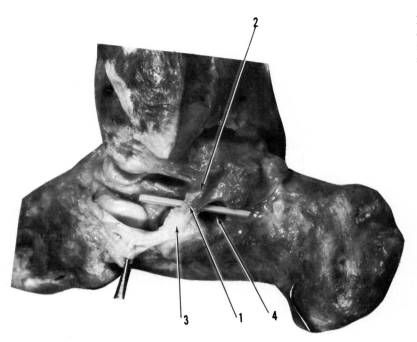

Fig. 4-50. Medial aspect of hindfoot. (1, Medial talocalcaneal ligament; 2, origin of [1] from talar posteromedial tubercle; 3, insertion of [1] on posterior aspect of sustentaculum tali; 4, medial opening of canalis tarsi.)

MEDIAL TALOCALCANEAL LIGAMENT

The medial talocalcaneal ligament (Fig. 4-50) is a short, strong ligament. It originates from the talar posteromedial tubercle, courses anteriorly and inferiorly, and inserts on the posterior border of the sustentaculum tali. It limits posteroinferiorly the medial opening of the tarsal canal. A second band may be present, originating from the same site but directed downward and posteriorly; this band inserts posterior to the sustantaculum tali and completes the groove lodging the flexor hallucis tendon.

TALONAVICULAR LIGAMENT

The talonavicular ligament (Fig. 4-51) occupies the dorsal interval between the superomedial calcaneonavicular ligament and the lateral calcaneonavicular ligament. It is a capsular thickening. Barclay-Smith recognized two components, superficial and deep.[11] The superficial component originates from the dorsum of the talar neck and is a thin, long, broad band that courses anteromedially and inserts on the dorsum of the navicular. It crosses the superomedial calcaneonavicular ligament in an X, and their fibers interlace. The deep component is shorter and deeper. It originates from the superomedial aspect of the talar neck, courses anterolaterally, passes under the superficial component, and inserts on the dorsum of the navicular.

Ligaments of the Calcaneocuboid and Cubonavicular Joints

MEDIAL CALCANEOCUBOID LIGAMENT

The medial calcaneocuboid ligament has already been described as the outer component of the bifurcate ligament (V ligament, ligament of Chopart) (see Fig. 4-43).

DORSOLATERAL CALCANEOCUBOID LIGAMENT

The dorsolateral calcaneocuboid ligament (see Fig. 4-43) originates from the dorsolateral corner of the anterior segment of the calcaneus close to the margin of the anterior articular surface of the calcaneus. It is directed, as a flat band, anteromedially and inserts on the dorsum of the cuboid at least 0.5 cm distal to the articular interline. Occasionally a smaller, more lateral band is present.

INFERIOR CALCANEOCUBOID LIGAMENT

The inferior calcaneocuboid ligament (long and short plantar ligaments) is a thick, powerful, longitudinally oriented ligament with two components: superficial or long and deep or short (Fig. 4-52). The superficial or long plantar ligament originates from the segment of the inferior surface of the os calcis extending from the anterior surface of the posterior tuberosities and their intertubercular segment to the anterior tuberosity. The strong longitudinal fibers pass over the calcaneocuboid joint and divide into two sets of fibers, deep and superficial. The deep fibers, representing the bulk of this component, insert on the oblique crest of the cuboid. The more superficial fibers form a thinner layer, cross the tunnel of the peroneus longus (contributing to its formation), and divide into four thinner slips inserting over the metatarsal bases 2 to 5. Paturet[7] describes the band directed to the base of the fifth metatarsal as a rectangular ligament 20 mm to 25 mm in width, called the *long cubo-fifth metatarsal ligament*.[7] This band is also well illustrated by Spalteholz (Fig. 4-53).[27] The deep or short calcaneocuboid ligament (Fig. 4-54) originates from the anterior tuberosity of the os calcis. The strong, fasciculated fibers fan out, course anteromedially, and insert over the entire triangular surface located posterior to the crest of the cuboid. A strong band oriented almost transversely inserts on the nonarticulating

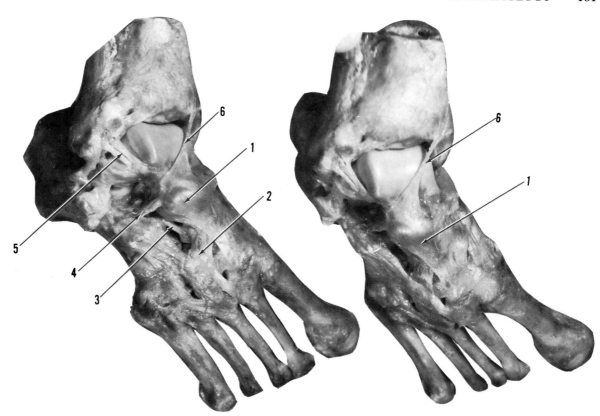

Fig. 4-51.   Talonavicular ligament. (1, Dorsal talonavicular ligament; 2, dorsal cuneo₃navicular ligament; 3, lateral calcaneonavicular ligament; 4, cervical ligament; 5, anterior talofibular ligament; 6, anterior tibiotalar ligament.)

Fig. 4-52.   Plantar aspect of foot. (1, Long plantar ligament; 2, superficial distal component of [1]; 3, deep insertion of [1] on cuboidal crest forming the long calcaneocuboid ligament; 4, short plantar ligament or deep, short, calcaneocuboid ligament; 5, plantar segment of tibialis posterior tendon; 6, reflected peroneus longus tendon.)

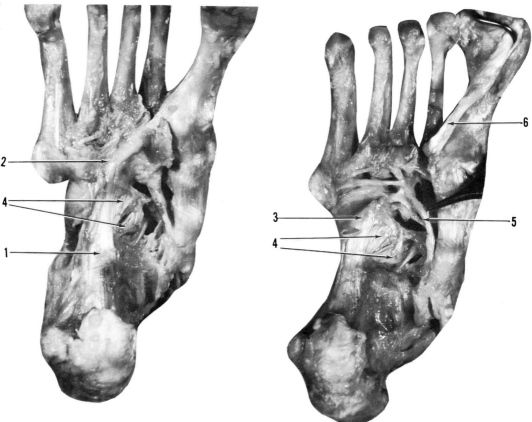

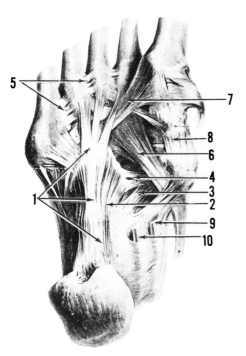

Fig. 4-53. Plantar aspect of foot. (1, Longitudinal plantar ligament; 2, short plantar calcaneocuboid ligament; 3, plantar calcaneonavicular ligament; 4, plantar cubonavicular ligament; 5, intermetatarsal ligaments M_5-M_4, M_4-M_3; 6, tibialis posterior tendon; 7, peroneus longus tendon; 8, plantar cuneo$_1$navicular ligament; 9, flexor digitorum longus tendon [cut through]; 10, flexor hallucis longus tendon [cut through].) (From Spalteholz W: Hand Atlas of Human Anatomy, Vol 1, p 219. Philadelphia, JB Lippincott, 1903)

Fig. 4-54. Plantar aspect of foot. (*A*) (1, Long calcaneocuboid ligament; 2, insertion of [1] on cuboidal crest; 3, short, deep calcaneocuboid ligament; 4, 5, 6, tibialis posterior tendon and insertions.) (*B*) (1, Deep calcaneocuboid ligament; 2, reflected long calcaneocuboid ligament.)

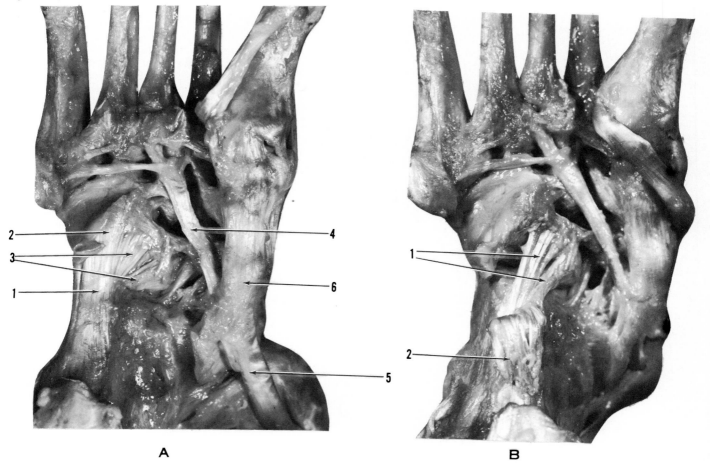

A

B

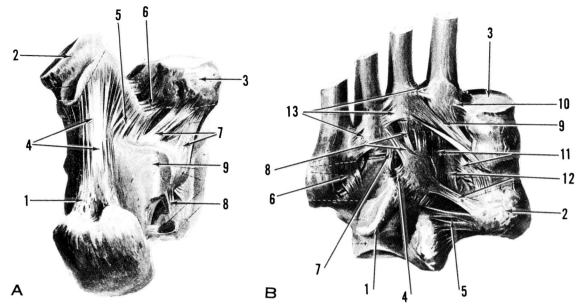

Fig. 4-55. (*A*) **Plantar view of hindfoot.** (1, Os calcis; 2, cuboid; 3, navicular; 4, long plantar or long calcaneocuboid ligament; 5, short or deep calcaneocuboid ligament; 6, plantar cubonavicular ligament; 7, plantar calcaneonavicular ligament; 8, medial talocalcaneal ligament; 9, sulcus of flexor hallucis longus tendon.)
(*B*) **Plantar view of tarsus.** (1, Cuboid; 2, navicular; 3, first cuneiform; 4, plantar cuneo$_3$-cuboid ligament; 5, plantar cubonavicular ligament; 6, plantar cubo-M$_5$ ligament; 7, plantar cubo-M$_4$ ligament; 8, plantar cuneo$_3$-M$_3$, M$_4$ ligaments; 9, long plantar cuneo$_1$-M$_3$, M$_2$ ligament; 10, short plantar cuneo$_1$-M$_2$ ligament; 11, plantar cuneo$_1$-cuneo$_2$, cuneo$_2$-cuneo$_3$ ligaments; 12, plantar cuneo$_{2,3}$ navicular ligaments; 13, intermetatarsal ligaments M$_5$-M$_4$, M$_4$-M$_3$, M$_3$-M$_2$.) (From Spalteholz W: Hand Atlas of Human Anatomy, Vol 1, p 219. Philadelphia, JB Lippincott, 1903)

surface of the beak of the cuboid. The deep component is covered by the longitudinal ligament only laterally and is in continuity medially with the inferior calcaneonavicular ligament.

CUBONAVICULAR LIGAMENTS

There are three cubonavicular ligaments: dorsal, plantar, interosseous.

The dorsal cubonavicular ligament (see Fig. 4-43) is a triangular ligament with a medial apex and a lateral base. It originates from the dorsal aspect of the navicular, anteromedial to the insertion of the lateral calcaneonavicular ligament. The fibers extend laterally and transversely, pass over the corner of the third cuneiform (wedged between the navicular and the cuboid), and insert on the dorsum of the cuboid in its distal half. Some fibers attach to the dorsum of the third cuneiform also.

The plantar cubonavicular ligament (Figs. 4-53 and 4-55, *A*) is a rectangular band that originates from the inferior surface of the cuboid along the medial border, posterior to the cuboid crest. It overlaps, in this segment, the insertional fibers of the deep calcaneocuboid ligament. The fibers course transversely and insert on the inferior surface of the navicular, distal to the insertion of the plantar calcaneonavicular fibers. Occasionally the plantar cubonavicular ligament is formed by two fascicles; these are more or less triangular, with the apex attached to the cuboid and the base

to the navicular. These bands are directed medially and posteriorly.

The interosseous cubonavicular ligament is a very short, strong ligament that originates from a narrow, vertical segment of the medial surface of the cuboid, posterior to the third cuneiform articular surface. When a small articular surface is present for the navicular (45%–55%), the fibers originate above and below this articular surface. The fibers are transversely oriented and insert on the anteroinferior segment of the lateral end of the navicular.

Ligaments of the Cuneonavicular and Cuneocuboid Joints

CUNEONAVICULAR LIGAMENTS

Each cuneiform is united to the navicular by a dorsal and a plantar ligament. In addition, the first cuneiform is united to the navicular by the medial cuneonavicular ligament.

There are three dorsal cuneonavicular ligaments (Figs. 4-56 and 4-57). Each ligament, in the form of a flat fibrous band, arises from the distal segment of the dorsal surface of the navicular. The first cuneonavicular ligament extends straight anteriorly and inserts on the dorsum of the first cuneiform; it is the strongest of the three. The second and third ligaments are thinner and oblique, are oriented anter-

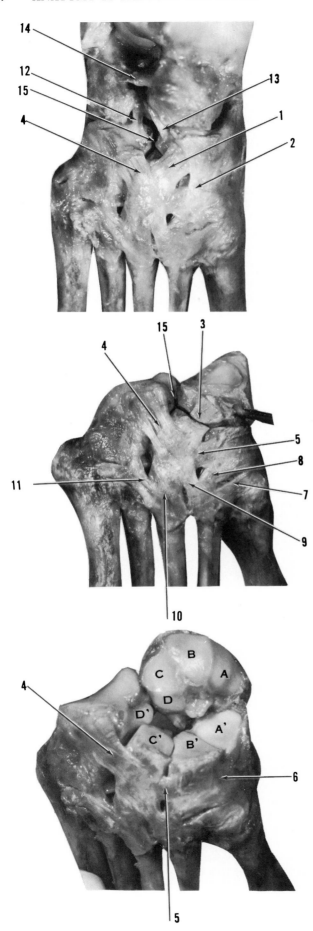

Fig. 4-56. Dorsal aspect of tarsus. (1, Dorsal cuneo₃-navicular ligament; 2, dorsal cuneo₂-navicular ligament; 3, incised dorsal cuneo₃-navicular ligament; 4, dorsal cubocuneo₃ ligament; 5, dorsal intercuneiform C₃-C₂ ligament; 6, dorsal intercuneiform C₂-C₁ ligament; 7, dorsal cuneo₁-M₂ ligament; 8, dorsal cuneo₂-M₂ ligament; 9, dorsal cuneo₃-M₂ ligament; 10, dorsal cuneo₃-M₃ ligament; 11, dorsal cubo-M₃ ligament; 12, dorsal, medial calcaneocuboid ligament; 13, dorsal, lateral calcaneonavicular ligament; 14, cervical ligament; 15, cubonavicular articular interline; A, A′, navicular and cuneiform₁ articular surfaces; B, B′, navicular and cuneiform₂ articular surfaces; C, C′, navicular and cuneiform₃ articular surfaces; D, D′, navicular and cuboid articular surfaces.)

omedially, and insert on the dorsum of the corresponding cuneiform. They are partially covered by an expansion from the talonavicular ligament. The third dorsal cuneonavicular ligament forms a triangular complex in association with the dorsal cuneocuboid ligament and the dorsal cubonavicular ligament (see Fig. 4-43).

There also are three plantar cuneonavicular ligaments (see Figs. 4-54 and 4-55, B). The first arises from the anterior and plantar aspect of the tuberosity of the navicular, extends anteriorly as a thick, rectangular, flat cuff, and inserts on the plantar tuberosity of the first cuneiform; this ligament is short and strong. The second and third ligaments arise from the inferior surface of the navicular, between the tuberosity and the beak. They are thin and deep and are masked by the expansions of the tibialis posterior tendon. Each ligament inserts on the posterior segment of the corresponding cuneiform crest. The third ligament is oriented anterolaterally and is the longest; the second ligament is the deepest.

The medial cuneonavicular ligament (Fig. 4-58) is a thick, strong ligament that extends from the medial aspect of the tuberosity of the navicular to the medial aspect of the first cuneiform and receives a few fibers from the tibialis posterior tendon.

CUNEO₃-CUBOID LIGAMENTS

There are three cuneocuboid ligaments: dorsal, plantar, and interosseous.

The dorsal cuneo₃-cuboid ligament (see Figs. 4-56 and 4-57) is a broad, flat ligament extending obliquely anteromedially from the dorsum of the cuboid to the dorsal aspect of the third cuneiform. As mentioned above, this ligament makes a triangular arrangement with the dorsal cubonavicular and the dorsal cuneo₃-navicular ligament. Occasionally this ligament is divided into two fascicles.

The plantar cuneo₃-cuboid ligament (see Figs. 4-54 and 4-55, B) is a short ligament extending from the medial aspect of the cuboid crest and the segment of the medial border immediately behind it to the posterior segment of the third cuneiform crest.

The interosseous cuneo₃-cuboid ligament is a very short but thick ligament binding the two bones and located anterior to their articular surfaces.

Intercuneiform Ligaments

There are two dorsal, two interosseous, and one plantar intercuneiform ligaments.

The dorsal intercuneiform ligaments (see Figs. 4-56 and 4-57) are small, rectangular bands transversely binding the cuneiforms, the first to the second and the second to the third.

There are two interosseous cuneiform ligaments. The medial interosseous (see Fig. 4-58) is a strong, thick, transverse ligament uniting the first cuneiform with the second. It is located in the angle of the intercuneiform articulating surfaces. Its origin on the first cuneiform is confined to the posterior half of the lateral surface, at least 8 mm posterior to the anterior border. The lateral interosseous ligament is also a short, strong band transversely uniting the second to the third cuneiform; it is located anterior to the intercuneiform articulating surfaces.

The plantar intercuneiform ligament (see Fig. 4-55, *B*), a short ligament, originates on the posterolateral corner of the plantar surface of the first cuneiform. It is directed anterolaterally and inserts on the deeply located crest of the second cuneiform.

Ligaments of the Tarsometatarsal Joint

The tarsometatarsal joint (Lisfranc's joint), connecting the cuneocuboid block to the bases of the metatarsals, has a complex joint interline configuration. The line is oblique, directed laterally and posteriorly, and presents a dorsolateral convexity corresponding to the transverse cubocuneiform arch (Fig. 4-59). A line drawn through the first metatarsal–cuneiform joint and extended laterally transects the shaft of the fifth metatarsal near the middle. A line drawn through the fifth metatarsal–cuboid joint and extended medially passes behind the head of the first metatarsal (Fig. 4-60).

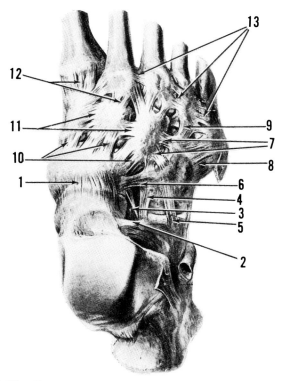

Fig. 4-57. Dorsum of foot. (1, Dorsal talonavicular ligament; 2, cervical ligament; 3, calcaneonavicular component of bifurcate ligament; 4, calcaneocuboid component of bifurcate ligament; 5, dorsolateral calcaneocuboid ligament; 6, dorsal cubonavicular ligament; 7, dorsal cubo-cuneo$_3$ ligaments; 8, dorsal cubo-M$_5$ ligament; 9, dorsal cubo-M$_4$ ligament; 10, dorsal cuneo$_{1-2-3}$- navicular ligaments; 11, dorsal intercuneiform ligaments C$_1$-C$_2$, C$_2$-C$_3$; 12, dorsal cuneometatarsal ligaments C$_1$-M$_1$, C$_1$-M$_2$, C$_2$-M$_2$, C$_3$-M$_2$; 13, dorsal intermetatarsal ligaments M$_2$-M$_3$, M$_3$-M$_4$, M$_4$-M$_5$.) (From Spalteholz W: Hand Atlas of Human Anatomy, Vol 1, p 219. Philadelphia, JB Lippincott, 1903)

Fig. 4-58. Medial aspect of foot. (1, Medial cuneo$_1$-navicular ligament; 2, medial cuneo$_1$-M$_1$ ligament; 3, reflected tibialis anterior tendon; 4, tibialis posterior tendon.)

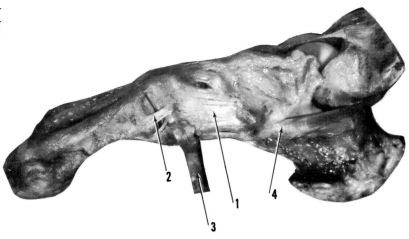

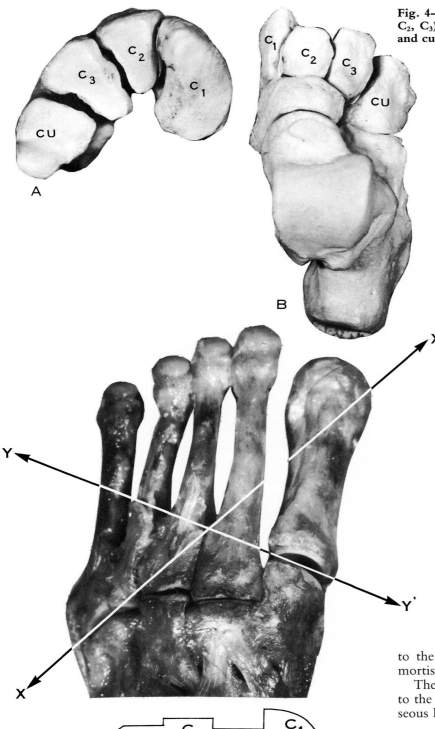

Fig. 4-59. (A) Transverse arch formed by cuneiforms (C_1, C_2, C_3) and cuboid (*CU*). (B) Contour of distal cuneiform and cuboid interline with recess of C_2.

Fig. 4-60. **Lisfranc's (tarsometatarsal) articular interline.** Cuneiform$_2$ (C_2) is in recess relative to cuneiform$_1$ (C_1) and cuneiform$_3$ (C_3). A line YY' extended from the cuneiform$_1$-metatarsal$_1$ transects the shaft of metatarsal$_5$ in its mid segment. A line XX' extended from the cubo-metatarsal$_5$ interline passes behind the head of the first metatarsal. The base of M_2 is locked in the intercuneiform recess at the level of C_2. The cuneiform$_3$ is locked, to a lesser degree, in the intermetatarsal recess at the level of M_3. (*Cu*, cuboid.)

The second cuneiform is in proximal recess of 8 mm relative to the first cuneiform and 4 mm relative to the third cuneiform; this creates the cuneiform mortise that will receive its tenon—the base of the second metatarsal. This arrangement enhances the stability of Lisfranc's joint. The cuboid is in slight proximal recess of at least 2 mm relative to the third cuneiform; this creates a shallow metatarsal mortise receiving its tenon—the third cuneiform.

The ligaments connecting the cuboid and the cuneiforms to the metatarsal bases are the dorsal, plantar, and interosseous ligaments.

DORSAL LIGAMENTS

There are seven dorsal tarsometatarsal ligaments (see Figs. 4-56 and 4-57).

The base of the first metatarsal is united by a large, thick ligament to the first cuneiform (see Fig. 4-57). This ligament is in a dorsomedial location and is the strongest.

The base of the second metatarsal is secured by three ligaments to the dorsum of the first, second, and third cuneiforms. The first two have an anterolateral obliquity, whereas the third is directed anteromedially.

The base of the third metatarsal is connected by a dorsal ligament to the dosum of the third cuneiform. An accessory cuboid–cuneiform$_3$–metatarsal$_3$ band may also be present, which is then in continuity with the ligament connecting the base of the fourth metatarsal to the cuboid.

The fifth metatarsal base is connected to the cuboid by a ligament that is in a dorsolateral location. Occasionally a transverse band extends from this ligament to the dorsum of the third cuneiform.

PLANTAR LIGAMENTS

The plantar cuneometatarsal ligaments (see Fig. 4-55, *B*) are always present on the medial aspect of Lisfranc's joint, but they are very variable in number and disposition on the lateral side.[28]

The cuneiform 1 is attached to the base of the metatarsal 1 by a broad, rectangular ligament. This ligament arises from the plantar aspect of the cuneiform 1 near the articular surface, extends slightly outward and distally, and inserts on the lateral half of the first metatarsal base.[28] Proximally, the fibers are seen to be in continuity with the fibers of the inferior cuneo$_1$-navicular ligament.

The cuneo$_1$-metatarsal$_{2,3}$ ligament is a very strong ligament, considered by Sappey to be the key of the tarsometatarsal arch.[12] The ligament originates from the inferolateral surface of the cuneiform 1 and soon divides into two bands.[28] The superficial band is the stronger and thicker; it courses obliquely outward and upward and makes a broad insertion on the base of the metatarsal 3. The deep band is less developed and inserts on the base of metatarsal 2.

There is no ligament between cuneiform 2 and matatarsal 2 on the plantar aspect.

The plantar ligament cuneiform$_3$-metatarsal$_{3,4}$ is inconstant. It originates from the inferolateral surface of the third cuneiform and inserts on the bases of metatarsals 3 and 4. In a study of eight feet, Welti found this ligament absent in three and present with two bands in three (two, cuneo$_3$-metatarsal$_3$, and one, cuneo$_3$-metatarsal$_4$)[28]. The plantar ligaments between the cuboid and metatarsals 4 and 5 are often absent. Welti finds these ligaments absent in five feet of eight, present as two bands (cubometatarsal$_4$, cubometatarsal$_5$) in one, and only one band present in two (cubometatarsal$_4$). The ligaments, when present, are small and rectangular. The long cubometatarsal$_5$ ligament, extending from the crest of the cuboid to the base of the fifth metatarsal as a quadrilateral ligament, is a component of the long plantar ligament.

INTEROSSEOUS LIGAMENTS

There are three sets of interosseous ligaments (Fig. 4-61), corresponding to the first, second, and third cuneometatarsal spaces. There are none in the fourth interspace. An extensive study of the interosseous ligaments, based on the dissection of 50 adult feet, is provided by Thomas.[29]

The first interosseous cuneometatarsal ligament (Lisfranc's ligament, medial interosseous ligament) is the strongest ligament of the three (Figs. 4-62 and 4-63). It

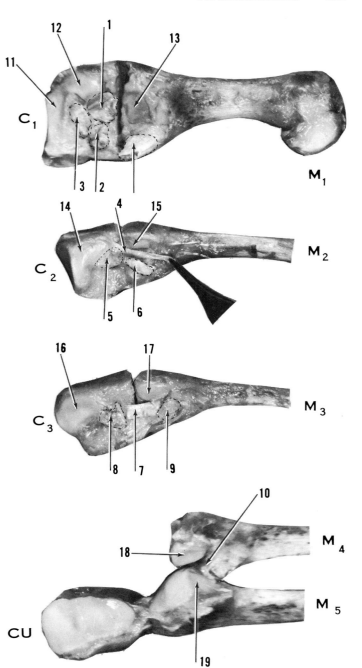

Fig. 4-61. Lateral aspect of metatarsocuneiform joints (M_1-C_1, M_2-C_2, M_3-C_3) and intermetatarsal (M_4-M_5) joints. (1, Surface of origin of Lisfranc's ligament [cuneiform$_1$-metatarsal$_2$]; 2, origin of accessory band of C_2-M_2 ligament; 3, origin of intercuneiform C_1-C_2 ligament; 4, cuneo$_2$-metatarsal$_3$ ligament; 5, origin on intercuneiform C_2-C_3 ligament; 6, origin of intermetatarsal M_2-M_3 ligament; 7, cuneo$_3$-metatarsal$_3$ ligament; 8, origin of cuneo$_3$-cuboid ligament; 9, origin of intermetatarsal M_3-M_4 ligament; 10, intermetatarsal ligament M_4-M_5; 11, articular surface of C_1 corresponding to C_2; 12, articular surface of C_1 corresponding to M_2; 13, articular surface of M_1 corresponding to M_2; 14, articular surface of C_2 corresponding to C_3; 15, articular surface of M_2 corresponding to M_3; 16, articular surface of C_3 corresponding to cuboid [CU]; 17, articular surface of M_3 corresponding to M_4; 18, 19, articular surfaces of M_4-M_5.)

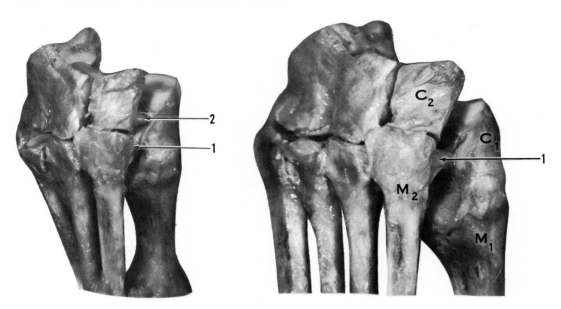

Fig. 4-62. Lisfranc's ligament. (1, Lisfranc's ligament [cuneiform$_1$-metatarsal$_2$]; 2, intercuneiform [C_1-C_2] ligament.)

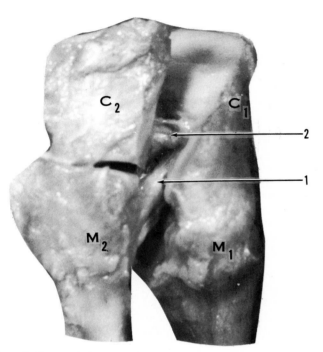

Fig. 4-63. Lisfranc's ligament. (1, Lisfranc's ligament [cuneiform$_1$-metatarsal$_2$]; 2, intercuneiform [C_1-C_2] ligament.)

arises from the lateral surface of the first cuneiform in front of the intercuneiform ligament and under the articular surface corresponding to the second metatarsal. The ligament is directed obliquely outward and slightly downward and inserts on the lower half of the medial surface of the second metatarsal base. The ligament measures nearly 1 cm in height and approximately 0.5 cm in thickness. In 22%, this ligament is formed by two bands, each band being 3 mm to 4 mm thick. In 18%, one band is anterior and the other posterior, and in 4%, there is an inferior and a superior fascicle. The anterior band is nearly always the thinner.

Some secondary fibers may be seen in the interspace running from the first cuneiform near the attachment of Lisfrancs ligament to the first metatarsal base. These fibers, seein in 30%, are less than 2 mm in size. In another 30%, small fibrous formations are present, 1 mm to 2 mm in thickness, extending from the metatarsal insertion of Lisfranc's ligament to the base of the first metatarsal.[29]

Lisfranc's ligament is separated by an interval of 1 mm to 2 mm from the dorsal surface of the peroneous longus tendon.

The second interosseous cuneometatarsal ligament (middle interosseous ligament) has a complex ligamentous arrangement. It is located between the cuneiforms and metatarsals 2 and 3. The ligamentous arrangement in this interspace is very variable. Thomas described the following possibilities, as seen on 50 feet (Fig. 4-64):

Type 1 (48%): The ligament forms a strong, obliquely placed triangular lamina extending from one cuneiform to the corresponding and opposite metatarsals. The origin on the cuneiform represents the apex of the triangle and is located anterior or inferior to the intercuneiform 2, 3 ligament. The metatarsal insertion or base of the triangle is in close connection with the intermetatarsal ligament 2, 3. The ligament divides the intespace into an upper and a lower segment. In 28% the origin of the ligament is on the second cuneiform and in 20%, on the third cuneiform.

Type 2 (22%): A single ligamentous band is present, connecting the cuneiform and the metatarsal of the same ray. The connection of the third cuneiform and the third metatarsal occurs more frequently. The insertions are located under the intercuneiform and intermetatarsal ligaments.

Type 3 (8%): A longitudinal band is present simultaneously, corresponding to each cuneometatarsal ray.

Type 4 (4%): A quadrilateral lamina fills the entire second interspace, dividing it completely into an upper and a lower segment.

Type 5 (8%): This represents a complex arrangement. Longitudinal bands are present along with each cuneo-metatarsal ray, and crossing fibers are present, forming an X. Fibers extend from the second cuneiform to the base of the third metatarsal. Other fibers unite the third cuneiform to the base of the second metatarsal.

Type 6 (10%): The ligament is absent.[29]

The third interosseous cuneometatarsal ligament (lateral interosseous ligament) has a variable morphology. The following arrangements are described by Thomas (Fig. 4-65):

Type 1 (32%; the most frequent arrangement): The ligament extends from the lateral aspect of the third cuneiform to the base of the third metatarsal. The origin is located anterior to the intercuneiform ligament. A similar unilateral arrangement may be present along the cubometatarsal$_4$ ray. This ligament is 2 mm to 3 mm in thickness.

Type 2 (14%): Two longitudinal bands are present, each corresponding to its cuneo$_3$-metatarsal$_3$ or cubometatarsal$_4$ ray.

Type 3 (20%): A V arrangement is present. The ligament originates from the lateral aspect of the third cuneiform (12%) or from the medial aspect of the cuboid (8%) and inserts on the third and fourth metatarsals. This ligament has very strong fibers.

Type 4 (16%): An oblique band extends from the lateral aspect of the third cuneiform to the base of the fourth metatarsal in 10%. In the remaining 6%, the oblique band originates on the cuboid and inserts on the base of the third metatarsal.

Type 5 (4%): This type is similar to the type 4, but a second band is also present, ascending in an oblique manner from the anteroinferior corner of the third cuneiform to the dorsal aspect of the fourth metatarsal.

Type 6 (4%): This ligament, similar to the oblique ligament of type 5 is the only one filling the interspace; it arises from the intercuneiform ligament.

Type 7 (4%): There is a V disposition of the ligament (as in type 3) arising from cuneiform 3, supplemented by a strong ligament originating from the inferior surface of the intercuneiform ligament, coursing parallel to the fourth metatarsal band.

Type 8 (6%): Weak ligamentous fibers are arranged in an X.[29]

Intermetatarsal Ligaments

The intermetatarsal ligaments are dorsal, plantar, and interosseous. There is no ligament between metatarsal 1 and metatarsal 2 on the dorsal or plantar aspect. The interosseous connection between metatarsals 1 and 2 is through poorly individualized weak fibers.

The dorsal intermetatarsal ligaments are three small, thin, flat bands located obliquely on the dorsum of the base of the metatarsals 2,3, metatarsal 3,4 and metatarsal 4,5. The middle band is the strongest.

The plantar intermetatarsal ligaments also are three in number with a similar distribution. They are stronger than the dorsal ligaments. They are oriented obliquely, medially and slightly anteriorly.

The three interosseous ligaments are very short and very strong, determining the intermetatarsal stability. They are located in the posterior aspect of the intermetatarsal space but anteroinferior to the articular surfaces. They are in close connection with the corresponding interosseous cuneo-metatarsal ligaments.

Ligaments of Metatarsophalangeal Joints and Proximal Phalangeal Apparatus

At the level of the metatarsophalangeal joint of the lesser toes, the proximal phalanx and the fibrocartilaginous plantar plate form an anatomic and functional unit. They are both suspended from the sides of the metatarsal head through the collateral and the suspensory glenoid ligaments. Furthermore, the plantar plate is connected on each side by the deep transverse intermetatarsal ligament and gives insertion on the plantar side to the fibrous flexor tendon sheath, the two longitudinal septae of the plantar aponeurosis, the transverse head of the adductor hallucis, and the vertical fibers extending to the superficial component of the plantar aponeurosis; some of these fibers are arciform and form a pre-flexor tendinous space retaining the premetatarsal adipose cushion (Figs. 4-66–4-68).[30] On the dorsal aspect, the plantar plate gives insertion to the accessory collateral ligament or the metatarsoglenoid suspensory ligament, the transverse lamina of the extensor aponeurosis, and the corresponding interossei muscles at the junction of the deep transverse intermetatarsal ligament with the plantar plate.[31]

The anatomic unit formed by the proximal phalanx, the plantar plate, and their insertional connections as described is called the *phalangeal apparatus;* this is the main articular unit of the ball of the foot.

METATARSOPHALANGEAL LIGAMENTS OF THE LESSER TOES

The lateral ligaments of the metatarsophalangeal joints are divided into metatarsophalangeal collateral ligaments and metatarsoglenoid suspensory ligaments. The lateral ligaments on the peroneal side are thicker and stronger than those on the tibial side.

The metatarsophalangeal ligament originates on the lateral tubercle of the metatarsal heads. It is directed downward and anteriorly and inserts on the lateral tubercle of the base of the proximal phalanx.

The metatarsoglenoid ligament or suspensory ligament originates from the posteroinferior aspect of the lateral metatarsal tubercle of the head. It is triangular (fan shaped), and the fibers descend vertically in the posterior part and obliquely in the anterior part and insert on the lateral border of the plantar plate. The fibers are also in continuity with the lower borders of the metatarsophalangeal collateral ligament.

(Text continues on p. 194.)

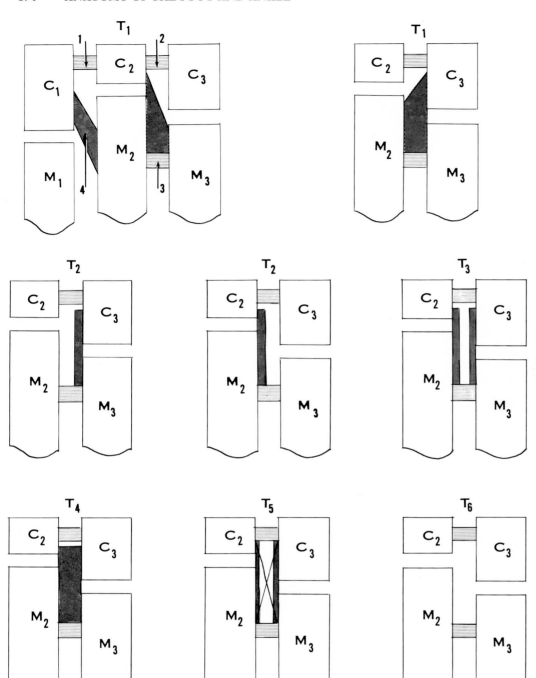

Fig. 4-64. Variations of cuneo-metatarsal ligaments. *Type 1* (T_1), 48%: the second interosseous cuneometatarsal ligament forming a triangular lamina originating from C_2 or C_3 and attached to the metatarsals M_2, M_3; *Type 2* (T_2), 22%: a single ligament present C_3-M_3 [more frequently] or C_2-M_2; *Type 3* (T_3), 8%: two ligaments are present (C_3-M_3 and C_2-M_2); *Type 4* (T_4), 4%: a quadrilateral ligamentous lamina fills the interosseous interspace; *Type 5* (T_5), 8%: longitudinal ligamentous bands C_2-M_2, C_3-M_3 supplemented by criss-crossing fibers C_2-M_3, C_3-M_2; *Type 6* (T_6), 10% : absent ligament. (C_1, cuneiform$_1$; C_2, cuneiform$_2$; C_3, cuneiform$_3$; M_1, metatarsal$_1$; M_2, metatarsal$_2$; M_3, metatarsal$_3$; 1, intercuneiform C_1-C_2 ligament; 2, intercuneiform C_2-C_3 ligament; 3, intermetatarsal M_2-M_3 ligament; 4, Lisfranc's ligament C_1-M_2.) (Redrawn after Thomas L: Recherches sur les ligaments interosseux de l'articulation de Lisfranc: Etude anatomique et embryologique. Arch Anat Histol Embryol 5: 110, 1926)

Fig. 4-65. Variations of the ligaments of the third interosseous space. *Type 1 (T_1), 32%: one ligament present (C_3-M_3 or CU-M_4); Type 2 (T_2), 14% : two ligaments present (C_3-M_3, CU-M_4); Type 3 (T_3), 20%: a V arrangement, the apex of the V being located on C_3 (12%) or on the CU (8%), the distal attachment being to M_3 and M_4. Type 4 (T_4), 16%: oblique ligament C_3-M_4 (10%) or CU-M_3 (6%); Type 5 (T_5), 4%: two oblique ligaments present (C_3-M_4); Type 6 (T_6), 4%: one short oblique band present, extending from the anteroinferior corner of C_3 to the dorsal aspect of M_4; Type 7 (T_7), 4%: a V disposition of the ligament with the apex attached to C_3 and the arms to M_3 and M_4, supplemented by an oblique C_3-M_4 ligament. Type 8 (T_8), 6%: weak ligamentous fibers arranged in X (C_3-M_4, CU-M_3). (C_3, cuneiform$_3$; CU, cuboid; M_3, metatarsal$_3$; M_4, metatarsal$_4$; 1, C_3-CU ligament; 2, M_3-M_4 ligament.)* (Redrawn after Thomas L: Recherches sur les ligaments interosseux de l'articulation de Lisfranc: Etude anatomique et embryologique. Arch Anat Histol Embryol 5: 110, 1926)

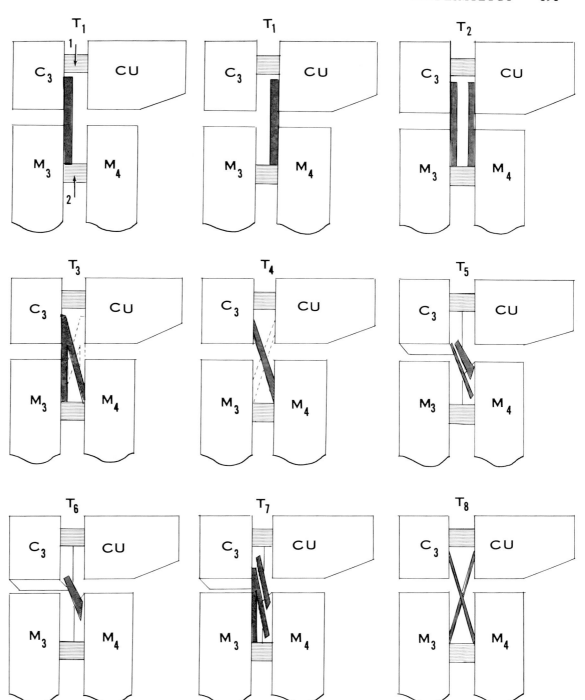

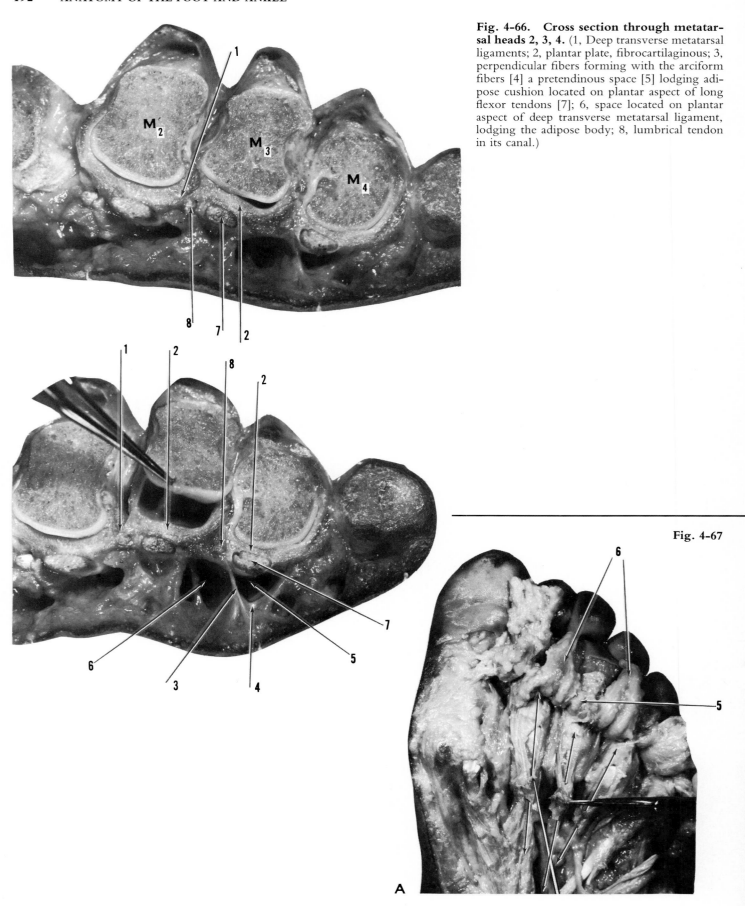

Fig. 4-66. Cross section through metatarsal heads 2, 3, 4. (1, Deep transverse metatarsal ligaments; 2, plantar plate, fibrocartilaginous; 3, perpendicular fibers forming with the arciform fibers [4] a pretendinous space [5] lodging adipose cushion located on plantar aspect of long flexor tendons [7]; 6, space located on plantar aspect of deep transverse metatarsal ligament, lodging the adipose body; 8, lumbrical tendon in its canal.)

Fig. 4-67

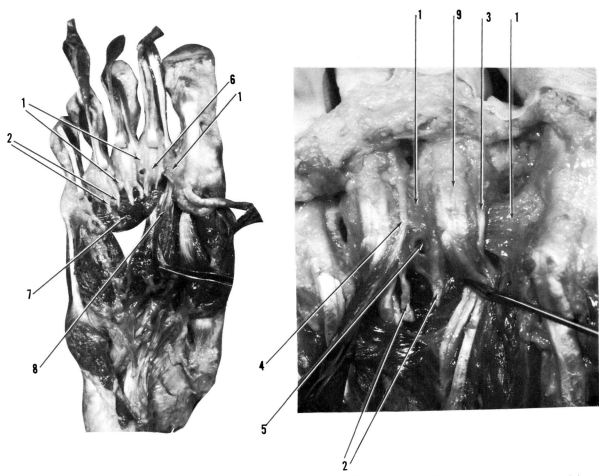

Fig. 4-68. Deep transverse metatarsal ligament. (1, Deep transverse metatarsal ligament; 2, insertion of longitudinal septae of plantar aponeurosis on plantar plate [6] and over aponeurosis covering transverse head of adductor hallucis muscle [7]; 3, lumbrical tendon crossing plantar aspect of [1]; 4 thin tunnel of lumbrical tendon; 5, foramina for passage of common digital artery; 8, oblique head of adductor hallucis muscle; 9, flexor digitorum longus and brevis tendons.)

Fig. 4-67 (*continued*)

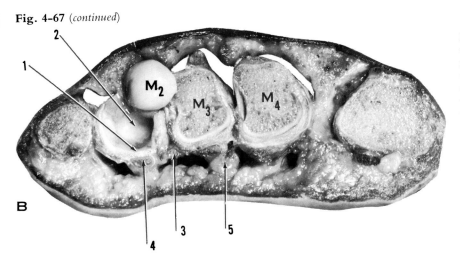

Fig. 4-67. (*A*) *Arrows* indicate the direction of the long flexor tendons passing through the foramina delineated by the longitudinal septae of the plantar aponeurosis. (5, Adipose pre-flexor tendon cushion, reflected; 6, adipose body, reflected from the intermetatarsal head space.) (*B*) Cross section through metatarsal heads $M_{2,3,4}$. (1, Plantar plate; 2, base of proximal phalanx; 3, lumbrical tendon and canal; 4, long flexor tendons and their fibrous tunnel; 5, pre-flexor fat cushion retained within preflexor space [see Fig. 4-66].)

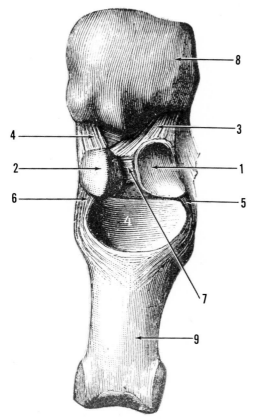

Fig. 4-69. Phalangeosesamoid apparatus of the big toe. (1, Medial sesamoid; 2, lateral sesamoid; 3, medial metatarsosesamoid ligament; 4, lateral metatarsosesamoid ligament; 5, medial phalangeosesamoid ligament; 6, lateral phalangeosesamoid ligament; 7, intersesamoid ligament; 8, head of first metatarsal; 9, proximal phalanx of big toe.) (From Gillette: Des os sésamoides. Anat Physiol Normal Pathol 8: 506, 1872)

INTERPHALANGEAL JOINT LIGAMENTS OF THE LESSER TOES

The collateral ligaments of the interphalangeal joints extend from the lateral aspect of the head of the corresponding phalanx to the base of the distally located phalanx. When sesamoid bones are present, as described in Chapter 2, they are then an integral part of the plantar plate and offer a small articular surface.

PROXIMAL PHALANGEAL APPARATUS OF THE LARGE TOE

The two sesamoids, embedded in the thick fibrous plantar plate and united to the proximal phalanx of the big toe, form an anatomic and functional unit called by Gillette the *sesamophalangeal apparatus* (Fig. 4-69).[32] The sesamophalangeal apparatus moves backward or forward relative to the fixed metatarsal head; in hallux valgus or in traumatic displacements, the sesamoids always follow the proximal phalanx and are displaced with the latter, not with the metatarsal head.

The smaller, upper portion of the metatarsal head is convex in the vertical and transverse direction and corresponds to the glenoid cavity of the proximal phalanx. The larger, inferior two thirds of the metatarsal head has a median crest separating two small, obliquely oriented trochlear surfaces, each corresponding to a sesamoid. The medial sesamoid is slightly larger than the lateral, and each sesamoid has an

Fig. 4-70. Phalangeosesamoid apparatus of the big toe. (Metatarsosesamoid ligaments, medial (1′)and lateral (1); 2, transverse band uniting the sesamophalangeal ligaments; sesamoids, medial (3′) and lateral (3); 4, proximal phalanx; 5, metatarsal head.)

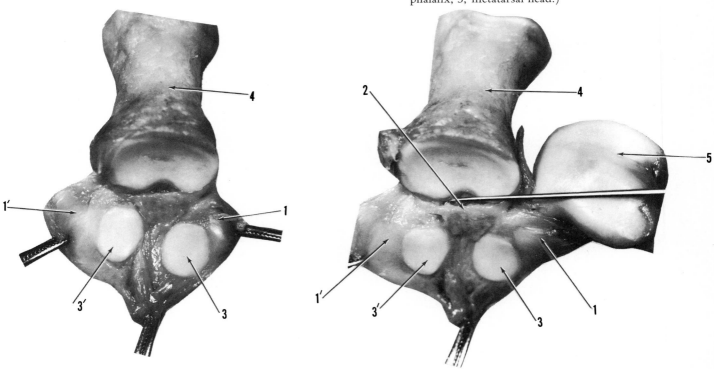

anteroposterior concavity, corresponding to the lateral contour of the metatarsal head, and a slight transverse convexity. Occasionally a definite smooth anteroposterior crest is recognizable, the mid axis of the sesamoid corresponding to the mid axis of the corresponding metatarsal trochlear surface.

The two sesamoids are united by a thick intersesamoid ligament (Fig. 4-70). Each sesamoid is united, by an ill-defined short sesamophalangeal ligament, to the base of the proximal phalanx, which makes the distal attachment to the plantar plate stronger on the sides and weaker centrally. On the intra-articular surface of the plantar plate, a transverse band extends from one sesamophalangeal ligament to the other, and the distal border of this band forms with the inferior concave border of the proximal phalanx a triangular small space lodging synovial tissue. The intersesamoid segment of the plantar plate corresponds to the crest of the metatarsal head, and longitudinally running fibers cover the area and blend with the more distal transverse band. Obliquely oriented fibers may be seen crossing the most proximal segment of the plate in a medial-to-lateral direction. Each side of the plantar plate receives the insertion of the corresponding metatarsosesamoid suspensory ligament.

The proximal border of the plantar plate is complex (Fig. 4-71). The central segment is in continuity proximally with synovial-type tissue and anchors on the neck of the first metatarsal. This central segment provides attachment to the two vertical septae of the plantar aponeurosis of the first ray and also blends with the proximal segment of the fibrous tunnel of the flexor hallucis longus tendon. The lateral and medial segments of the proximal border of the plantar plate give partial insertion to the lateral and medial heads of the flexor hallucis brevis, respectively (Fig. 4-72).

The plantar surface of the plantar plate is raised on each side by the medial and lateral sesamoids. Between the two, a groove for the flexor hallucis longus tendon is formed, converted into a fibrous tunnel by arcuate fibers. These fibers receive contributions from the two vertical septae of the plantar aponeurosis. The floor of the long flexor tunnel is formed by a transverse fibrocartilaginouslike ligament. Occasionally a smaller transverse subband is seen proximally. A triangular tendonlike structure extends from the distal border of the transverse ligament, and the apex fades away distally at the level of the proximal phalanx.

The sesamoids are foci of insertion. The proximal segment of each sesamoid gives insertion to the corresponding

Fig. 4-71. Plantar aspect of the big toe. (1, Proximal border of plantar plate; 2, insertion of longitudinal septae on plantar plate; 3, flexor hallucis longus tendon; 4, flexor hallucis longus tunnel; 5, flexor hallucis brevis muscle, lateral head; 6, flexor hallucis brevis muscle, medial head; 7, adductor hallucis muscle, oblique head; 8, adductor hallucis muscle, transverse head; 9, abductor hallucis muscle-tendon; 10, first metatarsal.)

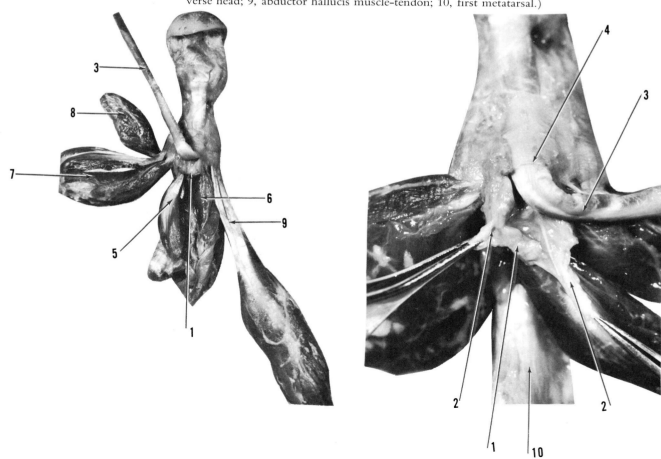

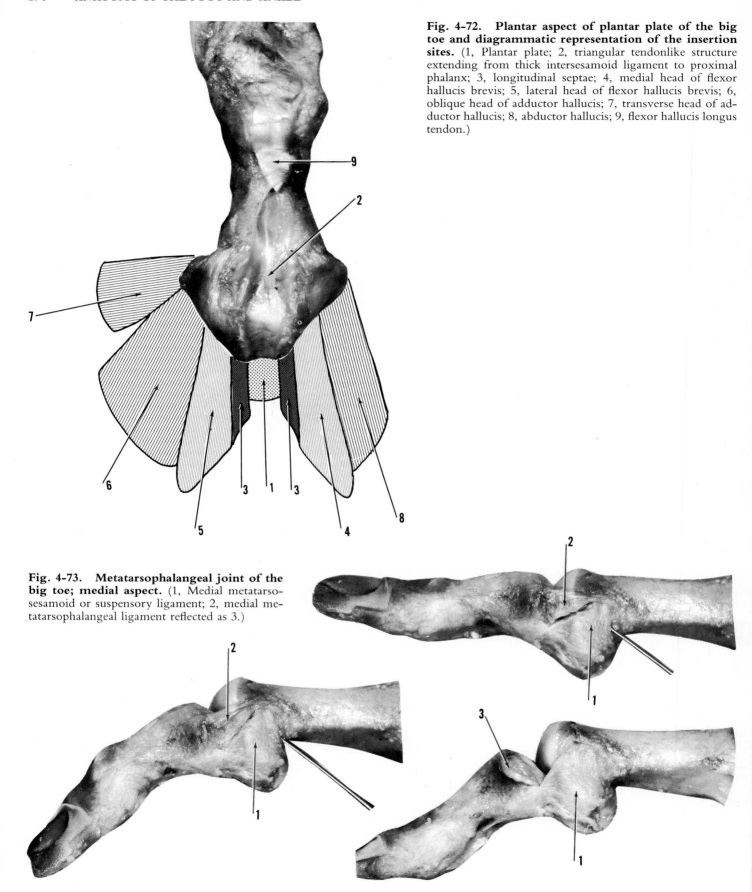

Fig. 4-72.   Plantar aspect of plantar plate of the big toe and diagrammatic representation of the insertion sites. (1, Plantar plate; 2, triangular tendonlike structure extending from thick intersesamoid ligament to proximal phalanx; 3, longitudinal septae; 4, medial head of flexor hallucis brevis; 5, lateral head of flexor hallucis brevis; 6, oblique head of adductor hallucis; 7, transverse head of adductor hallucis; 8, abductor hallucis; 9, flexor hallucis longus tendon.)

Fig. 4-73.   Metatarsophalangeal joint of the big toe; medial aspect. (1, Medial metatarsosesamoid or suspensory ligament; 2, medial metatarsophalangeal ligament reflected as 3.)

Fig. 4-74. Metatarsophalangeal joint of the big toe. (*A*) Medial aspect. (*B*) Lateral aspect. (1, Medial metatarsosesamoid ligament; 2, medial metatarsophalangeal ligament; 3, lateral metatarsosesamoid ligament; 4, lateral metatarsophalangeal ligament; 5, tendon of abductor hallucis muscle; 6, adductor hallucis muscle-tendon; 7, flexor hallucis brevis, lateral head; 8, flexor hallucis longus tendon.)

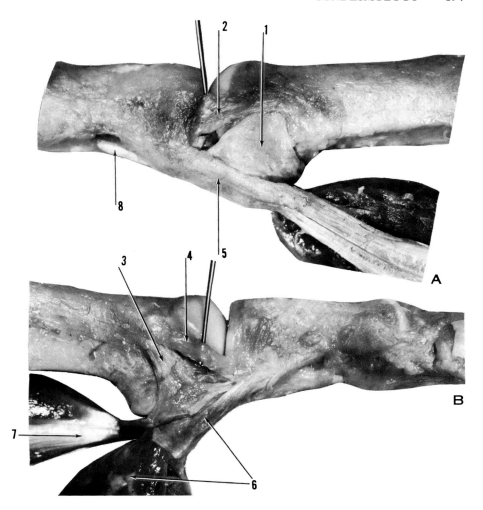

head of the flexor hallucis brevis. The lateral head of the flexor hallucis brevis enters into its own fibrous tunnel prior to the insertion on the sesamoid. The deep transverse metatarsal ligament attaches longitudinally along the lateral sesamoid. Dorsal to this ligament, the lateral sesamoid gives insertion to the oblique and transverse components of the adductor hallucis muscle. The medial sesamoid also receives insertional fibers from the abductor hallucis. Vertical fibrous bands extend from the sides of the sesamoids and the flexor hallucis longus tendon sheath and connect with the superficial band of the plantar aponeurosis. Some of these fibers curve over the fibrous flexor tunnel and form a pre-flexor tendon compartment retaining an adipose cushion, which also covers both sesamoids. From the dorsal aspect, the transverse lamina of the extensor hallucis longus aponeurosis inserts along the lateral and medial borders of the plantar plate.

METATARSOPHALANGEAL LIGAMENTS OF THE BIG TOE

The metatarsal head is united to the proximal phalangeal apparatus by two seats of ligaments: the lateral collateral ligaments and the metatarso-sesamoid suspensory ligaments (Figs. 4-73–4-75). These two sets originate from the lateral

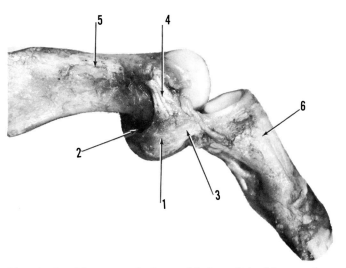

Fig. 4-75. Metatarsophalangeal joint of the big toe, lateral aspect. (1, Sesamoid; 2, proximal border of plantar plate; 3, sesamophalangeal ligament; 4, suspensory metatarsosesamoid ligament; 5, metatarsal; 6, proximal phalanx.)

tubercle of the metatarsal head, the origin of the lateral collateral ligament slightly covering the origin of the suspensory ligament. From their origin, the ligaments fan out in a triangular manner. The lateral collateral ligament is directed downward anteriorly and inserts on the tubercle at the base of the proximal phalanx. The thick metatarsosesamoid or suspensory ligament–descends vertically and inserts on the lateral and medial borders of the plantar plate. The posterior border of the lateral collateral ligament is in continuity with the suspensory ligament, and the anatomic separation is nearly artificial. These two ligaments are identified mostly by their insertions.

INTERPHALANGEAL JOINT LIGAMENTS OF THE BIG TOE

The interphalangeal joint of the big toe may possess a sesamoid bone, median and transversely oriented, embedded in the plantar plate and located above the flexor hallucis longus tendon. The superior articular surface of the sesamoid is divided by a transverse crest into two facets: one anterior, articulating with the distal phalanx, and one posterior, corresponding to the head of the proximal phalanx. The sesamoid is connected to the sides of the distal phalanx with two small ligaments.[32] Two collateral ligaments extend from the lateral aspect of the proximal phalangeal head to the tubercle at the base of the distal phalanx.

REFERENCES

1. Morris HL: The Anatomy of the Joints of Man, p 384. London, Churchill, 1879
2. Poirier P, Charpy A: Traité d'Anatomie Humaine, vol 1, pp 760–762. 756, Paris, Masson, 1899
3. Testut L: Traité d'Anatomie Humaine, vol 1, pp 630, 635–638. Paris, Doin, 1921
4. Prins JG: Diagnosis and treatment of injury to the lateral ligament of the ankle. Acta Chir Scand [Suppl] 486:23, 1978
5. Ruth CJ: The surgical treatment of injuries of the fibular collateral ligaments of the ankle. J Bone Joint Surg [Am] 43:229, 1961
6. Laidlaw PL: The varieties of the os calcis. J Anat Physiol 38:138, 1904
7. Paturet G: Traité d'Anatomie Humaine, vol. 2, pp 704–707, 726–727. Paris, Masson, 1951
8. Dujarier CH: Anatomie des Membres: Dissection—Anatomie Topographique, 2nd ed, pp 399, 403–407. Paris, Masson, 1924
9. Rouvière J, Canela Lazaro M: Le ligament péroneo-astragalo-calcanéen. Ann Anat Pathol Anat Normal 9:745, 1932
10. Beau A: Recherches sur le développement et la constitution morphologiques de l'articulation du cou-de-pied chez l'homme. Arch Anat Histol Embryol 26:238, 1939
11. Barclay-Smith E: The astragalo-calcaneo-navicular joint. J Anat Physiol 30:390, 1896
12. Sappey PC: Traité d'Anatomie Descriptive, 4th ed, Vol 1, pp 712–714, 728. Paris, Delahaye, Lecrosnier, 1888
13. Toldt C: Anatomischer Atlas für Studirende und Ärzte, 2nd ed, pp 242–243. Berlin, Wien, Urban und Schwarzenberg, 1900
14. Warwick R, Williams PL (eds): Gray's Anatomy, 35th ed, pp 460–461. Philadelphia, WB Saunders, 1973
15. Yashar J: Contribution à l'étude des ligaments des articulations tibiotarsienne et médio-tarsienne. Arch Anat Histol Embryol Normal Exp 44:25, 1961
16. Pankovich AM, Shivaram MS: Anatomical basis of variability in injuries of the medial malleolus and the deltoid ligament: I. Anatomical studies. Acta Orthop Scand 50:217, 1979
17. Fick R: Handbuch der Anatomie und Mechanik der Glenke, Vol 1, pp 410–414. Jena, Fischer, 1904
18. Bourgery, Jacob: Traité Complet de l'Anatomie de l'Homme, Vol 1. Paris, 1832
19. Henle J: Handbuch der Systematischen Anatomie des Menschen. Vol 3:160–163, Fig. 141, Braunschweig, 1856.
20. Lane AS: The causation, panthology and physiology of several of the deformities which develop during young life. Guy's Hosp Rep 44:254, 1887
21. Volkmann R: Ein ligamentum "neglectum" pedis (lig. calcaneonaviculare mediodorsale seu sustentaculo-naviculare). Verh Anat Ges 64:483, 1970
22. Köktürk: Remarques sur le ligament de Chopart (lig. bifurcatum). Comptes-Rendus Assoc Anat 44:380, 1957
23. Hovelacque A, Sourdin A: Note au sujet de quelques ligaments de l'articulation médio-tarsienne. Ann Anat Pathol Anat Normal 10:469, 1933
24. Jones WF: Structure and Function as Seen in the Foot, 2nd ed, p 120. London, Baillière, 1949
25. Cahill DR: The anatomy and function of the contents of the human tarsal sinus and canal. Anat Rec 153:1, 1965
26. Smith JW: The ligamentous structures in the canalis and sinus tarsi. J Anat 92:616, 1958
27. Spalteholz W: Hand Atlas of Human Anatomy, Vol 1, pp 219, 223. Philadelphia, JB Lippincott, 1903
28. Welti, H: Contribution a l'étude du ligament I cuneiforme II/III metatarsiens—etude d'anatomie comparée. Arch Histol Embryol 48:373, 1966
29. Thomas L: Recherches sur les ligaments interosseux de l'articulation de Lisfranc: Etude anatomique et embry. Arch Anat Histol Embryol 5:104, 1926
30. Bojsen-Møller F, Flagstad KE: Plantar aponeurosis and internal architecture of the ball of the foot. J Anat 121:599, 1976
31. Meyer P: Contribution à l'étude de la region métatarso-phalangienne. Comptes-Rendus Assoc Anat 44:500, 1958
32. Gillette: Des os sesamoides. J Anat Physiol Normal Pathol 8:506, 1872

5

Myology

In the anatomical position, the foot is in a transverse plane relative to the leg; all the extrinsic tendons destined for the midfoot and forefoot make the necessary turn around the ankle and are retained by their corresponding retinacular systems acting as pulleys. The detailed anatomy of these retaining systems has been dealt with in Chapter 3.

Anterior Aspect of the Ankle and Dorsum of the Foot

Four tendons are present on the anterior aspect of the ankle: the tibialis anterior, the extensor hallucis longus, the extensor digitorum longus, and the peroneus tertius.

TIBIALIS ANTERIOR

The flat tendon of the tibialis anterior acquires its first retaining tunnel under the superior extensor retinaculum (Fig. 5-1). From the anteromedial aspect of the ankle, the tendon courses toward the medial border of the foot. It makes a twist and inserts vertically over a tubercle on the inferomedial aspect of the first metatarsal base and on the medial aspect of the first cuneiform. Retaining tunnels are provided by the superomedial and inferomedial bands of the inferior extensor retinaculum. A terminal tunnel may be formed by the transverse retinacular band over the first metatarsal bone. The interretinacular segments of the tendon are covered by the thin dorsal aponeurosis of the foot.

Variations

The insertional variations of the tibialis anterior may be grouped under bifurcations, extensions of attachment, and loss of attachment.[1-3] Hallisy, in a comprehensive study of 290 feet, reported 90% with customary insertion of the tibialis anterior tendon on the base of the first metatarsal

and first cuneiform and 10% with insertional variations (Fig. 5-2).[3]

Bifurcation. The tibialis anterior tendon may be bifid.[1-5] The anterior tendon inserts on the base of the first metatarsal and the posterior tendon on the first cuneiform. The division of the tendon may extend 1 cm to 2 cm above the cuneometatarsal joint or may, rarely, reach the muscular fibers or even separate the muscle fibers a length of 1.5 cm.[1] Between these two extremes, all the intermediaries may exist.

Extensions of Attachment. The tibialis anterior tendon may insert additionally on the navicular, forming a fan-shaped tendon; on the base of the proximal phalanx of the big toe; on the distal dorsal part of the first metatarsal; on the adjacent parts of the first metatarsal head and proximal phalanx;[1] on the inferior extensor retinaculum and dorsal aponeurosis of the foot; on the talus and calcaneus with another band reaching the navicular and the first cuneiform; on the neck of the talus and the capsule of the ankle joint; on the plantar aponeurosis.[1-3, 5-7]

Loss of Attachment. There may be loss of attachment with insertion on the first metatarsal base only.[3]

Additional Muscle Variants

Three additional muscles may be present as variants of the tibialis anterior muscle: musculus tibioastragalus anticus of Gruber; musculus tibiofascialis anticus of Macalister or musculus tensor fasciae dorsalis pedis.[1-3, 8, 9]

Musculus Tibioastragalus Anticus of Gruber. Gruber describes three cases of a muscle located behind the tibialis anterior, originating from the tibia and the interosseous membrane and inserting on the lateral aspect of the

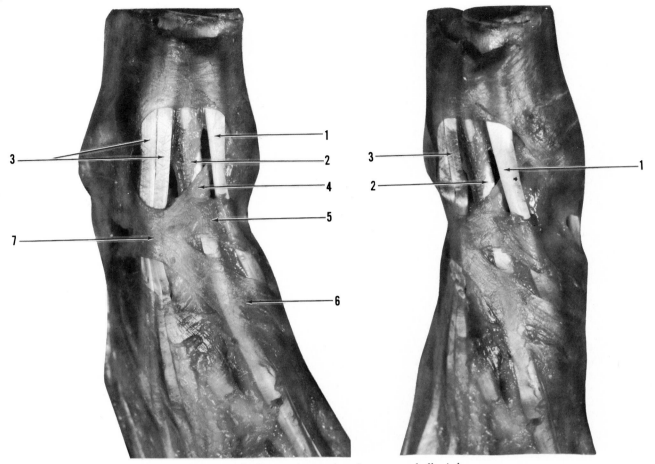

Fig. 5-1. Tibialis anterior tendon. (1, Tibialis anterior tendon; 2, extensor hallucis longus tendon; 3, extensor digitorum longus tendons; 4, 5, superior and inferior subdivisions of the superomedial band of the inferior extensor retinaculum, forming a tunnel for *1;* 6, inferomedial band of inferior extensor retinaculum; 7, stem of inferior extensor retinaculum.)

talar neck.[8] Two of the three muscles had additional attachment to the medial malleolus, and one also had an attachment into the talonavicular joint and the navicular.[8]

Seelaus describes a similar muscle originating from the anterior surface of the lower third of the tibia, lateral to the anterior tibial crest, from the interosseous membrane, and from an intermuscular septum intervening between the muscle and the tibialis anterior (Fig. 5-3).[9] The tendon of the muscle is first medial to the tendon of the tibialis anterior and then is located behind it; it passes with the tendon of the tibialis anterior through the same inferior extensor retinacular compartment. The tendon of the tibioastragalus anticus pierces the capsule of the ankle joint and inserts in a fanlike manner into the anterosuperior aspect of the talar neck.

Musculus Tibiofascialis Anticus of Macalister and Musculus Tensor Fasciae Dorsalis Pedis. These muscles originate from the lower third of the anterior edge or the lateral side of the tibia.[1-3] The muscle is located over the

tibialis anterior and inserts on the inferior extensor retinaculum over the extensor digitorum longus or on the dorsal aponeurosis of the foot.

EXTENSOR HALLUCIS LONGUS

At the level of the ankle the extensor hallucis longus tendon is deep and lateral to the tibialis anterior tendon, and the muscle fibers descend very low on the lateral aspect of the tendon, reaching the level of the inferior extensor retinaculum (Figs. 5-1 and 5-4). The tendon passes through its own fibrous tunnel and is directed anteriorly and slightly medially along the dorsum of the first metatarsal. It extends farther distally, gradually enlarges, and inserts on the dorsum of the base of the distal hallucal phalanx.

The extensor hallucis longus tendon is connected to the lateral aspect of the proximal phalanx by the extensor aponeurosis. The latter receives contributions laterally from the adductor tendon and medially from the abductor hallucis tendon.

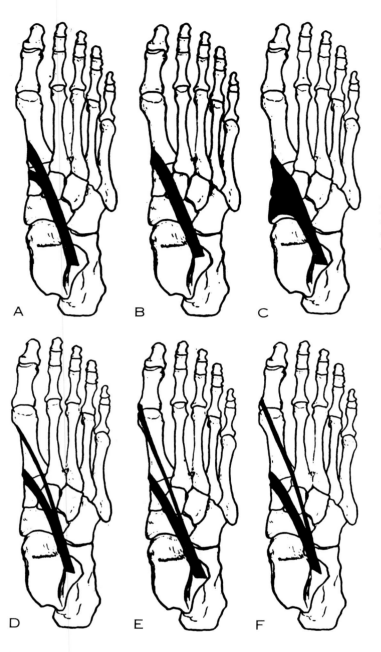

Fig. 5-2. Insertional variations of the tibialis anterior tendon. The customary insertion on the adjacent areas of the first metatarsal and the medial cuneiform occurs in 90%. The variations occur in 10%. (*A*) Splitting of tibialis anterior tendon at or near insertion but not more than 25 mm from the latter (1%). (*B*) Insertion of tibialis anterior tendon into first metatarsal only (1.5%). (*C*) Fan-shaped insertion of tibialis anterior tendon into navicular, cuneiform 1, metatarsal 1 (0.3%). (*D*) A slip of the tibialis anterior tendon inserting on the first metatarsal distally, representing in rudimentary form the musculus extensor ossis primi metatarsi (1%). (*E*) Accessory slip of tibialis anterior tendon inserting on the dorsum of the distal segment of the first metatarsal and the base of the proximal phalanx of the big toe (0.3%). (*F*) A slip of the tibialis anterior tendon inserting on the base of the proximal phalanx of the big toe, representing the musculus extensor primi internodii hallucis (2.3%). (From Hallisy JE: The muscular variations in the human foot: A quantitative study. Am J Anat 45, No. 3: 411, 1930)

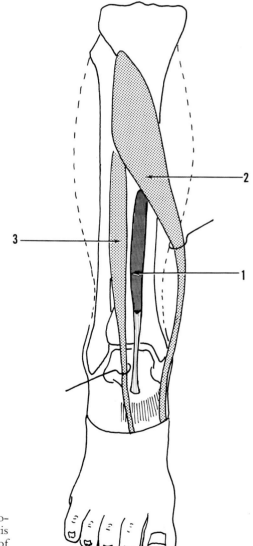

Fig. 5-3. Musculus tibio-astragalus anticus of Gruber. (1, Musculus tibio-astragalus anticus of Gruber; 2, tibialis anterior muscle; 3, extensor hallucis longus muscle.) (Redrawn from Seelaus HK: On certain muscle anomalies of the lower extremity. Anat Rec 35: 187, 1927)

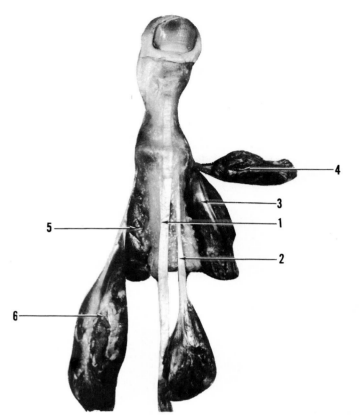

Fig. 5-4.   Dorsal aspect of big toe. (1, Extensor hallucis longus tendon; 2, extensor hallucis brevis; 3, adductor hallucis muscle, oblique head; 4, adductor hallucis muscle, transverse head; 5, flexor hallucis brevis, medial head; 6, abductor hallucis muscle.)

Fig. 5-5.   Insertional variations of the extensor hallucis longus tendon. (*A*) A slip from the extensor hallucis longus tendon to the base of the proximal phalanx of the big toe (23%), forming the musculus extensor primi internodii hallucis. (*B*) As in *A* but with two tendinous accessory insertional slips on the base of the proximal phalanx (1.5%). (*C*) A slip from the extensor hallucis longus tendon inserting on the distal segment of the first metatarsal (1.5%), representing the musculus extensor ossis primi metatarsi. (*D*) A slip from the extensor hallucis longus tendon joining the extensor hallucis brevis tendon (1%). (*E*) A slip from the extensor hallucis longus tendon joining the extensor digitorum longus tendon (0.3%). (*F*) Combined lateral expansion from the extensor hallucis longus tendon to a tendinous slip of the extensor digitorum longus inserting on the base of the proximal phalanx of the big toe and a second tendinous slip representing a musculus extensor primi internodii hallucis. (From Hallisy JE: The muscular variations in the human foot: A quantitative study. Am J Anat 45, No. 3:411, 1930)

Variations

There are a number of variations involving the insertion of the extensor hallucis longus (Fig. 5-5).[1, 2, 10-12] The most frequent variation is the tendinous attachment to the proximal phalanx. The percentage of occurrence of this variation, according to various sources, is as follows: in 290 feet, 23%; in 72 feet, 72%; in 50 feet, 54% (approximate average, 50%).[3, 10, 12]

A proximal hallucal phalangeal slip may also be provided by the tibialis anterior tendon (in 8%) and by the extensor digitorum longus.[12] Other rare insertional variations may occur in combination with the insertion to the distal phalanx: two tendinous slips inserting on the proximal phalanx;

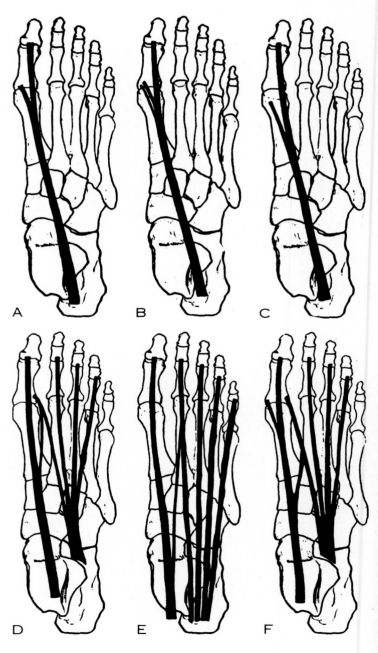

Fig. 5-6. Extensor digitorum longus. (1–4, Extensor digitorum longus tendon to toes 5, 4, 3, 2; 5, extensor hallucis longus tendon; 6, extensor hallucis brevis tendon; 7, extensor digitorum brevis tendons [none to the fifth toe]; 8, peroneus tertius tendon; 9, fat pad of prelateral malleolar fossa.)

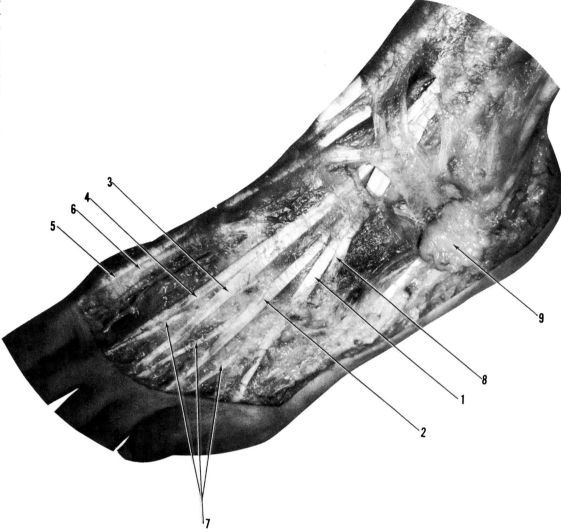

one tendinous slip attached into the distal part of the dorsal aspect of the first metatarsal; a small slip extended to the most medial tendon of the extensor digitorum brevis; a tendinous extension to the extensor digitorum communis of the second toe; a tendinous extension to the extensor digitorum brevis and to the base of the proximal phalanx (very rare).

Additional Muscle Variants

The division of the tendon of the extensor hallucis longus may extend proximally through the muscle fibers and form an additional muscle.[1] Two such muscles may be seen: extensor ossis metatarsi hallucis, when the insertion is on the dorsum of the first metatarsal, or extensor primi internodii hallucis, when the muscle inserts on the base of the proximal phalanx of the big toe. The latter muscle originates from the fibula and the interosseous membrane. Frequently the tendinous segment is traced proximally at the level of the ankle into an atrophic structure attached to the inter-

osseous membrane and formed by fibroadipose tissue intermingled with muscle fibers.

EXTENSOR DIGITORUM LONGUS

The muscle fibers of the extensor digitorum longus extend distally on the lateral border of the common tendon to a level 8 mm to 10 mm proximal to the inferior extensor retinaculum (Figs. 5-6 and 5-7).[13] Initially unique, the extensor digitorum longus tendon divides into two tendons under the superior extensor retinaculum. Both tendons enter the common tunnel under the inferior extensor retinaculum, and as they exit under the stem of the retinaculum, each divides into two tendons. The divided two lateral tendons reach the fifth and fourth toes and the medial two tendons reach the third and the second toe, respectively. At the level of the metatarsophalangeal joint, the long extensor tendons of the second to the fourth toe are joined from the peroneal side by the corresponding extensor brevis tendons.

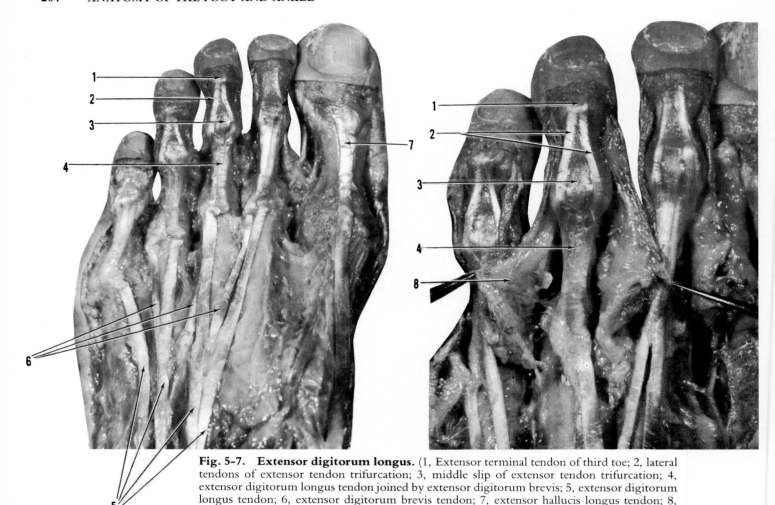

Fig. 5-7. Extensor digitorum longus. (1, Extensor terminal tendon of third toe; 2, lateral tendons of extensor tendon trifurcation; 3, middle slip of extensor tendon trifurcation; 4, extensor digitorum longus tendon joined by extensor digitorum brevis; 5, extensor digitorum longus tendon; 6, extensor digitorum brevis tendon; 7, extensor hallucis longus tendon; 8, adiporetinacular layer carrying superficial nerves and vessels.)

This extensor tendinous ensemble forms a trifurcation system over the dorsum of the proximal phalanx and divides into a middle or central slip and two lateral slips. The central slip inserts on the dorsum of the middle phalanx and the capsule of the proximal interphalangeal joint. The two lateral slips, after receiving tendinous contribution mostly from the lumbrical on the tibial side, form two lateral tendons. These two tendons gradually converge on the dorsum of the middle phalanx and form a common terminal tendon that inserts on the dorsal capsule of the distal interphalangeal joint and on the base of the distal phalanx. The corresponding tendon of the extensor digitorum brevis inserts on the common extensor tendon laterally or forms the entire lateral slip on the peroneal side.[14, 15]

The tendons of the extensor system are anchored at the level of the metatarsophalangeal joint and proximal phalanx by a fibroaponeurotic structure. The proximal segment of this aponeurosis has transversely oriented fibers originating from the lateral and medial borders of the flat aponeurotic tunnel surrounding the corresponding extensor tendons. The transverse aponeurotic fibers extend around the capsule of the metatarsophalangeal joint and blend on the plantar side with the plantar plate, the deep transverse metatarsal ligament, and the flexor tendon sheath. This firm insertion extends distally on the base of the proximal phalanx. The proximal segment of the extensor aponeurosis is termed the *transverse* or *quadrilateral lamina* or *extensor sling* (Figs. 5-8–5-10).[15]

Farther distally the extensor aponeurosis is formed by obliquely oriented fibers making up the extensor wing or extensor hood.[15] Tendinous expansions from the lumbrical or the minute expansion from the plantar interosseous to the middle slip forms the spiral fibers.[14, 15] The triangular space located between the lateral tendons is filled by an aponeurotic structure called the *triangular lamina*.[14, 15]

The fifth toe does not have a corresponding extensor brevis tendon; furthermore, beyond the base of the proximal phalanx there is an atrophy of the fibrous apparatus, and usually the spiral fibers and the triangular lamina do not exist at this level (Fig. 5-10).[14]

At the level of the proximal interphalangeal joint, transversely oriented fibers extend from the trifurcation tendons to the flexor tunnel.[14]

There are a number of variations involving the extensor digitorum longus.[1, 2]

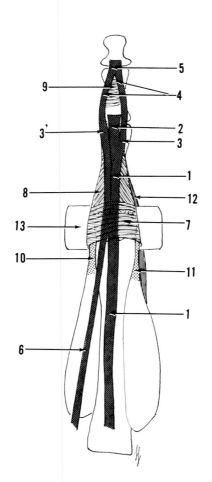

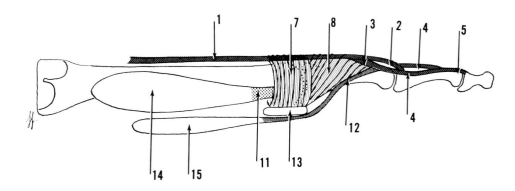

Fig. 5-8. Extensor complex of a lesser toe. (1, Extensor digitorum longus tendon; 2, middle slip of extensor tendon trifurcation; 3, 3′, lateral slips of extensor tendon trifurcation; 4, lateral tendons of extensor tendon trifurcation; 5, terminal extensor tendon; 6, extensor digitorum brevis tendon; 7, transverse lamina of extensor aponeurosis or extensor sling; 8, oblique component of extensor aponeurosis forming the extensor hood or wing; 9, triangular ligament; 10, 11, interossei tendons; 12, lumbrical tendon; 13, deep transverse metatarsal ligament; 14, interosseous muscle; 15, lumbrical muscle.)

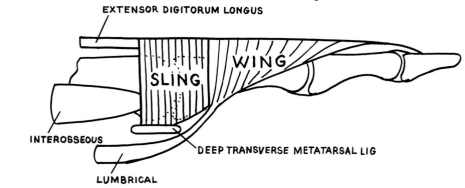

Fig. 5-9. Extensor aponeurosis of a lesser toe.

Individual Muscles

The level at which the common long extensor divides into the digital components proximally is very variable. The tendinous divisions may extend farther proximally and divide the muscle mass into separate muscle units. The following variations are possible:

Four muscle units followed by four tendons.
One muscle unit corresponding to the lateral three long extensor tendons and one muscle corresponding to the tendon of the second toe, thus forming the extensor proper of the second toe.
One muscle unit corresponding to the tendons of the second, third, and fourth toes and one muscle with a tendon to the fifth toe, the latter tendon combined with the peroneus tertius.

Bifid Tendons

Distally the long extensor tendon of a lesser toe may be bifid, with the following distributions:

Both tendons may insert on the same toe.
The additional tendons of the third and fourth toes may insert laterally or medially on the adjacent toes.
The additional tendon of the second toe may insert on the third toe, and that of the fifth toe may insert on the fourth toe.

Additional Slips

Additional tendinous slips from the extensor digitorum longus may insert on the metatarsal shaft, the extensor digitorum brevis tendon, the dorsal aponeurosis, the big toe. Anastomotic fibrous bands, variable in number and location, may also unite the long extensor tendons of the adjacent toes.

EXTENSOR DIGITORUM BREVIS

The extensor digitorum brevis muscle originates from the anterolateral aspect of the sinus tarsi (Fig. 5-11). The muscle is located between the lateral and intermediate roots of the

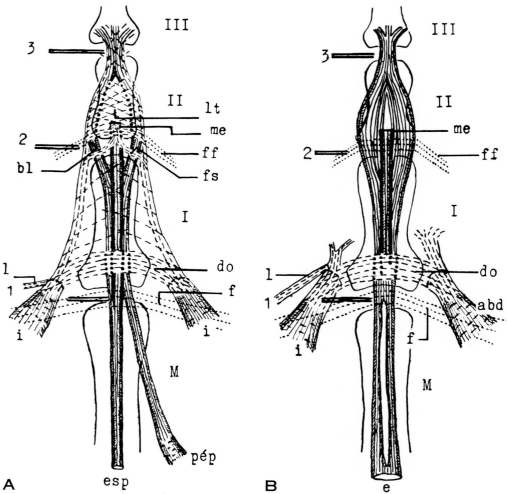

Fig. 5-10.   Internal structure of extensor mechanism of lesser toes. (*A*) Second toe, right foot. (*B*) Fifth toe, right foot. (*e, esp,* extensor digitorum longus tendon; *pep,* extensor digitorum brevis tendon; *i,* interossei; *l,* lumbrical; *do,* dorsal sling; *f,* perforating aponeurotic fibers arising from plantar aponeurosis; *fs,* spiral fibers; *ff,* fibers arising from sheath of long flexors; *lt,* triangular lamina; *bl,* lateral band of long extensor tendon; *me,* middle slip of long extensor tendon; *abd,* abductor of fifth toe; *M,* metatarsal; I, II, III, proximal, middle, and distal phalanges; 1,2,3, level of metatarsophalangeal and interphalangeal joints.) (From Baumann JA: Valeur, variations et équivalences des muscles extenseurs, interosseux, adducteurs et abducteurs de la main et du pied chez l'homme. Acta Anat 4:10, 1947–1948. By permission of S. Karger AG, Basel)

Fig. 5-12.   Variations of the extensor digitorum brevis—additional musculotendinous units. (1, Extensor digitorum brevis muscle; (*A*) 2, digastric muscle formed proximally by additional portion derived from extensor digitorum brevis of second toe and connected to an accessory muscle of first dorsal interosseous; (*B*) 3, digastric muscle derived proximally as in *2* but attached distally to an accessory muscle of second dorsal interosseous; (*C*) 4, trigastric muscle formed proximally by an additional muscle derived from extensor digitorum brevis to second toe and attached distally to accessory muscles of first and second dorsal interossei; (*D*) 5, two digastric muscles arising separately from extensor digitorum brevis and attached distally to accessory muscles of first and second dorsal interossei.) (Redrawn after Lucien M: Sur les connexions entre le pédieux et les muscles interosseur dorsaux chez l'homme: Considérations sur le developpement du muscle pédieux. Bibl Anat XIX:232, 1909)

Fig. 5-11.   Extensor digitorum brevis. (*A*) Extensor digitorum brevis tendon to toes 2, 3, 4; (*B*) extensor hallucis brevis tendon.) (From Meyer P: La morphologie du ligament annulair anterieur du cou-de-pied chez l'homme. Comptes-Rendus Assoc Anat 84: 281, 1955)

inferior extensor retinaculum and is lateral to the cervical ligament and posterior to the origin of the dorsal calcaneocuboid ligament. Occasionally a slip from the intermediary root divides the extensor hallucis brevis from the extensor digitorum brevis of the lesser toes.

The muscle divides into four fascicles that terminate in four tendons located on the peroneal side of the first four toes. There is no extensor brevis tendon to the fifth toe. As mentioned above, each extensor brevis tendon of the lesser toes joins the corresponding extensor digitorum longus tendon and may form the lateral slip of the trifurcation in its entirety. The extensor digitorum brevis to the first toe or extensor hallucis brevis is located deep under the extensor hallucis longus and its aponeurosis; it enlarges distally and inserts on the dorsum of the proximal phalanx.

Lucien, based on a study of 51 feet, reported that the normal division of the extensor digitorum brevis into four components occurs only in 26% and that in 72.5% an additional musculotendinous unit may be present.[16] The absence of a slip is rare.

Additional Musculotendinous Units

The additional musculotendinous units (Fig. 5-12) are of the following types: accessory medial head to the second, fourth, and third toes (in order of decreasing frequency); accessory digastric and trigastric muscles; extensions to the

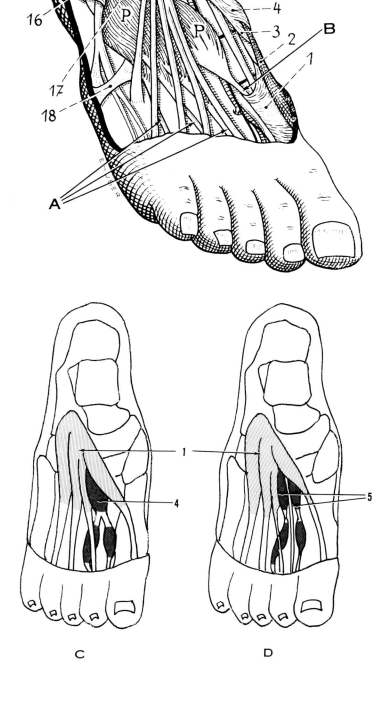

long extensor tendons; extensions to the metatarsal and midtarsal bones.

The *accessory medial head to the second toe* occurs quite frequently (in 34%), and the well-developed muscle ends with a tendon that inserts on the medial aspect of the head of the proximal phalanx of the second toe.[16] Occasionaly this tendon terminates on the first dorsal interosseous aponeurosis. The origin of this muscle is variable. In the majority it arises from the muscle fascicle to the second toe. It sometimes originates from the extensor hallucis brevis, the extensor hallucis brevis and the muscle fascicle to the second toe, or the middle cuneiform or cuboid.

The *accessory medial head of the fourth toe* originates from the corresponding muscle fascicle of the extensor digitorum brevis to the fourth toe. It is medial in location. Rarely the unit is completely developed, and most frequently the tendon terminates on the interosseous aponeurosis.

The *accessory medial head of the third toe* is very rare and originates from the fascicle to the second toe.

The *digastric muscle* is always formed by an accessory muscle arising from the second fascicle of the extensor digitorum brevis and is connected to an accessory muscle of the first or the second dorsal interosseous muscle. Two similar digastric muscles may be present, each connected separately to the accessory first and second dorsal interosseous muscles.

A *trigastric muscle* is formed when the accessory muscle arising from the second fascicle of the extensor brevis attaches simultaneously to the accessory first and second dorsal interosseous muscles.

Variations of Insertion and of Origin

The tendons of the extensor digitorum brevis of the lesser toes may insert on the corresponding base of the proximal phalanx, on the base of the metatarsal, or on the interosseous aponeurosis. The extensor hallucis brevis tendon may insert on the lateral aspect of the extensor hallucis longus tendon. The origin of the extensor digitorum brevis is also subject to variation, as this muscle may originate from the cuneiforms, the cuboid, or even the base of the metatarsals.[1, 17]

PERONEUS TERTIUS

The peroneus tertius tendon is lateral to the extensor digitorum longus tendon and passes in the same compartment or in a separate compartment under the inferior extensor retinaculum (Figs. 5-11 and 5-13). The tendon is directed anteriorly and laterally, fans out, and inserts on the superior surface of the fifth metatarsal base.

Absence

The peroneus tertius muscle may be absent; Ledouble provides the following data: in 102 feet, absent in 10; in 537 feet, absent in 44; in 120 feet, absent in 11 (759 feet total, absent in a total of 65 [8.5%]).[2]

Insertional Variations

There are insertional variations of an additional tendinous slip of the peroneus tertius.

> On the base of the fourth metatarsal. This additional slip seen frequently, and is usually smaller but occasionally equal to or even larger than the main tendon. It may also represent the sole insertion of the peroneus tertius tendon.
> On the fifth toe at the level of one of the phalanges or on the long extensor of the same toe.
> On the fifth metatarsal shaft or on the interosseous space.

Lateral Aspect of the Ankle and Foot and the Sole of the Foot

PERONEUS LONGUS

The peroneus longus is shown in Figures 5-14 and 5-15.[2, 18-20] The lateral surface of the fibula faces laterally in the middle third, becomes directed posteriorly in the distal fourth, and continues as the posterior surface of the lateral malleolus. The osseous twist is also followed by the peroneus longus tendon, which is lateral in the middle third, posterolateral in the distal fourth, and posterior to the peroneus brevis tendon behind the lateral malleolus.

The peroneus longus tendon is retained by three tunnels and makes three turns before reaching its destination. The first tunnel common to both peronei tendons is retromalleolar and is formed by the superior peroneal retinaculum. At the tip of the lateral malleolus, the tendon makes its first turn and is directed downward and anteriorly. It enters the inferior tunnel formed by the inferior peroneal retinaculum at the level of the processus trochlearis of the os calcis and makes its second turn; it is now directed inferiorly and medially. It makes its third turn around the lateral border of the foot between the cuboid and the base of the fifth metatarsal and enters the plantar tunnel. The tendon glides over the anterior convex slope of the cuboidal tuberosity (Fig. 5-16). It obliquely crosses the sole of the foot, oriented anteromedially, and inserts on the lateral tubercle of the base of the first metatarsal (Fig. 5-17). At times it sends an extension to the plantar aspect of the first cuneiform, the base of the second metatarsal, and the first dorsal interosseous. The plantar peroneal tunnel is fibrous at the level of the cuboid and is formed by arciform fibers extended from the crest of the cuboid tuberosity to the anterior ledge of the cuboid. These fibers are deep to the long cuboideometatarsals ligament. This plantar segment of the tunnel is also reinforced by the extensions of the long plantar ligament to the base of the fourth and third metatarsals. The inner segment of the peroneal tunnel is roofed by a thinner layer of fibrous tissue.

At the level of the cuboid tubercle, a near-constant sesamoid, osseous or fibrocartilaginous, is present in the substance of the peroneus longus tendon. Rarely a sesamoid is

Fig. 5-13. Peroneus tertius tendon.
(1, Peroneus tertius tendon; 2, peroneus brevis tendon; 3, supplementary slip of *2;* 4, extensor digitorum longus tendons; 5, extensor digitorum brevis tendons 2, 3, 4; 6, extensor digitorum brevis muscle origin; 7, stem of inferior extensor retinaculum occupying mid and anterior segments of sinus tarsi [8]; 9, peroneus longus tendon; 10, anterior talofibular ligament; 11, lower band of anterior tibiofibular ligament.)

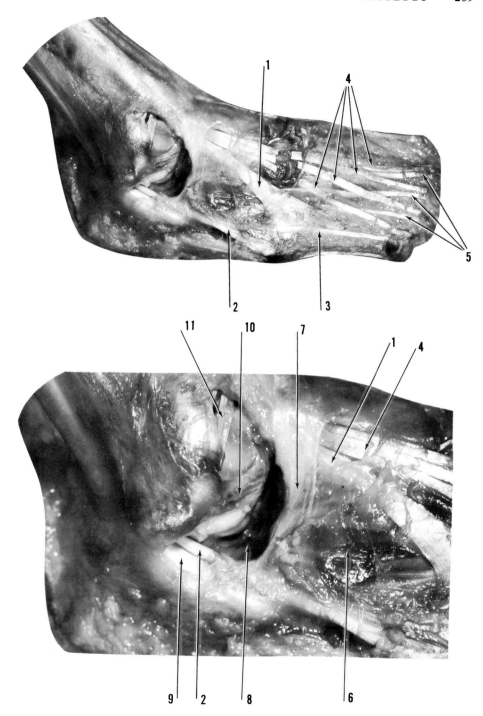

found in the retromalleolar portion of the tendon and very exceptionally in the calcaneal portion of the tendon.

Picou describes the normal insertions of the peroneous longus tendon as taking place on the first metatarsal base; the first cuneiform, plantar aspect; and the first metatarsal, behind the head, on the superolateral border (Fig. 5-18).[19, 20]

The slip to the first cuneiform is described by Picou as arising from the deep or dorsal surface of the peroneus longus tendon at the level of the sesamoid in the cuboid tunnel.[20] It is located near the posterior border and extends medially, and the fan-shaped end of the tendon terminates on the anterior aspect of the plantar surface of the first cuneiform (Fig. 5-19).

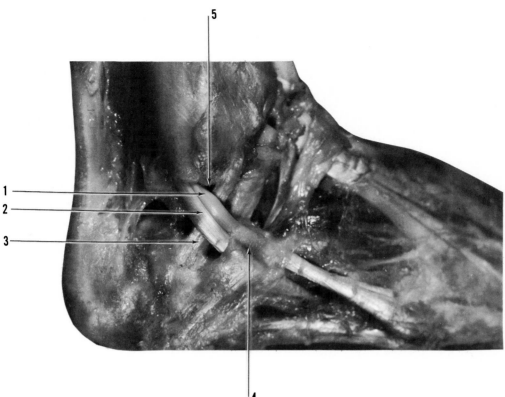

Fig. 5-14. Peroneus longus tendon. (1, Peroneus brevis tendon; 2, peroneus longus tendon; 3, calcaneofibular ligament; 4, inferior peroneal retinaculum; 5, tip of lateral malleolus, *free of insertion.*)

Fig. 5-15. Peroneus longus tendon. (*A*) Superior peroneal retinaculum split. (1, Peroneus brevis tendon; 2, peroneus longus tendon; 3, sulcus of peronei.) (*B*) Peroneus longus tendon reflected. (1, Peroneus brevis tendon; 2, reflected peroneus longus tendon; 3, septum dividing inferior peroneal retinacular tunnel into two; 4, deep surface of superior peroneal retinaculum; 5, sulcus of peronei.)

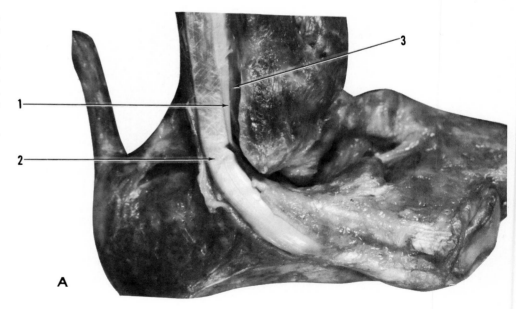

A

The slip to the anterior aspect of the first metatarsal arises from the anterior border of the tendon and is directed toward the base of the second metatarsal; it adheres very weakly to the second metatarsal but is braced against it by a transverse ligament acting as a fibrous bridge. The tendinous slip changes course and is directed toward the head of the first metatarsal. It passes through the first interosseous space and gives insertion from its two surfaces to the first dorsal interosseous muscle and inserts 10 mm behind the first metatarsal head on its lateral aspect. This tendinous slip forms an arcade with medial concavity that forms, with the lateral surface of the first metatarsal, an oval aperture filled with adipose tissue giving passage to the dorsal vessels going to the sole of the foot.

In a study of 54 feet, Picou gives the following information concerning the occurrence of the insertional slips of

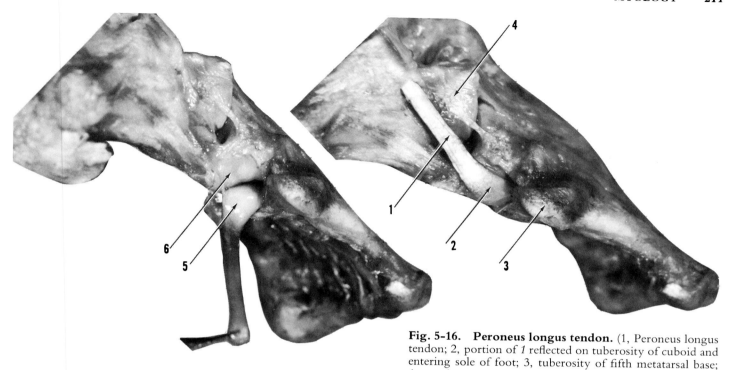

Fig. 5-15 (continued)

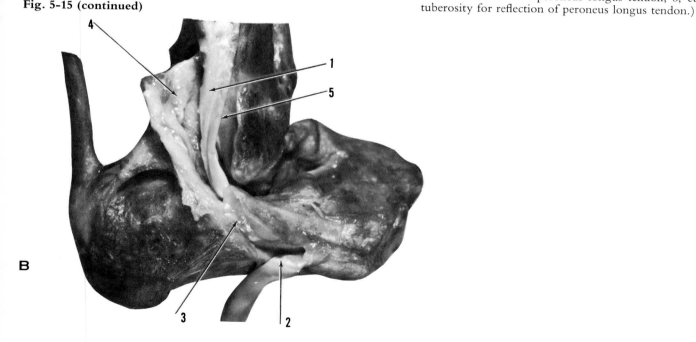

B

Fig. 5-16.   Peroneus longus tendon. (1, Peroneus longus tendon; 2, portion of *1* reflected on tuberosity of cuboid and entering sole of foot; 3, tuberosity of fifth metatarsal base; 4, anterior segment or greater apophysis of os calcis; 5, intra-articular sesamoid of peroneus longus tendon; 6, cuboidal tuberosity for reflection of peroneus longus tendon.)

the peroneus longus tendon: insertion on the cuneiform and metatarsal base, 95%; in the former group, insertion on the metatarsal head, 89%; insertion on the metatarsal base only, 5.5%.[18]

A fibrous expansion may connect the peroneus longus tendon at the level of the cuboidal sesamoid to the base of the fifth metatarsal and to the origin of the short flexor of the fifth toe and forms the anterior frenular ligament contained in the mesotenon. Occasionally the anterior ligament may be large and represent an insertion of the principal tendon on the base of the fifth metatarsal. A posterior frenular ligament, sesamocuboid, may also exist. The rate of occurrence of these frenular ligaments, according to different sources, is as follows: anterior ligament, 80% in 30 feet, 63% in 30 feet; posterior ligament, 13% in 30 feet, 10% in 30 feet.[2, 19] The peroneus longus may receive a slip from the tibialis posterior tendon in 22%.[20]

(Text continues on p. 214.)

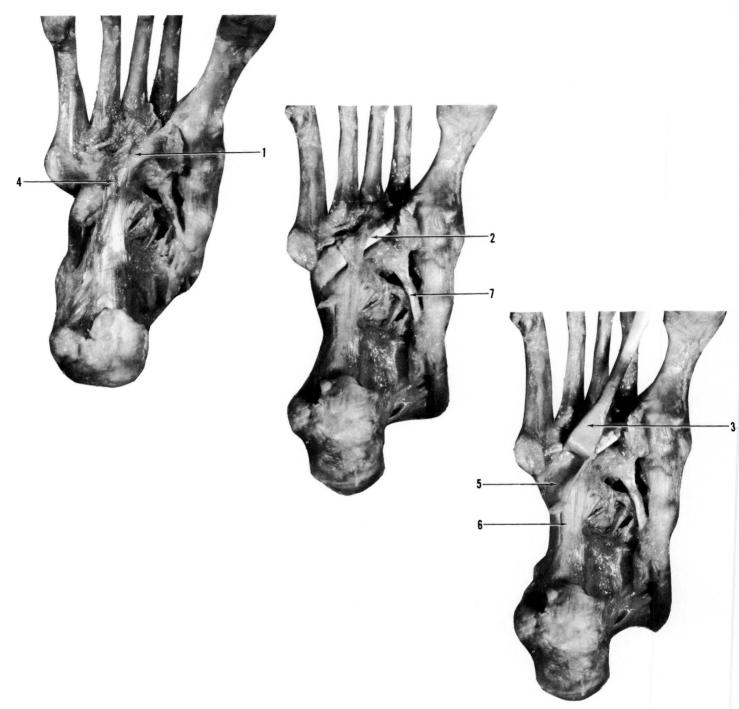

Fig. 5-17. Peroneus longus tendon. (1, Sheath of peroneus longus tendon; 2, peroneus longus tendon; 3, reflected peroneus longus tendon with intratendinous sesamoid; 4, distal segment of long plantar ligament contributing to formation of peroneus longus tunnel; 5, peroneus longus sulcus; 6, long calcaneocuboid ligament; 7, plantar portion of tibialis posterior tendon.)

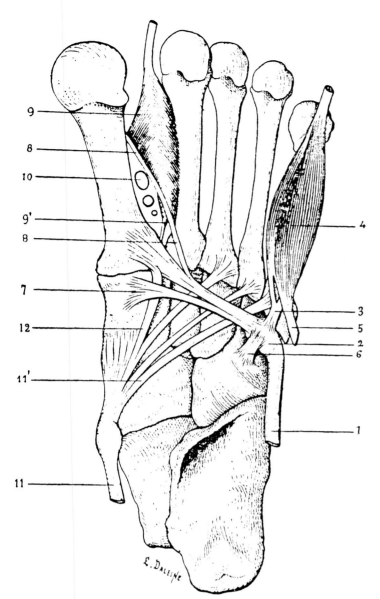

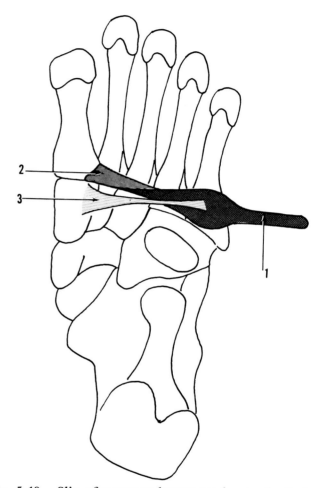

Fig. 5-18.   Normal insertions of peroneus longus tendon. (1, Peroneus longus tendon; 2, sesamoid of *1*; 3, anterior frenulum of sesamoid; 4, short flexor muscle of fifth toe; 5, expansion of *4* that inserts on fibrous tunnel of peroneus longus tendon; 6, posterior frenulum of sesamoid [inconstant]; 7, attachment of *1* on medial cuneiform; 8, expansion of *1* forming an arcade of origin to the first dorsal interosseous muscle (9) and inserting on the superolateral corner of the first metatarsal neck; 9′, origin of first dorsal interosseous from base of first metatarsal; 10, dorsalis pedis vessels; 11, tibialis posterior tendon; 11′, expansion of *11* to base of fifth metatarsal [inconstant]; 12, expansion of *11* to peroneus longus tendon [inconstant].) (From Picou R: Insertions inférieures du muscle long peronier lateral: Anomalie de ce muscle. Bull Soc Anat Paris 8, No. 7:160, 1894)

Fig. 5-19.   Slip of peroneus longus tendon to the first cuneiform. (1, Deep surface of peroneus longus tendon; 2, superficial surface of *1* inserting on base of first metatarsal; 3, deep slip arising from deep surface of *1* and inserting on first cuneiform.) (From Picou R: Insertions inférieures du muscle long peronier lateral: Anomalie de ce muscle. Bull Soc Anat Paris 8, No. 7:162, 1894)

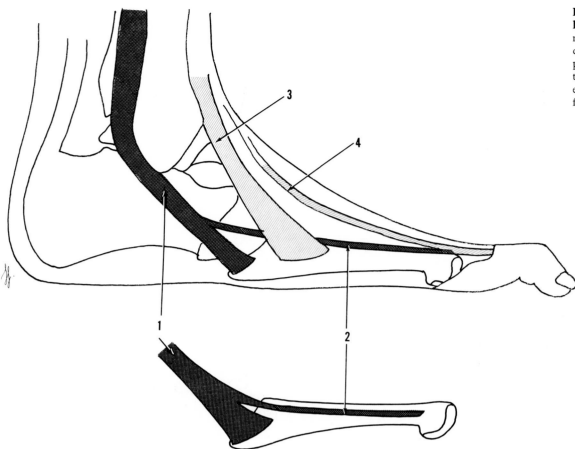

Fig. 5-20. Variation of lateral peronei. (1, Peroneus brevis tendon; 2, accessory slip passing through peroneus tertius [3] insertion and attaching to long extensor of fifth toe [4] or fifth metatarsal shaft.)

PERONEUS BREVIS

The peroneus brevis tendon is applied against the posterior surface of the lateral malleolus and glides in the retromalleolar canal (Figs. 5-14 and 5-15). Just below the tip of the lateral malleolus, the tendon makes a turn anteriorly, following the contour of the bone. It is retained by the fibrous sheath of the peronei. The tendon is then directed downward, anteriorly, and slightly laterally, crossing the calcaneofibular ligament superficially. It passes above the calcaneal processus trochlearis through the tunnel formed by the inferior peroneal retinaculum. It fans out and inserts on the styloid apophysis of the fifth metatarsal.

VARIATIONS OF THE LATERAL PERONEI

The variations of the lateral peronei are of the additional type and involve mostly the peroneus brevis.

A tendinous slip may extend from the peroneus brevis tendon to the fifth toe. This additional tendon originates distal to the inferior peroneal retinaculum and always pierces the terminal fanned-out tendon of the peroneus tertius and inserts on the fifth toe at the level of the proximal phalanx or the long extensor tendon of the fifth toe or its aponeurotic complex (Fig. 5-20). Occasionally the additional slip terminates on the fifth metatarsal shaft.

The following data are given on the frequency of occurrence of the fifth digital extension from the peroneus brevis: in 102 feet, the fifth digital slip was well developed in 22.5% and vestigial in 12.74% (total, 35.24%); in 100 feet, the slip was well developed in 21% and vestigial in 13% (total, 34%).[2] Occasionally this digital slip arises proximally from an independent muscle originating from the distal fourth of the fibula below the peroneus brevis. The tendon passes in the retromalleolar tunnel and inserts distally on the extensor aponeurosis of the fifth toe (peroneus quinti digiti, peroneus quartus).[1]

Hecker, in a comprehensive study of the variations of the lateral peronei, grouped under the heading of the lateral peronei of the tarsus, the different forms of variations: lateral peroneocalcaneal muscle, peroneocuboid muscle, peroneoperoneolongus muscle.[21] The frequency of occurrence of the lateral peronei of the tarsus has been stated as 13% in 47 adult feet and 20% in 16 embryonic feet.[21]

The majority of the variations are of the peroneocalcaneal type, forming the lateral peroneocalcaneus muscle. Hecker describes six types of variations (Fig. 5-21).[21]

Type I. The muscle originates from the peroneus longus and the peroneus brevis muscle mass. The strong tendon (4 mm) glides through the retromalleolar tunnel and divides into two slips below the tip of the lateral

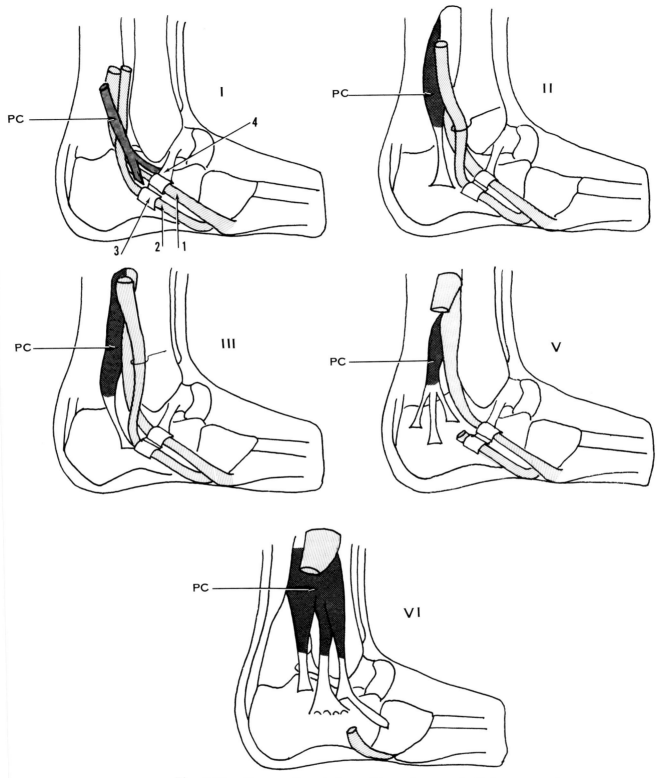

Fig. 5-21.   Types of variation of lateral peronei. (*PC*, peroneocalcaneal muscle; 1, peroneus brevis tendon; 2, peroneus longus tendon; 3, inferior peroneal retinaculum; 4, stem of inferior extensor retinaculum.) (Redrawn from Hecker P: Etude sur le péronier du tarse: Variations des péroniers latéraux. Arch Anat Histol Embryol 3:327, 1924)

malleolus. The thin anterior slip passes along the anterior border of the peroneus brevis tendon and inserts on the origin of the inferior extensor retinaculum and on the superolateral aspect of the os calcis. The thicker posterior slip diverges and inserts on the inferolateral aspect of the os calcis and on the septum separating the two compartments of the inferior peroneal retinaculum. With its diverging two slips, the lateral peroneocalcaneal tendon forms a buttonhole through which passes the tendon of the peroneus brevis.

Type II. The muscle derives from the peroneus brevis at the junction of the middle and lower thirds of the leg. The cylindrical tendon measures 2.5 mm in diameter and 5 cm in length and inserts on the lateral surface of the os calcis. The insertion is fan shaped and located posterior to the inferior peroneal retinaculum and posterior to the peroneus longus tendon.

Type III. The muscle arises from the peroneus brevis muscle at the level of the inferior third of the leg. The thin tendon attaches on the lateral surface of the os calcis in close connection with the lower component of the inferior peroneal retinaculum.

Type IV. The muscle is similar to type III distally. Proximally, however, the muscle is larger and extends higher on the fibula and on the posterolateral intermuscular septum.

Type V. The muscle arises from the peroneus brevis in the lower third of the leg. At a level three fingerbreadths proximal to the tip of the lateral malleolus, a few musculotendinous fascicles separate from the muscular portion and spread in the fibrous tissue, forming the peroneocalcaneal ligament. The true tendinous formation appears farther down and divides into three slips: anterior, middle, posterior. The stronger middle slip inserts on a tubercle on the lateral surface of the os calcis, the thin anterior slip fans out and inserts anterior to the middle slip, whereas the vertical posterior slip inserts posterior and slightly more proximal to the middle slip.

Type VI. This muscle represents a lateral peroneal of the tarsus replacing completely the peroneus brevis. The muscle arises from the middle third of the lateral surface of the fibula, the anterior crest of the fibula, and the lateral intermuscular septum. The large muscle divides into three parts. The anterior tendon inserts on the os calcis, the dorsal calcaneocuboid ligament, and the lateral surface of the cuboid. The middle tendon has a broad, fan-shaped insertion on the lateral surface of the os calcis. The posterior tendon is thin and inserts posteriorly below the lateral malleolus. This type of variation is extremely rare.

Three other rare types of variation may also occur: peroneocuboid muscle, bifid peroneus longus tendon, peroneoperoneolongus muscle. The peroneocuboid muscle originates from the lateral compartment in the inferior third, and the tendon inserts on the lateral surface of the cuboid. The bifid peroneus longus tendon forms a buttonhole through which passes the peroneus brevis tendon. The per-

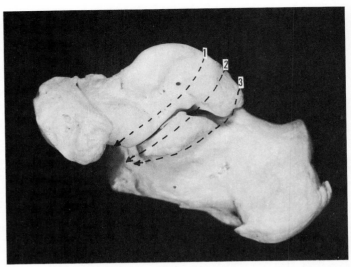

Fig. 5-22.   Medial aspect of the talocalcaneal joint. (*Dotted lines,* direction of 1, tibialis posterior tendon; 2, flexor digitorum longus tendon; 3, flexor hallucis longus tendon.)

oneoperoneolongus muscle originates from the inferior third of the lateral compartment, and the tendon inserts on the peroneus longus tendon.

Medial Aspect of the Ankle and Foot and the Sole of the Foot

On the posteromedial aspect of the ankle, the tendons of the tibialis posterior and of the flexor digitorum longus are behind the medial malleolus and nearly vertical in direction (Fig. 5-22). The tendon of the flexor hallucis longus is behind the talus and oriented obliquely downward and medially. All three tendons make their turn with anterior concavity and pass through the tarsal tunnel and the porta pedis and penetrate the sole of the foot.

On the posterior aspect of the medial malleolus and of the talus, each tendon is retained in a fibrous tunnel. The tunnel of the *tibialis posterior* crosses the medial aspect of the posterior talus, the medial aspect of the talar neck, and the inferior surface of the inferocalcaneonavicular ligament. The tibialis posterior tendon is thus transtalar during its course and crosses the tibiotalar and tibiocalcaneal components of the deltoid ligament. Farther distally it crosses the origin of the superomedial calcaneonavicular ligament and the inferior surface of the inferior calcaneonavicular ligament. The tibialis posterior tendon is located above the sustentaculum tali.

The tunnel of the *flexor digitorum longus* is adjacent to that of the tibialis posterior. The tendon of the flexor digitorum longus crosses the very posterior aspect of the medial talar surface, passes over the subtalar joint, and crosses the medial surface of the sustentaculum tali.

The tendon of the *flexor hallucis longus* passes through the fibrous retrotalar tunnel, which is at a distance from the fibrous tunnel of the flexor digitorum longus. Farther down, the interval between the tendons narrows as the flexor hallucis longus converges medially. The tendon crosses the posterior talocalcaneal joint and passes under the inferior surface of the sustentaculum tali.

The superficial and deep layers of the flexor retinaculum are in close connection with the fibrous sheath of the tibialis posterior and flexor digitorum longus tendons. The interval between these two tunnels and that of the flexor hallucis longus is bridged by the deep aponeurosis that inserts laterally on the tunnel of the peronei; this creates a third compartment for the posterior tibial neurovascular bundle. The neurovascular compartment is superficial to the intertendinous interval and to the tunnel of the flexor hallucis longus. Farther down, the neurovascular compartment is divided into an upper and a lower space by the interfascicular septum.

TIBIALIS POSTERIOR TENDON

On the inferior aspect of the inferior calcaneonavicular ligament, the tibialis posterior tendon is flat and contains a fibrocartilaginous or bony sesamoid (Figs. 5-22–5-26). Just in front of the tuberosity of the scaphoid, the tendon divides into the three components: anterior, middle, posterior.

The *anterior component* is the largest of the three, in direct continuity with the main tendon, and inserts on the tuberosity of the navicular, the inferior capsule of the $cuneo_1$-navicular joint, the inferior surface of the first cuneiform. This is a very broad insertion that engulfs the tuberosity of the navicular and reaches the first cuneiform, similar to a cuff.

The *middle component* is very deep and continues distally into the sole of the foot as a tarsometatarsal extension that inserts on the second cuneiform, the third cuneiform, the cuboid, laterally and over the peroneal canal. Beyond this point, the metatarsal extension of the tendon passes deep or dorsal to the peroneus longus tendon, the two crossing in an X. Three metatarsal tendinous slips are formed. The medial two slips make a twist, become sagittal in orientation, penetrate the narrow spaces between the bases of the corresponding metatarsals, and insert on the base of the second metatarsal laterally and the base of the third metatarsal medially and on the base of the third metatarsal laterally and the base of the fourth metatarsal medially. The third tendinous slip is oriented transversely and inserts on the base of the fifth metatarsal; at times this slip is absent.

The tarsometatarsal component of the tibialis posterior tendon also gives attachment to the Y-shaped origin of the flexor hallucis brevis. A detailed description of this Y-shaped or triangular component is provided by Lewis and by Martin.[22, 23] The medial limb of the Y is in continuity

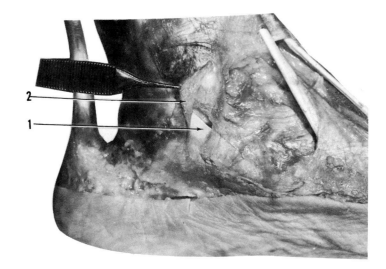
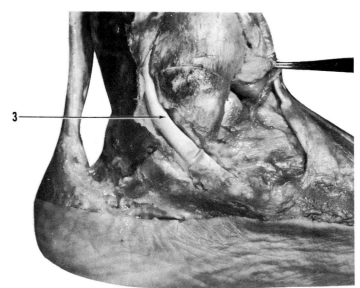
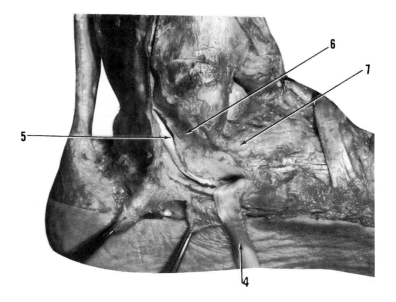

Fig. 5-23. Medial aspect of the ankle and calcaneal canal. (1, Tibialis posterior tendon; 2, reflected flexor retinaculum and fibrous sheath of *1;* 3, retro medial malleolar position of tibialis posterior tendon; 4, reflected tibialis posterior tendon; 5, flexor digitorum longus tendon exposed through incised fibrous tunnel; 6, sulcus of tibialis posterior tendon; 7, origin of superomedial calcaneonavicular ligament.)

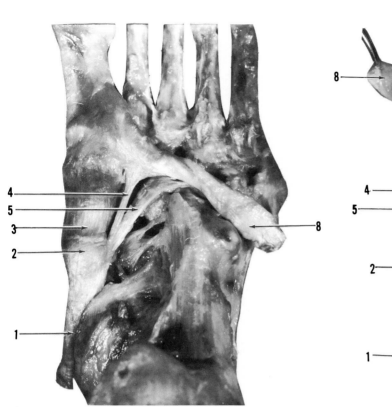

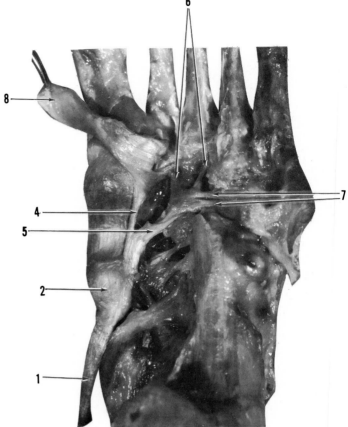

Fig. 5-24.

Fig. 5-25.

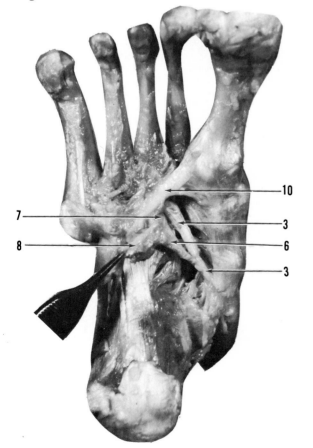

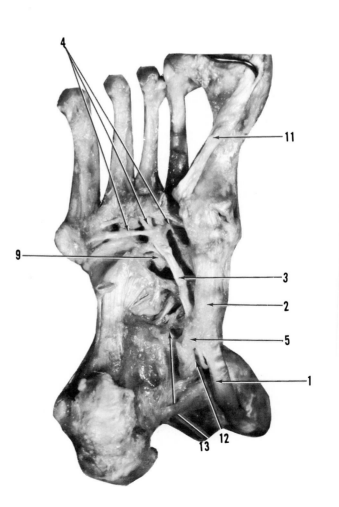

Fig. 5-24.   Tibialis posterior tendon. (1, Tibialis posterior tendon; 2, insertion of *1* on tuberosity of navicular; 3, insertion of *1* on medial cuneiform; 4, insertion of *1* on peroneus longus tendon; 5, plantar segment—cuneometatarsal—of *1*; 6, insertional slips of *1* on metatarsal 2–3, 3–4; 7, insertional slips of *1* on metatarsals 4, 5; 8, peroneus longus tendon.)

Fig. 5-25.   Tibialis posterior tendon. (1, Tibialis posterior tendon; 2, insertion of *1* on tuberosity of navicular; 3, plantar cuneometatarsal portion of *1*; 4, metatarsal insertions of *1*; 5, calcaneal, recurrent insertion band of *1*; 6, band from tibialis posterior tendon forming medial arm of Y stem of origin of flexor hallucis brevis; 7, lateral arm of Y stem of origin of flexor hallucis brevis muscle; 8, stem of origin of flexor hallucis brevis muscle; 9, lateral calcaneal insertion of *1*; 10, peroneus longus tendon within its thin fibrous tunnel crossing superficially the metatarsal insertional bands of tibialis posterior tendon; 11, reflected peroneus longus tendon; 12, direction of flexor digitorum longus tendon; 13, direction of flexor hallucis longus tendon.)

Fig. 5-26.   Insertion of tibialis posterior tendon. (1, Tibialis posterior tendon; 2, plantar cuneometatarsal component of *1*; 3, Y stem of origin of flexor hallucis brevis muscle; 4, medial arm of *3*; 5, lateral arm of *3*; 6, cuboidal insertion of *1*; 7, insertion of *1* on cuneiforms 3, 2; 8, insertion of *1* between metatarsals 2–3 and 3–4 and on metatarsal 5; 9, recurrent calcaneal band of *1*; 10, attachment slip of *1* to peroneus longus; 11, peroneus longus.)

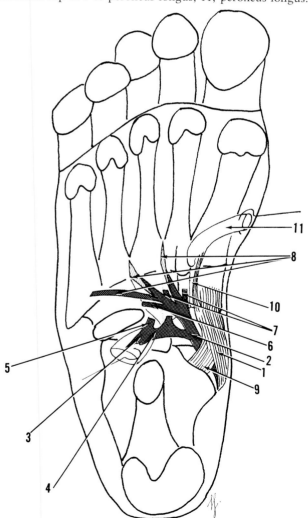

with the tibialis posterior tendon. The lateral limb inserts on the cuboid and the lateral cuneiform. The stem of the Y provides attachment to the flexor hallucis brevis (Fig. 5-27).[22] The arms of the Y component may be united, forming a triangular fold that bends medially and gives attachment to the flexor hallucis brevis (Fig. 5-28).[23] This brings forth the dynamic connection between the tibialis posterior tendon and the flexor hallucis brevis. Occasionally the tarsometatarsal component of the tendon sends a sizable tendinous slip to the peroneus longus tendon close to its insertion on the base of the first metatarsal.

The *posterior component* of the tibialis posterior is recurrent and originates from the main tendon prior to its insertion the tuberosity of the navicular. It is oriented laterally and posteriorly and inserts as a band on the anterior aspect of the sustentaculum tali. This complex insertion of the tibialis posterior tendon provides a firm grip on the planta pedis.

FLEXOR DIGITORUM LONGUS AND FLEXOR HALLUCIS LONGUS

In the upper compartment of the inferior segment of the calcaneal canal, above the interfascicular septum, the tendons of the flexor digitorum longus and the flexor hallucis longus converge (Figs. 5-22, 5-23, 5-29, and 5-30). Both tendons pierce the medial intermuscular septum in a medial-to-lateral direction and enter the middle compartment of the sole of the foot. They cross in an X as the tendon of the flexor digitorum longus continues its oblique course—anteriorly and laterally—and passes superficial or plantar to the tendon of the flexor hallucis longus, which remains oriented anteriorly and slightly medially. A tendinous slip extends from the lateral border of the flexor hallucis longus and anastomoses with the flexor digitorum longus tendon after its segmentation (Fig. 5-31). The lateral border of the flexor digitorum longus tendon gives insertion to the quadratus plantae muscle.

The tendon of the *flexor digitorum longus* divides into four diverging tendons directed anteriorly and laterally; all four tendons give origin to the lumbrical muscles. Each long flexor tendon with its accompanying and more superficially placed flexor brevis tendon pass through an arch formed by the deep septa of the plantar aponeurosis at the level of the

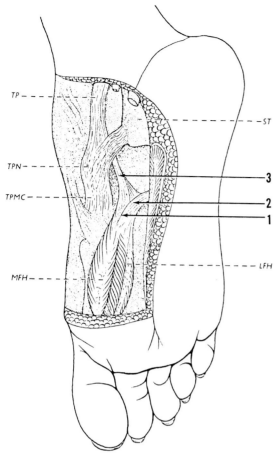

Fig. 5-27. Y-shaped origin of the flexor hallucis brevis muscle. (1, stem of origin of flexor hallucis brevis muscle; 2, lateral stem of origin; 3, medial stem of origin provided by tibialis posterior tendon; *MFH*, medial head of flexor hallucis brevis; *LFH*, lateral head of flexor hallucis brevis; *TPMC*, medial cuneiform insertion of tibialis posterior; *TPN*, navicular insertion of tibialis posterior; *TP*, tibialis posterior; *ST*, sustentaculum tali with attachment of recurrent band of *TP*.) (From Lewis OJ: The tibialis posterior tendon in the primate foot. J Anat 98, No. 2:209, 1964. By permission of Cambridge University Press)

transverse head of the adductor hallucis. At the level of the plantar plate, both tendons enter the osteofibrous tunnel, the flexor brevis tendon still more superficial (plantar) to the long flexor tendon. The flexor brevis tendon bifurcates at the level of the proximal phalanx. The tendon of the flexor digitorum longus passes through the bifurcation and continues its distal course, now located more superficial to the tendon of the brevis. A slit appears in the mid axis of the flexor digitorum longus tendon, which gradually enlarges transversely at the distal end and inserts on the base of the distal phalanx.

The tendon of the *flexor hallucis longus* remains in the middle compartment, lateral to the medial intermuscular septum, for a short distance. Farther distally, it passes through the medial septum into the medial compartment

and obliquely crosses the lateral belly of the flexor hallucis brevis.[23] It passes through the fibrous arch formed by the two septa emanating from the deep surface of the plantar aponeurosis and reaches the intersesamoid interval. The tendon penetrates the osteofibrous flexor tunnel and courses distally. The terminal end gradually spreads in a transverse direction and inserts on the base of the distal phalanx.

Tendinous Connections

The variations basically involve the tendinous connection between the flexor hallucis longus and the flexor digitorum longus; the connection occurs after the segmentation of the latter. In the majority, the tendinous connection extends from the flexor hallucis longus to the flexor digitorum longus tendons with the following distribution: in 50 feet— 22% insert on the second tendon, 40% insert on the second and third tendons, 36% insert on the second through fourth tendons, and 2% insert on the second through fifth tendons; in 100 feet—32% insert on the second tendon, 58% insert on the second and third tendons, and 10% insert on the second through fourth tendons.[1, 2, 22–24] The tendinous connection from the flexor digitorum longus to the flexor hallucis longus occurs less frequently: 12% in 50 feet, 29% in 100 feet, 20.5% in 29 feet.[1, 2, 24] The absence of the connecting tendon is rare; Martin has observed two such cases.[23]

Fig. 5-28. Attachment of the tibialis posterior tendon. (1, Y stem of origin of flexor hallucis brevis muscle; 2, lateral arm of *1*; 3, medial arm of *1* arising from tibialis posterior tendon.) (From Martin BF: Observations on the muscles and tendons of the medial aspect of the sole of the foot. J Anat 98, No. 3:437, 1964. By permission of Cambridge University Press)

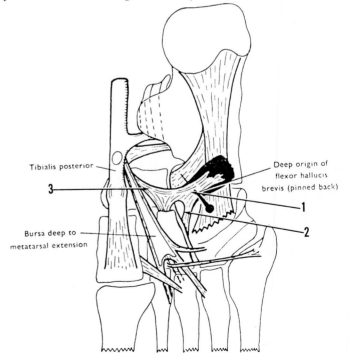

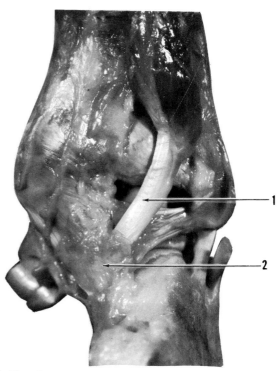

Fig. 5-29.   Posterior aspect of the ankle. (1, Flexor hallucis longus tendon; 2, fibrous tunnel of *1* on posterior aspect of talus.)

Additional Muscle

Three additional muscles may be seen on the medial aspect of the ankle and tarsal tunnel: peroneocalcaneus internus, tibiocalcaneus internus and accessory soleus, and long accessory of the long flexors or of the quadratus plantae.

Peroneocalcaneus Internus Muscle.   This muscle originates from the lower half of the medial surface of the fibula and partly by digitations from the flexor hallucis longus.[25–29] The tendon is directed downward and forward and enters the same compartment as the flexor hallucis longus. It inserts on the distal segment of the medial calcaneal surface (Fig. 5-32).

Tibiocalcaneus Internus and Accessory Soleus.
Hecker describes the tibiocalcaneo internus originating from the medial crest of the tibia, the site of attachment measuring 7 cm to 8 cm (Fig. 5-32).[21] The muscular portion measures 17 cm, followed by a tendinous portion of 4 cm, which inserts on the medial surface of the os calcis about 1 fingerbreadth anterior to the Achilles tendon. The posterior border of the muscle touches the soleus, and the separation is more or less artificial. This muscle is quite similar to the well-recognized variation of the accessory soleus muscle that arises from the oblique line of the tibia, the deep fascia of the leg, or the deep surface of the soleus and inserts on the medial surface of the os calcis through a distinct tendon. This muscle is always located posterior to the neurovascular bundle.[30]

Long Accessory of the Long Flexors or of the Quadratus Plantae.   The long accessory of the long flexors or of the quadratus plantae (accessorius of the accessorius of Turner, second accessorius of Humphrey) extends from the lower third of the leg into the flexor digitorum longus or the quadratus plantae. The variable origin may be from the fibula, tibia, deep aponeurosis of the leg, soleus, flexor hallucis longus, flexor digitorum longus in the leg, or peroneus brevis.[30] Nathan and co-workers confirm the variable origin of this muscle and describe the following sites of origin: tibia, fibula, fasciae covering the deep compartment of the leg, transverse intermuscular septum, calcaneus.[31] The attachment is fleshy, tendinous, or aponeurotic. The muscle may have a double head (long and short) or a single short head arising from the lower leg. The accessory muscle

Fig. 5-30.   Flexor digitorum longus and flexor hallucis longus tendons. (1, Flexor digitorum longus tendon; 2, flexor hallucis longus tendon; 3, extension slip of *2* to *1;* 4, lumbrical muscles; 5, lateral head of quadratus plantae muscle; 6, medial head of quadratus plantae muscle.)

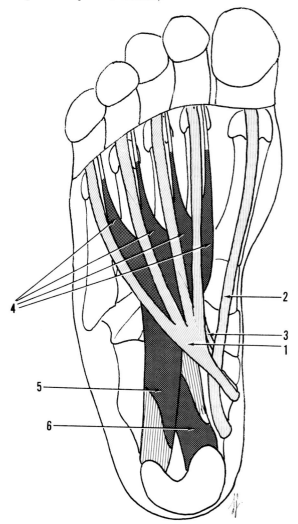

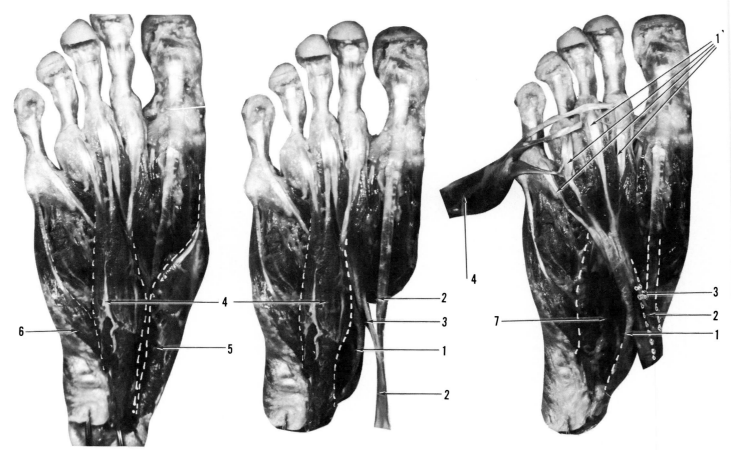

Fig. 5-31.   Plantar muscles, superficial layer. (1, 1', Flexor digitorum longus tendons; 2, flexor hallucis longus tendon; 3, extension slip from *2* to *1;* 4, flexor digitorum brevis muscle; 5, abductor hallucis muscle; 6, abductor of fifth toe; 7, quadratus plantae muscle.)

courses through the tarsal tunnel. It remains deep to the neurovascular bundle but occasionally may cross it superficially.[21] Frequently it descends into the tarsal tunnel as a fleshy structure and may become tendinous in the planta or may remain fleshy until its insertion.[31]

The tendon courses in the planta and inserts on the undivided portion of the flexor digitorum longus tendon. The tendon passes deep or superficial to the latter or joins the lateral head of the quadratus plantae for a combined insertion.[21, 30] The flexor digitorum accessorius longus occurs with the following frequency, according to various sources: 3.9% of legs, 7%, 8%.[12, 31–33]

FLEXOR DIGITORUM BREVIS

The flexor digitorum brevis arises from the posteromedial calcaneal tuberosity, the posterior third of the deep surface of the plantar aponeurosis, and the lateral and medial intermuscular septa (Figs. 5-31 and 5-33). The calcaneal origin extends to the posterolateral tuberosity and is sandwiched between the origin of the plantar aponeurosis posteriorly, the abductor hallucis anteromedially, and the abductor digiti quinti anterolaterally. The muscular attachment to the deep

surface of the plantar aponeurosis in the posterior third is dense, allowing separation only by sharp dissection. At this level, there is no potential space between the flexor digitorum brevis and the plantar aponeurosis. The muscle body is thick and narrow posteriorly and gradually spreads out transversely. In the mid segment of the foot, it divides into four muscular fascicles, each followed by a flat tendon centered on and superficial to the corresponding long flexor tendon. Both tendons pass through an arc formed by the vertical septa of the plantar aponeurosis and penetrate the osseofibrous tunnel. The flat tendon of the short flexor divides into two slips at the level of the base of the proximal phalanx. The slips contour the long flexor tendon on each side, pass underneath, decussate fibers, and insert on the inferior aspect of the middle phalanx near the borders. They form a tendinous groove through which passes the long flexor tendon. The medial two tendons are usually larger than the lateral two.

The variations involving the flexor digitorum brevis are frequent; Nathan and Gloobe provide the following data on 100 feet: 37% had a normal flexor digitorum brevis and 63% had variations involving mostly the fifth toe and less frequently the fourth toe.[34] The variations involve the origin or the insertion of the muscle or both.

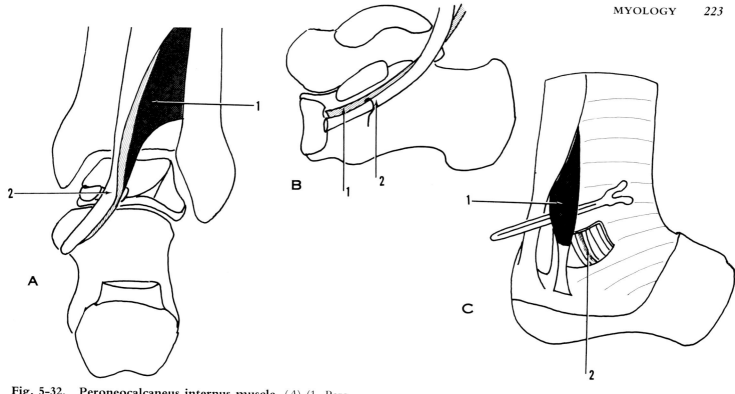

Fig. 5-32.   Peroneocalcaneus internus muscle. (*A*) (1, Peroneocalcaneus internus muscle; 2, flexor hallucis longus tendon.)
(*B*) (1, tendon of peroneocalcaneus in same compartment as flexor
hallucis longus tendon [2].) (*C*) (1, tibiocalcaneal muscle superficial
to medial neurovascular bundle [2] seen through a window in
flexor retinaculum.) (*A* redrawn from Perkins JD Jr: An anomalous
muscle of the leg: Peroneo-calcaneous internus. Anat Rec 8:21,
1914; *B, C* redrawn from Testut L: Les Anomalies Musculaires
Considérées du Point de Vue de la Ligature des Artères. Paris,
Doin, 1892)

Fig. 5-33.   Flexor digitorum brevis muscle. (1, Flexor
digitorum brevis; 1′, tendons of flexor digitorum brevis; 2,
abductor hallucis muscle; 3, abductor of fifth toe.)

Variations of Origin

In addition to the normal muscle, a second muscle may arise
from the flexor digitorum longus and join the tendon of the
brevis. Occasionally this additional muscle arises from the
tibialis posterior tendon. The flexor brevis to the fourth and
fifth toe may arise from the long flexor or the lateral intermuscular septum. This muscle is then deeper than the rest
of the flexor brevis.

The frequency of occurrence of these variations in 100
feet is as follows: An additional slip of the flexor digitorum
brevis from the flexor digitorum longus to the fifth toe is
present in 20% and from the flexor digitorum longus to the
fourth and fifth toes in 3%; an additional slip from the
tibialis posterior to the fifth toe occurs in 1%. A sole origin
of the flexor digitorum brevis from the flexor digitorum
longus to the fifth or fourth and fifth toes is present in 5%;
a sole origin from the lateral intermuscular septum to the
fifth toe occurs in 1%.[34]

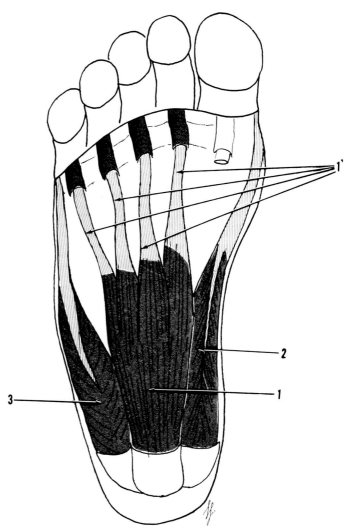

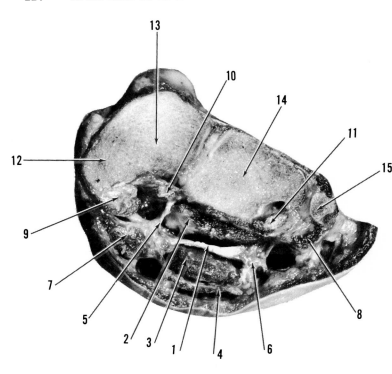

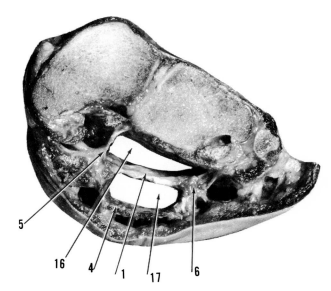

Fig. 5-34. **Cross section of left foot passing through the cuboid and the navicular—anterior view.** (1, Transverse septum extending from medial intermuscular septum to lateral intermuscular septum and dividing middle compartment of hindfoot into a deep compartment [16] for quadratus plantae muscle and a superficial compartment [17] for flexor digitorum brevis muscle; 2, quadratus plantae muscle with tendon of flexor digitorum longus; 3, flexor digitorum brevis muscle; 4, middle segment of plantar aponeurosis; 5, medial intermuscular septum; 6, lateral intermuscular septum; 7, abductor hallucis muscle; 8, abductor of fifth toe; 9, insertion of tibialis posterior tendon on navicular tuberosity; 10, flexor hallucis longus tendon; 11, peroneus longus tendon; 12, tuberosity of navicular; 13, navicular; 14, cuboid; 15, tuberosity of fifth metatarsal base.)

The unsplit tendon is seen in 5% (fifth or fourth toes) and runs parallel to the long flexor and inserts on the second phalanx.[1, 30] The short flexor tendon of the fifth may fuse to the long flexor tendon in 2%.[1, 30]

QUADRATUS PLANTAE OR FLEXOR ACCESSORIUS

The quadratus plantae (caro quadrata of Sylvius) is a flat, trapezoidal muscle formed by two heads: lateral and medial (Figs. 5-30 and 5-31).

The lateral head has a tendinous origin and arises from the posterolateral calcaneal tuberosity and from the lateral segment of the calcaneocuboid ligament up to the cuboidal crest. The medial head has a fleshy origin from the lower segment of the medial surface of the os calcis in the calcaneal canal, from the anterior aspect of the posteromedial calcaneal tuberosity, and from the inferior surface of the interfascicular septum of the calcaneal canal. The medial head of the muscle forms the lateral wall of the lower segment of the calcaneal canal and is inferior to the interfascicular septum. Both heads, initially separated by a triangular space with an anterior apex, gradually unite. Most of the muscular fibers of the medial head terminate in a narrow tendon that inserts into the deep surface of the common long flexor tendon. The remaining fibers join the lateral head, and both heads insert with the fleshy fibers on the segmented tendons of the long flexor, mostly of the fifth toe, and on the anastomotic tendon between the flexor digitorum longus and the flexor hallucis longus. The flexor hallucis longus may occasionally receive some direct insertional fibers from the accessory flexor.

The quadratus plantae is sandwiched posteriorly between the short flexor and the osseoligamentous frame. A thin transverse fascia, occasionally thick, is interposed between the superficial surface of the accessory flexor and the deep surface of the flexor brevis; this transverse band extends from the medial to the lateral intermuscular septum (Fig. 5-34).

Insertional Variations

The frequent connection between the quadratus plantae and the anastomotic band of the flexor digitorum longus with

Variations of Insertion

The variations of insertion of the flexor brevis are of three types: absence of tendon, unsplit tendon, or tendon fused to the long flexor.

The absence of the flexor brevis tendon to the fifth toe occurs with the following frequency, according to various sources: in 5 of 50 feet (10%), in 22 of 136 feet (16.1%), in 135 of 540 feet (25%), in 14 of 100 feet (14%), in 23 of 100 feet (23%) (total, 199 in 926 feet).[2, 34] The average of absence of the flexor digitorum brevis to the fifth toe is 21.5%.

The brevis tendons of the fifth and fourth toes may be absent in 3%.[30]

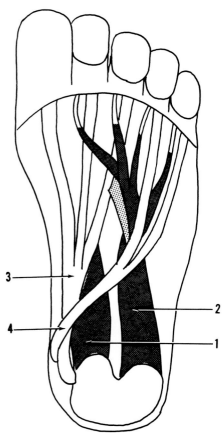

Fig. 5-35. Insertional variation of the long flexors and of the quadratus plantae. (1, Medial head of quadratus plantae inserting on a common long flexor tendon [3] for toes 1, 2, 3; 2, lateral head of quadratus plantae inserting on a common long flexor tendon [4] for toes 4, 5.) (Redrawn from Auvray M: Anomalies musculaires et nerveuses. Bull Soc Anat Paris 10:223, 1896)

the flexor hallucis longus or the connection with the latter has already been mentioned.[1] Further union may occur with the lumbricals or the short flexor of the toes; the quadratus plantae may even provide the entire absent component of the short flexor to the fifth toe.

Auvray reported an interesting variation of the long flexors of the toe also involving an insertional variation of the quadratus plantae (Fig. 5-35).[28] The long flexors of the second and third toe are provided by the flexor hallucis longus tendons. The flexor digitorum longus provides the long flexors only to the fourth and fifth toes. The quadratus plantae remains divided into two components: the medial head inserts on the long flexors of the second and third toes, and the lateral head inserts on the long flexors of the fourth and fifth toes.

Absence

The absence of the lateral head of the quadratus plantae is "far from being rare."[1] Ledouble mentions having observed ten such cases.[2] The absence of the medial head is rare, and

a bilateral case is reported by Morestin (Fig. 5-36).[35] The accessory flexor may be reduced in size or converted to a fibrous band.

Additional Muscle

The long accessory of the quadratus plantae has been dealt with previously. The muscle has a variable origin in the leg and terminates on the quadratus plantae.

Fig. 5-36. Absence of the medial head of the quadratus plantae muscle. (1, Flexor hallucis longus tendon; 2, flexor digitorum longus tendon; 3, lateral head of quadratus plantae.) (From Morestin H: Anomalie de l'accessoire du long fléchisseur commun des orteils. Bull Soc Anat Paris 11:46, 1895)

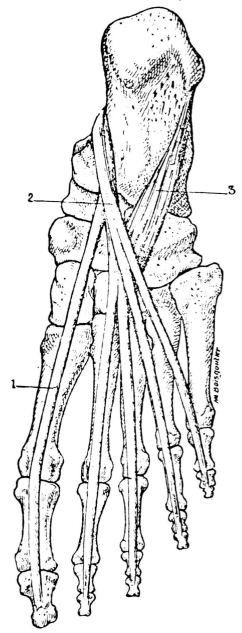

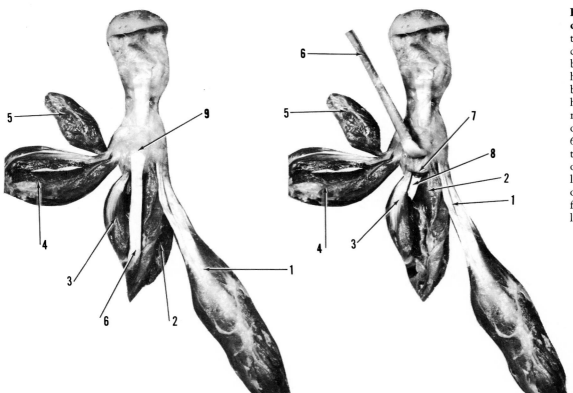

Fig. 5-37. Plantar aspect of the big toe. (1, Abductor hallucis muscle; 2, medial head of flexor hallucis brevis muscle; 3, lateral head of flexor hallucis brevis muscle; 4, oblique head of adductor hallucis muscle; 5, transverse head of adductor hallucis muscle; 6, flexor hallucis longus tendon; 7, proximal border of plantar plate; 8, triangular space between two heads of flexor hallucis brevis; 9, fibrous tunnel of flexor hallucis longus tendon.)

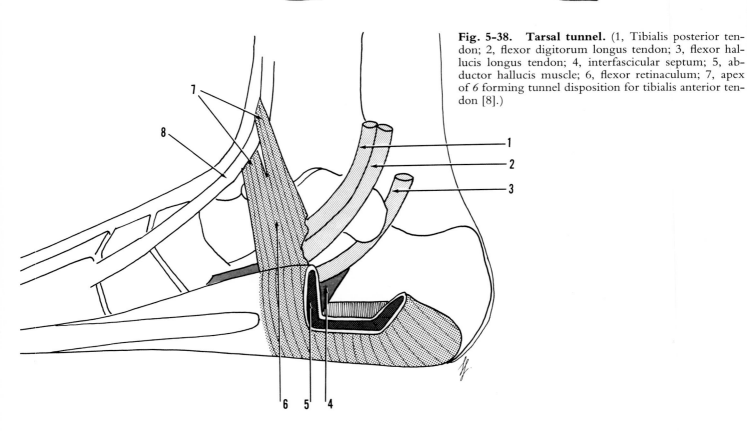

Fig. 5-38. Tarsal tunnel. (1, Tibialis posterior tendon; 2, flexor digitorum longus tendon; 3, flexor hallucis longus tendon; 4, interfascicular septum; 5, abductor hallucis muscle; 6, flexor retinaculum; 7, apex of *6* forming tunnel disposition for tibialis anterior tendon [8].)

INTRINSIC MUSCLES OF THE BIG TOE

There are four intrinsic muscles of the big toe: extensor hallucis brevis (described previously), abductor hallucis, flexor hallucis brevis with two heads, medial and lateral, and adductor hallucis with two heads, oblique and transverse (Fig. 5-37).

Abductor Hallucis

The abductor hallucis is a superficial, thick, flat elongated muscle extending from the tuberosity of the os calcis to the big toe (Figs. 5-31, 5-33, and 5-37). It is the muscle of the medial border of the foot and originates from the inferior and medial aspect of the posteromedial calcaneal tuberosity through mostly tendinous fibers (the main origin), the deep surface of the plantar aponeurosis, the posterior end of the medial intermuscular septum, and the flexor retinaculum, which invests the muscle.[36]

The abductor hallucis muscle bridges the calcaneal canal and with the flexor retinaculum converts it into a tunnel (Fig. 5-38). The deep investing aponeurosis of the muscle is anchored proximally to the medial surface of the os calcis through the attachment of the interfascicular septum (Figs. 5-39 and 5-40). Distally, the same investing aponeurosis makes fibrous connection with the common fibrous tunnel of the flexor digitorum longus and the flexor hallucis longus tendons. It also is adherent to the tunnel of the tibialis posterior tendon and to the tuberosity of the navicular. Poirier and Charpy described a frequently seen aponeurotic expansion detached from the superior border of the abductor muscle and in continuity with the inferior arm of the inferior extensor retinaculum.[37] The tendon of origin of the muscle is located on the deep or lateral aspect of the muscle. The tendon of insertion appears early on the superficial or medial aspect of the muscle. Distally the tendon is flat, slightly twisted, fasciculated, and more plantar in location. Its inferolateral fibers insert on the medial sesamoid, in conjunction with the fibers of the medial head of the flexor hallucis brevis, and on the medial plantar tubercle of the proximal phalanx of the big toe. The superomedial fibers connect with the transverse lamina of the extensor aponeurosis (Figs. 5-41 and 5-42).

The variations of the abductor hallucis are limited. An extension from the anterior part of the abductor to the proximal phalanx of the second toe may be seen in 7%.[2] Occasionally the entire muscle originates from the flexor hallucis longus.[2]

Flexor Hallucis Brevis

The flexor hallucis brevis has a Y-shaped fibrotendinous origin (Figs. 5-37, 5-41, and 5-43).[22, 23] The medial arm of the Y originates from the metatarsal component of the tibialis posterior tendon. The lateral arm originates from the lateral cuneiform and the cuboid, with some fibers inserting on the groove of the peroneus longus tendon and on the long and short plantar ligaments. The stem of the Y origin of the muscle resembles a triangular lamina or fold. The stem of the Y is considered by Martin as the deep origin of the muscle, whereas superficial fibers originate from the medial intermuscular septum, which creates an additional anchorage of the muscle to the medial calcaneal tubercle.[23] The Y-shaped origin of the muscle has been found in 46 of 50 feet (Fig. 5-44).[23]

A large bursa is interposed between the proximal part of the muscle and the underlying medial cuneiform, first tarsometatasal joint, and the terminal portion of the tunnel of the peroneus longus.[22] The flexor hallucis brevis muscle is oriented anteriorly and medially, crosses the first interosseous space and the first metatarsal, and divides into two parts, medial and lateral. The smaller lateral head is crossed obliquely by the tendon of the flexor hallucis longus, which imprints a groove. An insertional tendon appears on the plantar aspect of the lateral head and penetrates the plantar plate laterally through a flat tunnel at a distance from the adductor tendon (Fig 5-45). The fibers insert on the plantar plate laterally, on the central, medial aspect of the lateral sesamoid, and on the base of the proximal phalanx laterally in conjunction with the corresponding fibers of the adductor hallucis. The medial head of the flexor hallucis brevis is larger and courses on the inner side of the flexor hallucis longus tendon. The fibers insert on the medial aspect of the plantar plate, on the lateral, central aspect of the medial sesamoid, and on the base of the proximal phalanx medially in conjunction with the corresponding fibers of the abductor hallucis. The parting of the two heads of the flexor hallucis brevis delineates a triangle at the level of the first metatarsal neck.

The following variations are mentioned by Ledouble:

Lateral head of the short flexor more or less united to the oblique adductor and occasionally inseparable from it

Medial head inserting with the majority of its fibers on the tendon of the abductor hallucis

A small tendinous fascicle originating from the flexor hallucis and inserting on the first cuneiform (interosseous plantaris primus)

A tendon extending from the short flexor to the proximal phalanx of the second toe

Short flexor of the big toe reinforced by a tendinous extension from the flexor digitorum longus[2]

Adductor Hallucis

The adductor hallucis is formed by two muscles, oblique and transverse (Figs. 5-43, 5-46, and 5-47).

Oblique Head.   The fibrous tunnel of the peroneus longus tendon inserts laterally on the crest of the cuboid and the base of the fourth and fifth metatarsals and medially on the lateral two cuneometatarsal joints. The oblique head of the adductor hallucis originates from the midsegment of the peroneus longus tunnel. It is through this simple rela-

(Text continues on p. 233.)

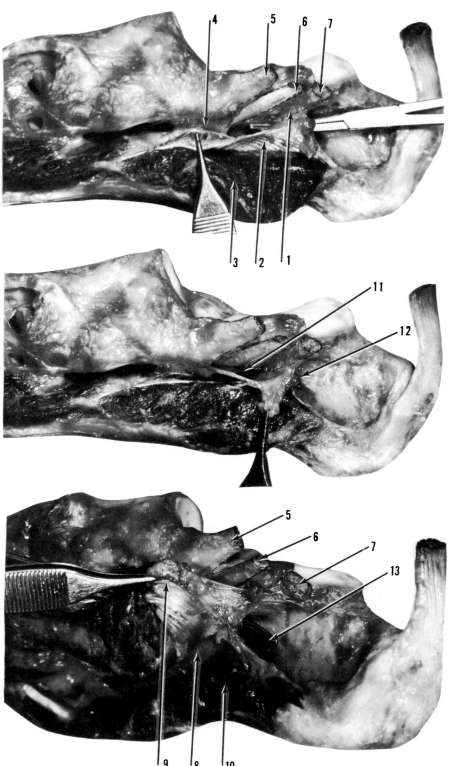

Fig. 5-39. Upper and lower chambers of the calcaneal canal. (1, Interfascicular septum; 2, deep investing aponeurosis of abductor hallucis muscle [3]; 4, navicular attachment of investing fascia of abductor hallucis muscle; 5, tendon of tibialis posterior; 6, tendon of flexor digitorum longus; 7, tendon of flexor hallucis longus; 8, medial intermuscular septum; 9, reflected calcaneal origin of abductor hallucis muscle; 10, flexor digitorum brevis muscle; 11, upper chamber of calcaneal canal; 12, lower chamber of calcaneal canal with hemostat [13] passing through.)

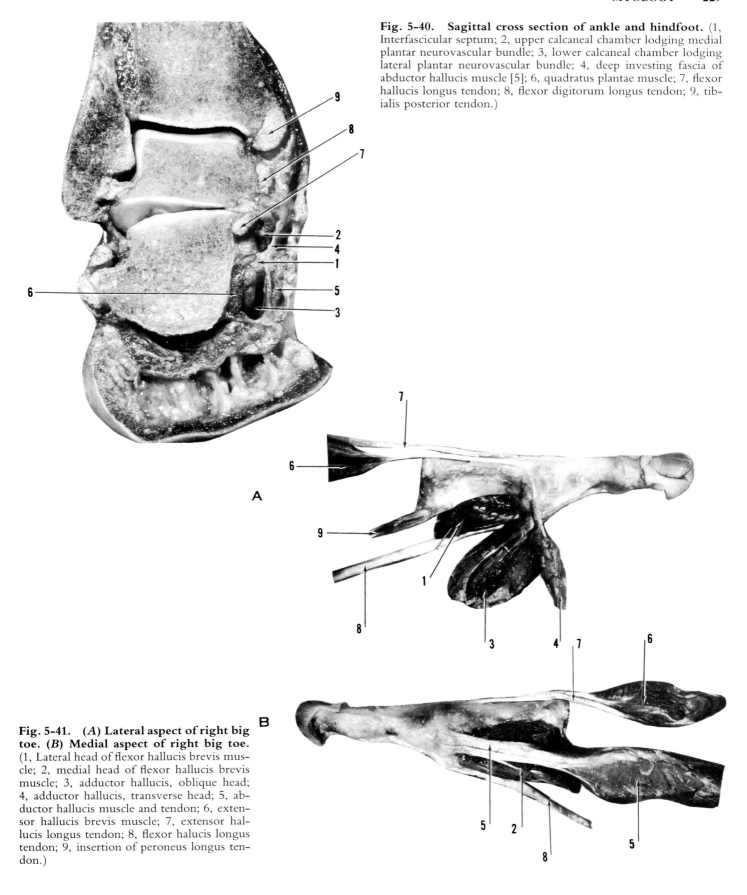

Fig. 5-40.   Sagittal cross section of ankle and hindfoot. (1, Interfascicular septum; 2, upper calcaneal chamber lodging medial plantar neurovascular bundle; 3, lower calcaneal chamber lodging lateral plantar neurovascular bundle; 4, deep investing fascia of abductor hallucis muscle [5]; 6, quadratus plantae muscle; 7, flexor hallucis longus tendon; 8, flexor digitorum longus tendon; 9, tibialis posterior tendon.)

Fig. 5-41.   (A) Lateral aspect of right big toe. (B) Medial aspect of right big toe. (1, Lateral head of flexor hallucis brevis muscle; 2, medial head of flexor hallucis brevis muscle; 3, adductor hallucis, oblique head; 4, adductor hallucis, transverse head; 5, abductor hallucis muscle and tendon; 6, extensor hallucis brevis muscle; 7, extensor hallucis longus tendon; 8, flexor halucis longus tendon; 9, insertion of peroneus longus tendon.)

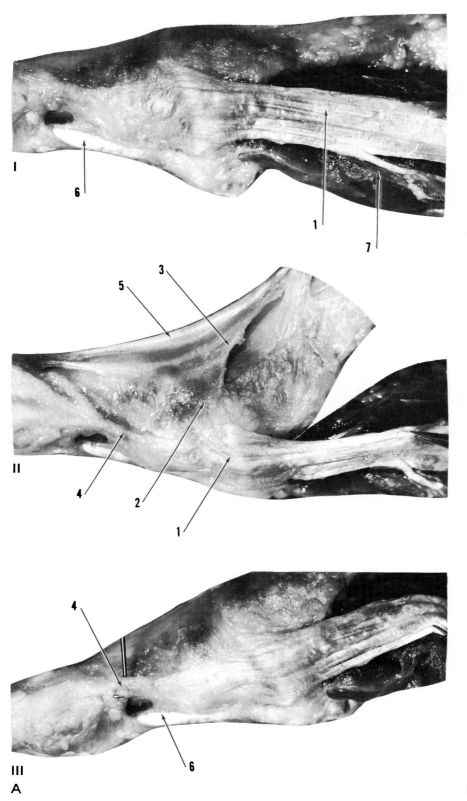

A

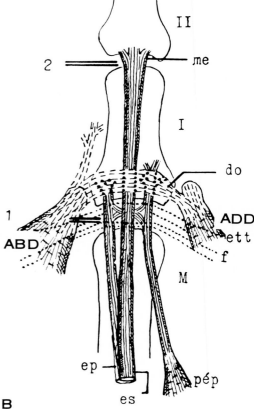

B

Fig. 5-42. **(A) Medial aspect of the metatarsophalangeal level of the right big toe.** (I) In neutral. (II) In hyperextension. (III) In flexion. (1, Tendon of abductor hallucis muscle; 2, transverse lamina of extensor aponeurosis; 3, proximal border of *2;* 4, phalangeal insertional band of *1;* 5, extensor hallucis longus tendon; 6, flexor hallucis longus tendon; 7, medial head of flexor hallucis brevis muscle.) **(B) Internal structure of the extensor apparatus of the right big toe.** (*es*, superficial fibers of extensor hallucis longus tendon; *ep*, deep fibers of extensor hallucis longus tendon; *pép*, extensor hallucis brevis tendon; *me*, insertion of extensor hallucis longus tendon; *ABD*, tendon of abductor hallucis tendon and insertion fibers contributing to extensor sling; *ADD*, tendon of adductor hallucis contributing to dorsal sling; *do*, dorsal sling; *f*, perforating fibers arising from plantar aponeurosis; *M*, metatarsal; I–II, proximal and distal phalanges; 1–2, level of metatarsophalangeal and interphalangeal joints.) (From Baumann JA: Valeur, variations et équivalences des muscles extenseurs, interosseux, adducteurs et abducteurs de la main et du pied chez l'homme. Acta Anat 4:10, 1947–1948. By permission of S. Karger AG, Basel)

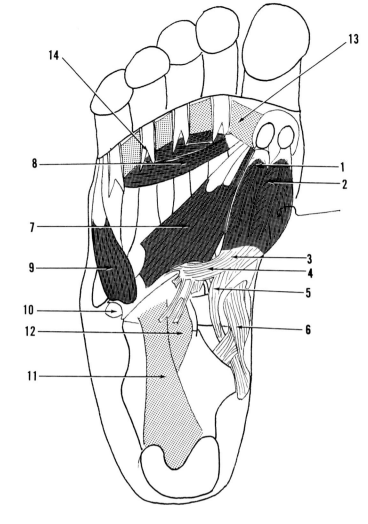

Fig. 5-43. Flexor hallucis brevis. (1, Lateral head of flexor hallucis brevis; 2, medial head of flexor hallucis brevis; 3, stem of Y origin of flexor hallucis brevis; 4, lateral arm of Y origin of flexor hallucis brevis; 5, medial arm of Y origin of flexor hallucis brevis provided by tibialis posterior tendon [6]; 7, oblique head of adductor hallucis muscle; 8, transverse head of adductor hallucis muscle; 9, short flexor of fifth toe; 10, peroneus longus tendon; 11, long calcaneocuboid ligament; 12, short calcaneocuboid ligament; 13, deep transverse metatarsal ligament; 14, deep insertional septa of plantar aponeurosis.)

Fig. 5-44. Origin of flexor hallucis brevis muscle. (From Martin BF: Observations on the muscles and tendons of the medial aspect of the sole of the foot. J Anat 98, No. 3:437, 1964. By permission of Cambridge University Press)

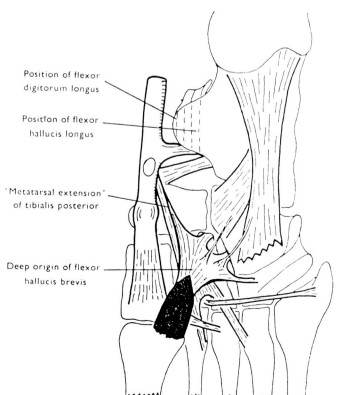

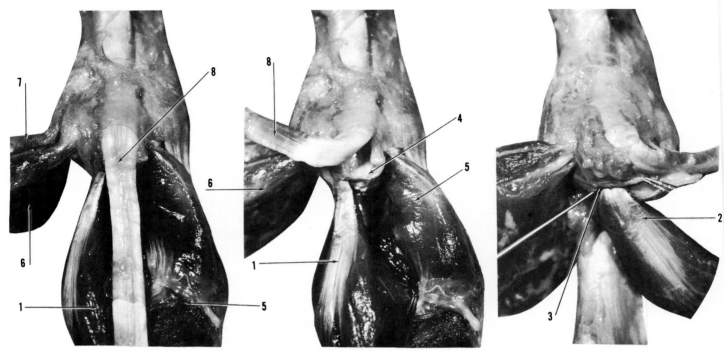

Fig. 5-45.   Plantar aspect of the metatarsophalangeal joint of the big toe. (1, Lateral head of flexor hallucis brevis; 2, tendon of *1* entering its own tunnel [3] before inserting on lateral sesamoid; 4, proximal border of plantar plate; 5, medial head of flexor hallucis brevis; 6, oblique head of adductor hallucis muscle; 7, transverse head of adductor hallucis muscle; 8, flexor hallucis longus tendon.)

Fig. 5-46.   Adductor hallucis. (1, Oblique head of adductor hallucis muscle, lateral component; 2, medial component of *1;* 3, transverse head of adductor hallucis muscle; 4, lateral head of flexor hallucis brevis muscle; 5, deep transverse metatarsal ligament; 6, plantar plate; 7, deep insertional septa of plantar aponeurosis; 8, foramen for common digital artery.)

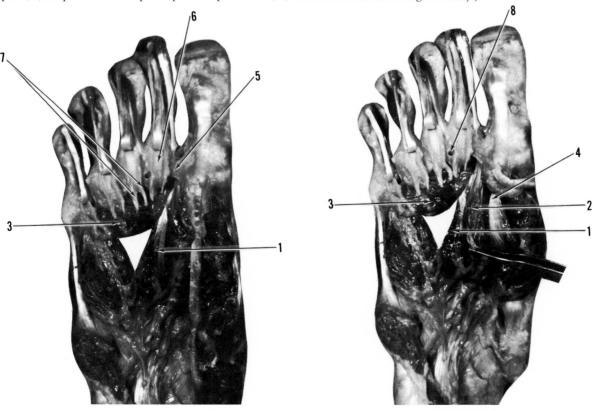

Fig. 5-47. Internal structure of plantar–lateral aspect of the right big toe. The specimen is fanned out for display of anatomic details. (1, medial component of oblique head of adductor hallucis muscle; 2, central component of oblique head of adductor hallucis muscle; 3, lateral component of oblique head of adductor hallucis muscle; 4, phalangeal insertion of *3;* 5, transverse head of adductor hallucis muscle with contribution to extensor aponeurosis [6] and insertion on flexor hallucis longus tendon tunnel [6′]; 7, extensor hallucis longus tendon; 8, extensor hallucis longus tendon; 9, lateral head of flexor hallucis brevis entering its own tunnel [10]; 11, insertion of deep transverse metatarsal ligament; 12, insertion of medial intermuscular septum; 13, deep insertional septa of plantar aponeurosis; 14, fibrous tunnel of flexor hallucis longus tendon; 15, fibrous bridge extending from metatarsal to proximal phalanx; diagram after dissection under magnification × 8.)

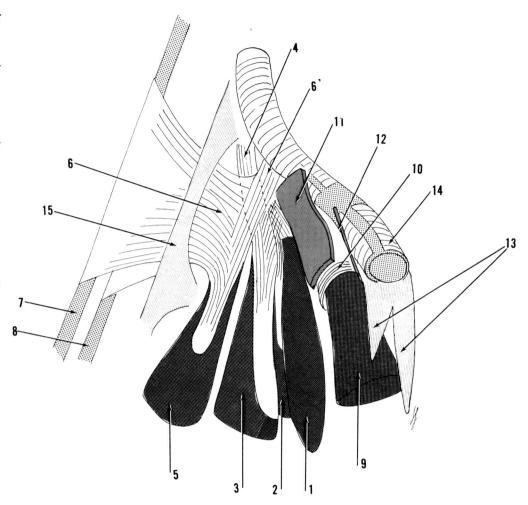

tionship that the oblique head is said to arise from the anterior segment of the inferior calcaneocuboid ligament, the crest of the cuboid, the base of metatarsals 4, 3, and 2, and the cuneiforms. The origin of the muscle may form a fibrous arc extended from the base to the inferior border of the fourth metatarsal bone. This arc gives passage to the lateral plantar neurovascular bundle in the middle compartment of the planta pedis.

The oblique head of the adductor hallucis courses obliquely (anteromedially) toward the lateral aspect of the metatarsophalangeal joint of the big toe. Its lateral border crosses the underlying metatarsals 4, 3, and 2 and the corresponding interossei along an oblique line drawn from the base of the fourth metatarsal to the base of the proximal hallucal phalanx. The medial border is apposed to the flexor hallucis brevis muscle. Three components are recognizable in the distal segment of the adductor hallucis obliquis—medial, central, lateral. All three components, prior to reaching their insertional destination, pass dorsal to the deep transverse metatarsal ligament (Figs. 5-48 and 5-49). The medial component with fleshy fibers inserts directly on the

lateral sesamoid. The central component is the deepest and presents a tendinous band that takes a firm grip on the plantar aspect of the lateral sesamoid. The lateral component has a broad plantar tendon that inserts on the lateral sesamoid and the plantar lateral aspect of the proximal phalanx and gives minor contribution to the extensor aponeurosis. The phalangeal tendinous component may be traced as a definite band (Fig. 5-50).

Transverse Head. The transverse head of the adductor originates from the proximal border of the plantar plate of the fifth, fourth, and third metatarsophalangeal joints; the proximal border of the deep transverse metatarsal ligament between toes 5 and 4, 4 and 3, 3 and 2; the longitudinal septa of the plantar aponeurosis to the fifth, fourth, and third toes; the medial crux of the lateral component of the plantar aponeurosis (Figs. 5-43, 5-46, and 5-51).[38]

Three transversely oriented muscular fascicles are formed. The most posterior is the longest and the most superficial. It arises from the fifth toe and the medial crux of the lateral plantar aponeurosis. It partially overlaps the

(Text continues on p. 236.)

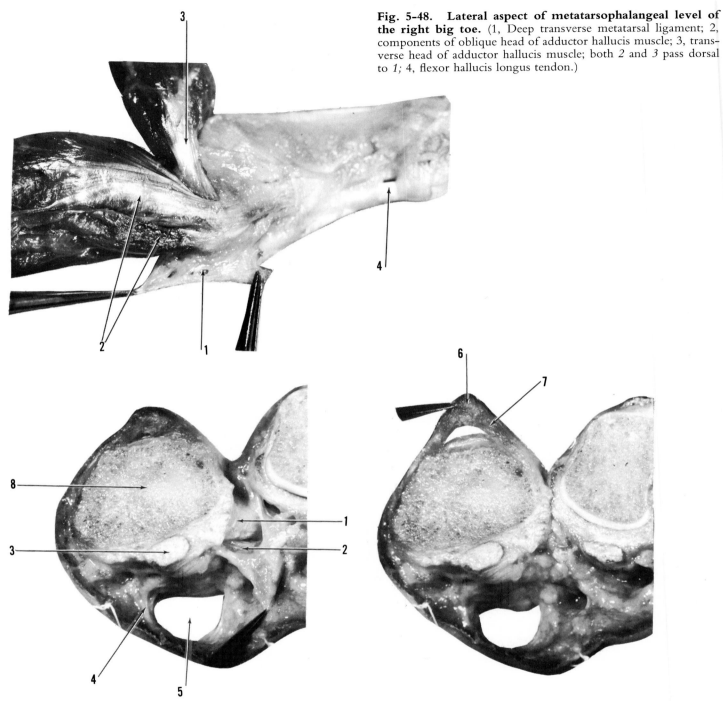

Fig. 5-48. **Lateral aspect of metatarsophalangeal level of the right big toe.** (1, Deep transverse metatarsal ligament; 2, components of oblique head of adductor hallucis muscle; 3, transverse head of adductor hallucis muscle; both 2 and 3 pass dorsal to 1; 4, flexor hallucis longus tendon.)

Fig. 5-49. **Cross section through proximal phalanx of the big toe.** (1, Adductor tendon passing dorsal to deep transverse metatarsal ligament [2]; 3, flexor hallucis longus tendon and its fibrous sheath attached to 1; 4, arciform fibrous fibers forming a pre-flexor chamber [5] retaining pre-flexor adipose cushion; 6, extensor hallucis longus tendon giving origin to transverse lamina [7].)

Fig. 5-50.   Insertion of adductor muscle of the big toe. (1, Medial component of oblique head of adductor hallucis; 2, central component of oblique head of adductor hallucis; 3, lateral component of oblique head of adductor hallucis; 4, transverse head of adductor hallucis; 5, phalangeal insertional band of *3*, retracted with a hook [6]; 7, flexor hallucis longus tendon.)

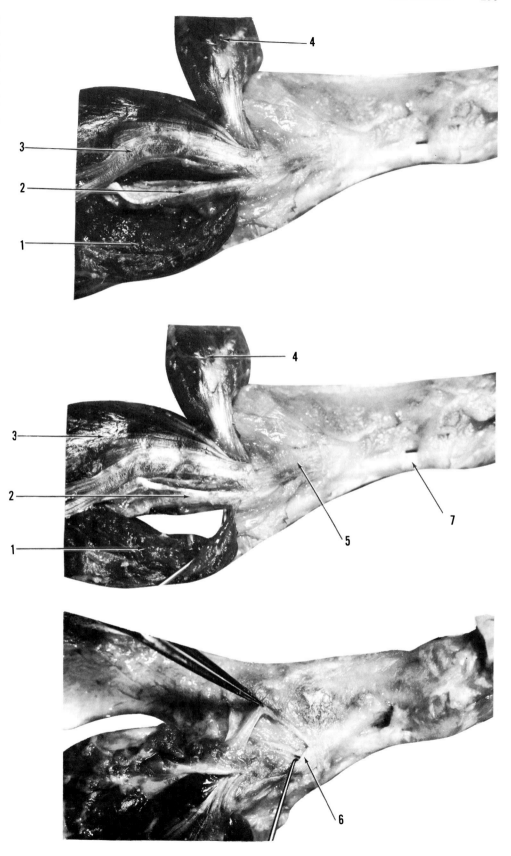

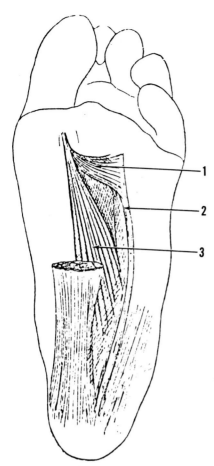

Fig. 5-51. Origin of the transverse head of the adductor hallucis from the medial crux of the lateral component of the plantar aponeurosis. (1, Transverse head of adductor hallucis muscle; 2, medial crux of lateral component of plantar aponeurosis; 3, oblique head of adductor hallucis muscle.) (From Loth E: Etude anthropoligique de l'aponevrose plantaire. Bull Mem Soc Anthropol Paris 4:606, 1913)

second fascicle, which in turn overlaps the shortest, deepest, and most anterior component arising from the third toe. The three fascicles unite at the level of the second metatarsophalangeal joint, and a short tendon appears, which passes dorsal to the deep transverse metatarsal ligament of the first toe and reaches the tendons of the oblique head of the adductor. At this level, some fibers of the tendon of the transverse head insert on the extensor aponeurosis; the remaining fibers pass over the fibers of the oblique head at the level of the lateral sesamoid, share their insertion, and terminate on the fibrous sheath of the flexor hallucis longus.

Leboucq emphasized the independent insertion of the transverse head of the adductor hallucis and its connection with the sheath of the flexor hallucis longus.[39] Furthermore, he mentioned some fibers inserting on the deep surface of the flexor tendon sheath of the second, third, and fourth toes and a bifurcation of the insertion at the level of the distal end of the fifth metatarsal, some fibers passing dorsal to the long flexor of the little toe and the remaining fibers

passing plantar and uniting with the superficial plantar aponeurosis.

The transverse head of the adductor hallucis has no insertion on the metatarsals.

Variations.   The following variations may be seen:[2]

Oblique adductor

Inseparable from the lateral head of the flexor hallucis brevis

Insertion on the tendon or the muscle of the lateral head of the short flexor

A fascicle extending from the lateral border of the oblique adductor to the lateral aspect of the proximal phalanx of the second toe at the base

Transverse adductor

Origin only from the fifth–fourth or fourth–third plantar plate and corresponding deep transverse metatarsal ligaments

Origin only from the joint of the fifth toe

Absent transverse component or replaced by an extremely thin contractile band

Proximal extension of the muscle reaching the anterior border of the oblique adductor

Additional muscle located in the first interosseous space. This is a small triangular muscle that measures about 1 cm and originates through its base from the distal third of the plantar border of the second metatarsal. It is located between the first dorsal interosseous and the oblique adductor, courses anteromedially, and inserts on the tendon of the transverse adductor.

INTRINSIC MUSCLES OF THE FIFTH TOE

There are five intrinsic muscles of the fifth toe: abductor, short flexor, opponens, and third plantar interosseous and fourth lumbrical (see Intrinsic Muscles of the Lesser Toes) (Figs. 5-31, 5-33, 5-43, and 5-46).

Abductor Digiti Minimi

The abductor digiti minimi is an elongated, fusiform muscle extending from the tuberosity of the os calcis to the base of the fifth toe. It is the muscle of the lateral border of the foot. It originates from the plantar aspect of the posterolateral tuberosity of the os calcis and extends to the adjacent posteromedial calcaneal tuberosity slightly anterior to the origin of the flexor digitorum brevis; from the deep surface of the fibular component of the plantar aponeurosis; and from the lateral intermuscular septum.

The fleshy fibers are directed forward and form an elongated muscle. The tendon appears in the substance of the muscle at the level of the calcaneocuboid joint and passes over the base of the fifth metatarsal. At this level, it may glide over the tuberosity of the metatarsal base, separated then by a bursa, or may (occasionally) receive fibers of attachment from it. From this point on, a substantial tendon appears, located in a lateral position. The tendon passes through the bifurcation arms or crux of the peroneal component of the plantar aponeurosis (Fig. 5-52). It still receives some fleshy fibers from its superior surface and extends distally, inserting on the plantar plate of the fifth metatarsophalangeal joint and the lateral aspect of the base of the proximal phalanx of the fifth toe. Frequently the terminal tendon sends an extension into the extensor aponeurosis.

The variations occur in the form of additional muscle components:

Muscle arising from the tuberosity of the fifth metatarsal and the overlying plantar aponeurosis, independent of the main component. It runs deep to the abductor (clear of its fibers) and inserts on the base of the proximal phalanx in conjunction with the abductor of the fifth toe, which may be then considered as a "biventral muscle."[40]

Abductor ossis metatarsi quinti. This is a fusiform long muscle that originates from the calcaneal posterolateral tuberosity and inserts on the apophysis of the fifth metatarsal. The muscle may be partially or totally adherent to the abductor of the fifth toe. Ledouble reported a frequency of 43% in 68 feet and 45% in 40 feet.[2]

Accessory abductor of the fifth toe. Ledouble described an independent muscle that originates from the posterolateral tuberosity of the os calcis and the plantar aponeurosis about 1 cm from the origin of the abductor of the fifth toe and inserts separately on the base of the proximal phalanx of the fifth toe or joins the tendon of the abductor at the level of the fifth metatarsal base.[2] In another variety, the accessory abductor arises from the sheath of the peroneus longus and inserts separately on the basal phalanx of the fifth toe.

Flexor Digiti Minimi Brevis

The short flexor of the fifth toe originates from the fibrous sheath of the peroneus longus, the crest of the cuboid, the base of the fifth metatarsal, and the plantar aponeurosis.

A small fusiform muscle forms that courses lateral to the converging long flexor tendon and inserts on the plantar plate of the fifth metatarsophalangeal joint and the base of the proximal phalanx of the fifth toe. This insertion is located between the attachment of the abductor tendon and the flexor tendon sheath.

The short flexor may be more or less united to the abductor of the fifth toe and is always fused—completely or incompletely—to the opponens of the fifth toe.[2, 37]

Opponens Digiti Quinti

The opponens digiti quinti is a flat, triangular muscle that originates from the sheath of the peroneus longus tendon and the crest of the cuboid. The tendon contours the base of the fifth metatarsal and gives origin to fleshy fibers that fan out and insert on the lateral border of the fifth metatarsal. The close connection of this muscle with the short flexor has been mentioned above.

Ledouble recognized this muscle in more than 50% of

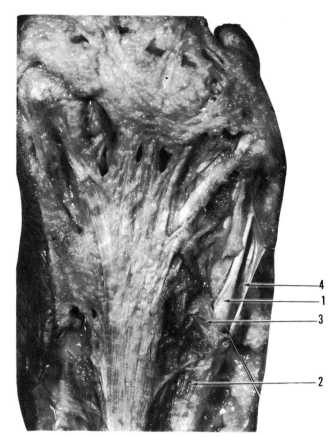

Fig. 5-52. Tendon of the abductor digiti minimi. (1, Tendon of abductor muscle of fifth toe; 2, lateral component of plantar aponeurosis; 3, medial crux of *2*; 4, lateral crux of *2*.)

his material.[2] Jones summarized the controversy surrounding this muscle very well: "the frequence of its occurrence as an independent muscle and the practically constant occurrence of fibers representing it, though partly incorporated in the short flexor, justifies its recognition as an entity entitled to its own name."[40]

The muscle is not listed in the *Nomina Anatomica* (PNA 1964).

INTRINSIC MUSCLES OF THE LESSER TOES

The intrinsic muscles of the lesser toes, excluding the muscles of the lateral compartment of the fifth toe, include four dorsal interossei, three plantar interossei, and four lumbricals (Figs. 5-53–5-55).

The functional axis of the foot passes through the second toe. The motions of abduction and adduction occur relative to this axis. The dorsal interossei are the abductors of the toes, the plantar interossei are the adductors, and the second toe possesses two dorsal interossei. The functional classification simplifies the location of the insertion of the interossei.

The first through the fourth dorsal interossei are inserted, respectively, on the tibial and the peroneal aspect of the second toe and the peroneal aspect of the third and fourth toes (acting as the abductors). The first through the third plantar interossei insert, respectively, on the tibial side of the third, fourth, and fifth toes (acting as adductors). The lumbricals are located on the tibial aspect of the corresponding toes.

Dorsal Interossei

The four dorsal interossei bipenniform muscles originate from the lateral surface of the metatarsals delineating the corresponding intermetatarsal space (Figs. 5-56 and 5-57).

The *first dorsal interosseous* attaches to the entire tibial surface of the second metatarsal bone and to the inferior surface of its base. Dorsally, the attachment of the peroneal component extends to the anterolateral corner of the first cuneiform. The medial or tibial head arises from a tendinous arch that originates from the anterior border of the peroneus longus tendon near its insertion, crosses the base of the second metatarsal, and inserts on the anterior segment of

the superolateral border of the first metatarsal (Fig. 5-18).[18] This fibrous arcade with posteromedial concavity delineates, with the lateral surface of the first metatarsal, an elliptic space that gives passage to the pedal vessels. The frequency of occurrence of the arcade, according to various sources, is 89% in 54 feet, 74% in 27 feet, 63.5% in 149 feet.[18, 41, 42]

The attachment of the medial head to the first metatarsal shaft may be by loose connective tissue only. If the fibrous arcade has a more proximal insertion on the base of the first metatarsal, the medial head of the interosseous may then attach to the lateral surface of the first metatarsal, not exceeding the proximal half of the surface or being limited to a few insertional fibers.[42]

The *second dorsal interosseous* originates from the entire peroneal surface of the second metatarsal and partially from the superior segment of the tibial surface of the third metatarsal. It may extend its origin to the dorsum of the lateral cuneiform.

The *third dorsal interosseous* originates from the entire peroneal surface of the third metatarsal and partially from the

Fig. 5-53. Insertion sites of lumbrical muscles.

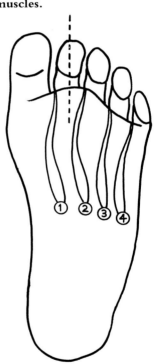

Fig. 5-54. Insertion sites of dorsal interossei muscles.

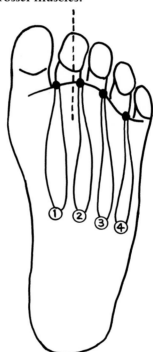

Fig. 5-55. Insertion sites of plantar interossei muscles.

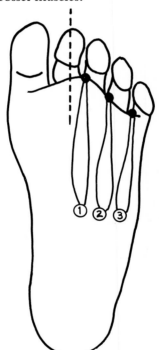

superior aspect of the tibial surface of the fourth metatarsal.

The *fourth dorsal interosseous* originates from the entire peroneal surface of the fourth metatarsal and partially from the superior aspect of the tibial surface of the fifth metatarsal.

The last two interossei receive some fibers from the plantar calcaneocuboid ligament.[40]

Plantar Interossei

The three plantar interossei are smaller than the corresponding dorsal interossei. They are single headed and fusiform and arise from the inferior segment and border of the tibial surface of the third, fourth, and fifth metatarsals (Figs. 5-56 and 5-57). Their origin extends to the base of the same metatarsals and to the metatarsal expansions of the inferior calcaneocuboid ligament.

Lumbricals

The lateral three lumbricals are bipenniform and arise from the intertendinous angle of the flexor digitorum longus tendons (Figs. 5-57 and 5-58). The first lumbrical has a single origin from the tibial side of the long flexor to the second toe. Distally, the muscle–tendon units are located on the tibial side of the corresponding toe.

Insertion

Interossei. The tendons of the dorsal and plantar interossei, in their path to the toes, pass dorsal to the deep transverse metatarsal ligament (Figs. 5-58 and 5-59), whereas the lumbrical tendons remain plantar (Fig. 5-60). Prior to their insertions, all the tendons of the toes are grouped and retained around the metatarsophalangeal joint by fibrous formations.

The long extensor tendon and the short extensor tendon are each located in a flat, independent tendon sheath and are centered over the corresponding metatarsal head. Within the tunnel, the deep surface of the tendon is connected to the sheath with fibrous bands, whereas on the dorsal aspect, a gliding or a bursal component is interposed between the tendon and the sheath.[43] The extensor tendon sheaths are formed by the distal segment of the common dorsal aponeurosis.

(Text continues on p. 242.)

Fig. 5-56. (*A*) **Origin of dorsal interossei muscles 1 to 4.** The first dorsal interosseous with an accessory origin from the first cuneiform. The second dorsal cuneiform with an accessory origin from the third cuneiform. The *arrow* indicates the axis of the foot passing through the second metatarsal. (*B*) **Metatarsal origin of the dorsal and plantar interossei muscles.** (M_1–M_5, metatarsals 1 to 5; D_1–D_4, dorsal interossei muscles 1 to 4; P_1–P_3, plantar interossei muscles 1 to 3.)

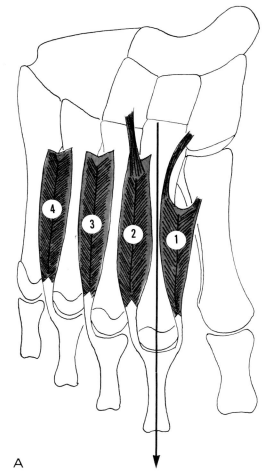

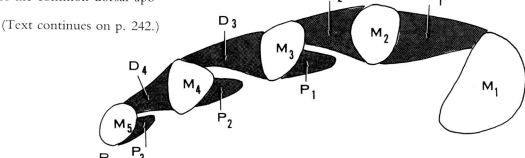

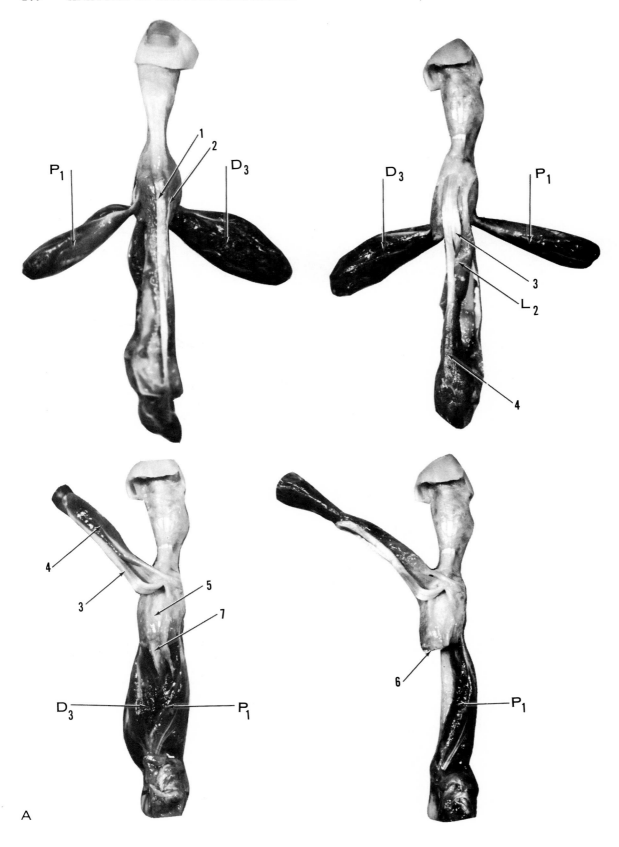

A

Fig. 5-57. **(A) Right third toe.** (*Left*) Dorsal aspect. (*Right*) Plantar aspect. (P₁, first plantar interosseous muscle; D₃, third dorsal interosseous muscle; L₂, second lumbrical muscle; 1, long extensor tendon; 2, extensor digitorum brevis tendon; 3, flexor digitorum longus tendon; 4, flexor digitorum brevis muscle; 5, plantar plate; 6, proximal border of plantar plate; 7, insertion of plantar aponeurosis septa.) **(B) Right third toe, peroneal aspect.** (1, Third dorsal interosseous muscle; 2, superficial phalangeal tendon of *1*; 3, deep phalangeal tendon of *1*; 4, flexor digitorum brevis muscle and tendon; 5, extensor aponeurotic lamina forming tunnel for tendon of *1*; 6, split transverse lamina of extensor aponeurosis; 7, flexor hallucis longus tendon; 8, extensor digitorum longus tendon; 9, extensor digitorum brevis tendon; 10, capsule of metatarsophalangeal joint.) **(C) Right third toe, tibial side.** (1, Lumbrical tendon and muscle; 2, first plantar interosseous muscle and tendon; 3, flexor digitorum brevis muscle and tendon; 4, flexor hallucis longus tendon; 5, extensor digitorum brevis tendon; 6, proximal border of transverse lamina; 7, proximal border of plantar plate; 8, metatarsophalangeal collateral ligament; 9, deep transverse metatarsal ligament.)

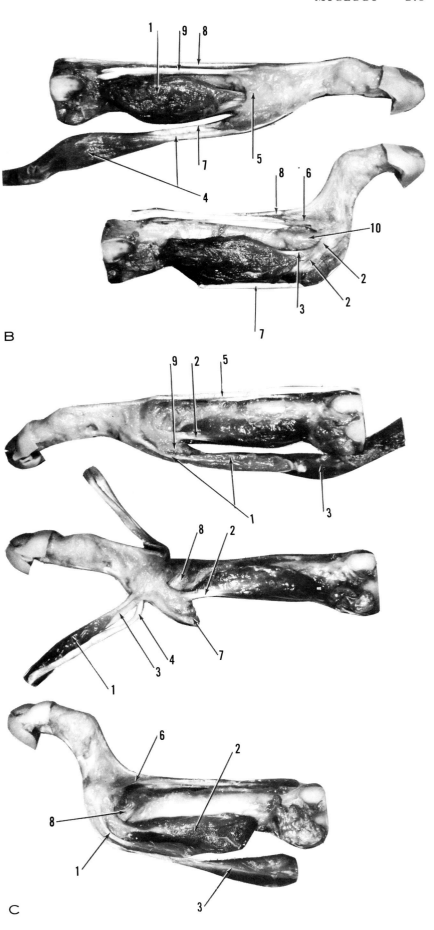

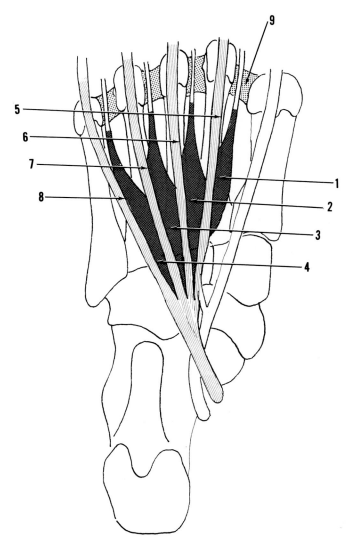

Fig. 5-58.   Lumbricals. (1–4, Lumbricals 1–4; 5–8, flexor digitorum longus tendons 2–5; 9, deep transverse metatarsal ligament.)

on each side by the corresponding lateral surfaces of the metatarsals. The dorsal aspect is limited by the dorsal interosseous aponeurosis and the plantar aspect by the proximal segment of the deep transverse intermetatarsal ligament. An oblique fibrous expansion divides this chamber into two sections: large for the dorsal interosseous tendon and smaller for the plantar interosseous tendon. It is at this level that the dorsal interosseous makes its first insertion on the deep transverse intermetatarsal ligament.

Farther distally, between the metatarsal heads, the extensor intertendinous aponeurosis advances plantarward as a wedge, carrying the dorsal adipose tissue and neurovascular structures, and unites with the dorsal interosseous aponeurosis (Fig. 5-63). Multiple fascial septa now extend vertically plantarward from the apex of the united aponeurosis. A vertical lamina passes over each interosseous tendon and inserts on the deep transverse intermetatarsal ligament. This arrangement corresponds to the transverse lamina or extensor sling. Some septa pierce the transverse intermetatarsal

(Text continues on p. 247.)

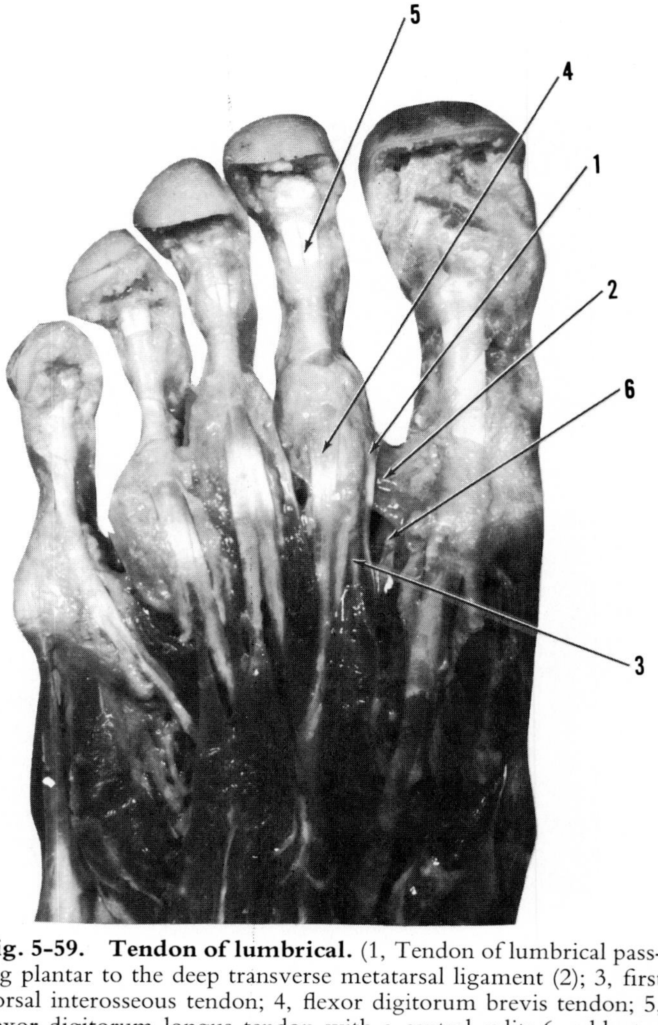

A fibrous annular formation originates from the sides of the extensor sheath, wraps around the metatarsophalangeal joint capsule (independent from it), and inserts on the plantar aspect along the sides of the plantar plate in conjunction with the deep transverse intermetatarsal ligament. This annular structure centralizes and stabilizes the extensor tendons. It represents the proximal segment of the digital extensor aponeurosis and is called the *transverse lamina* or *extensor sling* (Figs. 5-61 and 5-62). Meyer, in a cross sectional study of 15 adult feet and 20 fetal feet supplemented by sagittal sections of 10 adult feet, provided a detailed account of the formation and arrangement of the retaining fibrous structures.[43] Proximal to the metatarsal heads, the extensor sheaths of two adjacent rays are united by the intertendinous segment of the dorsal common aponeurosis, which is superficial to the underlying dorsal interosseous aponeurosis covering the intermetatarsal space (Fig. 5-63). At this level the quadrilateral intermetatarsal space is limited

Fig. 5-59.   Tendon of lumbrical. (1, Tendon of lumbrical passing plantar to the deep transverse metatarsal ligament (2); 3, first dorsal interosseous tendon; 4, flexor digitorum brevis tendon; 5, flexor digitorum longus tendon with a central split; 6, adductor hallucis tendon passing dorsal to the deep transverse metatarsal ligament [2].)

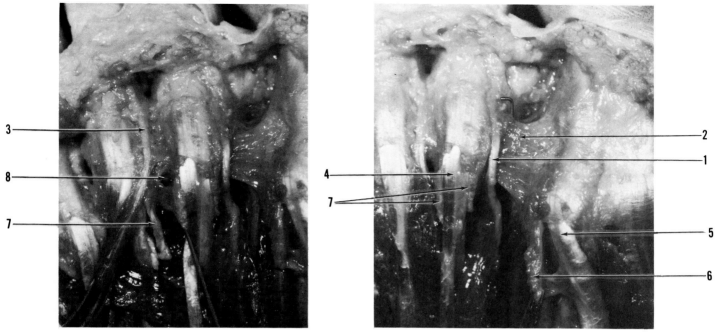

Fig. 5-60. Lumbrical tendons. (1, Lumbrical tendon; 2, deep transverse metatarsal ligament 1–2; 3, lumbrical fascia forming thin tunnel to tendon; 4, flexor digitorum brevis tendon; 5, flexor hallucis longus tendon; 6, 7, deep insertional septa of plantar aponeurosis; 8, foramen for common digital artery.)

Fig. 5-61. Cross section of the ball of the foot. (*M*, metatarsal head; 1, extensor digitorum longus tendon; 2, extensor digitorum brevis tendon; 3, transverse lamina of extensor aponeurosis; 4, capsule of metatarsophalangeal joint; 5, deep transverse metatarsal ligament; 6, plantar plate; 7, 7', interossei muscles located in narrow cleft formed by capsule and transverse lamina [7] or incorporated in split of transverse lamina [7']; 8, lumbrical tendon in its own tunnel on tibial side of joint; 9, long flexor tunnel; 10, long flexor tendons; 11, longitudinal band of plantar aponeurosis; 12, vertical thin fibrous band of plantar aponeurosis forming a pre-flexor tendon space lodging a pre-flexor adipose cushion [13]; 14, fat body on plantar aspect of *5* covering neurovascular bundle [16]; 15, transverse component of plantar aponeurosis; 17, triangular adipofascial complex filling intermetatarsal capitular space and carrying superficial nerves and vessels.)

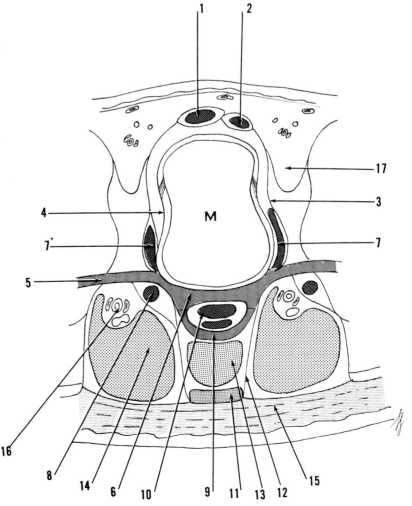

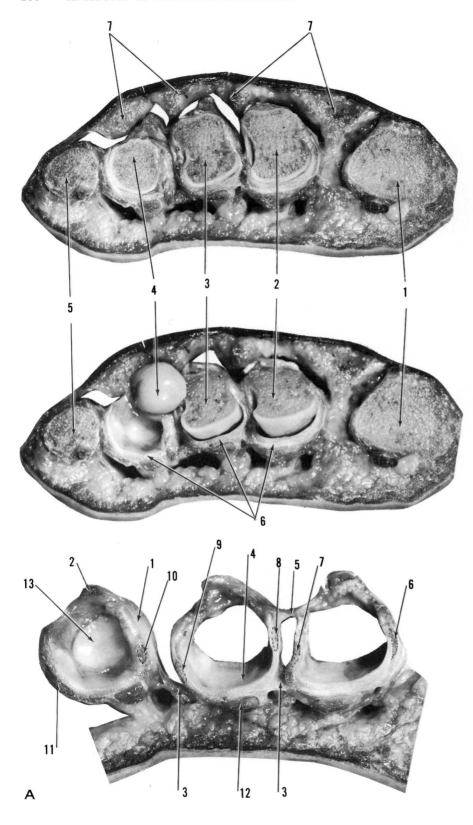

Fig. 5-62. (*A*) (*Top* and *middle*) Cross section passing through metatarsal heads *2, 3, 4* and phalanges *1* and *5*. *1* (6, Plantar plates 2, 3, 4; 7, adipofascial triangular pads filling interspaces.) (*Bottom*) Extensor ring complex formed around the metatarsal heads. (1, Transverse lamina of extensor aponeurosis; 2, extensor digitorum longus tendon of fourth toe; 3, deep transverse metatarsal ligament; 4, plantar plate; 5, superficial transverse metatarsal ligament; 6, insertional tendon of first dorsal interosseous; 7, insertional tendon of second dorsal interosseous; 8, insertional tendon of first plantar interosseous; 9, insertional tendon of third dorsal interosseous; 10, insertional tendon of second plantar interosseous; 11, insertional tendon of fourth dorsal interosseous; 12, long flexor tendons; 13, base of proximal phalanx of fourth toe.) (*B*) **Cross section through metatarsal heads.** (*Top*) (1, Transverse lamina; 2, capsule of metatarsophalangeal joint; 3, plantar plate; 4, fibrous tunnel for long flexors; 5, insertional tendon of third dorsal interosseous muscle; 6, second lumbrical; 7, long flexor tendons.) (*Bottom*) (1, Transverse lamina; 2, capsule of metatarsophalangeal joint; 3, point of junction of *1, 2,* plantar plate, and flexor tendon tunnel; 4, insertional tendon of first plantar interosseous muscle; 5, insertional tendon of third dorsal interosseous muscle; 6, insertional tendon of second dorsal interosseous muscle; 7, insertional tendon of first dorsal interosseous muscle.)

Fig. 5-62 (continued)

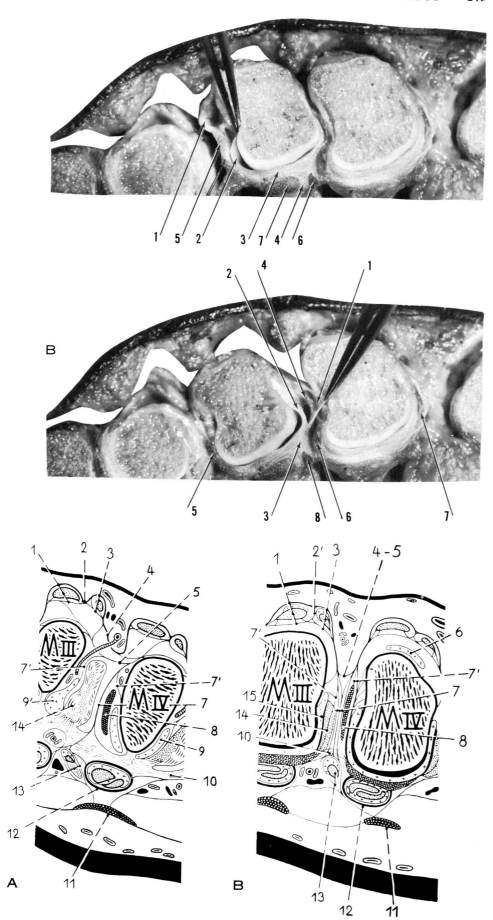

Fig. 5-63. Metatarsophalangeal region of the right foot. (*A*) Anterior segment of a vertical and transverse section of the metatarsophalangeal region of the right foot, passing through the articular interlines at the level of the big toe and the fifth toe and through the intermetatarsal spaces between metatarsals 2, 3, and 4. Segment of the section passing through the third intermetatarsal space. (*B*) Anterior segment of a vertical and transverse cross section of the metatarsophalangeal region of the right foot, passing through the metatarsal heads 3 and 4. (1. Tendinous portion of dorsal aponeurosis common to extensor tendons forming sheath to long extensor tendon; 2, 2′, axial intertendinous portion of dorsal aponeurosis; 3, tendinous portion of dorsal aponeurosis forming sheath to extensor digitorum brevis tendon; 4, intertendinous, interaxial portion of dorsal common aponeurosis; 5, dorsal interosseous aponeurosis [4 and 5 form dorsal transverse ligament]; 6, superior articular cul-de-sac; 7, interaxial lamina; 7′, vertical laminae arising from 5 and inserting on metatarsals, articular capsules, and tendons of interossei; 8, plantar interosseous tendon; 9, 9′, lateral and inferior articular cul-de-sac; 10, deep plantar transverse ligament; 11, pretendinous band of superficial plantar aponeurosis; 12, fibrous sheath of long flexor tendons; 13, fibrous sheath of lumbrical tendon; 14, dorsal interosseous tendon; 15, articular capsule.) (From Meyer P: Contribution a l'étude de la region métatarso-phalangienne. Bull Assoc Anat 99:500, 1958)

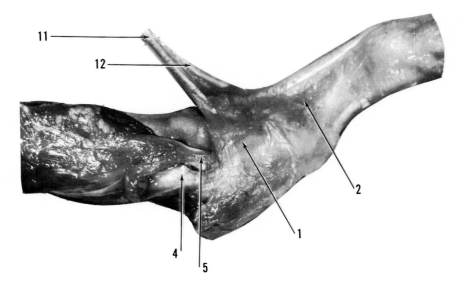

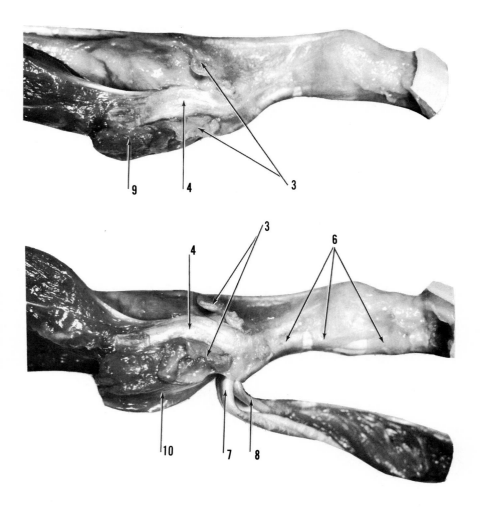

Fig. 5-64.   Metatarsophalangeal region of the right third toe, peroneal side. (1, Transverse lamina of extensor aponeurosis; 2, oblique segment of extensor aponeurosis; 3, split transverse lamina; 4, 5, superficial and deep tendons of third dorsal interosseous tendon; 6, pulleys of long flexor tendons; 7, long flexor tendon; 8, short flexor tendon; 9, deep transverse metatarsal ligament; 10, plantar plate; 11, extensor digitorum brevis tendon; 12, extensor digitorum longus tendon.)

ligament and connect with the deep longitudinal septa of the plantar aponeurosis. At this level the dorsal interosseous is strongly attached to the lateral lower aspect of the capsule and glenoid ligament of the metatarsophalangeal joint and also to the lateral aspect of the plantar plate; it is also attached to the deep surface of the transverse lamina.

Occasionally, and especially with the second dorsal interosseous, two definite tendons are seen, corresponding proximally to a subdivision of the same muscle into two units. One tendon inserts on the plantar plate, the proximal phalanx, whereas the second tendon terminates on the deep surface of the transverse lamina.[15]

The plantar interossei have insertions similar to those of the dorsal interossei.

At the level of the metatarsophalangeal joint, the tendons of the interossei are thus located in vertical clefts limited on one side by the capsule of the joint and on the other side by the transverse lamina (see Fig. 5-62, *B*). At the level of the proximal phalanx the interossei attach to the base of the corresponding phalanx and have no or very minimal contribution to the oblique component or extensor hood of the extensor mechanism (Fig. 5-64).

In summary, the interossei are inserted on:

The deep transverse intermetatarsal ligaments
The lateral capsule and the glenoid ligament of the metatarsophalangeal joint
The plantar plate of the metatarsophalangeal joint
The deep surface of the transverse lamina
The base of the proximal phalanx

Lumbricals. The lumbrical tendons are located on the plantar and tibial aspects of the corresponding deep transverse intermetatarsal ligaments. They are retained within a tunnel formed by a septum extending from the sagittal band of the plantar aponeurosis and inserting between the lumbrical tendon and the digital neurovascular bundle. At the distal end of the deep transverse intermetatarsal ligament, the lumbrical tendon is directed anteriorly and dorsally. It joins the extensor hood, and most of the fibers remain concentrated on the tibial border distally, reaching the extensor middle and lateral slips. Few fibers insert on the base of the proximal phalanx. Baumann, analyzing the microanatomy of the extensor aponeurosis, brings forth the participation of the interossei muscles to the constitution of the transverse proximal component and of the extensor hood.[14] In the fifth toe, however, the extensor hood is more or less atrophic and the spiral contributory fibers from the intrinsics are absent.[15]

Variations of the Interossei

A comprehensive study of the variations of the interossei muscles, based on 149 feet, has been reported by Manter.[42] These variations involve the origin, the insertion, and fusion or addition.

Variations of Origin. There are four variations of origin (Fig. 5-65).

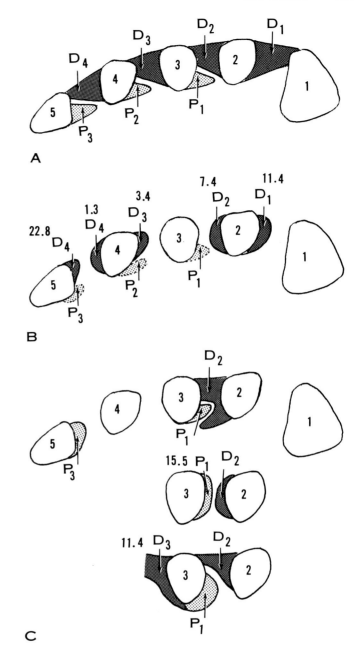

Fig. 5-65. Variations of origin of the interossei muscles. (*A*) Normal pattern of origin. (*B*) Variation with origin of dorsal interossei from a single metatarsal. (*C*) Variation with extension of origin of D_2, D_3, P_1, P_3. (1–4, Metatarsals; D_1–D_4, dorsal interossei; P_1–P_3, plantar interossei.) (Adapted from Manter JT: Variations of the interosseous muscles of the human foot. Anat Rec 93:117, 1945)

Dorsal Interossei with Single Head. The dorsal interossei may have one head of origin only and the frequency of occurrence is as follows: the fourth dorsal interosseous from the fifth metatarsal, 22.8%; the first dorsal interosseous from the second metatarsal, 11.4%; the second dorsal interosseous from the second metatarsal, 7.4%; the third dorsal interosseous from the fourth metatarsal, 3.4%; the fourth dorsal interosseous from the fourth metatarsal, 1.3%.[42] The first two dorsal interossei remain grouped along the second metatarsal. The third and fourth dorsal interossei shift their origin laterally (except for a small percentage of the fourth dorsal interossei).

Dorsal Extension of Plantar Interossei.
In the second intermetatarsal space, the second dorsal interosseous originates from the entire lateral surface of the second metatarsal and from the upper segment of the medial surface of the third metatarsal. In 15.5% the "origin of the first plantar interosseous had extended dorsally on the third metatarsal at the expense of the second dorsal muscle which had lost, wholly or in part, its attachment to that bone."[42] In one case, only the third plantar interosseous extended dorsally on the fifth metatarsal.

Accessory Origins.
The first and second plantar interossei and the second and third dorsal interossei may have plantar accessory origins.[42] The most frequently seen arrangement, occurring in 11.4 percent, is the presence of a plantar slip extending from the third dorsal interosseous to the first plantar interosseous. The second dorsal interosseous may extend plantarward, covering the first plantar interosseous without creating an attachment to it. The dorsal interossei may also receive tendinous slips from the extensor digitorum brevis, the peroneus brevis, and the peroneus tertius.

Fusion and Doubling of Muscle Bellies.
The fusion may occur between the muscle bellies of: the second plantar interosseous and the third dorsal interosseous (2.5%) or the first plantar interosseous and the second dorsal interosseus (1.3%). Doubling of the muscle was only observed with the second dorsal interosseous (1.3%).[42]

Variation of Insertion

Bifid Tendons.
Bifid tendons inserting each on the adjacent toe and involving mostly the second dorsal interosseous were observed with the frequency shown in Table 5-1.[42]

Table 5-1.   Frequency of Occurrence of Bifid Tendons

Intermetatarsal Space	Muscle With Bifid Tendon	Insertion on Digits	Frequency
2	Second dorsal interosseous	Digits 2 and 3	3.4%
	First plantar interosseous	Digits 2 and 3	0.7%
3	Third dorsal interosseous	Digits 3 and 4	1.4%
	Second plantar interosseous	Digits 3 and 4	0.7%
4	Fourth dorsal interosseous	Digits 4 and 5	0.7%
	Third plantar interosseous	Digits 4 and 5	1.4%

Additional Muscle.
Leboucq described a small triangular muscle located between the first dorsal interosseous and the oblique head of the adductor hallucis. This muscle originates with a 1-cm base from the distal third of the plantar border of the third metatarsal, is directed obliquely and anteriorly, and terminates by a tendon inserting on the deep surface of the transverse head of the adductor. In certain cases the muscle is replaced by an aponeurotic lamella having similar insertions and position. In a study of 60 feet, Leboucq observed such a muscle in 5%.[39]

Manter mentioned having observed "a tiny thread to a band about 4 mms wide" with similar position and insertion in 55.5% of 54 feet.[42]

Ledouble described an additional muscle originating from the midsegment of the inferior calcaneocuboid ligament or from the sheath of the peroneus longus.[2] It is separated from the plantar interossei by the deep branch of the lateral plantar nerve. It courses anteriorly and medially and inserts on the lateral aspect of the base of the proximal phalanx of the second toe.

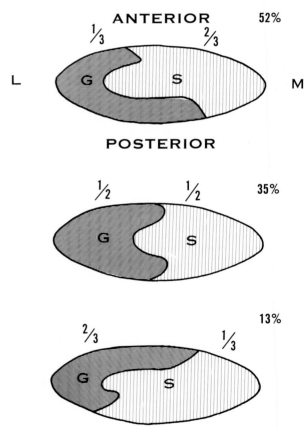

Fig. 5-66.   Degree of rotation of gastrocnemius-to-soleus portions of the calcaneal tendon (left extremity) at the level of insertion into the calcaneus. Occurrence in 100 specimens is indicated for each. (*G*, gastrocnemius; *S*, soleus; *L*, lateral; *M*, medial.) (Adapted from Cummins EJ, Anson JB, Carr WB, Wright RR, Hauser DWE: The structure of the calcaneal tendon [of Achilles] in relation to orthopedic surgery with additional observations on the plantaris muscle. Surg Gynecol Obstet 83:107, 1946)

Variations of the Lumbricals

Variation of Origin.   The first lumbrical may originate from the tibialis posterior tendon or from this tendon and the tendon of the flexor hallucis longus. The second, third, and fourth lumbricals may originate from the flexor digitorum brevis.

Absence.   The lumbrical may be absent. In a study of 100 feet (400 lumbricals), Schmidt and co-workers found 32 lumbricals absent (8%), with the following distribution: first lumbrical, 1 absent (0.25%); second lumbrical, 9 absent (2.25%); third lumbrical, 10 absent (2.5%); fourth lumbrical, 12 absent (3%).[44]

Duplicity and Bifidity.   The third and fourth lumbricals are sometimes double.[44] The fourth lumbrical may be bifid at the insertion.[44]

Calcaneal (of Achilles) and Plantaris Tendons

The *calcaneal tendon* is the conjoint tendon of the gastrocnemei and soleus. Large and strong, ovoid in contour, it measures 1.2 cm to 2.5 cm in width at the insertion and 5 mm to 6 mm in thickness at the level of the ankle.[45, 46]

Oriented nearly in the frontal plane, the tendon is invested by the superficial crural fascia. The tendon is larger at the insertion on the inferior half of the posterior calcaneal surface. Some of the insertional fibers are in continuity with the plantar aponeurosis.

Structurally, the fibers of the calcaneal tendon do not descend straight down but rotate to a variable degree in a spiral manner. This internal arrangement is analyzed by Cummins and co-workers and Jones.[40, 45] At the onset, the tendinous fibers of the gastrocnemius are posterior to the fibers contributed by the soleus component. At 12 cm to 15 cm from the insertion, the fibers rotate from a medial to a lateral direction, as observed posteriorly. The gentle twist of the fibers is progressive, reaching a maximum at 2 cm to 5 cm from the insertion.[46]

During their descent, the medial fibers of the gastrocnemius component reach a lateral position posteriorly, whereas the middle fibers are straight laterally and the most lateral fibers are anterolateral in location. The fibers of the soleus component are subjected to the same rotation, bringing some of the anteriorly located fibers into a posterior position (Fig. 5-66).

The degree of rotation of the calcaneal tendon is variable, and the grouping and distribution shown in Table 5-2 is provided by Cummins and co-workers.[45]

The *plantaris* arises in close association with the lateral head of the gastrocnemius. The flat fusiform muscle is fol-

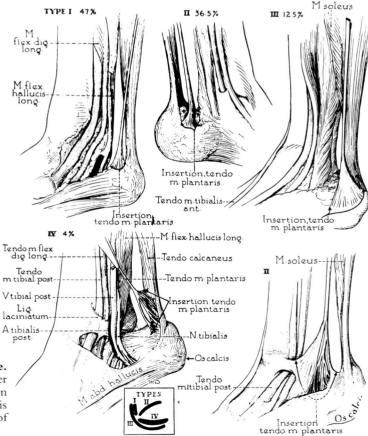

Fig. 5-67.   Types of tendinous insertion of plantaris muscle. (From Cummins EJ, Anson JB, Carr WB, Wright RR, Hauser DWE: The structure of the calcaneal tendon [of Achilles] in relation to orthopedic surgery with additional observations on the plantaris muscle. Surg Gynecol Obstet 83:107, 1946. By permission of Surgery, Gynecology & Obstetrics)

Table 5-2. Posterior Contribution to Calcaneal Tendon*

Group	Gastrocnemius	Soleus	%	Rotation
I	2/3	1/3	52	Minimum
II	1/2	1/2	35	
III	1/3	2/3	13	Maximum

*In 100 tendons. (From Cummins JE, Anson JB, Carr WB, Wright RR, Hauser DWE: The structure of the calcaneal tendon (of Achilles) in relation to orthopedic surgery with additional observations on the plantaris muscle. Surg Gynecol Obstet 83:107, 1946)

lowed by a slender and long tendon that courses obliquely downward and medially between the soleus and the gastrocnemei. The tendon locates itself along the medial border of the calcaneal tendon and has a variable insertion, as reported by Cummins and co-workers, based on the analysis of 200 plantaris tendons (Fig. 5-67):

Type I (47%). Fan-shaped expansion inserting into the medial aspect of the superior calcaneal tuberosity for the insertion of the calcaneal tendon

Type II (36.5%). Insertion on the os calcis, 0.5 cm to 2.5 cm anterior to the medial border of the calcaneal tendon. This insertion may radiate into the laciniate ligament and the fascia covering the medial aspect of the calcaneus.

Type III (12.5%). Broad insertion investing the dorsal and medial surfaces of the adjacent terminal calcaneal tendon.

Type IV (4%). Insertion on the medial border of the calcaneal tendon at a level 1 cm to 16 cm proximal to the insertion of the latter on the calcaneum. Occasionally a slip may reach the os calcis.[45]

The plantaris "is exceedingly variable in origin, structure and insertion" and is absent in 7.05%.[45]

REFERENCES

1. Testut L: Les Anomalies Musculaires Chez l'Homme Expliquées par l'Anatomie Comparée: Leur Importance en Anthropologie, pp 588–694, 705–732, 735–737, 741–744. Paris, Masson, 1884
2. LeDouble AF: Traité des Variations du Système Musculaire de l'Homme et de leur Signification au Point de Vue de l'Anthropologie et Zoologique, Vol II, pp 327–360, 374–397, 402–408, 413–421, 425–427. Paris, Schleicher Frères, 1897
3. Hallisy JE: The muscular variations in the human foot: A quantitative study. Am J Anat 45, No. 3:411, 1930
4. Chudzinski T: Contributions à l'étude des variations musculaires dans les Races Humaines. Rev Anthropol 5:613, 1882
5. Macalister A: Additional observations on muscular anomalies in human anatomy (3rd series) with a catalogue of the principal muscular variations hitherto published. Trans R Irish Acad 25:1, 1875
6. Knott JF: Muscular anomalies, including those of the diaphragm and subdiaphragmatic regions of the human body. Proc R Irish Acad 3:627, 1877–1883
7. Macalister A: Further notes on muscular anomalies in human anatomy and their bearing upon homotypical myology. Proc R Irish Acad 10:1866–1869
8. Gruber W: Ueber einen musc. tibio-astragalus anticus des Menschen. Arch Anat Physiol, p 663, 1871
9. Seelaus HK: On certain muscle anomalies of the lower extremity. Anat Rec 35:187, 1927
10. Gruber W: Ueber die Varietaeten des Musc. Extensor hallucis longus. Reich und DuBoise—Reymond's Arch., p 565, 1875
11. Gruber W: Ein neuer fall von Musc. Extensor hallucis longus tricaudatus. Reich und DuBoise—Reymond's Arch., p 746, 1876
12. Wood J: Variations in human myology observed during winter session of 1867–68 at King's College, London. Proc R Soc 16:438, 1867–1868
13. Paturet G: Traité d'Anatomie Humaine, Vol II, Membres Superieur et Inferieur, p 834. Paris, Masson et Cie, 1951
14. Baumann JA: Valeur, variations et équivalences des muscles extenseurs, interosseux, adducteurs et abducteurs de la main et du pied chez l'homme. Acta Anat 4:10, 1947–1948
15. Sarrafian SK, Topouzian LK: Anatomy and physiology of the extensor apparatus of the toes. J Bone Joint Surg [Am] 51, No. 4:669, 1969
16. Lucien M: Les chefs accessoires du muscle court extenseur des orteils chez l'homme. Bibl Anat 14:148, 1909
17. Ruge G: Entwicklungsvorgänge an der Musculatur des Menschlichen Fusses. Morphol Jahrbuch 4:117, 1875
18. Picou R: Insertions inférieures du péronier lateral. Bull Soc Anat Paris 8, No. 7:254–259, 1894
19. Picou R: Quelques considérations sur les insertions du muscle long péronier lateral à la plante du pied. Rev Orthop, pp 216–220, 1894
20. Picou R: Insertions inférieures du muscle long peronier lateral: Anomalie de ce muscle. Bull Soc Anat Paris 8, No. 7:160–164, 1894
21. Hecker P: Etude sur le péronier du tarse: Variations des péroniers latéraux, Arch Anat Histol Embryol 3:327, 1924
22. Lewis OJ: The tibialis posterior tendon in the primate foot. J Anat 98, No. 2:209, 1964
23. Martin BF: Observations on the muscles and tendons of the medial aspect of the sole of the foot. J Anat 98, No. 3:437, 1964
24. Turner: On variability in human structure with illustrations from the flexor muscles of the fingers and toes. Trans R Soc Edinburgh 24, 1865
25. Macalister A: Additional observations on muscular anomalies in human anatomy. Trans Roy Irish Acad 25:125, 1872
26. Curnow: Notes of some irregularities on muscles and nerves. J Anat Physiol 7:304, 1873
27. Hartmann H: Anomalie du fléchisseur propre du gros orteil (muscle peroneo-calcanéen interne). Bull Soc Anat Paris 2:1044, 1888
28. Auvray M: Anomalies musculaires et nerveuses. Bull Soc Anat Paris 10:223, 1896
29. Perkins JD Jr: An anomalous muscle of the leg: Peroneo-calcaneus internus. Anat Rec 8:21, 1914
30. Testut L: Les Anomalies Musculaires Considérées du Point de Vue de la Ligature des Artères, pp 38–40. Paris, Doin, 1892
31. Nathan H, Gloobe H, Yosipovitch Z: Flexor digitorum accessorius longus. Clin Orthop Rel Res 113:158, 1975
32. Driver JR, Denison AB: The morphology of the long accessorius muscle. Anat Rec 8:341, 1914
33. Lewis OJ: The comparative morphology of m. flexor accessorius and the associated long flexor tendons. J Anat 96, No. 3:321, 1962
34. Nathan H, Gloobe H: Flexor digitorum brevis: Anatomical variations. Anat Anz 135:295, 1974
35. Morestin H: Anomalie de l'accessoire du long fléchisseur commun des orteils. Bull Soc Anat Paris 11:46, 1895
36. Baumann J: La région de passage de la loge posterieure de la jambe a la plante du pied. Ann Anat Pathol Anat Normal Medico-Chirurg 7, No. 2:201, 1930
37. Poirier P, Charpy A: Traité d'Anatomie Humaine, 2nd ed, Vol 2, pp 279, 284. Paris, Masson et Cie, 1901
38. Loth E: Etude anthropologique de l'aponevrose plantaire. Bull Mem Soc Anthropol Paris 4:606, 1913
39. Leboucq H: Les muscles adducteurs du pouce et du gros orteil. Bull Acad R Med Belg 7, No. 1:26, 1893
40. Jones FW: Structure and Function as Seen in the Foot, 2nd ed, pp 134–135, 176–177, 181. London, Baillière, 1949
41. Harbeson AE: The origin of the first dorsal interosseous muscle of the foot. J Anat 68:116, 1934
42. Manter JT: Variations of the interosseous muscles of the human foot. Anat Rec 93:117, 1945
43. Meyer P: Contributions a l'étude de la region metatarso-phalangienne. Bull Assoc Anat 99:500, 1958
44. Schmidt VR, Reissig D, Heinrichs HJ: Die Mm. lumbricales am Fuss des Menschen. Anat Anz 113:450, 1963
45. Cummins JE, Anson JB, Carr WB, Wright RR, Hauser DWE: The structure of the calcaneal tendon (of Achilles) in relation to orthopedic surgery with additional observations on the plantaris muscle. Surg Gynecol Obstet 83:107, 1946
46. Testut L: Traité d'Anatomie Humaine, Vol I, p 992. Paris, Doin, 1921

6

Tendon Sheaths and Bursae

Synovial Tendon Sheaths

The tendons of the leg at the level of the ankle and the plantar aspect of the foot engage in fibrous, fibro-osseous tunnels acting as pulleys or as retention systems. Within these tunnels the tendons are surrounded by synovial sheaths to facilitate their gliding.

Structurally, a synovial tendon sheath has a parietal layer lining the deep surface of the fibrous or fibro-osseous canal, a visceral layer covering the tendon, and a mesotenon connecting the latter to the parietal lining. The synovial sheath forms a cavity closed at both ends, and proximally, synovial folds permit the play of the tendon through the sheath.

TIBIALIS ANTERIOR

The synovial tendon sheath of the tibialis anterior (Figs. 6-1 and 6-2) extends from above the proximal arm of the inferior extensor retinaculum to the level of the talonavicular interline. Hartman mentions that the synovial sac extends 5.75 cm proximal to a line joining the center of the malleoli.[1] The length of this synovial sheath is given as 6 cm to 8 cm or 8 cm to 10 cm.[2, 3] Hartman reports that the distal end of the synovial sac reaches the talonavicular joint in 60%, is shorter in 22%, and is longer in 18%.[1] There is a complete mesotenon to the tibialis anterior tendon throughout the length of the sheath, located on the deep surface of the tendon.

EXTENSOR HALLUCIS LONGUS

The synovial tendon sheath of the extensor hallucis longus (Figs. 6-1 and 6-2) starts lower than the synovial sac of the tibialis anterior tendon but extends more distally. It originates slightly above the upper arm of the inferior extensor retinaculum, at 1.75 cm proximal to the intermalleolar interline, just above the talotibial articular interline.[1, 4] The lower limit of this synovial sac is more difficult to delineate;

it usually reaches the level of the first cuneometatarsal joint. Less frequently, this distal end of the synovial sheath extends distal to the cuneometatarsal joint interline and advances more or less on the dorsum of the first metatarsal bone.[2] Hartman mentions that the synovial sac terminates at the level of the $cuneo_1$-$metatarsal_1$ joint in 34%, proximal to it in 34%, and distal to it in 32% and that it may reach the lower third of the first metatarsal in 24%.

EXTENSOR DIGITORUM LONGUS

The synovial tendon sheath of the extensor digitorum longus (Figs. 6-1 and 6-2) is a large but short synovial sac that enlarges as it extends distally and also covers the tendon of the peroneus tertius. It starts 2 cm to 3 cm above the ankle joint, about 1 cm above the upper limit of the extensor hallucis longus tendon sheath.[3] The synovial sac passes under the undivided segment of the inferior extensor retinaculum, enlarges to cover the diverging tendons, and ends at the level of the cuneonavicular joint in a large blind sac that is subdivided into small saclike projections, 0.5 cm in length, located on the superficial aspect of the tendons.[3] There is no prolongation over the tendon of the peroneus tertius.

EXTENSOR DIGITORUM BREVIS

Lovell and Tanner describe synovial sheaths to the tendons of the extensor digitorum brevis (see Fig. 6-1) when the tendons are well developed.[3] The synovial sheath of the extensor digitorum brevis to the big toe is the longest, measuring 5.5 cm; it originates under the fascial band extending from metatarsal 1 to 2 and terminates at the proximal end of the proximal phalanx.

The synovial sheaths of toes 2, 3, and 4 are 3 cm to 4 cm in length; they start from close to where the tendons originate, pass under the digital extensor aponeurosis, and terminate at the level of the proximal phalanges.[3]

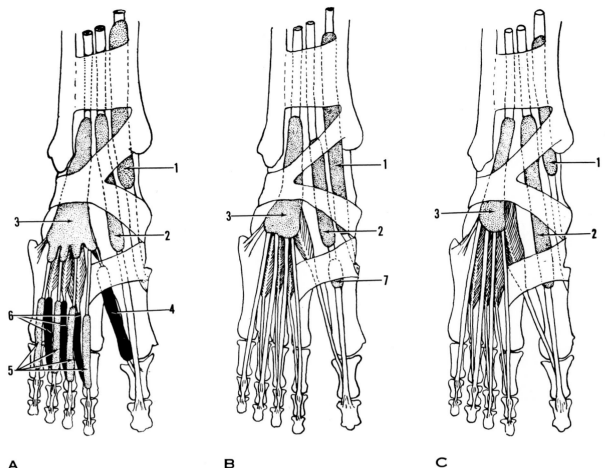

Fig. 6-1. Extensor tendon sheaths. (*A*) According to Lovell and Tanner.[3] (*B*) According to most French anatomists. (*C*) According to most German anatomists. (1, Tendon sheath of tibialis anterior; 2, tendon sheath of extensor hallucis longus; 3, tendon sheath of extensor digitorum longus; 4, tendon sheath of extensor hallucis brevis; 5, tendon sheath of extensor digitorum longus, digital portion; 6, tendon sheath of extensor digitorum brevis; 7, distal segment of extensor hallucis longus tendon sheath.) (After Jones FW: Structure and Function as Seen in the Foot, 2nd ed, pp 229–245. London, Baillière, Tindall & Cox, 1949)

PERONEUS LONGUS AND PERONEUS BREVIS

The synovial sheath of the peroneus longus and peroneus brevis is complex (Figs. 6-3 and 6-4). It is common to both tendons behind the lateral malleolus, and bifurcates for a short distance above and for a longer distance below the malleolus. The common synovial sheath extends 2.5 cm to 3.5 cm above the tip of the lateral malleolus.[3] The proximal bifurcation extends 2.5 cm on the peroneus longus and 1.5 cm on the peroneus brevis.[3] Inferiorly, the synovial sac bifurcates at the level of the peroneal tubercle of the calcaneus, which separates the two tendons. The bifurcation extension of the peroneus brevis is located above the tubercle and extends up to within 2 cm of the insertion of the tendon on the base of the fifth metatarsal or to the level of the calcaneocuboid joint.

The synovial sac of the peroneus longus terminates in the region of the groove of the cuboid. On the superficial surface of the tendon, the sac extends for about 1 cm distal to the peroneal tubercle, whereas on the osseous surface, it extends into the groove of the cuboid entering the planta pedis.[3]

In the sole of the foot the peroneus longus tendon receives a second synovial sheath, which extends from the groove of the cuboid to the insertion of the tendon on the base of the first metatarsal. At the level of the cuboid, this synovial sac extends laterally less on the superficial surface of the tendon and more on the deep surface; this brings the two sacs close to one another on the osseous surface of the tendon. At this level the two synovial sacs of the peroneus longus tendon are separated only by a thin, cellular, transparent lamella, or they may even communicate (about one third of the cases).[2]

According to Brostrom and Prins and based on their arthrographic assessment of injured ankles in healthy individuals, there is no communication between the synovial sheath of the peronei and the synovial cavity of the ankle joint.[5, 6] The data provided by investigators is as follows: *post mortem*—in 18 ankles, 0 communications; in 40 ankles, 0 communications; *in vivo*—in 45 ankles, 0 communications; in 68 ankles, 0 communications; in 17 ankles, 14% had communications; in 95 ankles, 26% had communications.[5-10]

TIBIALIS POSTERIOR

The synovial sheath of the *tibialis posterior* tendon (Fig. 6-5; see Fig. 6-7) is 7 cm to 9 cm in length and starts 6 cm proximal to the tip of the medial malleolus. It descends along the tendon in the retromalleolar groove and terminates close to the tuberosity of the navicular, extending more on the osseous surface and less on the superficial surface. The tibialis posterior tendon has no mesotenon.

The synovial sheath sometimes communicates with that of the flexor digitorum longus or with the synovial cavity of the ankle joint (in 5.8%).[3, 6]

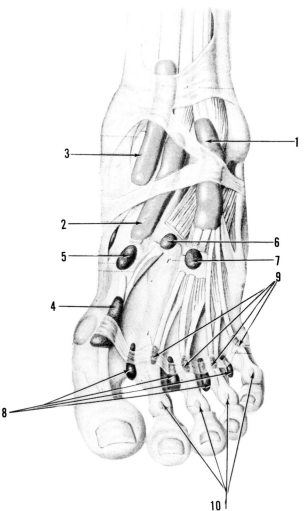

Fig. 6-2. Tendon sheaths and bursae of the dorsum of the foot. (1, Tendon sheath of extensor digitorum longus and peroneus tertius; 2, tendon sheath of extensor hallucis longus; 3, tendon sheath of tibialis anterior; 4, distal synovial space of extensor hallucis longus [may be tendon sheath or bursa]; 5, bursa between metatarso$_1$-cuneiform$_1$ joint and extensor hallucis longus tendon; 6, 7, bursae between tarsometatarsal joint and extensor digitorum brevis, extensor hallucis brevis; 8, intermetatarsophalangeal bursae seen in upper and anterior parts; 9, bursae between extensor digitorum longus tendons and dorsal extensor aponeurosis at level of metatarsophalangeal joint; 10, subcutaneous bursae over proximal interphalangeal joints.) (From Hartman H: Die Sehnenscheiden und Synovialsäcke des Fusses. Morphol Arbeit 5:214, 1896)

Fig. 6-3. Tendon sheaths and bursae of the lateral aspect of the ankle and foot. The combined tendon sheath of the peronei tendons splits into two: peroneus longus and peroneus brevis above and peroneus longus and peroneus brevis below. (1, Peroneus longus above; 2, peroneus brevis above; 3, peronei tendons; 4, peroneus longus below; 5, peroneus brevis below; 6, tendon sheath of extensor digitorum longus and peroneus tertius; 7, bursa between peroneus longus tendon and abductor digiti quinti; 8, bursa between metatarsal 5 and abductor digiti quinti; 9, pre-Achilles bursa; 10, lateral malleolar subcutaneous bursa.) (From Hartman H: Die Sehnenscheiden und Synovialsäcke des Fusses. Morphol Arbeit 5:214, 1896)

Behind the lateral malleolus the common synovial sheath of the peronei tendons is in close contact with the synovium of the ankle joint above and below the posterior talofibular ligament. The peronei tendon sheath and the calcaneofibular ligament cross each other in an X and are in intimate contact. The possible communication of the common synovial sheath of the peronei with the ankle joint is of importance in the arthrographic assessment of ligamentous injuries of the ankle joint.

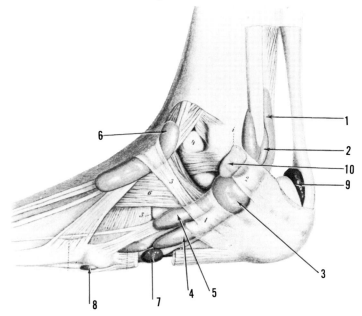

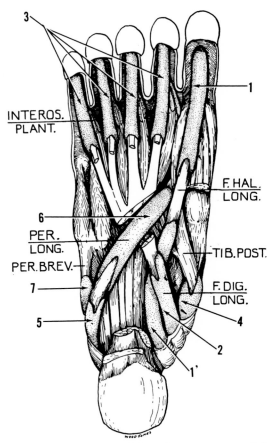

Fig. 6-4.   Tendon sheaths of the plantar aspect of the foot. (1, Distal tendon sheath of flexor hallucis longus; 1′, proximal tendon sheath of flexor hallucis longus; 2, proximal tendon sheath of flexor digitorum longus; 3, distal digital tendon sheath of flexor digitorum longus; 4, tendon sheath of tibialis posterior; 5, proximal tendon sheath of peroneus longus; 6, distal tendon sheath of peroneus longus; 7, tendon sheath of peroneus brevis.) (From Jones FW: Structure and Function as Seen in the Foot, 2nd ed, pp 229–245. London, Baillière, Tindall, & Cox, 1949)

FLEXOR DIGITORUM LONGUS

The synovial sheath of the flexor digitorum longus (Figs. 6-5–6-7) has two components, malleolar and digital.

The malleolar synovial sac starts about 5 cm above the tip of the medial malleolus, slightly lower than the sac of the tibialis posterior. The synovial sac accompanies the tendon of the flexor digitorum longus in the calcaneal canal and terminates in the sole of the foot where the flexor digitorum longus tendon crosses that of the flexor hallucis longus. On the superficial aspect of the tendon, the sheath falls 1 cm short of this crossing point, and a mesotenon is present on its entire length.[3] The synovial sheath of the flexor digitorum longus may communicate with those of the tibialis posterior and flexor hallucis longus tendons.

The digital synovial sacs of the lesser toes envelop the tendons of the flexor digitorum longus and the flexor digitorum brevis. These synovial sheaths are independent and lie within the fibrous tunnels extending from the heads of

the metatarsals to the bases of the distal phalanges. A comprehensive study of the vincular system within the tenosynovial tube is provided by Harman, Lovell and Tanner, and Ziegler.[1, 3, 11]

At the level of the proximal third of the proximal phalanx, the tendon of the flexor digitorum brevis is still superficial and it bifurcates. The slips of the divided tendon slide on each side of the long flexor tendon, decussate fibers under the tendon at the level of the middle phalanx, and insert on the sides of the middle third of the middle phalanx. The flexor digitorum longus tendon courses through the bifurcation and inserts on the base of the distal phalanx. The distal segments of the flexor tendons are connected to the parietal layer of the tenosynovial membrane with short triangular mesomembranes, the vincula brevis. The vinculum brevis of each short flexor tendon slip has a free concave proximal border (Fig. 6-8) and has a variable location. Ziegler provides the following data on the location of the proximal border of the triangular vinculum of the flexor digitorum brevis in 300 toes: on the base of the shaft of the proximal phalanx, 52%; more proximal, 18%; distal to the middle of the proximal phalanx, 28.3%; more distal, 1.3%; on the base of the middle phalanx, 0.3%.[11]

The distal triangular vinculum brevis connecting the flexor digitorum longus tendon to the parietal tenosynovial sheath extends from the middle or base of the middle phalanx to the distal phalanx. Proximal to the chiasma ten-

Fig. 6-5.   Tendon sheaths and bursae of the medial aspect of the ankle and foot. (1, Tendon sheath of tibialis posterior; 2, tendon sheath of flexor digitorum longus; 3, tendon sheath of flexor hallucis longus; 4, bursa between abductor hallucis and tibialis posterior tendon; 5, bursa under tibialis anterior tendon near its insertion; 6, subcutaneous medial malleolar bursa.) (From Hartman H: Die Schnenscheiden und Synovialsäcken des Fusses. Morphol Arbeit 5:214, 1896)

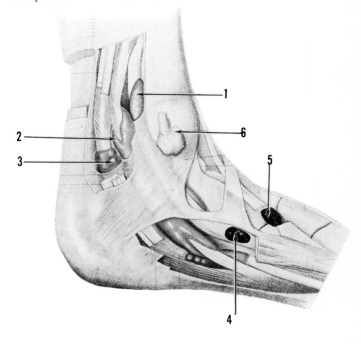

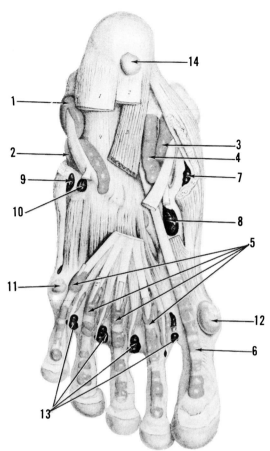

Fig. 6-6. Tendon sheaths and bursae of the sole of the foot. (1, 2, Proximal and distal segment of sheath of peroneus longus; 3, tendon sheath of flexor digitorum longus, proximal segment; 4, tendon sheath of flexor hallucis longus, proximal segment; 5, digital segment of flexor digitorum longus tendon sheath; 6, digital segment of flexor hallucis longus tendon sheath. 7, bursa between abductor hallucis and tibialis posterior; 8, bursa under origin of flexor hallucis brevis; 9, bursa between metatarsal 5 and abductor of fifth toe; 10, bursa under origin of flexor brevis and opponens of fifth toe; 11, subcutaneous bursa under head of metatarsal 5; 12, subcutaneous bursa under head of metatarsal 1; 13, intermetatarsophalangeal bursae; 14, plantar calcaneal subcutaneous bursa.) (From Hartman HO: Die Schnenscheiden und Synovialsäcke des Fusses. Morphol Arbeit 5:214, 1896)

dinum, the flexor digitorum brevis tendinous slips are united by a horizontal synovial membrane that forms with the chiasma a bed for the flexor digitorum longus tendon. A transverse mesosynovial membrane connects the same tendons at the level of the proximal borders of the vincula brevis. This arrangement contributes to the formation of a closed space (Fig. 6-8).

The vinculum longus connecting the above-described tenosynovial floor to the dorsal aspect of the flexor digitorum longus tendon has two parts, proximal and distal. The proximal vinculum longus originates on the midline of the long flexor tendon; it then splits into two sagittal plates, which gradually diverge, forming a tent, and insert along the horizontal tenosynovial membrane connecting the slips

of the flexor digitorum brevis. This insertion is proximal to the chiasma tendinum. The form of this proximal vinculum longus is variable, and Ziegler provides the following data in 300 toes: tent form (Fig. 6-8), 22.7%; one sagittal plate (Fig. 6-9), 16.7%; cordlike (Fig. 6-9), 28%; one filament (Fig. 6-9), 9.6%; multiple filaments (Fig. 6-9), 5.7%; meshlike, very narrow, 4%; absent vinculum longus, 10%; absent vinculum longus and horizontal connecting membrane, 3.3%.[11] The distal vinculum longus extends from the midline of the dorsal surface of the flexor digitorum longus to the level of or distal to the chiasma tendinum. It may be present as a sagittal plate, a filiform structure, or a multifilamentous complex (Fig. 6-9). Accessory vincula may be present in toes 2 to 4.

FLEXOR HALLUCIS LONGUS

The synovial sheath of the flexor hallucis longus (see Figs. 6-4–6-7) has two components, proximal and distal. The proximal synovial sheath extends 1 cm proximal to the ankle joint and accompanies the tendon in the fibro-osseous tunnel of the talus, over the calcaneus, under the sustentaculum tali, and past the crossing of the flexor digitorum longus tendon and ends usually in the region of the cuneonavicular joint on the plantar aspect of the tibialis posterior tendon. This proximal synovial sheath measures 10 cm to

Fig. 6-7. Tendon sheath of the posterior aspect of the lower leg and the ankle. (1, Tendon sheath of peronus longus; 2, tendon sheath of peroneus brevis; 3, tendon sheath of tibialis posterior; 4, tendon sheath of flexor digitorum longus; 5, tendon sheath of flexor hallucis longus.) (From Hartman H: Die Schnenscheiden und Synovialsäcke des Fusses. Morphol Arbeit 5:214, 1896)

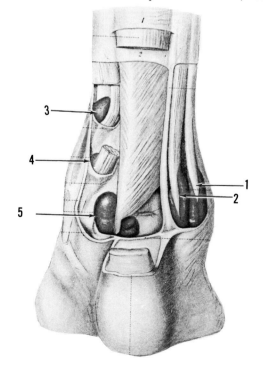

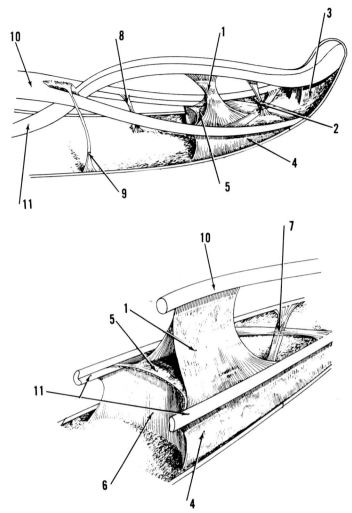

Fig. 6-8. Vincula of the flexor tendons of the lesser toes. (1, Proximal segment of long vinculum of flexor digitorum longus forming a tentlike arrangement; 2, distal segment of long vinculum of flexor digitorum longus; 3, short vinculum of flexor digitorum longus; 4, vinculum of flexor digitorum brevis; 5, horizontal mesomembrane; 6, transverse mesomembrane forming with *4* and *5* a closed space; 7, chiasma tendineum; 8, 9, accessory vincula; 10, flexor digitorum brevis tendon; 11, flexor digitorum longus tendon.) (From Ziegler EM: Zur Morphologie der Vincula Tendinum Menschlichen Zehen Erwachsener. Anat Arz Bd 130:404, 1972)

12 cm in length, has no mesotenon, and may communicate with the sheath of the flexor hallucis longus (in 20%) and the sheath of the tibialis posterior tendon.[2, 3, 12] A communication may exist normally between the posterior aspect of the ankle joint and the synovial sheaths of the long flexor tendons and the tibialis posterior tendon; according to Prins, the posterior aspect of the ankle joint communicates with the sheath of the flexor hallucis longus in 13%, with the sheath of the flexor digitorum longus in 7%, and with the sheath of the tibialis posterior in 6%.[6]

The distal or digital segment of the flexor hallucis longus sheath is longer than the sheath of the lesser toes and extends from near the base of the first metatarsal to the insertion of the tendon on the base of the distal phalanx. Commu-

nication between the proximal and the distal digital sheath is exceedingly rare; one case has been described by Chemin.[3, 13]

In 34% of the big toes, the proximal vinculum is in the form of two quadrangular simple mesomembranes extending from the shaft of the proximal phalanx to the dorsal surface of the flexor hallucis tendon.[11] The proximal border of this mesomembrane reaches the level of the base of the proximal phalanx in 8% and the level of the head of the proximal phalanx or the interphalangeal joint in 25%.[11] In 42%, a triangular mesomembrane extends from the parietal tendon sheath to the dorsal surface of the flexor hallucis longus tendon, up to its insertion.[11] The distal vinculum of the flexor hallucis longus tendon is a very weak structure but regularly present; an accessory vinculum to the same tendon is rarely present.

Synovial Bursae

The synovial bursae are flat pouches present where there is excess pressure of friction (see Figs. 6-2, 6-3, 6-6, and 6-10). They are subject to considerable variation in both location and size.

SUBCUTANEOUS

Subcutaneous bursae are found over the medial and the lateral malleoli of the ankle joint, the former being the larger. Subcutaneous retro-Achilles tendon bursae may be present, one or three in number, forming a superior, a middle, and a lower bursa.[14] A subcalcaneal bursa may be present between the tuberosity of the os calcis and the subcutaneous fat pad; this bursa occurs in 50% of the cases.[1] Subcutaneous bursae may be found over the dorsomedial aspect of the head of the first metatarsal and the dorsolateral aspect of the fifth metatarsal head. Plantar subcutaneous bursae may be located over the head of the first and fifth metatarsals.[1] Frequently, subcutaneous bursae are seen over the dorsum of the proximal interphalangeal joints.[1, 15]

SUBFASCIAL

Subfascial synovial bursae may be classified as follows:

Group I: Bursae located between the origin or insertion of a tendon and the bone
Group II: Bursae located
Under the tendon or the muscle crossing a bony prominence
Between tendons and ligaments
Between tendons and muscles gliding over each other or running close to each other[1]

Group I

The bursae of this group are comprised of the following:

Pre-Achilles tendon, retrocalcaneal bursa
Bursae corresponding to the insertion of the tibialis anterior tendon

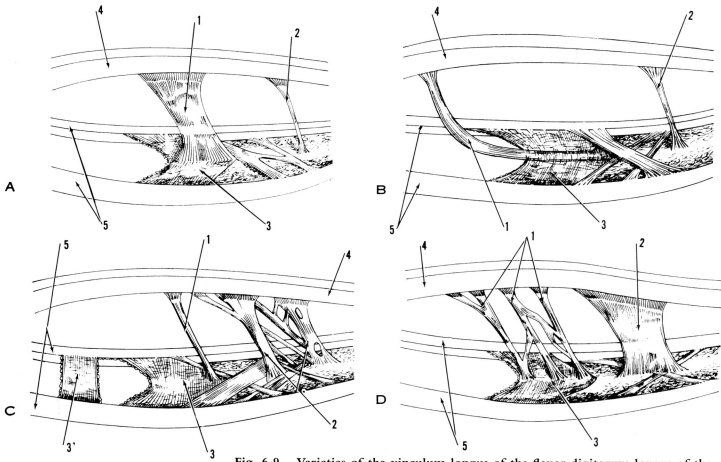

Fig. 6-9.   Varieties of the vinculum longus of the flexor digitorum longus of the lesser toe. (*Type A*) *1* is in sagittal plate configuration; *2* is filiform. (*Type B*) *1* is cordlike; *2* is filiform. (*Type C*) *1* is filiform; *2* is meshlike. (*Type D*) *1* is meshlike; *2* is in sagittal plate configuration. (1, Proximal segment of vinculum longus of flexor digitorum longus; 2, distal segment of vinculum longus of flexor digitorum longus; 3, horizontal mesomembrane; 3', proximal horizontal membrane; 4, flexor digitorum longus tendon; 5, flexor digitorum brevis tendon.) (From Ziegler EM: Zur Morphologie der Vincula Tendinum Menschlichen Zehen Erwachsener. Anat Arz Bd 130:404, 1972)

Bursae corresponding to the insertion of the tibialis posterior tendon

Bursae located between the tendons of the interossei and the metatarsophalangeal joint

Bursa located between the common origin of the tendons of the short flexor and opponens of the fifth toe and the base of the fifth metatarsal

Bursa located between the flexor hallucis brevis and the first cuneiform

The retrocalcaneal tendon bursa is a large, constant bursa situated between the smooth upper part of the posterior end of the calcaneus and the deep surface of the Achilles tendon. The bursa is in the form of a triangle, with the apex inferior and the base superior. The upper border carries synovial fringes and extends 8 mm to 10 mm above the os calcis.[14]

The bursae in association with the terminal portion of the tibialis anterior tendon are often three in number.[12] A bursa is present between the tendon and the cuneo$_1$-metatarsal$_1$ joint. A second bursa is located between the tendon and the first cuneiform bone. The third bursa is superficial, located between the tendon and the overlying extensor retinaculum.

The bursa corresponding to the insertion of the tibialis posterior tendon is found between the plantar component of the tibialis posterior tendon and the second cuneiform. This bursa is 2 cm long and may communicate with the second cuneometatarsal joint.[1]

The bursae of the interossei are located between the tendons of the interossei and the collateral ligaments of the metatarsophalangeal joints. Hartman provides the following data in regard to their occurrence in 38 feet: toe 2—dorsal interosseous 1, 4%; dorsal interosseous 2, 2%; toe 3—plantar interosseous 1, 38%; dorsal interosseous 3, 7%; toe 4—plantar interosseous 2, 55%; dorsal interosseous 4, 9%; toe 5—plantar interosseous 3, 16%.[1]

A pea-sized bursa may be present between the common origin of the tendons of the short flexor and opponens of

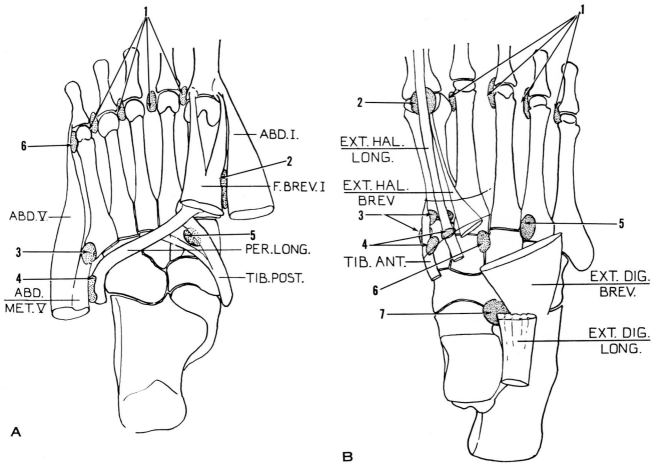

Fig. 6-10. Bursae. (*A*) Plantar aspect of the foot. (1, Intermetatarsophalangeal bursae; 2, bursa between flexor hallucis brevis and abductor hallucis; 3, bursa between abductor of fifth toe and base of metatarsal 5; 4, bursa between abductor of fifth toe and peroneus longus tendon; 5, bursa between tibialis posterior tendon and first cuneiform 6, bursa between abductor of fifth toe and fifth metatarsal head.) (*B*) Dorsal aspect of the foot. (1, Lumbrical bursae; 2, bursa under extensor hallucis longus tendon at metatarsophalangeal joint level; 3, bursae under tibialis anterior tendon near its insertions; 4, bursae superficial to tibialis anterior and extensor hallucis longus tendons; 5, 6, bursae under extensor digitorum brevis and extensor hallucis brevis; 7, bursa of sinus tarsi of "bursae mucosa Grüberi" inserting between deep surface of extensor digitorum longus and neck of talus.) (From Jones FW: Structure and Function as Seen in the Foot, 2nd ed, pp 229–245. London, Baillière, Tindall, & Cox, 1949)

the fifth toe and the base of the fifth metatarsal.[1] A bursa may be also seen between the tendon of the flexor hallucis brevis near its origin and the first cuneiform.

Group II

Under Tendon or Muscle Crossing Bony Prominence. The bursa of the sinus tarsi is located between the neck of the talus dorsolaterally and the inferior extensor retinaculum. This bursa is present in 56% of the cases and may extend anteriorly to the talonavicular joint and posteriorly to the ankle joint.[1] It may communicate with these joints or with the sheath of the extensor digitorum longus.[1]

The bursae of the extensor digitorum brevis are usually two in number. One bursa is located between the extensor hallucis brevis and the $cuneo_2$-$metatarsal_2$ base. The second bursa is situated more laterally under the extensor digitorum brevis to the lesser toes.

The bursa of the extensor hallucis longus is found between the tendon and the $cuneo_1$-$metatarsal_1$ joint. This bursa does not communicate with the joint but frequently opens, with a superficial bursa present on the dorsal aspect of the tendon at that level. Occasionally the bursa may communicate with the sheath of the extensor hallucis longus, which then seems to extend up to the base of the first metatarsal.

A bursa is also found between the abductor of the fifth toe and the tuberosity of the fifth metatarsal.

Between Tendons and Aponeurosis. Bursae are described as being present between the long extensor tendons of the toes and the dorsal aponeurosis of the toes at the level of the metatarsophalangeal joints. When well developed, these could be considered as the distal sheaths of the long extensor tendons of the lesser toes. The bursa of the big toe is the largest and covers over one third of the first metatarsal; at times it is difficult to differentiate this bursa from a vaginal sheath.[1]

Between Close Tendons and Muscles. A bursa is present between the tendon of the peroneus longus and the abductor digiti minimi where the former turns into the sole of the foot in the groove on the cuboid. Another bursa may be seen between the tibialis posterior tendon and the abductor hallucis at the level of the navicular and the first cuneiform.

INTERMETATARSOPHALANGEAL

Intermetatarsophalangeal bursae are located in the narrow intermetatarsal head space between the tendons of the corresponding interossei. They cover the dorsal aspect, the distal border, and partially the plantar aspect of the deep transverse metatarsal ligament. Bursae 1 to 3 are constant, whereas bursa 4 is missing in 80%.[1] Communication between the joint and the adjacent bursa may occur.

REFERENCES

1. Hartman H: Die Sehnenscheiden und Synovialsäcke des Fusses. Morphol Arbeit 5:214, 1896
2. Poirier P, Charpy A: Traité d'Anatomie Humaine, Vol II, pp 302–305. Paris, Masson, 1901
3. Lovell AGH, Tanner HH: Synovial membranes with special reference to those related to the tendons of the foot and ankle. J Anat 42:414, 1908
4. Testut L: Traité d'Anatomie Humaine, 7th ed, Vol II, pp 1006–1007. Paris, Doin, 1921
5. Brostrom L: Sprained ankles: II. Arthrographic diagnosis of recent ligament ruptures. Acta Chir Scand 129:485, 1965
6. Prins JG: Diagnosis and treatment of injury to the lateral ligament of the ankle: A comparative clinical study. Acta Chir Scand [Suppl] 486:81, 1978
7. Arner O, Ekengren K, Hulting et al: Arthrography of the talo-crural joint: Anatomic, roentgenographic and clinical aspects. Acta Chir Scand 113:253, 1957
8. Mehrez M, Elgeneidy S: Arthrography of the ankle. J Bone Joint Surg [Br] 52:309, 1970
9. Gordon RB: Arthrography of the ankle joint: Experience in one hundred seven studies. J Bone Joint Surg [Am] 52:1623, 1970
10. Pascoet G: L'arthrografie tibio-tarsienne dans la traumatologie capsuloligamentaire du coup de pied. Rev Chir Orthop [Suppl] 2:142, 1975
11. Ziegler EM: Zur Morphologie der Vincula Tendinum an Menschlichen Zehen Erwachsener. Anat Anz Bd 130:404, 1972
12. Jones FW: Structure and Function as Seen in the Foot, 2nd ed, pp 229–245. London, Baillière, Tindall & Cox, 1949
13. Chemin: Recherches sur les gaines synoviales tendineuses du pied. Soc Biol Comptes Rendus 3:237, 1896
14. Testut L, Jacob O: Traité d'Anatomie Topographique avec Applications Médico-Chirurgicales, Vol II, pp 1032–1033, 1036. Paris, Doin, 1909
15. Schreger: De Bursis Mucosis Subcutaneis. Erlangen, 1825

Angiology

Arteries

The arterial blood supply to the ankle and the foot (Fig. 7-1) is provided by three arteries: posterior tibial, anterior tibial, and peroneal.

The tibial arteries are the major suppliers of the foot, but the peroneal artery may predominate when the anterior and posterior tibial arteries are atrophic or absent in their distal segments. As described by Dubreuil-Chambardel, the anterior branch of the peroneal artery or perforating branch may supply the dorsalis pedis artery, or the posterior branch of the peroneal artery may be the only supplier of the plantar arteries.[1] When the terminal segments of the posterior and anterior tibial arteries are absent simultaneously, the peroneal artery with its anterior and posterior branch is the sole supplier of the dorsal and plantar arterial network (Fig. 7-2).

The posterior tibial artery may be greatly attenuated or absent (Table 7-1). Adachi reports the absence of the posterior tibial artery as being nearly 2% (ten cases in 486 feet).[2] Dubreuil-Chambardel has never encountered a complete absence of the posterior tibial artery.[1]

The anterior tibial artery may be a very thin vessel distally or may terminate in the mid leg, thus leaving the entire supply of the dorsum of the foot to the perforating branch of the peroneal artery. Such a variation occurs with the frequency shown in Table 7-2.

The peroneal artery is diminished in volume with the frequency shown in Table 7-3. Dubreuil-Chambardel has never seen this artery completely absent.[1] Edwards mentions "that either of its two terminal branches—the perforating or the posterior lateral malleolar—may be missing."[8]

DORSAL ARTERIAL NETWORK OF THE FOOT AND ANKLE

The dorsal arterial network of the foot is extremely variable, but these variations can be superimposed almost constantly on a general pattern termed as a "very constant pattern," a "potential arterial pattern," or a "grundform."[1, 2, 5, 8] As mentioned by Huber, "any part of that network might be encountered as a vessel of significant size."[5]

General Pattern

The general pattern of this network is shown in Figure 7-3.[5] At the ankle joint interline, the anterior tibial artery is continued by the dorsalis pedis artery, which extends along an axis drawn from the middle of the transverse bimalleolar axis to the tip of the first intermetatarsal space. The dorsalis pedis artery gives origin at the level of the ankle to the anterior malleolar arteries, medial and lateral. During its pedal course the dorsalis pedis artery provides the following branches from its lateral side: artery to the sinus tarsi, lateral tarsal artery, artery to the proximal segment of the second intermetatarsal space, arcuate artery, and artery to the first intermetatarsal space.

The artery of the sinus tarsi may arise directly from the dorsalis pedis artery at the level of the talar neck. Directed transversely, it enters the sinus tarsi.

The lateral tarsal artery also originates at the level of the talar neck; it courses obliquely laterally and distally to the dorsum of the cuboid, and divides into three longitudinal branches reaching the proximal segments of intermetatarsal spaces 2, 3, and 4.

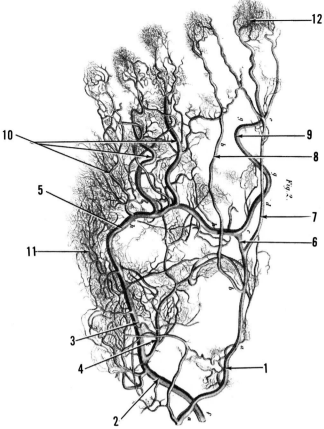

Fig. 7-1.   Arterial tree of the foot, corrosion study. (1, Dorsalis pedis artery; 2, posterior tibial artery; 3, lateral plantar artery; 4, medial plantar artery; 5, plantar arc, deep; 6, first proximal perforating artery; 7, first dorsal interosseous artery; 8, second dorsal interosseous artery; 9, first plantar interosseous artery; 10, plantar metatarsal arteries; 11, dense arterial network of lateral border of foot; 12, anastomotic network at level of pulp of big toe.) (From Hyrtl J: Die Corrosions—Anatomie und Ihre Ergebnisse, p 249. Wien, Braumüller, 1873)

TABLE 7-1   Frequency of Absent or Very Thin Posterior Tibial Artery

Author	Number of feet	Frequency (%)	
Adachi[2]	486	4.9±	0.98
Quain[3]	211		
Manno[4]	66	380	
Dubreuil-Chambardel[1]	103	8.4±	1.42
Total	866	6.35	

TABLE 7-2   Frequency of Absent or Very Thin Anterior Tibial Artery

Author	Number of Feet	Frequency (%)
Dubreuil-Chambardel[1]	165	2.4
Adachi[2]	1239	7.1
Huber[5]	200	3
Salvi[6]	200	3
Schwalbe and Pfitzner[7]	213	3.8
Quain[3]	199	5.5
Total	2216	5.27

TABLE 7-3   Frequency of Very Thin Peroneal Artery

Author	Number of feet	Frequency (%)
Quain[3]	208	2.8
Dubreuil-Chambardel[1]	103	3.8

The artery to the proximal segment of the second intermetatarsal space takes off at the level of the middle cuneiform. It crosses the base of the second metatarsal and reaches the second intermetatarsal space. This longitudinal branch is connected to the first division branch of the lateral tarsal artery with a transverse branch on the dorsum of the lateral cuneiform.

The arcuate artery originates at the level of the first tarsometatarsal joint and transversely crosses the bases of the second, third, and fourth metatarsals. The arterial arcade is joined by the previously described longitudinal branches of the lateral tarsal artery. The arcuate artery gives origin to the proximal perforating arteries in intermetatarsal spaces 2, 3, and 4 and to the second, third, and fourth dorsal metatarsal arteries. The latter give a set of perforating branches proximal to the corresponding metatarsal heads, and farther distally in the web space, they divide into the dorsal digital arteries. They give a perforating branch in the axis of the web space and a dorsoplantar anastomotic branch on the side of the corresponding proximal phalanx.

The first intermetatarsal artery or the first dorsal metatarsal artery continues the direction of the dorsalis pedis artery. At the base of the first intermetatarsal space, it plunges plantarward and forms the first proximal perforating artery. The first dorsal metatarsal artery provides two lateral branches to the first metatarsal and one anastomotic branch to the medial aspect of the second metatarsal neck. Farther distally, at the level of the web space, the artery divides into the dorsal digital artery of the big toe—providing both its dorsolateral and dorsomedial branches—and the dorsomedial artery of the second toe. The first dorsal metatarsal artery finally gives the first distal perforating artery. From its medial side, the dorsalis pedis artery provides two medial tarsal arteries taking off at the level of the navicular and the first cuneiform.

The perforating branch of the peroneal artery crosses the distal segment of the tibiofibular interspace, passes over the anterior aspect of the tibiofibular syndesmosis, contours the anterior border of the lateral malleolus, and establishes communication with the lateral malleolar and lateral tarsal arteries.

The above-described standard pattern of distribution of the branches of the dorsalis pedis artery occurs in 5.5%.[5] Huber, in a study of 200 feet, grouped the possible variations of pattern according to the level of origin of the arcuate

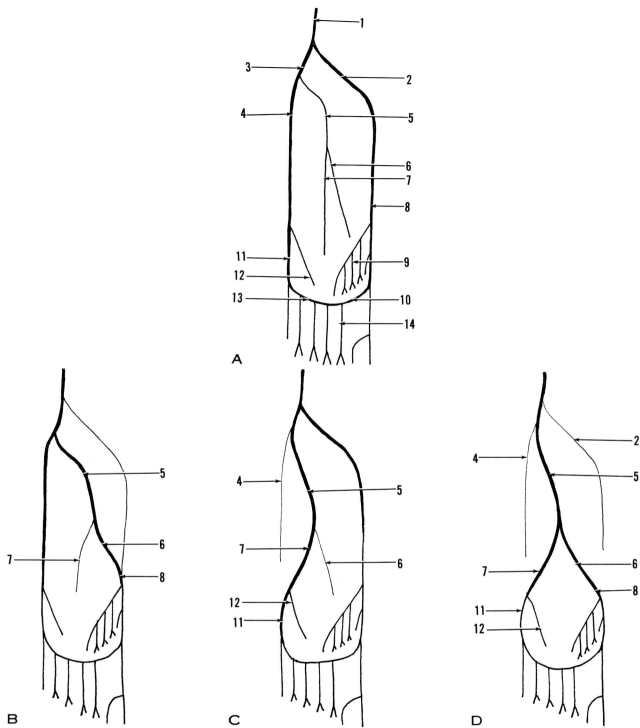

Fig. 7-2.   Variations of the arteries of the leg and foot. (*A*) Habitual pattern. (1, Popliteal artery; 2, anterior tibial artery; 3, tibioperoneal arterial trunk; 4, posterior tibial artery; 5, peroneal artery; 6, anterior peroneal artery; 7, posterior peroneal artery; 8, dorsalis pedis artery; 9, dorsal metatarsal arteries; 10, perforating artery of first interspace; 11, lateral plantar artery; 12, medial plantar artery; 13, deep plantar arterial arc; 14, first plantar metatarsal artery.) (*B*) The dorsalis pedis artery (*8*) is provided by the anterior peroneal artery (*6*). (5, Peroneal artery; 7, posterior peroneal artery.) (*C*) The posterior peroneal artery (*7*) supplies the lateral and medial plantar arteries (*11* and *12*). (4, Posterior tibial artery, incomplete; 5, peroneal artery, well developed; 6, anterior peroneal artery.) (*D*) The peroneal artery (*5*) supplies the dorsalis pedis artery (*8*) through the anterior peroneal artery (*6*) and the plantar arteries (*11* and *12*) through the posterior peroneal artery (*7*). The anterior tibial artery (*2*) and the posterior tibial artery (*4*) are incomplete or absent. (From Dubreuil-Chambardel L: Variations des Artères du Pelvis et du Membre Inferieur, p 246. Paris, Masson et Cie, 1925)

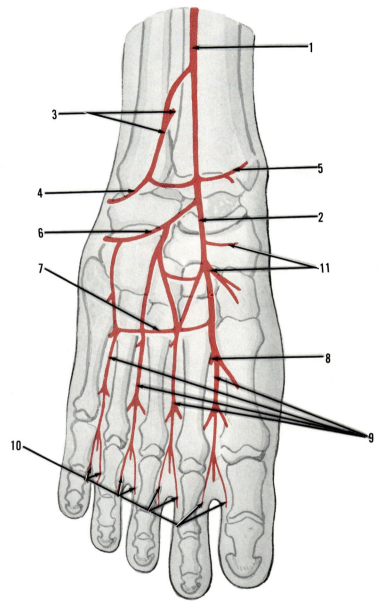

Fig. 7-3.   The arterial network of the dorsum of the foot, general or potential pattern. (1, Anterior tibial artery; 2, dorsalis pedis artery; 3, anterior or perforating peroneal artery; 4, anterior lateral malleolar artery; 5, anterior medial malleolar artery; 6, lateral tarsal artery; 7, arcuate artery; 8, first proximal perforating artery; 9, dorsal metatarsal arteries; 10, dorsal digital arteries; 11, medial tarsal arteries.) (From Huber JF: The arterial network supplying the dorsum of the foot. Anat Rec 80:373, 1941. By permission of Alan R. Liss, Inc., Publisher)

artery and the number of dorsal metatarsal arteries provided by the latter. The individual arrangements are classified into four categories.

> *Group A* (35%; Fig. 7-4): Arcuate artery arising at about the level of the first tarsometatarsal joint and giving rise to the following dorsal metatarsal arteries:
> Group A_1 (16.5%): Dorsal metatarsal arteries 2, 3, 4
> Group A_2 (9%): Dorsal metatarsal arteries 2, 3
> Group A_3 (9.5%): Dorsal metatarsal artery 2
> *Group B* (19%; Fig. 7-4): Arcuate artery arising at about the level of the cuneonavicular joint, with the subgroups similar to those of group A.
> Group B_1 (9%)
> Group B_2 (6.5%)
> Group B_3 (3.5%)
> *Group C* (34%; Fig. 7-5): No arcuate artery present
> *Group D* (12%; Fig. 7-5): Dorsalis pedis artery practically absent

Adachi describes the "grundform" of the rete of the dorsalis pedis (Fig. 7-6) as formed transversely by the proximal lateral tarsal artery, the distal lateral tarsal artery, and the arcuate artery. These transverse or oblique components are anastomosed by three sagittal or longitudinal arteries, forming a complex network. The longitudinal arteries run parallel to the dorsalis pedis artery; they may be very thin, or one or two branches may be missing. These arteries continue as the dorsal metatarsal arteries and give off the proximal or posterior perforating arteries. The distal lateral tarsal artery is usually insignificant in size. When the sagittal arteries are thin, the supply to the dorsal metatarsal arteries is provided by the proximal perforating arteries. When the dorsal metatarsal arteries are thin, the proximal perforating arterial branches are also rudimentary.

Dorsalis Pedis Artery

At the level of the ankle joint interline, the anterior tibial artery is continued by the dorsalis pedis artery, which runs along a line extending from the middle of the transverse malleolar line to the proximal end of the first intermetatarsal space. During its course, the artery passes across the talus, the navicular, the second cuneiform, and the base of the second metatarsal. It penetrates the first intermetatarsal space limited anteriorly by the arch formed by the first dorsal interosseous muscle and posteriorly by the base of the first and second metatarsals. It terminates by inosculation with the lateral plantar artery after making two 90° turns—one vertical and one horizontal–lateral. This standard course of the artery occurs in 73.5%.[5]

35 %

19%

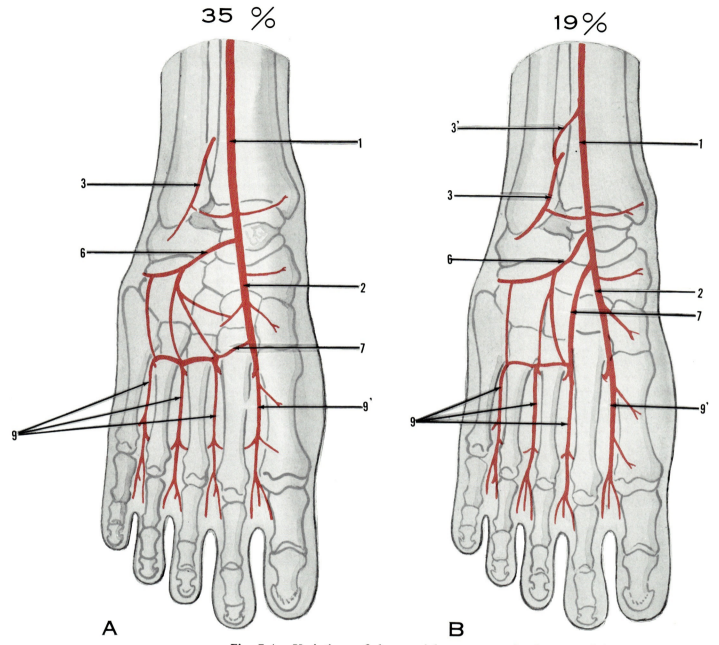

A

B

Fig. 7-4.   Variations of the arterial pattern on the dorsum of the foot. (*Group A*) Arcuate artery (*7*) arising at about the level of the first tarsometatarsal joint and giving rise to the dorsal metatarsal arteries 2, 3, 4 (*9*). (1, Anterior tibial artery; 2, dorsalis pedis artery; 3, anterior peroneal artery; 6, lateral tarsal artery; 9′, first dorsal metatarsal artery.) (*Group B*) Arcuate artery (*7*) arising at about the level of the cuneonavicular joint and providing the dorsal metatarsal arteries 2, 3, 4 (*9*). (1, Anterior tibial artery; 2, dorsalis pedis artery; 3, anterior peroneal artery; 3′, anastomotic branch between anterior tibial artery and anterior peroneal artery; 6, lateral tarsal artery; 9′, first dorsal metatarsal artery.) (From Huber JF: The arterial network supplying the.dorsum of the foot. Anat Rec 80:373, 1941. By permission of Alan R. Liss, Inc., Publisher)

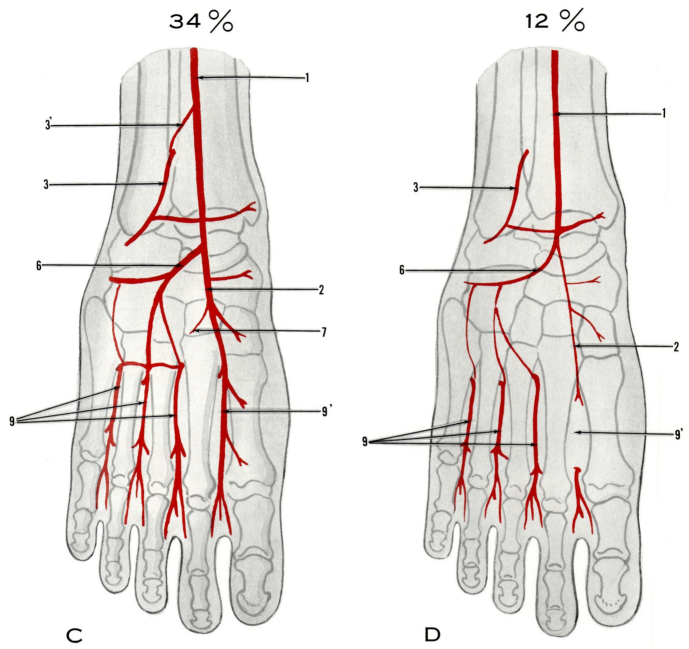

Fig. 7-5.   Variations of the arterial pattern on the dorsum of the foot. (*Group C*) Absent arcuate artery (*7*). (1, Anterior tibial artery; 2, dorsalis pedis artery; 3, anterior peroneal artery; 3′, anastomotic branch between anterior tibial artery and anterior peroneal artery; 6, lateral tarsal artery providing dorsal metatarsal arteries 2, 3, 4 (*9*); 9′, first dorsal metatarsal artery.) (*Group D*) Practically absent dorsalis pedis artery (*2*). (1, Anterior tibial artery; 3, anterior peroneal artery; 6, lateral tarsal artery; 9, dorsal metatarsal arteries 2, 3, 4; 9′, absent first dorsal metatarsal artery.) (From Huber JF: The arterial network supplying the dorsum of the foot. Anat Rec 80:373, 1941. By permission of Alan R. Liss, Inc., Publisher)

Variations. From a study of 200 feet, Huber reports the absence of the dorsalis pedis artery in 12% (Fig. 7-5).[5] Adachi, from a group of 230 feet, reports a very thin dorsalis pedis artery in 3% (Fig. 7-7).[2]

Lateral deviation of the artery occurs in 5.5%.[5] Such cases are also described by Adachi (0.4%) and Dubreuil-Chambardel (1.8%) (Fig. 7-8A).[1, 2]

Medial deviation of the artery occurs in 3.5%.[5]

In about 5% (as mentioned previously), the tibialis anterior artery is absent or filiform in the distal segment and the dorsalis pedis artery is supplied by the perforating branch of the peroneal artery (Fig. 7-9A).

The lower end of the anterior tibial artery is in the position of the perforating peroneal artery in 1.5% (Fig. 7-9B).[5]

The artery arises equally from the anterior tibial and the perforating peroneal artery in 0.5% (Fig. 7-10A).[5]

In very rare instances, the dorsalis pedis artery is formed by a branch of the posterior tibial artery passing around the medial malleolus and reaching the dorsum of the foot. This vessel is anastomosed by a transverse branch on the dorsum of the scaphoid, with the perforating branch of the peroneal

(Text continues on p. 270.)

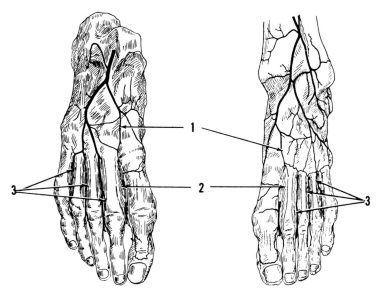

Fig. 7-7.   Very thin dorsalis pedis artery (*1*) and absent first dorsal metatarsal artery (*2*). (3, Dorsal metatarsal arteries 2, 3, 4.) (From Adachi B: Das Arteriensystem der Japaner, pp 246, 248. Kyoto, Maruzen, 1928)

Fig. 7-8.   (*A*) Lateral deviation of the dorsalis pedis artery. (*B*) General pattern of arterial distribution on the dorsum of the foot. (1, Anterior tibial artery; 2, dorsalis pedis artery; 3, first dorsal interosseous artery; 4, arcuate artery; 5, medial tarsal artery; 6, lateral tarsal artery; 7, dorsal metatarsal arteries 2, 3, 4; 8, first proximal perforating artery; 9, anterior peroneal artery; 10, anterior lateral malleolar artery; 11, anterior medial malleolar artery.) (From Adachi B: Das Arteriensystem der Japaner, p 243. Kyoto, Maruzen, 1928)

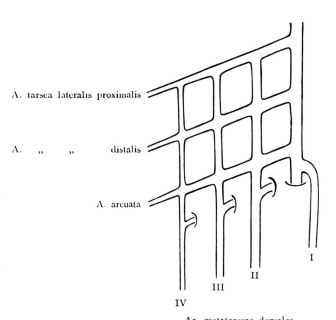

A. tarsea lateralis proximalis

A.   „   „   distalis

A. arcuata

I

II

III

IV

Aa. metatarseae dorsales

Fig. 7-6.   "Grundform" of the rete of the dorsalis pedis artery formed by the transversely oriented proximal, distal, and lateral tarsal arteries and the arcuate arteries connected by longitudinally oriented anastomotic branches and the dorsalis pedis artery. (From Adachi B: Das Arteriensystem der Japaner, p 251. Kyoto, Maruzen, 1928)

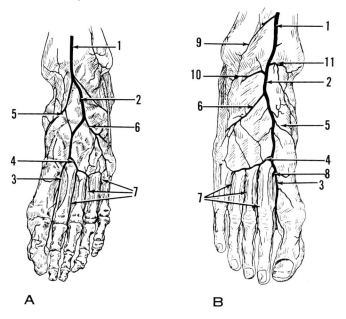

A   B

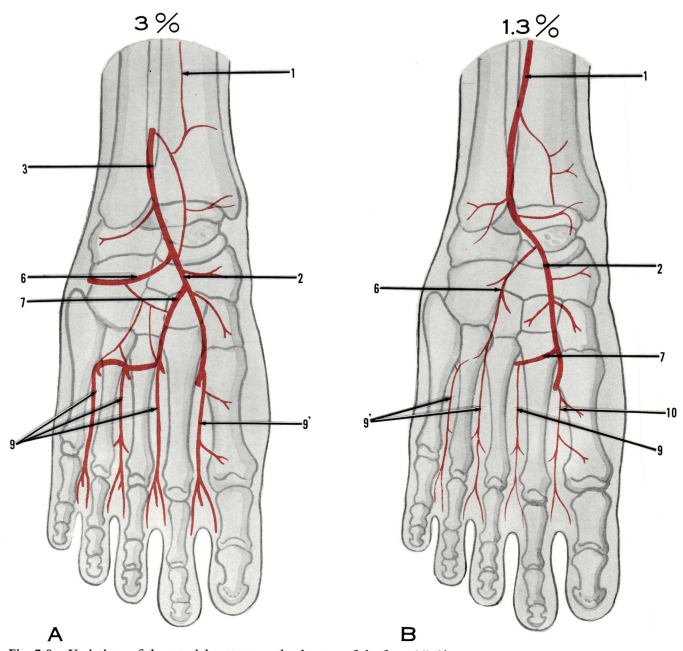

A   **B**

Fig. 7-9.   Variations of the arterial pattern on the dorsum of the foot. (*A*) Absent or filiform anterior tibial artery (*1*). The dorsalis pedis artery (*2*) is supplied by the anterior peroneal artery (*3*). (6, Lateral tarsal artery; 7, arcuate artery supplying the dorsal metatarsal arteries 2, 3, 4 (*9*); *9′*, first dorsal metatarsal artery.) (*B*) The lower end of the anterior tibial artery (*1*) is in the position of the perforating peroneal artery. (2, Dorsalis pedis artery; 6, lateral tarsal artery supplying the dorsal metatarsal arteries 3, 4; 7, arcuate artery supplying second dorsal metatarsal artery (*9*); 10, first dorsal metatarsal artery.) (From Huber JF: The arterial network supplying the dorsum of the foot. Anat Rec 80:373, 1941. By permission of Alan R. Liss, Inc., Publisher)

.5 %

.5 %

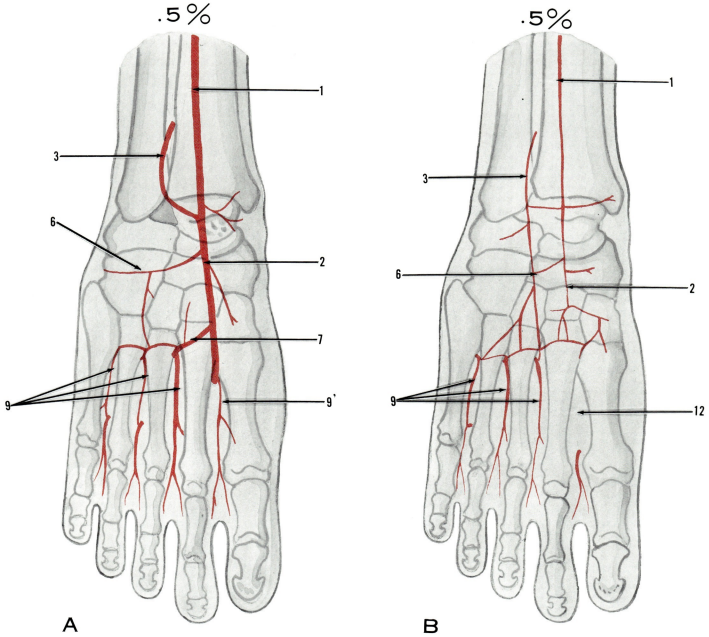

A

B

Fig. 7-10.   Variations of the arterial pattern on the dorsum of the foot. (*A*) The dorsalis pedis artery (*2*) arises equally from the anterior tibial artery (*1*) and the perforating peroneal artery (*3*). (6, Lateral tarsal artery; 7, arcuate artery; 9, dorsal metatarsal arteries 2, 3, 4; 9', first dorsal metatarsal artery.) (*B*) The lateral tarsal artery (*6*) is in continuity with the perforating peroneal artery (*3*). (2, Incomplete dorsalis pedis artery; 9, dorsal metatarsal arteries 2, 3, 4 supplied by *6;* 12, absent first dorsal metatarsal artery.) (From Huber JF: The arterial network supplying the dorsum of the foot. Anat Rec 80:373, 1941)

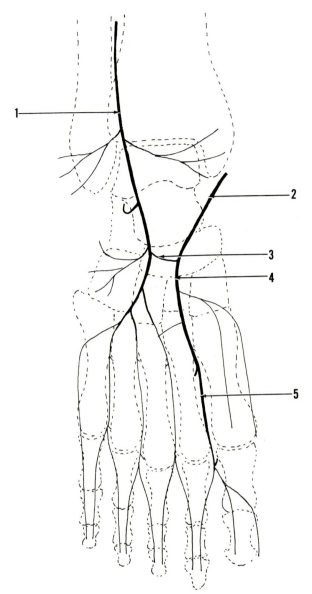

Fig. 7-11.   Dorsalis pedis artery (4) formed by a branch of the posterior tibial artery (2) passing around the medial malleolus and reaching the dorsum of the foot. (1, Anterior peroneal artery; 3, anastomotic branch between 1 and 4; 5, first dorsal metatarsal artery.) (From Dubreuil-Chambardel L: Variations des Artères du Pelvis et du Membre Inferieur, p 225. Paris, Masson et Cie, 1925)

artery supplying, in turn, the second, third, and fourth dorsal metatarsal arteries (Fig. 7-11).[1]

Caliber.   The usual diameter of the dorsalis pedis artery is 2 mm to 3 mm, and in 6% of 50 feet it was very small, not exceeding 1.5 mm.[9] The average diameter of the same artery at the upper limit of the extensor retinaculum is given as 2.79 mm.[10]

The continuation of the dorsalis pedis artery after giving off the lateral tarsal artery is reported by Adachi (230 feet)

as being larger than the latter in 86.5%, equal in 8.3%, and smaller in 5.2%.[2] Huber describes the lateral tarsal artery as being larger in 7% (200 feet).[5]

Lateral Tarsal Arteries

The lateral tarsal arteries are two, rarely three; it is the exception to have more than three.[2] The proximal lateral tarsal artery is the strongest. The second lateral tarsal artery is not significant and may be represented only by a connecting thin artery extending from the proximal lateral tarsal artery to the dorsalis pedis artery (Fig. 7-12).

Proximal.   The proximal lateral tarsal artery originates from the dorsalis pedis at the level of the talar head, 0.5 cm proximal to this level (occasionally), or 0.5 cm distal (rarely).[2] This arterial branch courses obliquely in a lateral and distal direction, crosses the calcaneonavicular junction and the dorsum of the cuboid, reaches the lateral border of the cuboid, passes under the peroneous brevis tendon, and anastomoses with the lateral plantar artery. At the level of the talar head, the proximal lateral tarsal artery provides arterial branches to the talar head and to the lateral anterior aspect of the talar body. In 21.7% to 32%, the artery provides direct origin to the artery of the sinus tarsi or forms with the perforating peroneal artery an arterial loop that gives origin to the artery of the sinus tarsi.[1, 2, 14] The artery forms an arterial anastomotic network in the tarsal sinus with contributions from the anterior lateral malleolar artery and the perforating peroneal artery. It also participates in the formation of the lateral malleolar arterial rete. At the level of the cuboid, the proximal lateral tarsal artery provides two, rarely three, longitudinal anastomotic branches with the arcuate artery; in some cases, these branches are large enough to continue distally as the fourth and third dorsal metatarsal arteries or, rarely, as the fourth, third, and second metatarsal arteries. The origin of the proximal lateral tarsal artery is variable and occurs at the following sites as reported by Huber in 200 feet: from the level of the junction of the talar head and neck, 58%; almost at the level of the ankle joint, 19.5%; from below the talonavicular joint, 19%; absent artery, 1.5%; extremely small artery, 1.5%; a continuation of the perforating peroneal artery, 0.5%.[5]

Distal.   The origin of the distal lateral tarsal artery is very variable; it is often found on the dorsum of the second cuneiform or, occasionally, more proximal at the level of the cuneo$_2$-navicular joint.[2] The proximal lateral tarsal artery is usually larger than the distal, and Adachi provides the following information concerning their sizes in 230 feet: in 84%, the proximal lateral tarsal artery is larger; in 6%, the distal lateral tarsal artery is larger; in 10%, both are equal.[2]

Arcuate Artery

The arcuate artery originates from the dorsalis pedis usually at the level of the first tarso-metatarsal joint, crosses the base of the second, third and fourth metatarsals almost transversely and provides the dorsal metatarsal arteries 2, 3, 4 and, occasionally, the artery metatarsi dorsalis fibularis (see Fig. 7-3 and Fig. 7-8*B*).[2] The artery is present in only 54%, and the variable origin of the artery occurs at the following sites as reported by Huber in 200 feet: at the $\text{cuneo}_1\text{-metatarsal}_1$ level, 35% (group A); at the cuneonavicular level, 17% (group B); below the cuneonavicular level, 2%. The dorsal metatarsal arteries provided by the arcuate artery occur with the following frequency in 200 feet: dorsal metatarsal arteries 2, 3, and 4—16.5% group A, 9% group B (25.5% total); dorsal metatarsal arteries 2 and 3—9% group A, 6.5% group B (15.5% total); dorsal metatarsal artery—9.5% group A, 3.5% group B (13% total).[5]

First Dorsal Metatarsal Artery, First Plantar Metatarsal Artery, and Arterial Supply of the Big Toe

The first dorsal metatarsal artery originates from the dorsalis pedis artery when the latter dives plantarward at the base of the first intermetatarsal space.

As described by Poirier and Charpy, the artery courses over the dorsum of the first dorsal interosseous muscle and divides into two branches—medial and lateral—at the level of the metatarsophalangeal joint of the big toe (Fig. 7-13).[11] The medial branch provides two dorsolateral collaterals to the big toe. The lateral branch terminates as the dorsomedial branch of the second toe.

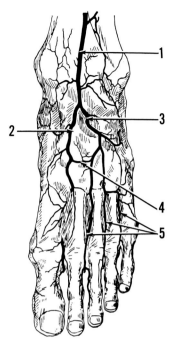

Fig. 7-12. Lateral tarsal arteries. (1, Anterior tibial artery; 2, dorsalis pedis artery; 3, proximal lateral tarsal artery; 4, distal lateral tarsal artery; 5, dorsal metatarsal arteries 2, 3, 4.) (From: Adachi B: Das Arteriensystem der Japaner, p 245. Kyoto, Maruzen, 1928)

Fig. 7-13. Arterial supply of the big toe. (1, Dorsalis pedis artery; 2, first proximal perforating artery or vertical descending portion of *1;* 3, transverse segment or deep plantar arterial arc; 4, first dorsal metatarsal artery; 5, first distal perforating artery or vertical descending portion of *4;* 6, medial division branch of first dorsal metatarsal artery, providing two dorsal collateral branches to big toe [*8*]; 7, lateral division branch of first dorsal metatarsal artery, providing tibial dorsal collateral branch to second toe; 9, first plantar metatarsal artery; 10, lateral division branch of first plantar metatarsal artery; 11, medial division branch of first plantar metatarsal artery; 12, medial plantar division branch of vertical portion of first dorsal metatarsal artery, providing medial [*13*] and lateral [*14*] hallucal plantar arteries; 15, lateral plantar division branch of vertical portion of first dorsal metatarsal artery, providing tibial plantar artery of second toe; 16, arterial branch arising from medial plantar artery joins first plantar metatarsal artery; 17, cruciate anastomosis formed by first plantar metatarsal artery and its two division branches joined by hallucal branch of medial plantar artery; 18, deep transverse metatarsal ligament; 19, first dorsal interosseous muscle arising from second metatarsal shaft.) (Diagram drawn in accordance with Poirier and Charpy's description.[11])

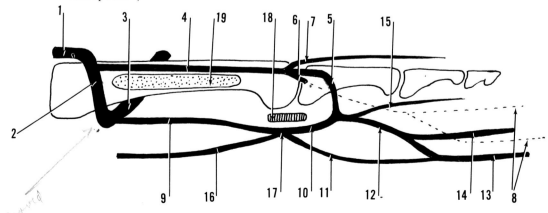

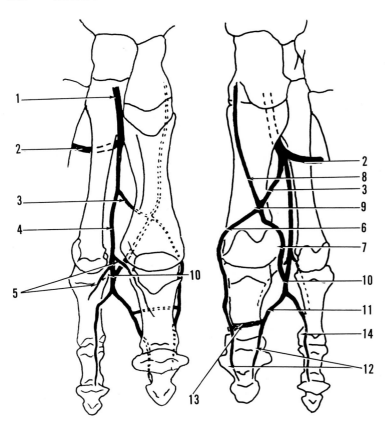

Fig. 7-14. Most common disposition of the first dorsal metatarsal artery. (1, Dorsalis pedis artery; 2, transverse plantar arterial arc; 3, first plantar metatarsal artery; 4, first dorsal metatarsal artery; 5, lateral and medial dorsal division branches of first dorsal metatarsal artery, forming dorsotibial collateral branch of second toe and dorsoperoneal collateral branch of big toe; 6, medial division branch of first plantar metatarsal artery; 7, lateral division branch of first plantar metatarsal artery; 8, hallucal branch arising from medial plantar artery and forming cruciate anastomosis [9] with first plantar metatarsal artery and its division branches [6, 7]; 10, descending vertical portion of first dorsal metatarsal artery joined by lateral division branch of first plantar metatarsal artery; 11, common plantar hallucal artery; 12, plantar hallucal arteries, medial and lateral, with their transverse anastomotic branch [13]; 14, tibial and plantar collateral artery of second toe.) (From Gilbert A: In Tubiana R [ed]: La Main. Paris, Masson et Cie, 1976)

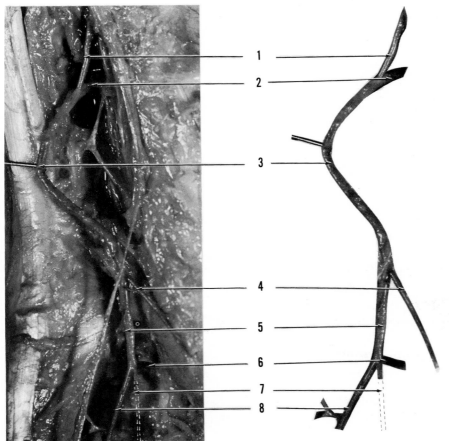

Fig. 7-15. Dorsal aspect of the first web space of the left foot. The big toe is on the left side. (1, Thin dorsalis pedis artery; 2, first proximal perforating artery provided from deep plantar arc and supplying first dorsal metatarsal artery [3]; 4, dorsal collateral arterial branch to second toe; 5, distal portion of first dorsal metatarsal artery; 6, vertical descending portion of first dorsal metatarsal artery; 7, 8, dorsal collateral branches of second and first toes.)

Distally, in the webspace, the first dorsal metatarsal artery plunges plantarward and bifurcates into its terminal branches, medial and lateral. The medial plantar branch forms the plantar hallucal arteries, fibular and tibial, whereas the lateral branch terminates as the medial plantar artery of the second toe. The lateral branch of the first plantar metatarsal artery joins the first dorsal metatarsal artery at the level of its plantar bifurcation. The plantar tibial hallucal artery crosses transversely between the mid segment of the proximal phalanx and the flexor hallucis longus tendon to reach the medial plantar aspect of the big toe, where it is joined by the medial bifurcation branch of the first plantar metatarsal artery (Fig. 7-14). Poirier and Charpy clearly state that "it is the dorsal interosseous (metatarsal$_I$) and not the plantar interosseous (metatarsal$_I$) that provides the three inner plantar collaterals of the toes" (first and second; Figs. 7-15 and 7-16).[11]

The first plantar metatarsal artery is considered a branch of the dorsalis pedis or as a terminal branch of the lateral plantar artery. It arises at the level of the inferior border of the second metatarsal from the dorsalis pedis arterial arc during its vertical course in the first intermetatarsal space.[9] It is directed medially and anteriorly, separated from the first dorsal metatarsal artery by the first dorsal interosseous muscle. It is located deep to the level of the oblique head of the adductor hallucis and the flexor hallucis brevis. Initially applied against the lateral surface of the first metatar-sal, the artery passes between the bone and the flexor hallucis brevis muscle. At the level of the distal bifurcation triangle of this muscle, the first plantar metatarsal artery divides into two branches, lateral and medial. The lateral branch courses between the two heads of the flexor hallucis brevis and then passes plantar to the lateral head of the short flexor. It turns around the lateral sesamoid, pierces the deep lateral sagittal septum of the plantar aponeurosis for the big toe, courses on the plantar aspect of the deep transverse metatarsal ligament, and joins the first dorsal metatarsal artery at the point of bifurcation in the first web space. The medial branch of the first plantar metatarsal artery also emerges between the two heads of the short flexors of the big toe, passes around the medial sesamoid or between the two sesamoids, and terminates in the tibial plantar hallucal artery. This medial branch is joined by a thin branch from the medial plantar artery (Figs. 7-13 and 7-14).

The more-recent description by Gilbert (Fig. 7-14) of the arterial blood supply of the big toe and second toe is quite similar to that provided by Poirier and Charpy except for some further details and minor variations in interpretation.[9, 11] The first dorsal metatarsal artery arises from the dorsalis pedis artery as the latter enters the intermetatarsal space "limited anteriorly by the arch formed by the first dorsal interosseous muscle and posteriorly by the base of the two first metatarsals and their ligaments."[9] The first dorsal metatarsal artery passes under a muscular tunnel

Fig. 7-16. Relationship of the first dorsal metatarsal artery and the deep terminal branch of the deep peroneal nerve. Dorsal aspect of the first web space of the left foot; the big toe is on the left. (1, Medial and lateral branches of deep peroneal nerve innervating first web space, crossing first dorsal metatarsal artery [2] superficially; 3, proximal dorsal collateral arterial branch to second toe; 4, vertical descending branch of first dorsal metatarsal artery; 5, 6, dorsal collateral arterial branches to second and first toe supplied by first dorsal metatarsal artery; dorsal collateral artery to second toe is thin.)

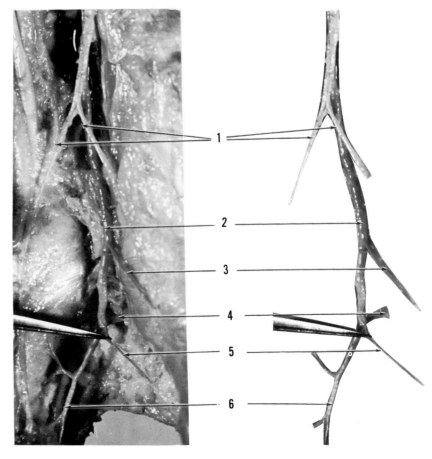

(about 15 mm long) formed by a belly of the first dorsal interosseous muscle and runs toward the web space in a subcutaneous position dorsal to the interosseous muscle.[9] In the web space the artery provides a dorsal branch to the big toe and a dorsal branch to the second toe and dives plantarward. It branches into the larger lateral plantar digital artery of the big toe and the thinner medial plantar digital artery of the second toe. By means of a transverse anastomotic branch located between the proximal phalanx of the big toe and the flexor hallucis longus tendon, the lateral plantar artery of the big toe unites with the distal segment of the medial plantar artery and provides the major blood supply to the big toe. At the level of the first metatarsal neck, the first plantar metatarsal artery is joined by the thin medial plantar artery. Two arteries arise from this junction and a "vascular cross" is formed. As described above, the lateral branch joins the first dorsal metatarsal artery in the web space. The distal medial branch forms the plantar tibial hallucal artery. Occasionally the latter is formed solely by the medial plantar artery.

The plantar fibular hallucal artery and the dorsal tibial artery of the second toe are the predominating vessels.[8, 9, 12]

The dorsal hallucal arteries derive from the first dorsal metatarsal artery, and the medial branch is present only in the distal segment.[8, 11] The medial branch may be supplied by the plantar medial hallucal artery through a vertical ascending branch.[8]

The first dorsal metatarsal artery provides muscular branches to the first dorsal interosseous muscle, articular branches to the metatarsophalangeal joints of the big toe and second toe, and cutaneous branches to the skin of the dorsum of the foot. The cutaneous branches arise from three

main sites: proximal to the dorsal muscular arch of the first dorsal interosseous, distal to the same arch, and at the anterior aspect of the first web space.[9]

The caliber of the first dorsal metatarsal artery is 1 mm to 1.5 mm. The first plantar metatarsal artery is of similar size or smaller.[9]

Variations of the First Dorsal Metatarsal Artery. The variations of the first dorsal metatarsal artery have been analyzed according to the origin and principal source of supply and the relationship with the first dorsal interosseous muscle.[2, 5, 9, 13]

Variations Relative to the Source of Supply. With regard to the main source of the first dorsal metatarsal artery, in 230 feet it is reported to be dorsal in 80.8% and plantar in 19.1%; in 200 feet, it is reported as dorsal in 76.5%, plantar in 8.5%, dorsal and plantar in 0.3%, and absent in 12%.[2, 5]

Variations Relative to the First Dorsal Interosseous Muscle and to the Insertion of the Adductor of the Big Toe. Murakami, in a study of 40 feet, groups the variations of the first dorsal and first plantar metatarsal arteries into eight types (Fig. 7-17).[13]

Type Ia (5%): The first dorsal and first plantar metatarsal arteries have a common trunk passing deep to the first dorsal interosseous muscle. The trunk reaches the plantar aspect of the first metatarsal bone and divides into the dorsal and plantar branches just proximal to the tendon of the adductor hallucis.

Type Ib (5%): The common trunk is more dorsal and

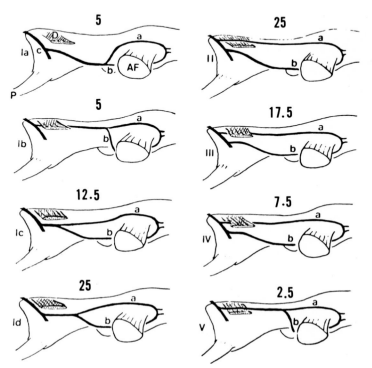

Fig. 7-17. **Variations in the origin and proximal course of the dorsal and plantar arteries in the first intermetatarsal space.** (*a*, first dorsal metatarsal artery; *b*, first plantar metatarsal artery; *c*, deep plantar branch of dorsalis pedis artery; *D*, medial head of first dorsal interosseous muscle; *AF*, adductor hallucis and flexor hallucis brevis muscles; *P*, tendon of peroneus longus muscle.) (From Murakami T: On the position and course of the deep plantar arteries, with special reference to the so-called plantar metatarsal arteries. Okajimas Folia Anat Jpn 48:295, 1971)

passes close to the plantar aspect of the first dorsal interosseous muscle, and the division occurs just proximal to the adductor hallucis tendon.

Type Ic (12.5%): The common trunk is short, is located under the first dorsal interosseous muscle, and bifurcates, proximal to the distal border of the origin of the muscle, into the first dorsal and first plantar metatarsal arteries.

Type Id (25%): The common trunk bifurcates just distal to the origin of the distal border of the first dorsal interosseous muscle origin.

Type II (25%): The dorsal and plantar arteries arise independently. The first dorsal metatarsal artery passes superficially to the first dorsal interosseous muscle, whereas the plantar artery passes deep to the same muscle.

Type III (17.5%): Both arteries arise independently. The dorsal artery passes just under the first dorsal interosseous muscle; the plantar artery descends on the plantar aspect of the first metatarsal bone.

Type IV (7.5%): The first dorsal metatarsal artery pierces the first dorsal interosseous muscle. The plantar artery is more plantar in location.

Type V (2.5%): The common trunk of both arteries passes dorsal to the first dorsal interosseous muscle and bifurcates just proximal to the adductor hallucis insertion.

Variations Relative to the First Dorsal Interosseous Muscle and to the Deep Transverse Metatarsal Ligament.
Gilbert, in a study of 50 feet, groups the variations of the first dorsal metatarsal artery into five types (Fig. 7-18).[9]

Types Ia and Ib (66%): Both metatarsal arteries arise independently. In Type Ia the first dorsal metatarsal

artery passes under the small posterior belly of the first dorsal interosseous muscle but remains superficial to the main muscle and to the deep transverse metatarsal ligament. In Type Ib the dorsal artery passes through the first dorsal interosseous muscle.

Types IIa and IIb (22%): The dorsal and plantar metatarsal arteries have a common trunk located under the first dorsal interosseous muscle. The first dorsal metatarsal artery courses deep to the muscle and passes dorsal to the deep transverse metatarsal ligament. In Type IIa a slender superficial branch is present passing superficially to the muscle and uniting at the anterior part of the web space with the dorsal metatarsal artery. In Type IIb the superficial arterial branch is not present.

Type III (12%): The first dorsal interosseous artery is slender and passes through the first dorsal interosseous muscle. The first plantar metatarsal artery is well developed.

Variations of the First Plantar Metatarsal Artery.
The variations of the first plantar metatarsal artery, as described by Gilbert, involve mainly the origin.[9] The artery may branch off from the dorsalis pedis or the dorsal metatarsal artery. In one case in 50 feet the artery branched from the plantar arterial arch, and in another, from the terminal segment of the medial plantar artery.

The distal segment of the artery is fairly constant in its course and anatomical location at the level of the lateral sesamoid bone.

Variations of the Tibial Plantar Hallucal Artery.
The tibial plantar hallucal artery has a variable origin. The artery may arise from the first dorsal metatarsal artery, the

Fig. 7-18. Anatomic variations of first dorsal metatarsal artery found in 50 specimens. (1, Descending branch of dorsalis pedis artery; 2, first dorsal metatarsal artery; 3, first plantar metatarsal artery; 4, common trunk to *2* and *3;* 5, thin superficial first dorsal metatarsal artery; 6, 7, origin of first dorsal interosseous muscle; 8, deep transverse metatarsal ligament.) (From Gilbert A: In Tubiana R [ed]: La Main. Paris, Masson et Cie, 1976)

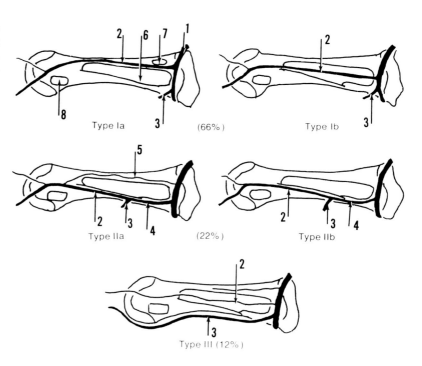

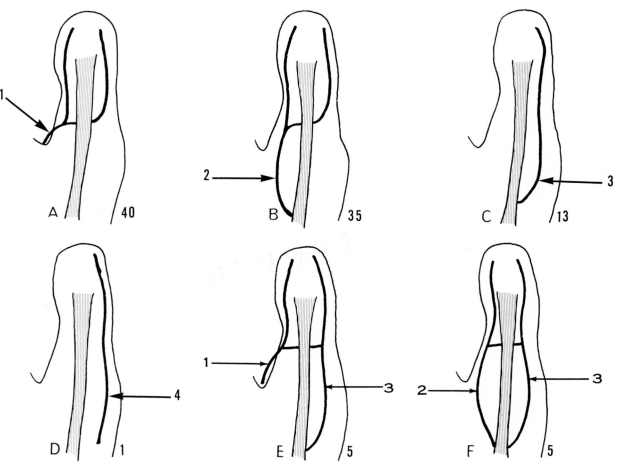

Fig. 7-19.   Variations of the origin of the tibial plantar hallucal artery. The tibial plantar hallucal artery is provided by (*A*) the first dorsal metatarsal artery (*1*); (*B*) the fibular branch of the first plantar metatarsal artery (*2*); (*C*) the tibial branch of the first plantar metatarsal artery (*3*); (*D*) the tibial superficial artery (*4*);.(*E*) the first dorsal metatarsal artery (*1*) and the tibial branch of the first plantar metatarsal artery (*3*); (*F*) both branches of the first plantar metatarsal artery (*2, 3*); (*G*) the first dorsal metatarsal artery (*1*) and the tibial superficial metatarsal artery (*4*). (From Adachi B: Das Arteriensystem der Japaner, p 281. Kyoto, Maruzen, 1928)

TABLE 7-4   Source of Dorsal Metatarsal Arteries

	Dorsal Metatarsal Arteries (%)		
	II	III	IV
Adachi[2]			
Plantar	56.5	56.9	63.4
Dorsal	36	35.6	33.9
Plantar and dorsal	7.3	7.3	2.6
Huber[5] **(200 western feet)**			
Dorsal	55	59	40.5
Plantar	33.5	23	37.5
Plantar and dorsal	6.5	10.5	0.5
Not present or classified	5	7.5	17

TABLE 7-5   Sources of Supply to Dorsal Digital Arteries

	Dorsal Digital Arteries (%)			
	1 & 2	2 & 3	3 & 4	4 & 5
Source				
Dorsal	82.5	89	79	39
Plantar	10.5	8.5	10.5	53.5
Dorsal and plantar	0	2	3.5	2.5
Not classified	7	0.5	2	5

(From Huber JF: The arterial network supplying the dorsum of the foot. Anat Rec 80:373, 1941)

first plantar metatarsal artery, or the tibial superficial plantar artery.

In a study of 100 feet, Adachi found that the tibial plantar hallucal artery originates from the first dorsal metatarsal artery in 40%; from the first plantar metatarsal artery, fibular branch in 35%, tibial branch in 13%, both branches in 5%; from the tibial superficial plantar artery in 1%; from the first dorsal metatarsal and first plantar metatarsal (tibial branch) arteries in 5%; from the first dorsal metatarsal artery and the tibial superficial plantar artery in 1% (Fig. 7-19).[2]

Dorsomedial Hallucal Artery and Variations. The artery dorsalis hallucis tibialis or dorsal medial hallucal artery has a plantar or dorsal origin. As mentioned by Adachi, the artery originating from the first dorsal metatarsal artery and oriented toward the dorsotibial aspect of the big toe does not extend distally beyond the first metatarsophalangeal joint. The distal segment of the dorsomedial aspect of the big toe is supplied by a plantar branch arising from the plantar medial hallucal artery, turning around the proximal phalanx, and reaching the dorsotibial aspect of the big toe.[8] Poirier and Charpy describe the distal segment of the dorsotibial hallucal artery as being provided by the first dorsal metatarsal artery.[11] The principal source of the dorsomedial hallucal artery is described as plantar in 98.7% of 200 feet and 4.3% of 140 feet; as dorsal in 0.9% of 200 feet and 95.7% of 140 feet; and as plantar and dorsal in 0.4% of 200 feet and 0 of 140 feet.[1, 2] The extreme differences are explained by the ethnic background: Japanese versus European.

Dorsal Metatarsal Arteries 2 to 4

The dorsal metatarsal arteries 2 to 4 have a double origin: dorsal and plantar (see Fig. 7-3). The dorsal source arises from the dorsal rete and the plantar source from the proximal or posterior perforating artery. According to the caliber of the supply vessel, one source may be considered to predominate or both sources may be of equal importance.

The respective sources of the dorsal metatarsal arteries II–IV are as shown in Table 7-4. The dorsal source is provided predominantly by the arcuate artery, followed in frequency by the proximal lateral tarsal artery. The plantar source is provided by the proximal or posterior perforating artery.

Dorsal Digital Arteries

The dorsal digital arteries arise close to the metatarsophalangeal joints from the dorsal metatarsal artery, a branch of the plantar metatarsal artery passing dorsally through the distal part of the intermetatarsal space and forming the distal part of the dorsal metatarsal artery, or equally from the dorsal and plantar sources. The incidence of these sources of supply in 200 Western feet is shown in Table 7-5.

Posterior Perforating Arteries

The posterior perforating arteries (proximal perforating arteries, posterior communicating arteries) pass through the proximal end of the corresponding intermetatarsal spaces and join the dorsal metatarsal arteries.[5] They are important contributors to the latter, especially when the dorsal source is deficient. They may be absent in 3% to 5%.[5]

Anterior Perforating Arteries

The dorsal metatarsal artery (distal perforating artery, inferior communicating artery) gives origin to two dorsal digital arteries in the web space, plunges plantarward, forming the anterior perforating artery, supplies the plantar digital arteries, and is joined by the plantar metatarsal artery.[5] In the distal segment of the intermetatarsal space and in the web space, there are five communicating branches between the dorsal and plantar arteries: two arteries that arise from each side of the dorsal metatarsal artery at the metatarsal neck and course plantarward obliquely to unite with the corresponding plantar metatarsal arteries; one artery that is the continuation of the dorsal metatarsal artery and called habitually the *anterior perforating artery;* and two small arteries that connect on each side the dorsal and plantar digital arteries at the level of the side of the corresponding proximal phalanx.[5] Huber groups all five branches under the heading "anterior communicating branches."[5] The connections between the first dorsal metatarsal artery and the first plantar metatarsal artery are indicated in Figure 7-20.

Arteries of the Sinus Tarsi

The artery of the sinus tarsi (perforating vessel of the sinus tarsi, arteria anastomotica tarsi, ramus anastomicus tarsi) has a very variable origin (Figs. 7-21 and 7-22). Frequently it arises from the lateral aspect of the dorsalis pedis artery at the level of the talar neck or from an anastomotic loop between the proximal lateral tarsal artery and the perforating peroneal artery.[14] The artery is always present. At the level of the talar neck, it gives off a few branches to the head, enters the sinus tarsi, supplies multiple branches to the talar body, and anastomoses with the artery of the tarsal canal emanating from the posterior tibial artery.

The caliber of the artery at the entrance of the sinus tarsi is reported by Adachi as being 1 mm to 1.5 mm, never more than 2 mm.[5] The origin of the artery of the sinus tarsi is reported to occur from the dorsalis pedis artery in 52% of 305 feet and 39.2% of 120 feet; from the lateral tarsal (proximal) artery in 32% of 305 feet and 21.7% of 120 feet; from the anterior lateral malleolar artery in 9% of 305 feet and 11.7% of 120 feet; from two equally strong arteries in 15.8% of 120 feet (proximal—dorsalis pedis, perforating branch of peroneal artery, 10%; distal—lateral tarsal artery [proximal], 5.8%).[1, 2]

Medial Tarsal Arteries

The medial tarsal arteries are very variable in size and number (see Fig. 7-3). They might be two of equal size arising from the dorsalis pedis, one at the level of the middle of the navicular and the other just below the cuneonavicular articulation.[5] At times there is only one proximal or one distal branch. Rarely are three branches present. These

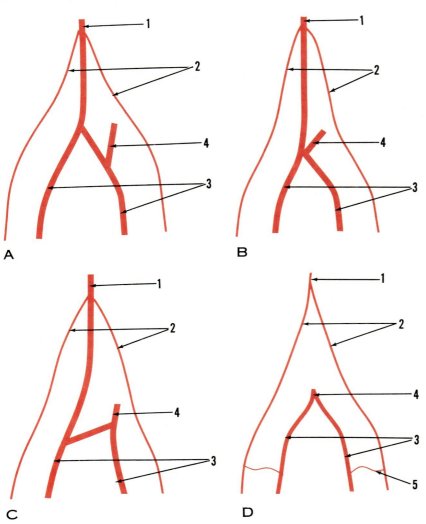

A

B

C

D

Fig. 7-20. Anastomoses between the dorsal and plantar arteries in the interdigital spaces. (*A–C*) Examples of the ways in which the continuation of the dorsal metatarsal artery may contribute to the plantar digital arteries. (*D*) There is a connection between the dorsal and plantar digital arteries. (1, Dorsal metatarsal artery; 2, dorsal digital arteries; 3, plantar digital arteries; 4, plantar metatarsal artery; 5, connection between dorsal and plantar digital arteries.) (From Huber JF: The arterial network supplying the dorsum of the foot. Anat Rec 80:373, 1941. By permission of Alan R. Liss, Inc., Publisher)

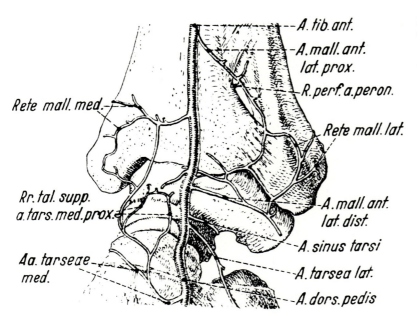

Fig. 7-21. Artery of the sinus tarsi arising from the dorsalis pedis artery. The calcaneus has been removed. (From Wildenauer E: Die Blutvesorgung des Talus. Z Anat Entwicklungs 115:32, 1950)

branches occur with the following frequency in 200 feet: two equal, 42%; one proximal, 13%; one distal, 13.5%; short common stem at the level of the proximal medial tarsus, divided into two branches, proximal and distal, 15%; minute branches, 16.5%.[5]

The medial tarsal arteries anastomose on the medial margin of the foot with the medial plantar artery. Adachi describes a significant anastomosis located on the medial margin of the foot between the first cuneiform and the muscles.[2]

Anterior Medial Malleolar Artery

The anterior medial malleolar artery originates from the dorsalis pedis artery just below the ankle joint (see Fig. 7-3 and Fig. 7-21). As mentioned by Huber, it is "not possible to decide in all cases on any one artery which should be called the anterior medial malleolar artery."[5]

The artery is directed transversely medially, passes under the tibialis anterior tendon, and at the level of the anterior border of the medial malleolus divides into two branches, superficial and deep. The superficial branch crowns the base of the medial malleolus and anastomoses with the terminal thin branch of the posterior medial malleolar artery arising from the posterior tibial artery. The anastomotic network or medial malleolar rete provides small branches penetrating the medial malleolus near the base and coursing in a proximodistal direction. The deep branch of the anterior medial malleolar artery disappears in the deltoid ligamentous complex.

The variations occur relative to the origin, number, and size of the artery. The variations of origin are listed in Table 7-6. The anterior medial malleolar artery is absent in 16%, and occasionally it is very insignificant.[1] It is usually smaller than the anterior lateral malleolar artery, and according to Adachi, the anterior lateral malleolar artery is larger in 69%, the anterior medial malleolar artery is larger in 7%, and both are equal in 24%.[2]

Anterior Lateral Malleolar Artery

The anterior lateral malleolar artery originates from the dorsalis pedis just below the ankle joint articular interline, usually 1 mm to 2 mm below the most common point of origin for the anterior medial malleolar artery (see Figs. 7-3 and 7-21).[5]

The artery is directed transversely laterally and passes under the tendons of the extensor digitorum longus and the

peroneus tertius. At the level of the anterior border of the lateral malleolus, it descends vertically along the anterior border of the lateral malleolus and the lateral border of the tarsus and anastomoses with the proximal lateral tarsal artery and the lateral plantar artery.

The transverse segment of the anterior lateral malleolar artery anastomoses proximally with branches from the perforating peroneal artery and sends a transverse branch over the lateral malleolus. The latter anastomoses with a similar transverse branch emanating from the peroneal artery and contributes to the formation of the perimalleolar transverse arterial loop. The descending retromalleolar branch of the peroneal artery unites with the descending segment of the anterior lateral malleolar artery, forms a sagittal arterial loop, and contributes to the formation of the lateral malleolar arterial rete.

The variations occur relative to the origin, number, and size of the artery. The variations of origin are shown in

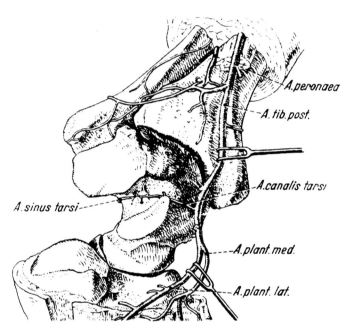

Fig. 7-22. Artery of the sinus tarsi and artery of the canalis tarsi arising from the posterior tibial artery. (From Wildenauer E: Die Blutvesorgung des Talus. Z Anat Entwicklungs 115:32, 1950)

TABLE 7-6   Variations of Origin of the Anterior Medial Malleolar Artery

Origin	%		
	Adachi (59 feet)[2]	Dubreuil-Chambardel (235 feet)[1]	Huber (200 feet)[5]
At the level of the ankle joint articular interline	44		55–60 (or just below)
Below the interline	36	52	3–4 (about 1 cm)
Above the interline	20	32	8 (2 cm–3 cm)
			13–15 (just above)

TABLE 7-7   Variations of Origin of the Anterior Lateral Maleolar Artery

Origin	%		
	Adachi (52 feet)[2]	Dubreuil-Chambardel (235 feet)[1]	Huber (200 feet)[5]
At the level of the ankle joint articular interline	31		60–65 (or 1 mm–2 mm below)
Below the interline	61	52	
Above the interline	8	40	3 (just above)

Table 7-7. The anterior lateral malleolar artery is absent in 8%, may be double in 16%, and in 29% originates not from the dorsalis pedis but from the perforating branch of the peroneal artery.[1, 2]

Perforating Branch of the Peroneal Artery

In the inferior segment of the leg the peroneal artery divides into two branches, posterior and anterior. The anterior branch or perforating branch obliquely pierces the interosseous membrane, passes anteriorly, and courses over the anterior aspect of the distal tibiofibular syndesmosis behind the peroneous tertius tendon. It anastomoses with the transverse segment of the anterior lateral malleolar artery and contributes to the lateral malleolar sagittal and transverse perimalleolar arterial loops. Variations of termination are multiple, and according to Huber, the perforating peroneal artery may continue as the dorsalis pedis artery in 3% (see Col. Fig. 7-9), contribute equally with the anterior tibial artery to the dorsalis pedis artery in 0.5% (see Fig. 7-10), or continue as the lateral tarsal artery in 0.5% (see Fig. 7-10).[5]

Huber also describes in 50% of the cases an unrecognized artery branching from the anterior tibial artery about 5 cm above the ankle joint. This artery courses obliquely laterally and inferiorly and unites with the peroneal perforating branch as it pierces the interosseous membrane. This artery is a small branch in 13% or is equal to the perforating artery in about 20%; in 17%, it occupies the position of the latter.[5] When the distal segment of the anterior tibial artery is missing (1.5%), this oblique artery may be considered as the link between the proximal segment of the anterior tibial artery and the perforating peroneal artery.

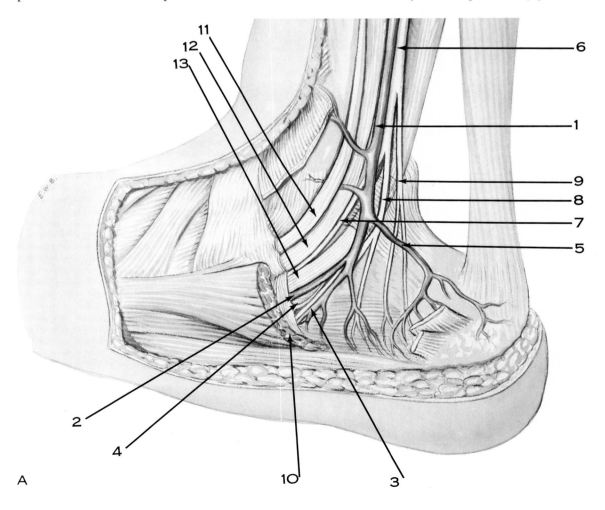

A

POSTERIOR AND PLANTAR ARTERIAL NETWORK OF THE FOOT AND ANKLE

Posterior Tibial Artery

On the posterior aspect of the ankle at the level of the tibial plafond, the tendons of the tibialis posterior, the flexor digitorum longus, and the flexor hallucis longus are applied against the posterior aspect of the tibia and are retained by their individual tunnels. The tunnels of the tibialis posterior and of the flexor digitorum longus are side by side and narrow and are separated from the larger tunnel of the flexor hallucis muscle–tendon unit by an interval. The neurovascular tunnel or fourth compartment is superficial to the intertendinous interval and to the tunnel of the flexor hallucis longus. At this level, the posterior tibial artery with its two accompanying veins is located in the tunnel, medial to the posterior tibial nerve (Figs. 7-23 and 7-24). As de-

scribed previously, the neurovascular compartment is covered by the deep fascia cruris.

In the retromedial malleolar area, the passage zone curves anteriorly and the tendinous and neurovascular elements previously located in a frontal plane are in a nearly sagittal oblique plane. The neurovascular compartment is now posterior to the tunnel of the flexor digitorum longus and is superficial and medial to the intertendinous interval and to the tunnel of the flexor hallucis longus tendon. The posterior tibial artery follows the anterior concavity of its compartment and is accompanied by its two veins. The posterior tibial nerve is divided into the lateral and the medial plantar nerve. The medial plantar nerve has already given the branch to the abductor digiti minimi muscle. The posterior tibial artery is not yet divided and is medial to the plane of the nerves.

The lower segment of the passage zone corresponds to

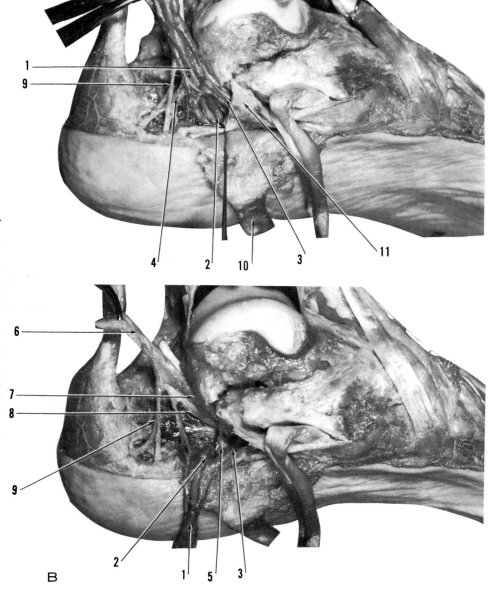

Fig. 7-23.   (A) Medial tibiotalocalcaneal tunnel. (1, Posterior tibial artery; 2, medial plantar artery passing above interfascicular ligament [4]; 3, lateral plantar artery passing under interfascicular ligament [4]; 5, posterior and medial arterial calcaneal branch; 6, posterior tibial nerve; 7, medial plantar nerve; 8, lateral plantar nerve giving branch to abductor hallucis muscle; 9, medial calcaneal nerve arising above bifurcation point of posterior tibial nerve; 10, abductor hallucis muscle; 11, tibialis posterior tendon; 12, flexor digitorum longus tendon; 13, flexor hallucis longus tendon.) **(B) Left foot, medial aspect.** The deltoid ligament is excised, exposing the talus, the medial malleolus, and the sustentaculum tali. (1, Posterior tibial artery; 2, lateral plantar artery; 3, medial plantar artery; 4, posteromedial calcaneal arterial branch; 5, interfascicular septum; 6, posterior tibial nerve; 7, medial plantar nerve; 8, lateral plantar nerve giving branch to abductor hallucis; 9, medial calcaneal nerve; 10, reflected flexor retinaculum; 11, deep investing aponeurosis contributing to formation of porta pedis.)

B

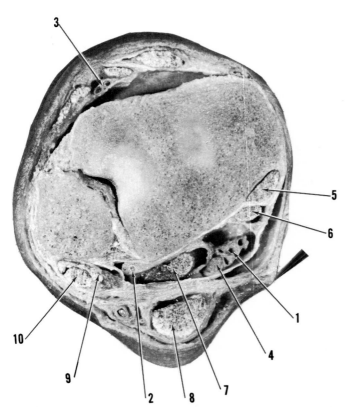

Fig. 7-24.   Cross section of the left ankle 2 cm proximal to the anterior colliculus of the medial malleolus. (1, Posterior tibial artery and accompanying veins; 2, posterior peroneal artery and veins; 3, anterior tibial artery and veins; 4, posterior tibial nerve; 5, tibialis posterior tendon; 6, flexor digitorum longus tendon; 7, flexor hallucis longus tendon and muscle; 8, Achilles tendon; 9, peroneus brevis tendon; 10, peroneus longus tendon.)

the calcaneal canal and the porta pedis. The sustentaculum tali is the landmark. The tunnel of the tibialis posterior is located above the sustentaculum tali and is applied against the deltoid ligament. The tunnel of the flexor digitorum longus passes over the medial border of the sustentaculum tali, crossing the tibiocalcaneal portion of the deltoid ligament. The tunnel of the flexor hallucis longus is located over the inferior surface of the sustentaculum tali. The lateral wall of the calcaneal canal is further formed by the quadratus plantae applied against the medial concave surface of the os calcis and the medial wall by the abductor hallucis muscle and its investing fascia. The interfascicular transverse septum (Fig. 7-25) originates from the fascia of the abductor hallucis and extends almost transversely laterally and inserts along the inferior border of the flexor hallucis longus tunnel, just above the superior border of the quadratus plantae muscle. This transverse septum divides the lower part of the calcaneal canal into a superior and an inferior chamber. The posterior tibial artery bifurcates into the medial and lateral plantar arteries just proximal to the posterior border of the transverse septum. The medial plantar artery is the anterior branch and passes above the transverse septum. The lateral plantar artery is directed obliquely below the

transverse septum. Relative to the sustentaculum tali, the bifurcation of the posterior tibial artery occurs at its posterior border, occasionally more proximal and rarely more distal.

According to various sources, the bifurcation level of the posterior tibial artery occurs with the following variations: under the posterior border of the sustentaculum tali, 67% and 61%; proximal to the posterior border of the sustentaculum tali (as far as 9 mm to 10 mm), 29% and 30%; distal to the posterior border of the sustentaculum tali (about 2 mm to 5 mm), 4% and 9%.[2, 4] The level of arterial bifurcation may also vary relative to the level of bifurcation of the posterior tibial nerve. According to Adachi, in a study of 208 feet, the division of the posterior tibial artery occurs distal to the division of the posterior tibial nerve (usually 1 cm to 2 cm) in 86.5%; proximal to the division of the posterior tibial nerve (usually up to 0.5 cm) in 2%; and at the same level as the division of the posterior tibial nerve in 11.5%.[2]

The lateral plantar artery is usually larger than the medial plantar artery. The following frequencies of variations have been given: lateral plantar artery larger, 80.7% of 223 feet and 62.1% of 58 feet; medial plantar artery larger, 2.7% of 223 feet and 22.4% of 58 feet; both equal, 16.6% of 223 feet and 15.5% of 58 feet.[2, 4]

In its distal segment, the posterior tibial artery provides four collateral branches:

An anastomotic branch, which passes transversely under the flexor hallucis longus tendon and unites with a similar branch of the posterior peroneal artery and forms the posterior half of the perimalleolar arterial circle

The posteromedial malleolar artery, which courses transversely over the tendons of the flexor digitorum longus and the tibialis posterior. This branch anastomoses anteromedially with the anterior medial malleolar artery and contributes to the formation of the medial malleolar rete. It also anastomoses with the medial tarsal arteries and provides cutaneous branches to the medial malleolar area.

Calcaneal rami, which reach the calcaneus and the medial and posterior aspects of the heel

The artery of the tarsal canal (Figs. 7-21 and 7-22).[14, 15]
This artery arises from the posterior tibial artery about 1 cm proximal to the bifurcation into the medial and lateral plantar arteries. It passes between the flexor digitorum longus and flexor hallucis longus tendon sheaths and enters the tarsal canal, where it anastomoses with the artery of the sinus tarsi. The size of the anastomosis varies, and the anastomosis may take place only in the talus.[14] In the sinus canal the artery lies closer to the talus and provides larger branches to the talar body and smaller branches to the calcaneus. A deltoid branch takes off from the artery to the tarsal canal at 5 mm from its origin.[14] This artery passes between the calcaneotibial and talotibial components of the deltoid ligament, supplies the medial aspect of the talus, and anastomoses with the dorsalis pedis artery over the talar neck.[14] According to Mulfinger and

Fig. 7-25.   Chambers of the calcaneal tunnel.
(1, Interfascicular septum dividing calcaneal tunnel into upper [2] and lower [3] chamber; 4, tibialis posterior tendon; 5, flexor digitorum longus tendon; 6, flexor hallucis longus tendon.)

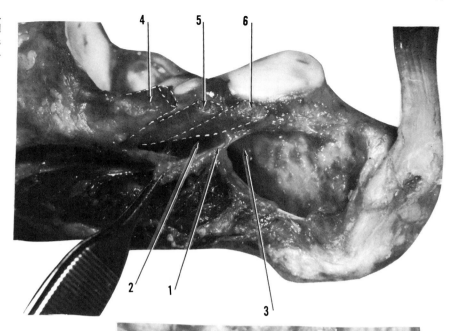

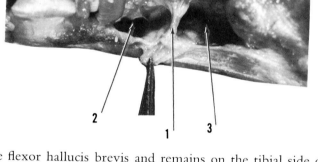

Trueta, in 30 feet, the artery of the tarsal canal originates from the medial plantar artery in 16.6% and is duplicated in 3.3% and absent in 3.3%; in 30% the deltoid branch originates from the posterior tibial artery, and it is duplicated in 6.6%.[14]

Medial Plantar Artery

The medial plantar artery continues anteriorly and remains initially in the medial compartment of the sole of the foot on the inner side of the medial intermuscular septum (Fig. 7-26; Fig. 7-27; see Fig. 7-32). It is covered by the abductor hallucis muscle and crosses the tendon of the flexor digitorum longus at an acute angle; it runs parallel to the tibial side of the flexor hallucis longus tendon. It divides into two branches, superficial and deep. The stem may give origin to the deltoid arterial branches.[14]

Superficial Branch.   The superficial branch emerges through the interval between the abductor hallucis and the flexor digitorum brevis and divides into two branches: the medial marginal plantar artery of the big toe (superficial tibial plantar artery) and the common plantar digital artery. The origin of the common plantar digital artery may be 1 cm to 1.5 cm or 5 cm to 6 cm from the origin of the medial plantar artery.[2]

The superficial tibial plantar artery runs constantly on the plantar aspect of the flexor hallucis brevis muscle, along the tibial side of the flexor hallucis longus. At the level of the first metatarsal neck, the artery passes between the bone and the flexor tendons and anastomoses with the first plantar metatarsal artery. The mode of termination of the superficial tibial plantar artery is variable. It may anastomose directly with the medial plantar hallucal artery or be the sole supplier of the latter;[11] in these cases the superficial tibial plantar artery courses on the plantar aspect of the medial head of

the flexor hallucis brevis and remains on the tibial side of the flexor hallucis longus tendon until anastomosing with the medial plantar hallucal artery. The superficial tibial plantar artery also may be very strong and replace the first plantar metatarsal artery.[2]

The stem of the common plantar digital arteries passes obliquely between the flexor digitorum brevis and the central plantar aponeurosis and provides the common superficial plantar digital arteries that unite with the first, second, and third plantar metatarsal arteries. The lateral terminal segment of the common superficial plantar digital artery may unite with the superficial branch of the lateral plantar artery and form the superficial plantar arch.

The superficial plantar arch formed by very slender arterial branches is present with the following frequency according to various sources: in 165 feet ("capillary caliber" arch), 28%; in 101 feet, 5%; in 66 feet, 30%; in 50 feet, 12% (well developed in 4%, frail in 8%).[1, 2, 4, 16] A superficial branch—the medial superficial artery of the foot of Henle—is always quite large and arises from the medial plantar artery close to its origin. It crosses the deep surface of the abductor hallucis, emerges above the muscle, follows the superior border of the muscle, and terminates at the level of the metatarsophalangeal joint of the big toe.[11]

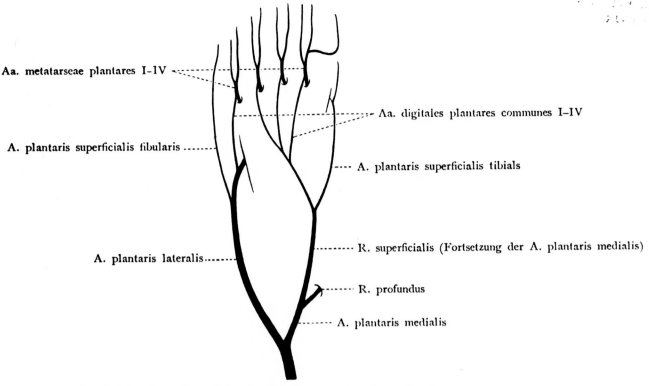

Aa. metatarseae plantares I–IV

Aa. digitales plantares communes I–IV

A. plantaris superficialis fibularis

A. plantaris superficialis tibials

R. superficialis (Fortsetzung der A. plantaris medialis)

A. plantaris lateralis

R. profundus

A. plantaris medialis

Fig. 7-26. The division branches of the medial plantar artery into the ramus superficialis and the ramus profundus. The ramus superficialis provides the plantar superficial tibial branch and the superficial common digital plantar arteries 1, 2, 3. (From Adachi B: Das Arteriensystem der Japaner. Kyoto, Maruzen, 1928)

Deep Branch.   The ramus profundus branches from the tibial side of the medial plantar artery near its origin, remains deep, and divides into two branches, tibial and lateral.[2]

The tibial branch courses distally along the tibial skeletal margin of the foot, reaches the base of the first metatarsal, and anastomoses with the first plantar metatarsal artery (Figs. 7-28 and 7-29). In rare cases, it may even substitute for the latter. The same branch also occasionally continues into the dorsal tibial hallucal artery after emerging between the base of the first metatarsal bone and the abductor hallucis muscle. Further connections are established on the dorsomedial margin of the foot between branches of this artery and the dorsal arterial system.

The fibular branch penetrates even deeper into the planta pedis, passes dorsal to the peroneous longus tendon near its insertion on the base of the first metatarsal, and terminates on the tibial segment of the deep plantar arch (Figs. 7-28 and 7-29). The fibular branch may arise directly from the medial plantar artery.

In a study of 100 feet, Adachi provides the following variations of the origin of the branches of the medial plantar artery: ramus profundus arising independently from the medial plantar artery, 63%; ramus profundus and superficial tibial plantar artery arising from the medial plantar artery through a short common trunk, 28%; medial plantar artery trifurcating into the superficial tibial plantar artery, ramus

profundus, common trunk of the plantar digital arteries, 9%.[2]

Lateral Plantar Artery

The lateral plantar artery passes under the interfascicular septum of the calcaneal canal and enters the middle compartment of the foot (Fig. 7-30). It courses obliquely and anterolaterally, under the fascia of the quadratus plantae muscle, and remains posterolateral to the lateral plantar nerve. It continues toward the base of the fifth metatarsal bone, pierces the lateral intermuscular septum, and extends forward between the lateral septum and the sheath of the abductor digiti quinti. On the medial aspect of the base of the fifth metatarsal and just distal to the latter, it gives off the superficial fibular plantar artery of the little toe. At about 2.5 cm distal to the fifth metatarsal base, the lateral plantar artery passes deep on the medial side of the flexor digiti quinti brevis, pierces again the lateral intermuscular septum, and enters the fascial space M_3 of the middle compartment. On the lateral border of the adductor hallucis obliquis, the artery penetrates the fascial space M_4 located between the adductor hallucis obliquis and the interossei muscles. The artery now has a nearly transverse course and crosses the base of the metatarsals 4, 3, and 2 and terminates by inosculation with the perforating branch of the dorsalis pedis at the proximal end of the first intermetatarsal space. This

Dr. T. Derek V. Cooke
La Salle Building
146 Stuart Street
Kingston, Ont. K7L 3N6
Tel: 549-6414

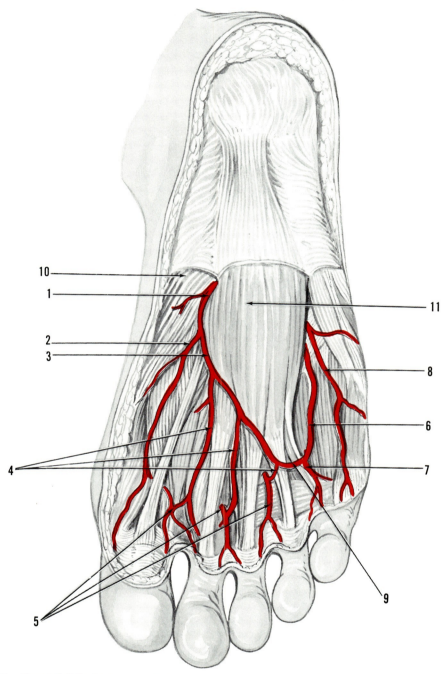

Fig. 7-27. Superficial plantar arterial arc. (1, Superficial branch of medial plantar artery; 2, tibial plantar superficial artery; 3, common digital plantar superficial artery; 4, superficial plantar digital arteries joining corresponding plantar metatarsal arteries [5]; 6, superficial plantar digital artery to fourth web space joining plantar metatarsal artery to same place [7]; 8, fibular plantar superficial artery; 9, superficial plantar arcade formed when 3 and 6 are anastomosed superficial to flexor digitorum brevis [11]; 10, abductor hallucis muscle.) (Adapted from Aschner B: Zur Anatomie der Arterien der Fussshole. Anat Hefte Beit Ref Anat Entwicklungs 27:345, 1905)

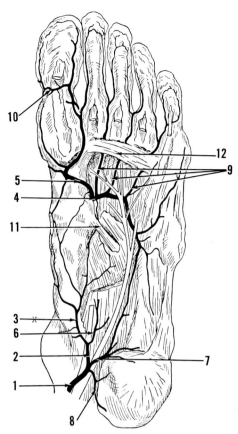

Fig. 7-28.   The deep branch of the medial plantar artery. (1, Posterior tibial artery; 2, medial plantar artery; 3, deep branch of medial plantar artery, which passes under peroneus longus tendon [*11*] and joins deep plantar arc [*4*]; 5, first plantar metatarsal artery; 6, superficial branch of medial plantar artery; 7, lateral plantar artery; 8, medial calcaneal artery; 9, plantar metatarsal arteries passing dorsal to transverse head of adductor hallucis muscle [*12*]; 10, transverse plantar hallucal anastomotic branch passing on dorsal aspect of flexor hallucis longus tendon.) (From Adachi B: Das Arteriensystem der Japaner. Kyoto, Maruzen, 1928)

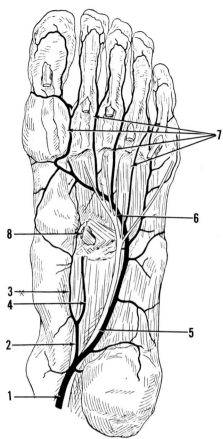

Fig. 7-29.   The deep branch of the medial plantar artery. (1, Posterior tibial artery; 2, medial plantar artery; 3, deep branch of medial plantar artery passing on dorsum of peroneus longus tendon [*8;* cut in this specimen]; 4, superficial branch of medial plantar artery; 5, lateral plantar artery; 6, deep plantar arterial arc; 7, plantar metatarsal arteries.) (From Adachi B: Das Arteriensystem der Japaner. Kyoto, Maruzen, 1928)

deep arterial arch provides the proximal or posterior perforating arteries of the second to fourth intermetatarsal space communicating with the dorsal metatarsal arterial system and the second to fourth plantar metatarsal arteries. The first plantar metatarsal artery is considered as a branch of the dorsalis pedis artery.

Deep Plantar Arch

The deep plantar arch is formed by inosculation of the deep plantar branch of the dorsalis pedis artery with the deep transverse component of the lateral plantar artery. The site of union of the two arteries is indicated by the thinnest portion of the arterial arch. This point of junction is not constant, indicating the variable contribution of each arterial component (Table 7-8; Fig. 7-31). Vann, in a study of 361 feet related to the formation of the deep plantar arch, reports the dorsalis pedis contribution to predominate in 80.8% and the lateral artery in 15.23%.[17]

Plantar Metatarsal Arteries

The four plantar metatarsal arteries arise from the deep plantar arch, and their blood supply is provided by the deep plantar branch of the dorsalis pedis or by the lateral plantar artery. The frequency of contribution of these two arterial sources to the individual plantar metatarsal artery is shown in Table 7-9. Figure 7-31 provides further information concerning the number of plantar metatarsal arteries supplied in each type of foot by these two arterial sources.

The plantar metatarsal arteries may be missing, as reported by Adachi, in the following percentages: 1, 2.3%; 2, 2.3%; 3, 0; 4, 6.1%, or they may be rudimentary and substituted for by the superficial plantar arterial system in the following frequency: 1, 16%; 2, 3%; 3, 0; 4, 19%.[2] The first plantar metatarsal artery may be substituted for by the tibial superficial plantar artery and the first common plantar digital artery. The second plantar metatarsal artery may be substituted for by the second common plantar digital artery and the fourth by the fibular superficial plantar artery or the fourth common plantar digital artery.

Fig. 7-30. Plantar arteries. (1, Posterior tibial artery; 2, medial plantar artery; 3, lateral plantar artery; 4, superficial branch of medial plantar artery; 5, deep branch of medial plantar artery; 6, deep arterial plantar arc; 7, first proximal perforating artery or vertical descending segment of dorsalis pedis artery; 8, first plantar metatarsal artery; 9, lateral division branch of first plantar metatarsal artery; 10, medial division branch of first plantar metatarsal artery; 11, common digital artery 1; 12, first distal perforating artery or vertical descending segment of first dorsal interosseous artery; 13, transverse plantar hallucal anastomotic branch passing dorsal to flexor hallucis longus tendon; 14, lateral plantar hallucal artery; 15, medial plantar hallucal artery; 16, superficial common digital artery 1; 17, proximal perforating arteries; 18, plantar metatarsal arteries 2, 3, 4; 19, bifurcation of metatarsal arteries forming an arcade [in more usual form, medial limb of bifurcation is absent]; 20, common digital arteries 2, 3, 4; 21, distal perforating arteries; 22, plantar digital arteries; 23, fibular plantar superficial artery.) (Adapted from Edwards EA: Anatomy of the small arteries of the foot and toes. Acta Anat 40:81, 1960)

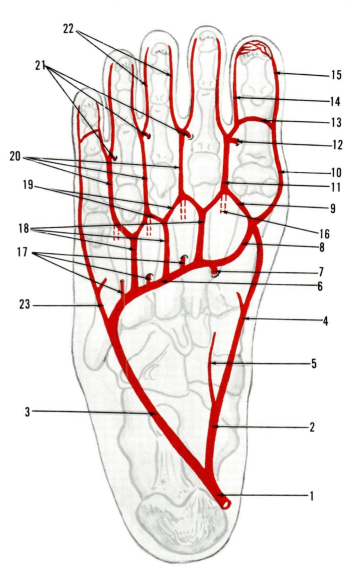

TABLE 7-8 Frequency of Contribution of Arterial Components

	Dubreuil-Chambardel (203 feet)[1]	Manno (66 feet)[4]	Adachi (130 feet)[2]
Deep Plantar Arterial Arch Formed by %			
Type I: Only deep plantar branch of dorsalis pedis artery	40.2	48.4	25.3 (Type A)
Type II: Union of deep plantar branch of dorsalis pedis artery and lateral plantar arteries	55.8	51.6	67.6 (Type B,32.3; Type C, 14.6; Type D, 14.6; Type E, 6.1)
Type III: Only lateral plantar artery	4		7 (Type F)

TABLE 7-9 Contributions to Individual Plantar Metatarsal Arteries

Plantar Metatarsal Artery	Deep Plantar Branch of Dorsalis Pedis Artery (%)		Lateral Plantar Artery (%)	
	Adachi[2]*	Manno[4]†	Adachi[2]*	Manno[4]†
1	90.8	89.4	6.9	7.6
2	84.6	84.8	13.1	12.1
3	72.3	75.8	27.7	21.2
4	54.6	48.5	39.2	48.5

*130 feet
†66 feet

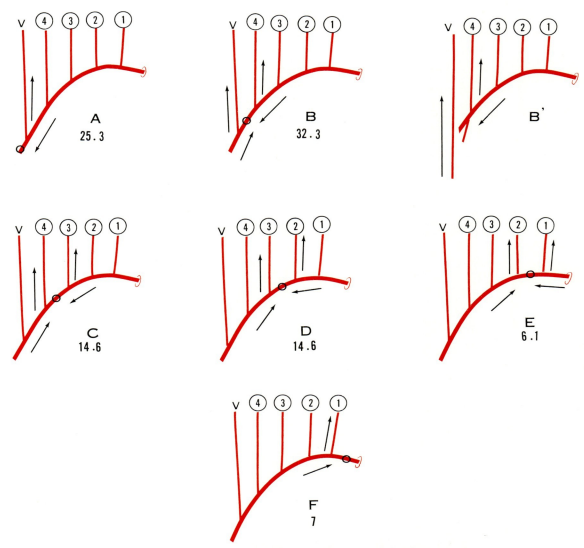

Fig. 7-31.   Deep plantar arterial arch—variable contribution of the deep transverse component of the lateral plantar artery and of the deep plantar branch of the dorsalis pedis. The site of union of the two arteries is indicated by a black circle representing the thinnest portion of the arterial arch. (*Type A*) The arch is formed only by the deep plantar branch of the dorsalis pedis and supplies the plantar meta-arteries 1 to 4 and the fibular plantar marginal artery *V.* (*Type B*) The point of junction is located between the plantar metatarsal artery 4 and the fibular plantar marginal artery *V.* The deep plantar branch of the dorsalis pedis supplies the plantar metatarsal arteries 1 to 4. (*Type B'*) The deep plantar arch is supplied only by the deep plantar branch of the dorsalis pedis artery. The fibular plantar marginal artery *V* is provided by the lateral plantar artery. (*Type C*) The point of junction is located between the plantar metatarsal arteries 3 and 4. The deep plantar branch of the dorsalis pedis artery provides the plantar metatarsal arteries 1 to 3. The lateral plantar artery provides the fibular plantar marginal artery *V* and the plantar metatarsal artery 4. (*Type D*) The point of junction shifts farther medially and is located between the plantar metatarsal arteries 2 and 3. The deep plantar branch of the dorsalis pedis supplies the plantar metatarsal arteries 1 and 2. The lateral plantar artery supplies the fibular plantar marginal artery and the plantar metatarsal arteries 4 and 3. (*Type E*) The point of junction is located between the plantar metatarsal arteries 1 and 2. The deep plantar branch of the dorsalis pedis supplies only the first plantar metatarsal artery. The lateral plantar artery supplies the fibular plantar marginal artery *V* and the plantar metatarsal arteries 4, 3, and 2. (*Type F*) The deep plantar arterial arch is formed entirely by the lateral plantar artery. (The numbers indicate the percentage of occurrence of the indicated variations.) (From Adachi B: Das Arteriensystem der Japaner. Kyoto, Maruzen, 1928)

The four lateral plantar metatarsal arteries course "along the midline of the shafts of the medial four metatarsals not, as is usually stated, along the interosseous space."[8] These arteries course forward and remain superficial or plantar to the interossei muscles. The plantar metatarsal arteries 2 and 3 pass without exception deep or dorsal to the transverse head of the adductor hallucis muscle (Fig. 7-32). In 102 feet, Adachi reports only one case in which the second and third plantar metatarsal arteries divide into two branches at the proximal border of the muscle;[2] one branch passes plantar and the other dorsal to the muscle, forming an arterial loop, and they join again distally (Fig. 7-33). The plantar metatarsal artery 4 passes dorsal (75%) or plantar (25%) to the same muscle.[2] Distally the plantar metatarsal artery bifurcates into two metatarsodigital branches. This division occurs at the level of a triangle centered on the head–neck of the metatarsal and is limited on each side by the corresponding interossei muscles (Fig. 7-34).[18] The base of the triangle is distal, corresponding to the entrance of the flexor tunnel and the plantar plate. The apex is proximal. The bifurcation branches pass on each side of the corresponding flexor tunnel through an aperture located between the transverse head of the adductor hallucis muscle and the deep transverse metatarsal ligament. They course on the plantar aspect of the latter and join distally the corresponding plantar digital artery formed in the web space by the bifurcation of the distal perforating branch of the dorsal metatarsal artery. The medial limb of the lateral three bifurcations of the plantar metatarsal artery may be missing.[8] Also, the adjacent

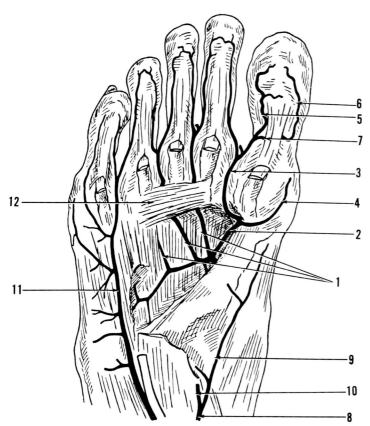

Fig. 7-32.   The plantar metatarsal arteries 2, 3, and 4 pass dorsal to the transverse head of the adductor hallucis muscle. (1, Plantar metatarsal arteries 2, 3, 4; 2, first plantar metatarsal artery; 3, lateral bifurcation branch of *2;* 4, medial bifurcation branch of *2;* 5, lateral plantar hallucal artery; 6, medial plantar hallucal artery; 7, transverse or anastomotic segment of plantar hallucal artery; 8, medial plantar artery; 9, tibial marginal plantar artery; 10, deep branch of medial plantar artery; 11, fibular marginal plantar artery; 12, transverse head of adductor hallucis muscle.) (From Adachi B: Das Arteriensystem der Japaner, p 288. Kyoto, Maruzen, 1928)

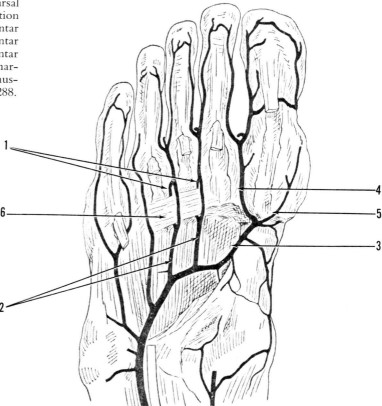

Fig. 7-33.   The second and third plantar metatarsal arteries (*2*) form an arterial loop (*1*) around the transverse head of the adductor hallucis muscle (*6*). (3, First plantar metatarsal artery; 4, lateral division branch of *3;* 5, medial division branch of *3.*) (From Adachi B: Das Arteriensystem der Japaner, p 289. Kyoto, Maruzen, 1928)

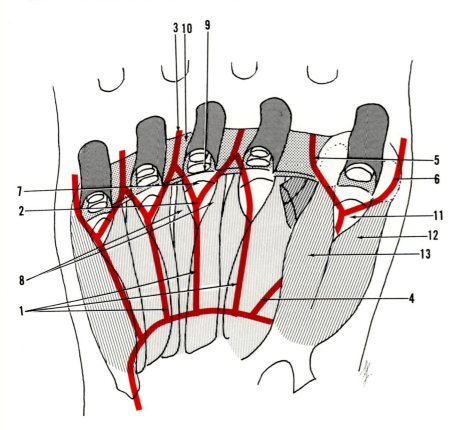

Fig. 7-34. The vascular triangle (7) overlies the plantar aspect of the metatarsal head. The apex is proximal and the base distal, corresponding to the distal segment of the plantar plate (9). The sides are formed by the corresponding interossei muscle (8). Plantar metatarsal arteries (1) bifurcate at the level of the vascular triangle (2) and form at the level of the deep transverse metatarsal ligament (10) the common digital artery (3). The first plantar metatarsal artery (4) passes dorsal to the lateral head of the flexor hallucis brevis muscle (13) and reaches the vascular triangle (11) of the big toe, where it bifurcates into the lateral (5) and medial (6) branches. (12, medial head of flexor hallucis brevis muscle.)

branches of the same bifurcation may unite and form an arterial arcade.[8]

Murakami describes two sets of plantar metatarsal arteries: superficial and deep (Fig. 7-35).[13] The superficial branches are located on the plantar aspect of the interossei muscles and are subdivided into two groups—the superficial metatarsal arteries (2–5) and the superficial intermetatarsal arteries (2–4). They all originate from the deep plantar arch, and almost all (38 of 40) are covered initially by the "accessory slips of the lateral two or three interosseous muscles arising from the lateral border of the plantar aponeurosis."[13]

The superficial metatarsal arteries course distally along the long axis of the corresponding metatarsals and reach the triangular space described above. Except for the superficial metatarsal artery 2, they are separated from the bone by the interossei muscles.

The superficial intermetatarsal arteries course over the interossei in the intermetatarsal space in the direction of the web space and reach the proximal border of the deep transverse metatarsal ligament.

Any of the superficial arteries may take an oblique course when the deep plantar arch is formed entirely or almost completely by the deep plantar artery of the dorsalis pedis artery (see Fig. 7-31).

The deep branches arise from the deep plantar arch or from the proximal perforating arteries. They penetrate the interossei muscles and are divided into two groups: deep metatarsal arteries (2–5) and deep intermetatarsal arteries (2–4).

The deep metatarsal arteries course distally on the plantar aspect of the metatarsal bones, between the plantar and dorsal interossei, and reach the triangular space at the neck of the corresponding metatarsal. The deep intermetatarsal arteries course distally between the plantar and dorsal interossei muscles in the intermetatarsal space. They descend on the medial surface of the lateral three metatarsal bones and enter the triangular space from the medial side. Any of the deep plantar arteries may also take an oblique course when the contribution of the dorsalis pedis to the deep plantar arch predominates.

Murakami's description, based on a study of 40 feet, provides the basis for the potential forms of the plantar metatarsal arteries, similar to the potential arterial system described on the dorsum of the foot.[5] Furthermore, it explains clearly that a "metatarsal" artery may be in a metatarsal or intermetatarsal position, the latter being the accepted location in most of the anatomy textbooks.

A fifth superficial plantar metatarsal artery is described by Murakami as the artery running distally between the third plantar interosseous muscle and the flexor digiti minimi brevis.[13] This artery may share a common trunk with the lateral marginal artery (Adachi's arteria plantaris superficialis lateralis). The lateral marginal artery, which may also arise independently from the lateral plantar artery, pierces the lateral intermuscular septum and courses distally between the flexor digiti minimi brevis and the abductor minimi muscles; it is present in 22.5%.[18]

The presence of the different components of the plantar "metatarsal" arteries is variable. The most commonly occurring arteries are the superficial plantar metatarsal arteries. Murakami provides data concerning these variations (Table 7-10).[13]

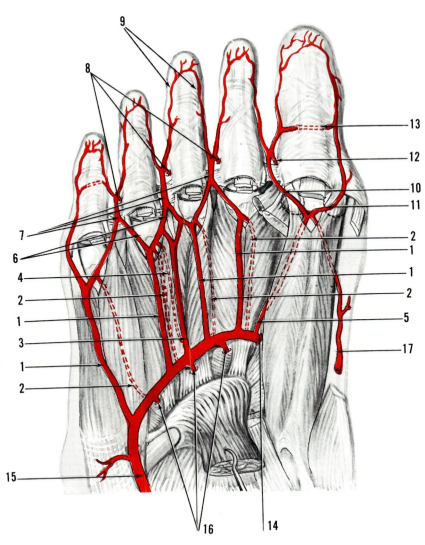

Fig. 7-35. Potential pattern of the plantar metatarsal arteries. The first superficial plantar metatarsal artery, not represented in this diagram, passes plantar to the flexor hallucis brevis. It originates from the tibial plantar marginal artery and connects with the medial bifurcation branch of the first deep plantar metatarsal artery at the level of the vascular triangle of the big toe. In the first metatarsal interspace, Murakami considers the first dorsal interosseous artery as the first superficial plantar intermetatarsal artery and describes another slender branch, more plantar in position, as the first deep plantar intermetatarsal artery; the latter arises from the first deep plantar metatarsal artery. (1, Superficial plantar metatarsal arteries, second to fifth; 2, deep plantar metatarsal arteries, second to fifth; 3, superficial plantar intermetatarsal artery; 4, intermediary plantar metatarsal artery; 5, first deep plantar metatarsal artery; 6, lateral and medial bifurcation branches of plantar metatarsal artery; 7, common plantar digital arteries; 8, distal perforating arteries; 9, plantar digital arteries, lateral and medial; 10, lateral bifurcation branch of first deep plantar metatarsal artery; 11, medial bifurcation branch of first deep plantar metatarsal artery; 12, first distal perforating artery or descending segment of first dorsal interosseous artery; 13, transverse anastomotic branch between plantar hallucal arteries; 14, first proximal perforating artery or vertical descending segment of dorsalis pedis artery; 15, lateral plantar artery; 16, proximal perforating arteries; 17, tibial plantar marginal artery, a superficial branch of medial plantar artery.) (Adapted from Murakami T: On the position and course of the deep plantar arteries, with special reference to the so-called plantar metatarsal arteries. Okajimas Folia Anat Jpn 48:295, 1971)

TABLE 7-10   Frequency of Occurrence (%) of Plantar "Metatarsal" Arteries

Plantar "Metatarsal" Arteries	Metatarsal Arteries		Intermetatarsal Arteries	
	Superficial	Deep	Superficial	Deep
Second	85★	22.5	32.5	32.5
Third	82.5	30	25	57.5
Fourth	62.5	57.5	22.5	67.5
Fifth	80	37.5	Mag† = 22.5	

★Includes the intermediate plantar metatarsal artery, which descends directly on the plantar surface of the second metatarsal bone.
† Mag, lateral marginal plantar artery

Plantar Digital Arteries of Lesser Toes

The plantar metatarsal arteries are the major source of blood supply to the lesser toes except the tibial aspect of the second toe. As described by Murakami, the superficial plantar metatarsal, the deep plantar metatarsal, and the deep plantar intermetatarsal arteries enter the triangular spaces located on the plantar aspect of the second to fifth metatarsal necks (Figs. 7-35 and 7-36).[13] The sides of the triangular space formed by the interossei muscles and the plantar aspect are crossed by the transverse head of the adductor hallucis muscle. In the triangular space the superficial plantar metatarsal, deep plantar metatarsal, and deep plantar intermetatarsal arteries anastomose and form a common trunk. A pair of transversely directed anastomotic branches take off from the latter; these branches pass between the sides of the metatarsal neck and the interossei and form two dorsally directed perforating arteries that then anastomose with similar branches arising from the dorsal metatarsal artery.[5] The common plantar arterial trunk bifurcates into two terminal branches at the level of the triangular space. Each branch bends sharply and passes between the distal border of the

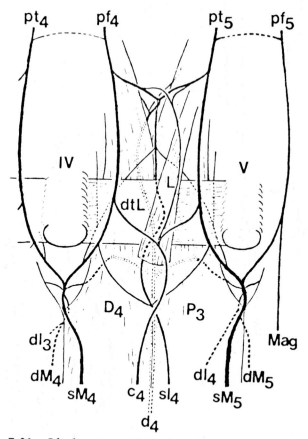

Fig. 7-36.   Ideal pattern of the branching and anastomosis of the deep metatarsal descending arteries. (*IV*, ray of fourth toe; *V*, ray of fifth toe; *L*, lumbrical muscle; *dtL*, deep transverse metatarsal ligament; D_4, fourth dorsal interosseous muscle; P_3, third plantar interosseous muscle; sM_4, sM_5, superficial plantar metatarsal arteries; dM_4, dM_5, deep plantar metatarsal arteries; sI_4, superficial plantar intermetatarsal artery; dI_3, dI_4, deep plantar intermetatarsal arteries; c_4, common superficial digital artery; d_4, dorsal interosseous artery; *Mag*, lateral marginal plantar artery; pt_4 and pf_4, tibial and fibular plantar arteries to the fourth toe; pt_5 and pf_5, tibial and fibular plantar arteries to the fifth toe.) (From Murakami T: On the position and course of the deep plantar arteries, with special reference to the so-called plantar metatarsal arteries. Okajimas Folia Anat Jpn 48:295, 1971)

transverse head of the adductor hallucis and the deep transverse metatarsal ligaments. The artery courses on the plantar aspect of the latter, along the flexor tendon sheath, and terminates as the corresponding proper plantar digital artery, which is joined by the bifurcation branch of the distal perforating branch of the corresponding dorsal metatarsal artery.

The superficial plantar intermetatarsal artery extends distally in the intermetatarsal space, passes dorsal to the deep transverse metatarsal ligament, and unites with the distal perforating branch of the dorsal metatarsal artery. The superficial plantar intermetatarsal artery may give two branches at the distal segment of the intermetatarsal space. These two branches are inconstant and, when present, join

the terminal branches of the superficial plantar metatarsal, deep plantar metatarsal, and deep plantar intermetatarsal arteries to form an arterial arcade.

Adachi provides the following information with regard to the blood supplied by the plantar metatarsal artery to the toes in 100 feet: in web space 2 (toes 2–3), 84.8%; in web space 3 (toes 3–4), 96%; in web space 4 (toes 4–5), 76%.[2] The substitutions are provided by the dorsal metatarsal arteries, the common plantar digital arteries, and the superficial plantar fibular artery or lateral marginal artery.

The major blood supply to the lesser toes except for the tibial side of the second toe is provided by the proper plantar digital arteries. The dorsal digital arteries may be thin or short, ending in the proximal part of the dorsum of the proximal phalanx. In a lesser toe, one proper plantar digital artery may predominate.

Levame, in an arteriographic study of 11 feet (9 adult, 2 fetuses of 4 months), reports the tibial-sided proper plantar digital artery to predominate in the toes 2 to 4.[12] The corresponding plantar digital artery on the fibular aspect of the toe is absent or always frail (Fig. 7-37).

The proper plantar digital arteries terminate in a tuft, and this "terminal arborization is a major and constant site of communication between each pair of plantar digitals."[8] In the "adult" form of arborization, a proximal arcade is present at the level of the tuft.[8]

A transverse anastomotic branch may be seen passing between the plantar aspect of the proximal phalanx of the little toe and the flexor tendons.[8, 13] Murakami cites the frequency of the occurrence of this anastomosis as 32.5% in 40 feet.[13]

Posterior Peroneal Artery

The posterior peroneal artery is the posterior bifurcation branch of the peroneal artery. It descends vertically along the posterior tibiofibular ligament and is located in the compartment of the flexor hallucis longus muscle–tendon, which is covered by the deep crural aponeurosis. The artery is anterior in the narrow interval between the flexor hallucis longus and the peroneus brevis. Farther distally, the flexor hallucis longus tendon parts medially, thus enlarging the posterior intertendinous interval that would give access to the artery. During its downward course, the artery traces a curve with an anterior concavity behind the peronei tendons and terminates on the lateral surface of the os calcis. To reach its destiny the artery perforates the deep crural fascia but remains under the superficial fascia.

The posterior peroneal artery provides proximally two transverse anastomotic branches: medial and anterolateral. The medial transverse branch passes anterior to the tendon of the flexor hallucis longus and anastomoses with a similar branch emanating from the posterior tibial artery. The anterolateral branch is also transverse, passes between the peronei tendons and the lateral malleolus, and connects with the anterior lateral malleolar artery. These two transverse branches contribute to the formation of the transverse perimalleolar arterial circle. A third collateral branch takes off from the artery below the tip of the lateral malleolus, passes deep to the peronei tendons, and anastomoses anteriorly with the descending branch of the anterior lateral malleolar artery, forming a sagittal lateral malleolar arterial loop. Other small terminal branches anastomose with branches from the lateral tarsal artery and contribute to the formation of the lateral malleolar arterial rete.

Cutaneous branches are provided to the lateral aspect of the heel, and recurrent calcaneal branches ascend to the dorsal surface of the os calcis, anastomose with similar branches provided by the posterior tibial artery, and form an anastomotic arcade that contributes to the formation of the calcaneal arterial rete.

CUTANEOUS ARTERIAL SUPPLY TO THE FOOT AND ANKLE

To the Dorsum of the Foot and Ankle

The skin of the dorsum of the foot and ankle is supplied by the distal segment of the tibialis anterior artery, the dorsalis pedis artery, and the first dorsal metatarsal artery. Further contribution is given by the anterior peroneal artery, the dorsal arterial rete, and the marginal anastomotic branches along the medial and lateral borders of the foot. The dorsalis pedis artery and the first dorsal metatarsal artery form the arterial axis and are the major providers of the blood supply to the dorsal skin. The anterior peroneal artery furnishes most of the cutaneous vessels of the sinus tarsi, which are carried through the fat pad. The skin covering the extensor digitorum brevis has the poorest blood supply.[18] A quantitative study of the contribution of the dorsalis pedis and the first dorsal metatarsal arteries to the blood supply of the skin of the dorsum of the foot and ankle in 23 feet is presented by Man and Acland.[10] The dorsal skin is divided into three zones (Fig. 7-38):

Zone 1: Extends from the superior border to the inferior border of the inferior extensor retinaculum
Zone 2: Extends from zone 1 to the proximal border of the first dorsal interosseous muscle
Zone 3: Extends from zone 2 to the distal tip of the first web space

In zone 1, the arterial branches pass between the arms of the extensor retinaculum. There are 5.4 arterial branches, with a diameter of 0.15 mm to 0.7 mm (average, 0.3 mm) and a mean total cross sectional area of 0.53 mm.[2] Two thirds of the branches pass between the tendons of the extensor digitorum longus and the extensor hallucis longus; one third of the branches course more medially and then pass between the extensor hallucis longus tendon and the tibialis anterior tendon.

In zone 2, the dorsalis pedis artery is crossed obliquely by the extensor hallucis brevis. The purely cutaneous branches are 1.9 in number, with a mean total cross sectional area of 0.16 mm.[2] If the arterial branches supplying the extensor hallucis brevis also are included with the assumption that they might reach the skin, the number of the arterial branches is 3.8, with a diameter of 0.15 mm to 0.7 mm (mean, 0.29 mm) and a mean total cross sectional area of 0.30 mm.[2]

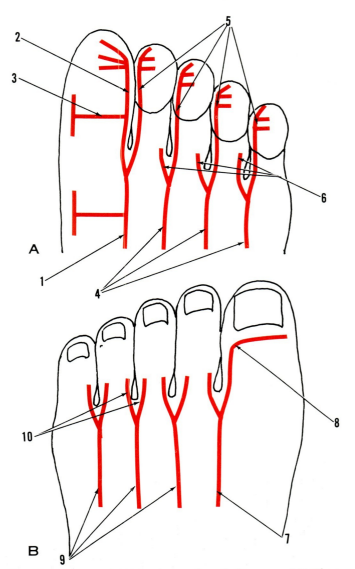

Fig. 7-37. Arterial blood supply of the toes. (*A*) Plantar aspect. Five plantar digital collateral arteries are constant: the peroneal hallucal plantar artery (*2*) and the four tibial plantar digital arteries (*5*). The peroneal plantar digital arteries (*6*) are not well developed. (1, First plantar metatarsal artery; 3, anastomotic transverse plantar hallucal artery; 4, plantar metatarsal arteries.) (*B*) Dorsal aspect. One dorsal peroneal hallucal artery (*8*) is constant. The dorsal collateral arteries of the lesser toes (*10*) are not well developed. (*7*, First dorsal intermetatarsal artery. 9, dorsal metatarsal arteries of lesser toes.) (Redrawn from Levame JH: Les artères des orteils: Etude anatomique et arteriographique: Conclusions chirugicales. J Chir 86, No. 6:651, 1963)

In zone 3, the provider is the first dorsal metatarsal artery. The cutaneous branches are 6.7 in number, with a diameter ranging from 0.15 mm to 0.33 mm (mean, 0.27 mm) and a mean total cross sectional area of 0.45 mm.[2] When the first dorsal metatarsal artery is missing (14% in this study), the cutaneous branches are absent and "the cutaneous blood supply in such cases presumably comes from the subdermal plexus."[10]

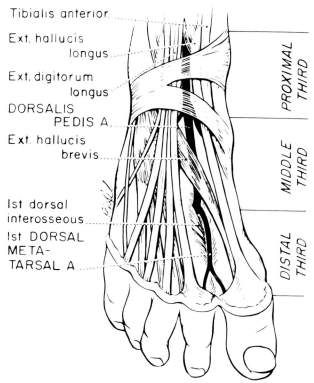

Tibialis anterior
Ext. hallucis
      longus
Ext. digitorum
      longus
DORSALIS
      PEDIS A.
Ext. hallucis
      brevis
Ist dorsal
interosseous
Ist DORSAL
META-
TARSAL A

PROXIMAL THIRD

MIDDLE THIRD

DISTAL THIRD

Fig. 7-38. Zones of the skin of the dorsum of the foot. (From Man D, Acland RD: The microarterial anatomy of the dorsalis pedis flap and its clinical applications. Plast Reconstr Surg 65, No. 4:419, 1980)

To the Malleolar Skin

The blood supply of the malleolar skin is provided by the malleolar rete. The *lateral malleolar rete,* a fine-meshed subcutaneous network, is formed by arterial twigs emanating from the sagittal and the transverse perilateral malleolar arterial loops and the lateral tarsal artery. Small recurrent branches from the lateral plantar artery may reach the network. The *medial malleolar rete* over the medial malleolus has finer arterial branches, and the loose network is formed by the anterior and posterior medial malleolar branches and the medial tarsal artery.

To the Heel

The skin of the medial aspect of the heel possesses more arteries than that of the lateral aspect.[8] The medial calcaneal branches provided by the lateral plantar artery stem from two or three main branches, which then divide, pass through the flexor retinaculum, and reach the skin of the heel. Several other smaller branches originate farther distally. The first medial calcaneal branch may emanate from the end of the posterior tibial artery. The lateral calcaneal branches are provided by the posterior peroneal artery above and by the lateral tarsal artery below.

As mentioned by Edwards, the upper lateral calcaneal branch may stem from the posterior tibial artery and the lower calcaneal branches may arise from the lateral plantar artery or the anterior peroneal artery.[8]

To the Planta Pedis

The skin of the planta pedis is as well vascularized as the skin of the scalp.[18] In the midtarsal area, the small perforating vessels are numerous and are provided by the medial and, to a larger degree, the lateral plantar arteries. The medial vertical branches pass through the medial plantar sulcus between the abductor hallucis and the flexor digitorum brevis. The lateral perforating branches pass through the lateral plantar sulcus between the flexor digitorum brevis and the abductor digiti quinti.

At the anterior segment of the planta pedis the skin is supplied by the cutaneous branches emanating from the common plantar digital arteries. These branches perforate the plantar aponeurosis to reach the skin.

ARTERIAL BLOOD SUPPLY TO THE SUPERFICIAL MUSCLES OF THE SOLE AND DORSUM OF THE FOOT

The *extensor digitorum brevis* muscle receives two arterial branches from the proximal lateral tarsal artery.[20] The branches penetrate the muscle from the posteromedial aspect of the proximal segment. Small arterial branches arise from the dorsalis pedis artery and penetrate the extensor hallucis brevis component at the level at which the latter crosses the artery distally.[18] Branches are also supplied to the muscle by the arcuate artery.

The *abductor hallucis* muscle is supplied by three to four arterial pedicles arising from the medial plantar artery as it crosses the interval between the abductor hallucis and the flexor digitorum brevis.[20] The arteries penetrate the muscle from the muscle's posterolateral aspect.

The *flexor digitorum brevis* receives arterial branches proximally from the lateral plantar artery.[20] The branches penetrate the dorsal surface of the muscle. The middle segment of the muscle is supplied from the medial side by branches arising from the medial plantar artery.

The *abductor digiti minimi* receives two to three arterial branches from the lateral plantar artery.[20] The branches penetrate the posterior segment of the muscle.

OSSEOUS ARTERIAL BLOOD SUPPLY TO THE FOOT AND ANKLE

Distal End of the Tibia and Fibula

The transverse perimalleolar arterial anastomotic circle, the medial and lateral malleolar rete, and the lateral malleolar sagittal arterial loop provide the blood to the distal tibia and fibula (Fig. 7-39). The anterior and posterior tibial and peroneal arteries are the providers of this arterial network. As described by Crock, "radiate epiphyseal arteries penetrate the distal tibial epiphysis" circumferentially and are located in a grid fashion near the epiphyseal plate or its remnant in the adult.[21] From this network, "branches drop vertically downward to end in the subchondral capillary bed" and a

Fig. 7-39. Osseous blood supply of the distal end of the tibia—a coronal section through the center of the lower ends of the tibia and fibula. The gridlike arrangement of the arterial network formed by the radiate arteries (*1*) is shown together with their vertically descending branches (*2*), which form the subchondral capillary bed. A medial malleolar descending artery (*3*) is indicated. (From Crock HV: The Blood Supply of the Lower Limb Bones in Man—Descriptive and Applied, p 74. Edinburgh, Churchill Livingstone, 1967)

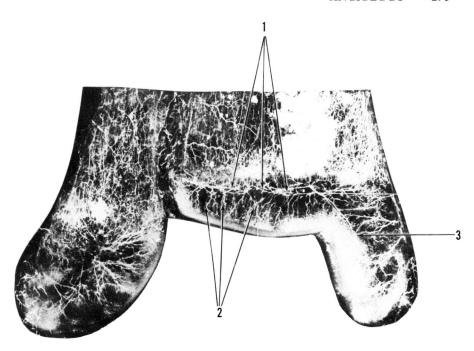

vertical branch penetrates the mid segment of the medial malleolus, which also receives radiate vessels from the nonarticular medial surface.[21] The lateral malleolus possesses a profuse arterial intraosseous network.

Talus

The arterial blood supply to the talus is provided by the three major arteries: dorsalis pedis or anterior tibial, posterior tibial, and peroneal (Figs. 7-40–7-42).[14, 15, 22, 23] More specifically, the providers are as follows:

> *The artery of the sinus tarsi.* As described previously, this artery arises more frequently from the dorsalis pedis artery or from any of the following—the proximal lateral tarsal artery, the anterior lateral malleolar artery, the perforating peroneal artery, or the ansa formed between the proximal lateral tarsal artery and the perforating peroneal artery.
>
> *The artery of the tarsal canal,* a branch of the posterior tibial artery or, less frequently, a branch of the medial plantar artery[14]
>
> *The deltoid artery,* a branch of the artery of the tarsal canal or, less frequently, a branch of the posterior tibial artery[14, 15]
>
> *Superomedial direct branches,* provided by the dorsalis pedis artery
>
> *Posterior direct branches,* provided by the peroneal artery

The artery of the sinus tarsi and the artery of the tarsal canal anastomose in the canalis tarsi and form the major arterial axis of the talus. This arterial line is located posterior to the talar neck level. There is a large anastomosis between the deltoid branch of the artery of the tarsal canal and the arteries of the superior aspect of the neck, and this anastomotic periosteal network continues into the sinus tarsi and

ends at the anterior edge of the talar articular surface of the lateral malleolus.[22]

Intraosseous Territory. The intraosseous territory of each artery is defined by Mulfinger and Trueta as follows.[14]

Head. The superomedial half of the talar head is supplied by direct branches from the dorsalis pedis artery or from the anterior tibial artery that penetrate the upper surface of the neck. The inferolateral half of the talar head is supplied by branches from the artery of the sinus tarsi and its anastomosis or by direct branches from the lateral tarsal artery.

Body. The artery of the tarsal canal and its anastomosis provide four or five main branches, which are directed posterolaterally. They supply the lateral two thirds of the talar body except for a small superior area in the middle third (supplied by the superior neck arteries), the lateral aspect of the posterior facet, and a variable amount of the lateral edge of the talar body.

The arteries from the anastomotic network in the tarsal sinus enter through the lateral anterior surface of the talar body and supply the lateral inferior segment and most of the posterior facet. The medial third or fourth of the talar body is supplied by the deltoid branches entering from the medial surface of the talus. The posterior tubercle is supplied by small branches from the posterior anastomotic network formed by the peroneal artery and the posterior tibial artery.

Variations. Mulfinger and Trueta report the following intraosseous territorial variations in 30 feet: lateral branches from the anstomotic network of the tarsal sinus supplying the lateral quarter of the body, 33.3%; superior neck vessels supplying approximately one third of the body, 6.6%; superior neck vessels not penetrating the bone, 23.3%.[14]

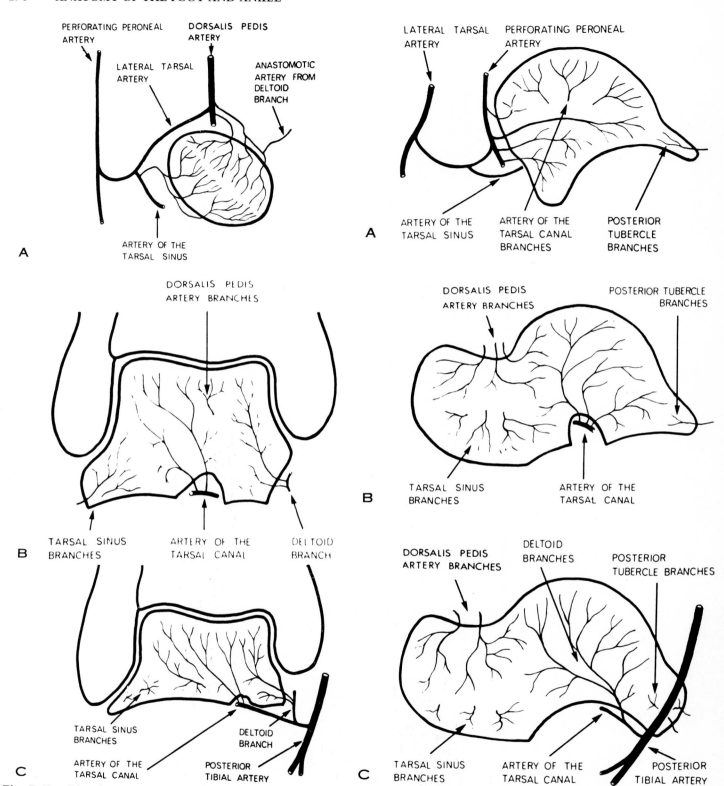

Fig. 7-40. Blood supply to the talus in coronal sections. (*A*) Blood supply to the head of the talus. (*B*) Blood supply to the middle third of the talus. (*C*) Blood supply to the posterior third of the talus. (From Mulfinger GL, Trueta J: The blood supply of the talus. J Bone Joint Surg [Br] 52, No. 1:160, 1970)

Fig. 7-41. Blood supply to the talus in sagittal sections. (*A*) Blood supply to the lateral third of the talus. (*B*) Blood supply to the middle third of the talus. (*C*) Blood supply to the medial third of the talus. (From Mulfinger GL, Trueta J: The blood supply of the talus. J Bone Joint Surg [Br] 52, No. 1:160, 1970)

Anastomosis. The intraosseous arteries may anastomose with each other. The anastomotic types and the frequency of their occurrence is reported by Mulfinger and Trueta in 30 feet as follows: between the superior neck arteries and the branches from the artery of the tarsal canal, 26.6%; between the inferior and superior branches in the head, 13.3%; between the branches from the artery of the sinus tarsi and the artery of the tarsal canal within the bone, 13.3%; between the posterior tubercle branches and the artery of the tarsal canal, 3.3%; between the deltoid branches and the artery of the tarsal canal, 3.3% (approximate total, 60%).[14]

Zchakaja, in a chronological study of the arterial blood supply in 68 feet, describes the following number of intraosseous talar arterial branches:

Newborn: 6 to 7 arterial branches penetrate the perichondrium from the lateral, inferior, superior, and medial surfaces and reach the ossification center, where they branch out.

Age group 13 to 14 years: 25 to 26 arterial branches are present, of which 17 are constant and 8 to 9 are of the supplementary type. The distribution of the branches is as follows:

Upper surface: 6 to 7 branches with 3 permanent branches

Lower surface: 4 permanent branches and 2 to 3 supplementary

Medial surface: 4 to 6 branches, of which 4 are permanent

Lateral surface: 1 to 2 branches entering through the anterior aspect of the lateral talar process

Posterior surface: 2 to 4 branches penetrating from each side of the posterior talar process

Age group 25 to 60 years: With aging the supplementary arterial branches decrease in number (25-year-old age group) and disappear later (65-year-old age group), but the permanent arterial branches remain unchanged in number. However, the number of branches extending from the central anastomotic zone to the periphery decreases gradually with age, and only a few remain by age 65.[23]

Calcaneus

The calcaneus is supplied by a rich arterial network that yields branches penetrating from all the surfaces not covered by the articular surface (Fig. 7-43). The arteries providing the blood supply are the following:

Medial calcaneal artery, branch of the posterior tibial artery

Lateral calcaneal artery, branch of the peroneal artery

Peroneal artery

Posterior transverse calcaneal anastomotic arcade formed between the posterior tibial artery and the peroneal artery

Lateral and medial plantar arteries

Artery of the sinus tarsi and artery of the tarsal canal

Direct branches from the proximal lateral tarsal artery and from the perforating peroneal artery

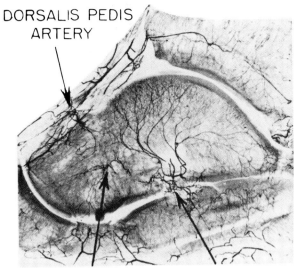

A

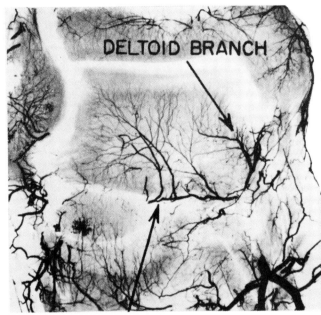

B

TARSAL CANAL ARTERY

Fig. 7-42. Blood supply to the talus. (*A*) Blood supply to the middle third of the talus through a sagittal section. (*B*) Blood supply to the middle third of the talus through a coronal section. (From Mulfinger GL, Trueta J: The blood supply of the talus. J Bone Joint Surg [Br] 52, No. 1, 1970)

Zchakaja describes the blood supply to the os calcis (age group 13 to 14 years) as follows.[23]

Superior Surface. The *frontal part* of the superior surface is supplied by the arteries of the sinus tarsi and canalis tarsi supplemented by direct branches from the proximal

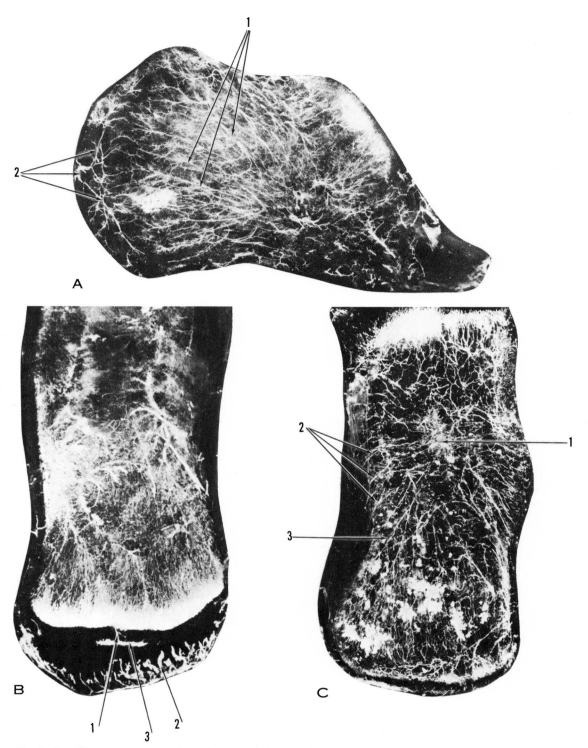

Fig. 7-43.   Blood supply to the calcaneus. (*A*) Sagittal section from the calcaneus viewed from the lateral side. Arteries penetrate the outer surface of the bone over a wide "waist area." Most of these give rise to recurrent branches (*1*), which pass backward to the epiphyseal zone of the heel, where they anastomose with epiphyseal arteries (*2*) across the site of the former growth plate. (*B*) Posterior half of a horizontal section through the middle of the calcaneus of a female child aged 11 years. The metaphyseal arteries (*1*) pass across the growth plate into the epiphysis (*3*). (*2*, Vertical peripheral epiphyseal arteries.) (*C*) Horizontal section from the calcaneus of a female aged 59 years. Peripheral penetrating arteries (*2*) converge to the center (*1*) and then sweep backward through recurrent branches (*3*) to the epiphyseal zone of the calcaneus. The periosteal network provides the radiate arteries that supply the facet areas and their subchondral capillary beds. (From Crock HV: The Blood Supply of the Lower Limb Bones in Man—Descriptive and Applied. Edinburgh, Churchill Livingstone, 1967)

lateral tarsal artery and the peroneal artery. These branches are small and 6 to 9 in number, of which 6 branches are permanent and penetrate the bone at the following sites: 2 branches enter at 0.5 cm from the anterior articular surface for the cuboid, 2 branches enter at 0.5 cm anterior to the posterior calcaneal articular surface, and 2 branches enter at the base of the sustentaculum tali. The three supplementary arteries penetrate the bone in the inner half of the calcaneal canal.

The *posterior part* of the superior surface is supplied by the calcaneal anastomotic arcade between the tibialis posterior artery and the peroneal artery and by the peroneal artery proper. There are 4 to 7 arterial branches, of which 4 branches are permanent and penetrate the bone at the following sites: 2 branches enter the bone at 0.5 cm to 1 cm posterior to the posterior calcaneal articular surface and 2 branches enter at 0.5 cm to 1 cm anterior to the posterior surface of the calcaneus.

Lateral Surface.   The *anterior segment* of the lateral surface is supplied by a branch of the proximal lateral tarsal artery and the *posterior segment* by the lateral calcaneal branches arising from the peroneal artery. Fifteen to 18 branches penetrate the bone almost at 90°, and 15 of these branches are permanent. Six of the permanent arteries are large and penetrate the bone at the following sites: 1 branch enters the bone at 0.5 cm to 1 cm posterior to the articular surface of the cuboid, 1 branch enters at the level of the posterior articular calcaneal surface, 1 branch penetrates at 0.5 cm to 1 cm posterior to the peronei tubercle, and 3 branches enter on the outer surface of the calcaneal tuberosity.

Medial Surface.   The medial calcaneal surface is supplied anteriorly by the medial plantar artery and posteriorly by the medial calcaneal branches.

The medial surface is supplied by 12 to 16 arteries; of these, 7 are of the permanent type. The 5 larger ones penetrate at the following sites: 1 penetrates the bone at 1 cm from the articular surface of the cuboid, 1 enters the bone at the base of the sustentaculum tali, 2 penetrate at the level of the posterior calcaneal tuberosity, and 1 enters the bone at 1 cm from the posterior rim. The foraminae of the remaining 5 to 9 supplementary arteries are aligned parallel to the sulcus of the flexor hallucis longus tendon at 1 cm below the latter.

Plantar Surface.   The plantar calcaneal surface is supplied by the lateral and medial plantar arteries. The surface is penetrated by 5 to 6 branches; of these 4 branches are permanent and penetrate at the following sites: 3 branches enter the medial and lateral calcaneal tuberosities and 1 branch enters the bone at 1 cm from the articular surface of the cuboid. The supplementary 1 to 2 branches penetrate the bone in the middle of the plantar surface.

Posterior Surface.   The posterior calcaneal surface is supplied by the branches from the calcaneal anastomotic arcade between the posterior tibial artery and the peroneal artery, by the branches from the lateral and medial calcaneal arteries, and by the branches from the lateral and medial plantar arteries. This arterial network forms the calcaneal rete.

The arterial branches, 5 to 8 in number (4 permanent and 1 to 3 supplementary), penetrate the posterior surface between the insertion of the Achilles tendon and the origin of the plantar aponeurosis. These branches are grouped in the middle of the posterior strip and represent the epiphyseal arteries.

The calcaneal intraosseous arteries, after penetrating the bone, turn anteriorly toward the center and anastomose. Many branches take a recurrent course posteriorly and reach the zone of the epiphysis.[16, 21] The epiphyseal plate is perforated by 5 to 6 metaphyseal arterial branches.

In the newborn, Zchakaja describes arterial branches penetrating the perichondrium of the calcaneus from the medial surface (2 to 3 branches), from the lateral surface (2 branches), and from the superior surface (1 to 2 branches).[23] These arterial arteries converge on the ossification center and anastomose with each other. By 25 years of age, the supplementary arteries have decreased in number, and by 65 years of age, these arteries and the peripheral 5 arterial branches have disappeared.

Navicular

The navicular receives its blood supply from the dorsal and plantar aspects and from the tuberosity. Velluda describes an artery on the dorsal side, a branch of the dorsalis pedis, that crosses the dorsum of the navicular and provides 3 to 5 branches.[24] Occasionally there are direct branches to the dorsum from the dorsalis pedis. The plantar surface receives vessels from the medial plantar artery and the tuberosity from an anastomotic network formed by the union of these two source arteries.

Waugh, in a study of 21 injected naviculars, describes at 8 weeks and 8 months a dense perichondral network of vessels that yield numerous arteries penetrating the cartilage and aiming toward the center (Figs. 7-44–7-46).[25] At 21 months the ossification nucleus appears near the center and is fed by 1 nutrient artery. At 5 years of age, the ossification nucleus receives 5 to 6 arteries, but less commonly, it may be totally supplied by a single plantar or dorsal artery. With further growth, the multiple peripheral radial vessels are anastomosed and incorporated by the ossific nucleus. Zchakaja describes in the 4- to 5-year age group 8 to 10 vessels that penetrate the perichondrium and reach the ossification nucleus.[23] By 13 to 14 years of age, the navicular receives 15 to 21 arteries, of which 12 are permanent and 3 to 9 supplementary; they penetrate the bone at the following sites: dorsal surface—2 to 8 arteries, of which 4 are permanent, and 1 of these enters the tuberosity of the navicular; plantar surface—8 to 9 arteries, of which 5 are permanent, and 1 of these enters the tuberosity of the navicular; medial margin—3 to 4 arteries, of which 3 are permanent. Between 20 and 65 years, the supplementary arteries decrease in number.

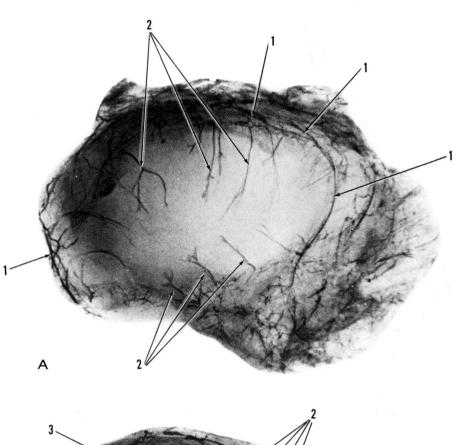

Fig. 7-44.   Blood supply to the navicular. (*A*) Fine-grain radiograph of an injected navicular from a girl aged 21 months. There is a rich perichondrial arterial network (*1*) with numerous radial penetrating arteries aiming to the center of the navicular (*2*). (*B*) Fine-grain radiograph of an injected navicular from a girl aged 21 months. The distribution is similar to *A* but a single artery–vein (*3*) reaches the ossifying nucleus (*4*). (From Waugh W: The ossification and vascularisation of the tarsal navicular and their relation to Köhler's disease. J Bone Joint Surg [Br] 40, No. 4:765, 1958)

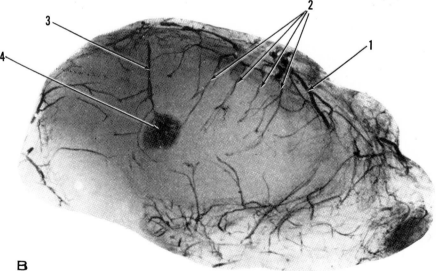

Cuneiforms

The cuneiforms receive their blood supply from their dorsal, medial, and lateral surfaces.[23] These vessels are provided mostly by the dorsal arterial rete. According to Zchakaja, in the 13- to 14-year age group the first cuneiform receives a total number of 21 to 24 arteries (17 permanent); the second cuneiform, 10 to 12 arteries (8 permanent); the third cuneiform, 14 to 16 arteries (11 permanent).[23] Between 21 and 65 years the number of supplementary arteries decreases.

Cuboid

The cuboid receives its blood supply from the plantar arterial rete formed by the deep branches of the lateral and medial plantar arteries, with contribution from the dorsal arterial rete. The bone is penetrated by 25 to 27 arterial branches (12 permanent) from the dorsal, medial, lateral, and plantar surfaces. The plantar arterial branch predominates, and the larger vessel on the plantar aspect enters at the level of the cuboid tuberosity and the remainder through the sulcus for the tendon of the peroneus longus.

Fig. 7-45.   Blood supply to the navicular. (*A*) Fine-grain radiograph of an injected and decalcified navicular from a girl aged 3.5 years. Radiate penetrating vessels (*1*) (six vessels counted from a study of the Spalteholz specimen) enter the central bony nucleus (*2*). (*B*) Fine-grain radiograph of an injected and decalcified navicular from a youth aged 19 years. Numerous radiate penetrating vessels (*1*) anastomose with each other (*2*) at the center and its periphery. (From Waugh W: The ossification and vascularisation of the tarsal navicular and their relation to Köhler's disease. J Bone Joint Surg [Br] 40, No. 4:765, 1958)

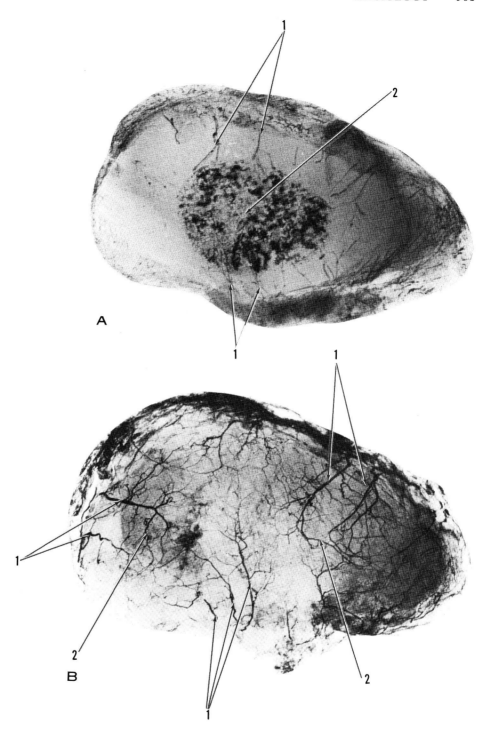

Metatarsals

The *metatarsals 2, 3, and 4* have a similar pattern of arterial supply provided by the dorsal and plantar metatarsal arteries. As described by Zchakaja, in the age group 13 to 14 years the diaphysis is supplied by 13 to 14 arterial branches entering the bone from the dorsal (5 to 6 branches), the medial (3 to 4 branches), and the lateral (3 to 4 branches) surface. The nutrient artery penetrates the lateral diaphyseal surface near the base and divides into 2 branches, distal and proximal. The distal branch is the strongest; it runs toward the epiphysis and divides into 6 to 7 branches that anastomose with the metaphyseal vessels. The proximal branch is smaller, maintains the oblique direction of the mother stem, and reaches the base of the metatarsal. The metaphysis is supplied by 7 arterial branches. Four to 6 arterial branches penetrate the epiphysis from the lateral and medial surfaces.

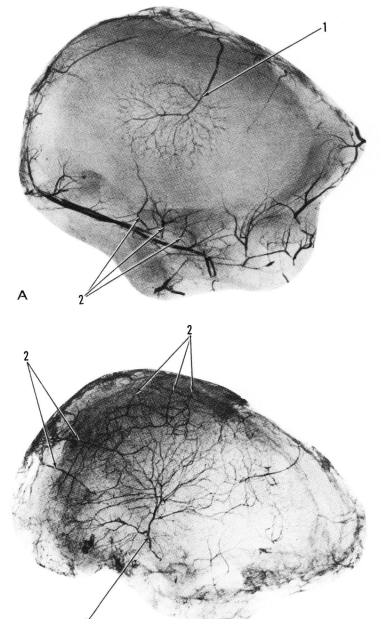

Fig. 7-46.   Blood supply to the navicular. (A) Fine-grain radiograph of an injected and decalcified navicular from a girl aged 4 years. A single main artery (1) from the dorsal surface branches and outlines the whole of the central bony nucleus. A few penetrating radiate vessels (2) are seen but take little part in the anastomotic network. (B) Fine-grain radiograph of a decalcified navicular from a boy aged 13 years. A large part of the bone is supplied by a single plantar artery (1). Other radial vessels (2) contribute to the blood supply of the bone. (From Waugh W: The ossification and vascularisation of the tarsal navicular and their relation to Köhler's disease. J Bone Joint Surg [Br] 40, No. 4:765, 1958)

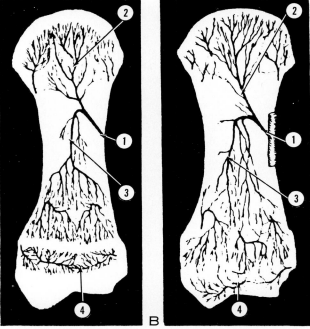

Fig. 7-47.   Blood supply to the first metatarsal bone. (A) In an adolescent aged 12–13 years. The nutrient artery (1) divides into a short distal (2) and a long proximal (3) branch. The distal branch anastomoses with the distal metaphyseal and capital vessels. The proximal branch is stronger and is directed proximally toward the epiphysis, which in turn is supplied by arterial branches entering from its medial and lateral sides; (4) epiphyseal vessels. (B) In the adult. (1, Nutrient artery; 2, distal division branch of 1; 3, proximal division branch of 1 anastomosing with the epiphyseal vessels [4].) (From Anseroff NJ: Die Arterien des Skelets der Hand und des Fusses des Mensche. Z Anat Entwicklungs 106:204, 1937)

The *metatarsal 5* receives its nutrient artery from the medial surface of the diaphysis and also receives arterial branches from the plantar aspect of the proximal diaphysis (3 to 5 branches) in addition to the arterial supply from the dorsal (5 to 6 branches) and medial (2 to 3 branches) surfaces. Two arterial branches penetrate the lateral aspect of the tuberosity. Distally the metaphysis is supplied by 3 to 4 small arterial branches and the epiphysis by 2 to 3 branches entering from the medial and lateral aspects. At times, the lateral epiphyseal vessel is missing.

The *metatarsal 1* has an arterial supply pattern similar to that of the proximal phalanx of the lesser toes (Fig. 7-47). The nutrient artery penetrates the diaphysis in the middle of the lateral surface at an angle of 90° and divides into 2 branches, proximal and distal. The distal branch is weaker; it runs distally and anastomoses with the arteries of the metaphysis and of the head. The metaphysis receives 4 to 5 arterial branches and the head, 12 to 16 small arteries penetrating from its medial and lateral aspects. The proximal, stronger branch is directed proximally toward the epiphysis, which is supplied by 4 to 8 arterial branches entering through the medial and lateral surfaces.

Phalanges

The proximal phalanges receive their blood supply predominantly from the dorsal digital arteries, the middle phalanges are supplied by the plantar and dorsal digital arteries, whereas the distal phalanges have predominantly a plantar supply.[23]

In the age group 13 to 14 years, the nutrient artery of the *proximal phalanges* penetrates the diaphysis from the lateral surface except for the artery of the fifth toe, which enters from the medial surface. In the bone, the nutrient artery divides into a distal, relatively weak and a proximal, stronger branch. The diaphysis receives 13 to 16 smaller branches entering mostly from the dorsal surface, to a lesser degree from the lateral and plantar surfaces, and minimally from the medial side. The epiphysis is supplied by 4 arterial branches.

The *middle phalanges* receive diaphyseal vessels from the periosteal network. These vessels penetrate the bone from the dorsal and plantar aspects. The epiphysis receives 2 arterial branches from the lateral and medial aspects.

The *distal phalanx of the big toe* has a large nutrient artery that penetrates the bone from the lateral rim of the mid diaphyseal segment; another large artery penetrates the bone from the plantar aspect. The metaphyseal area receives dorsal (6 to 8) and plantar (4 to 6) branches. The epiphysis is penetrated by 4 to 6 branches from the dorsal and plantar aspects. As the nutrient artery enters the bone, it divides into a weak distal and a stronger proximal branch. The distal branch runs distally and anastomoses with the artery entering the tuft.

The *distal phalanges of toes 2 through 5* have a similar pattern of blood supply. The diaphyseal vessel penetrates from the plantar surface in the middle third. The tuft is entered on each side by a branch, and the epiphysis receives 2 dorsal and 2 plantar arteries.

Sesamoids of the Big Toe

The two sesamoids of the metatarsophalangeal joint of the big toe receive their blood supply from the first plantar metatarsal artery. Two to 3 arteries penetrate the sesamoids from the sides and 1 to 2 branches from the center. These multiple branches anastomose in the center of the sesamoid.

Veins

The veins of the foot are divided into a dorsal and a plantar system. Contrary to the rest of the lower extremity, the flow in the foot is bidirectional, or when valves are present, the flow is from the depth of the planta to the superficial dorsal system.[26]

DORSAL VEINS OF THE FOOT

There are two superficial venous networks and one deep venous network in the dorsum of the foot, separated by the superficial and the deep dorsal fascias (Figs. 7-48 and 7-49).

Fig. 7-48.   Dorsal and plantar veins of the foot. (*A*) Veins of the dorsal aspect of the foot. (1, Anterolateral malleolar veins; 2, lateral marginal vein; 3, proximal interosseous perforating veins; 4, distal perforating interdigital veins; 5, communicating vein of first interosseous space; 6, medial marginal vein; 7, dorsalis pedis veins; 8, anteromedial malleolar vein.) (*B*) Deep veins of the plantar aspect of the foot. (1, Medial plantar vein; 2, periscaphoid venous circle receiving articular veins; 3, lateral plantar vein receiving plantar interosseous veins; 4, peroneus longus tendon; 5, peroneal communicating veins; 6, calcaneocuboid ligament.) (From Winckler G: Les veines du pied. Arch Anat Histol Embryol 37:175, 1954–1955)

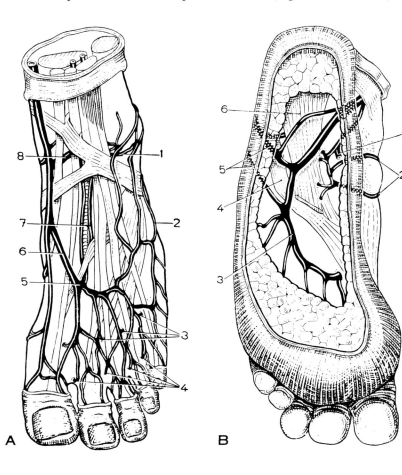

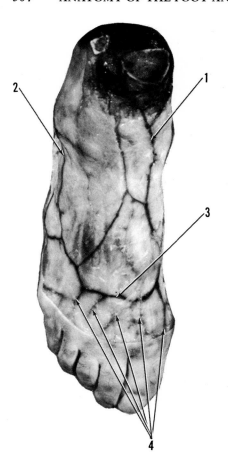

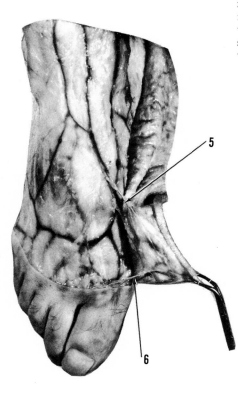

Fig. 7-49. Veins of the dorsum of the foot. (1, Greater saphenous vein; 2, branch forming lesser saphenous veins; 3, dorsal venous arc; 4, dorsal superficial interosseous veins; 5, 6, superficial subcuticular venous branches.)

Superficial Dorsal Venous Networks

The superficial dorsal veins and the greater and lesser saphenous veins with the dorsal venous arch constitute the superficial venous networks.

Superficial Dorsal Veins. The superficial dorsal veins are located immediately under the skin, superficial to the superficial dorsal aponeurosis of the foot.[27] They form a thin-meshed venous network with branches measuring up to 2 mm in diameter. The branches arise from the skin of the dorsum of the toes and from the superficial plantar veins. Other roots originate from the major dorsal venous arcade. The branches converge longitudinally to the anterior aspect of the ankle and join the saphenous venous system proximally. The superficial dorsal veins may take over the lesser saphenous vein when the latter does not reach the forefoot or they may be connected to the deep venous system (dorsalis pedis or plantar) through a perforating vein.[26]

Greater and Lesser Saphenous Veins and the Dorsal Venous Arch. This superficial venous network starts with the dorsal veins of the toes, which represent the major drainage route of the toes. As described by Winckler, these veins are formed at the level of the distal and middle phalanges of the toe by a median vein draining the nail matrix and two collateral dorsal veins (Figs. 7-50 and 7-51).[27] The

median vein bifurcates and joins the two dorsal veins in an M configuration. On the dorsum of the proximal phalanx, a transverse branch unites the two dorsal veins, and the network forms a vascular circle centered on the dorsum of the proximal interphalangeal joint. The adjacent dorsal veins of the toe unite in the web space and constitute the superficial dorsal metatarsal vein, which courses posteromedially to join the dorsal venous arch. Prior to the union in the web space, the medial dorsal digital vein receives the perforating interdigital vein that originates from the plantar superficial venous arch. The proximal end of the superficial dorsal metatarsal vein in turn is connected to the distal intermetatarsal perforating vein. The venous plexus on the plantar aspect of the pulp of the toe drains into two thin plantar digital veins, which end either in the interdigital vein or in the plantar superficial venous arch.

The dorsomedial vein of the big toe and the dorsolateral vein of the fifth toe, after receiving the medial and lateral ends of the superficial plantar venous arch, join the dorsal venous arch on the medial and lateral sides, respectively, forming the greater saphenous vein on the anterior aspect of the medial malleolus and the lesser saphenous vein on the posterior aspect of the lateral malleolus. The dorsal venous arcade is convex anteriorly; it crosses the metatarsals at a variable level, 4 cm to 5 cm posterior to the web space, or may reach the level of the metatarsal heads.

On the dorsomedial aspect of the foot, the greater saphenous vein and the corresponding medial marginal vein

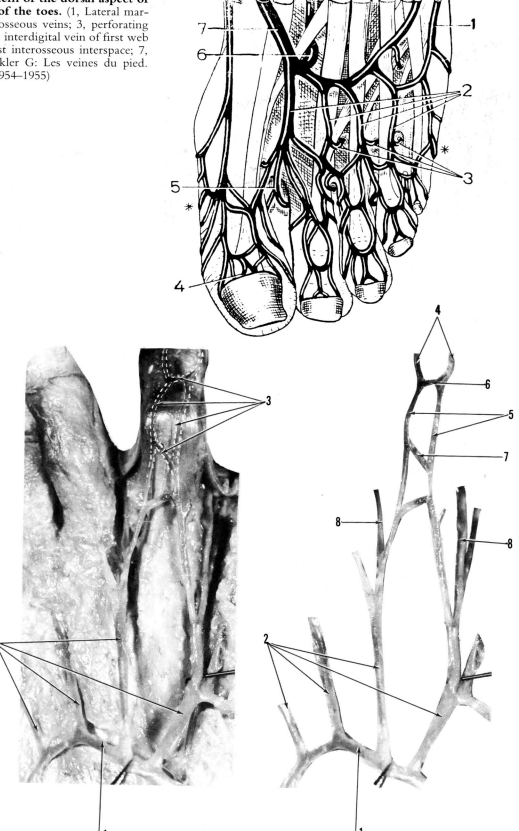

Fig. 7-50. Superficial venous system of the dorsal aspect of the web spaces and dorsal aspect of the toes. (1, Lateral marginal vein; 2, superficial dorsal interosseous veins; 3, perforating interosseous veins; 4, ungual veins; 5, interdigital vein of first web space; 6, communicating vein of first interosseous interspace; 7, medial marginal vein.) (From Winckler G: Les veines du pied. Arch Anat Histol Embryol 37:175, 1954–1955)

Fig. 7-51. Venous drainage system on the dorsum of the toe. (1, Dorsal venous arc; 2, dorsal metatarsal [or interosseous] veins; 3, venous circle centered on dorsum of proximal interphalangeal joint and formed by two dorsal collateral veins [5] anastomosed proximally [7] and distally [6] by transverse venous branches; dorsal ungual branches [4] continue with dorsal collateral veins; 8, interdigital veins penetrating corresponding web space.)

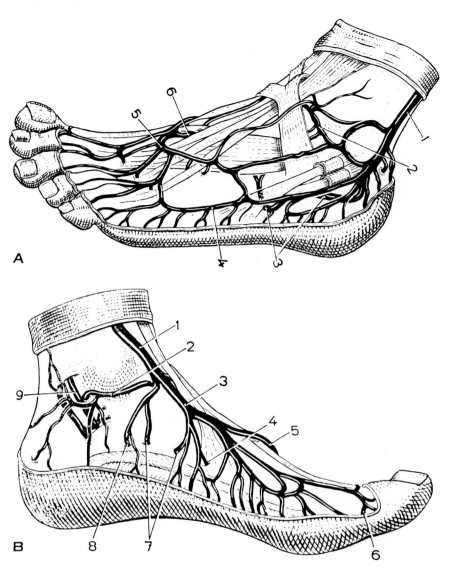

Fig. 7-52. *(A)* **Veins of the dorsolateral aspect of the foot.** (1, Lesser saphenous vein; 2, anterolateral malleolar vein; 3, communicating peroneal veins; 4, lateral marginal vein; 5, dorsal superficial venous arc; 6, communicating vein of first interosseous space.) *(B)* **Veins of the medial aspect of the foot.** (1, Major saphenous vein; 2, medial malleolar vein; 3, medial marginal vein; 4, articular vein arising from $cuneo_1$–$metatarsal_1$ joint; 5, superficial dorsal venous arc, 6, hallucal marginal communicating vein; 7, periscaphoid venous circle; 8, anastomosis between medial plantar vein and beginning of greater saphenous vein; 9, posterior tibial veins.) (From Winckler G: Les veines du pied. Arch Anat Histol Embryol 37:175, 1954–1955)

of the dorsal venous arch receive the dorsal veins of the toes, plantar veins of the toes through the interdigital veins and the superficial plantar venous arch, superficial dorsal metatarsal veins, plantar metatarsal veins through the distal intermetatarsal perforating vein, and superficial plantar venous system through the superficial marginal connecting vein.

The greater saphenous vein and its root from the dorsal venous arch are also connected with the plantar system through perforating veins. These veins are mostly articular veins and course between the abductor hallucis and the tarsus. Winckler describes the following specific perforating veins draining into the greater saphenous vein or the medial marginal vein (Figs. 7-52 and 7-53):

A vein arising from the $cuneo_1$-$metatarsal_1$ joint level
Two periscaphoid veins arising from the scaphocuneiform and the calcaneocuboid joints. These veins form a periscaphoid venous circle.

A vein uniting the medial plantar vein and the greater saphenous vein
A medial malleolar vein uniting the posterior tibial vein and the greater saphenous vein. This vein passes under the malleolus and receives superficial branches from the medial aspect of the heel and of the Achilles tendon.
The communicating vein of the first interosseous space, a perforating vein connecting the dorsal venous arcade with the medial end of the deep plantar venous arch[27]

On the dorsal side, the greater saphenous vein and the dorsalis pedis or the anterior tibial veins are united by the anteromedial malleolar vein, which is located between the bifurcation arms of the inferior extensor retinaculum under the tendons of the extensor hallucis longus and the tibialis anterior.

On the dorsolateral aspect, the lateral marginal vein is of a smaller caliber and more variable than the corresponding medial marginal vein. It courses along the lateral border of

Fig. 7-53. Veins of the medial aspect of the foot. (1, Greater saphenous vein; 2, superficial dorsal venous arc; 3, periscaphoid venous circle; 4, articular vein arising from cuneo$_1$-metatarsal$_1$ joint area.)

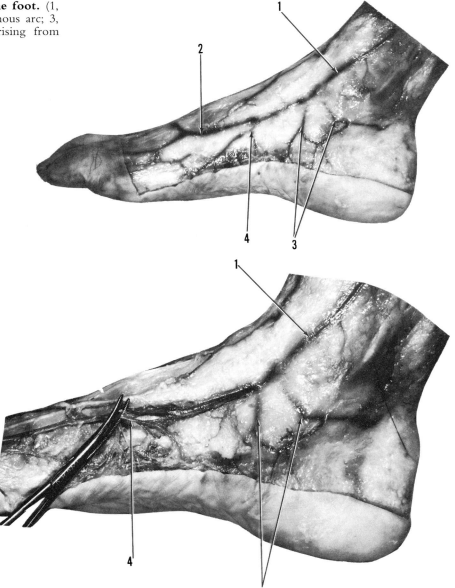

the foot, crosses the peronei tendons, and passes behind the lateral malleolus, where it forms the lesser saphenous vein (Figs. 7-52 and 7-54). It receives multiple (about 15) marginal, parallel veins arising from the superficial plantar venous system. These collaterals are distributed between the base of the fifth metatarsal and the heel. Two peroneal communicating veins, proximal and distal, are located on each side of the peroneus longus tendon as the latter makes its turn around the cuboid; these veins unite the lateral marginal vein with the lateral plantar veins. The distal communicating peroneal vein receives a branch that courses under the extensor digitorum brevis muscle and the tendon of the peroneus brevis and drains the dorsal calcaneocuboid joint. The proximal communicating peroneal vein receives a large vein from the plantar aspect of the calcaneocuboid joint.

The medial aspect of the lateral marginal vein is connected to the dorsal venous system through an oblique venous network extending to the greater saphenous vein. These veins are variable in distribution. A set of anterolateral malleolar veins is almost constantly present, connecting the lesser saphenous vein and the anterior tibial vein and contributing to the formation of a lateral malleolar venous circle; they drain the ankle joint and the tibiofibular syndesmosis.

Kuster and co-workers, in a study of 10 feet, describe 6 to 12 perforating veins connecting the deep plantar venous systems with the dorsal venous system (Fig. 7-55).[26] In 53.8% of the 91 perforators, no valves were found; in 41.7%, one valve was present; and in 4.3%, two valves were found. The valves, when present, face toward the superficial venous system, thus determining a plantar-to-

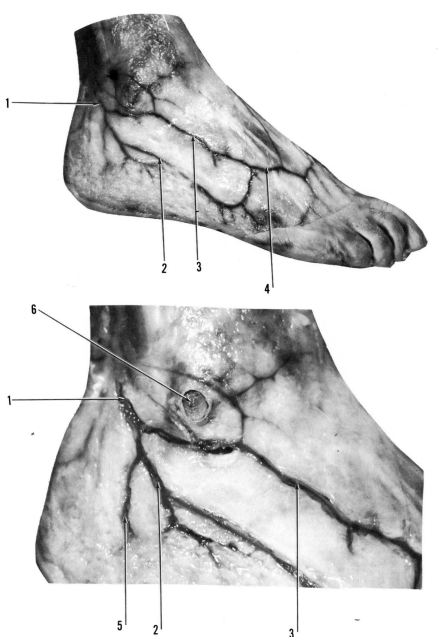

Fig. 7-54.   Veins of the lateral aspect of the foot. (1, Lesser saphenous vein; 2, lateral marginal vein; 3, anastomotic branch between dorsal superficial venous arc [4] and 1; 5, lateral calcaneal vein; 6, bursa of lateral malleolus.)

dorsal venous flow. In the perforators with no valves and in the marginal superficial connecting veins uniting the superficial plantar venous system to the dorsal veins, the blood flow is bidirectional. The perforators have a diameter ranging from 0.9 mm to 1.8 mm.

Deep Dorsal Venous Network

The deep dorsal venous network is located under the deep fascia of the foot and consists of the veins accompanying the dorsalis pedis artery and its tributaries. There are two veins for one artery. This deep venous system communicates with the greater saphenous vein through the anteromedial malleolar vein, the lesser saphenous vein through

the anterolateral malleolar vein, and the plantar metatarsal veins through the proximal and the distal perforating veins.

PLANTAR VEINS OF THE FOOT

The plantar venous network is formed by a superficial and deep plantar system (Fig. 7-48).

Superficial Plantar Venous Network

The superficial plantar venous network is formed by an extremely superficial, intradermal, and subdermal mesh (very thin) covering the sole of the foot and forming at the foot borders the medial and lateral marginal veins ending

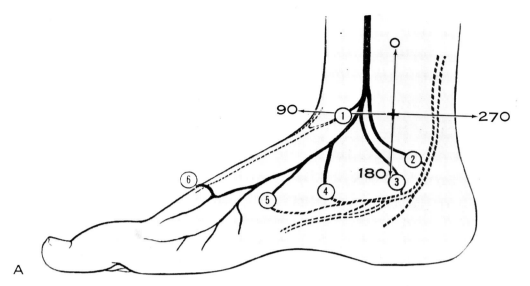

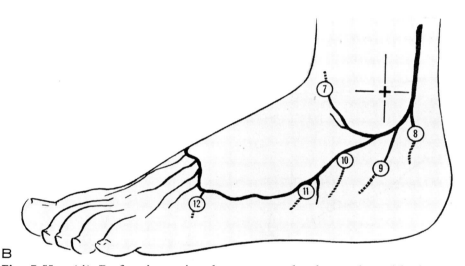

Fig. 7-55. *(A)* **Perforating veins that connect the deep veins with the greater saphenous vein.** The circled numbers indicate the places at which the perforators pierce the fascia. *Perforator 1* pierces the fascia 2.6 cm from the tip of the medial malleolus at 90°. It connects the greater saphenous vein with the dorsalis pedis vein and runs under the tendons of the extensor hallucis longus and tibialis anterior. *Perforator 2* is inconstant. It appears 2.8 cm from the medial malleolus at 200° and communicates with the medial plantar veins. *Perforator 3* pierces the fascia 3.4 cm from the medial malleolus at 180° and opens in the greater saphenous vein. It communicates with the deep plantar venous arch. *Perforator 4* pierces the fascia 5.33 cm from the malleolus at 136°. *Perforator 5* pierces the fascia 7.64 cm from the malleolus at 125°. Perforators 4 and 5 communicate with the medial plantar veins. *Perforator 6* connects the dorsalis pedis vein with the dorsal veinous arch and pierces the fascia between the first and second metatarsal bones at about 11 cm from the medial malleolus. **(B) Perforating veins that connect the deep veins with the lesser saphenous vein.** *Perforator 7* perforates the fascia 2.64 cm from the lateral malleolus at 90°. It originates from the dorsalis pedis vein, passes deep to the extensor digitorum longus tendons, and connects with the lesser saphenous vein behind the lateral malleolus. *Perforator 8* is inconstant. It pierces the fascia 2.8 cm from the tip of the lateral malleolus at 232°. *Perforator 9* pierces the fascia 4.41 cm from the lateral malleolus at 180° and opens in the lesser saphenous vein. *Perforator 10* pierces the fascia 3.42 cm from the lateral malleolus at 146°. *Perforator 11* pierces the fascia at 6.1 cm from the lateral malleolus at 138.5° just behind the tuberosity of the fifth metatarsal. *Perforator 12* is uncommon. It pierces the fascia at 9.2 cm from the lateral malleolus at 116°. The cross marks indicate the tips of the lateral and medial malleoli. (From Kuster G, Lofgren EP, Hollinshead WH: Anatomy of the veins of the foot. Surg Gynecol Obstet 127: 817, 1968. By permission of Surgery, Gynecology & Obstetrics)

in the dorsal venous system as described above. These veins are valveless. The superficial mid plantar region drains in a superficial venous arcade at the base of the toes. The medial and lateral ends of the venous arcade end dorsally by joining, respectively, the corresponding dorsal medial and lateral marginal veins of the first and fifth toes. The interdigital perforating veins originate from the superficial venous arcade, pass through the web space, and unite with the dorsal vein of the toe.

The superficial plantar system communicates also with the deep plantar veins. Ascar and Abdulah describe plantar communicators (lateral, medial, intermediary) that pierce the plantar aponeurosis and connect correspondingly with the medial and lateral plantar veins.[28]

Deep Plantar Venous Network

The deep veins of the planta are represented by the veins accompanying the medial and lateral plantar arteries. The larger lateral plantar vein, single or double at the origin, forms distally the deep plantar venous arch.[27] It receives two communicating peroneal veins, the first proximal perforating interosseous or intermetatarsal vein, and the plantar metatarsal veins that connect with the dorsal metatarsal veins through the proximal and distal perforating (interosseous) veins. The medial plantar vein is thinner and communicates on the medial margin of the foot with the periscaphoid veins and distally with the first perforating interosseous (intermetatarsal) vein.

Lymphatics

The lymphatics of the foot are divided into superficial and deep channels.

SUPERFICIAL LYMPHATICS OF THE FOOT

The superficial lymphatic vessels originate mainly from the skin of the toes, the skin of the sole of the foot, and the skin of the heel (Figs. 7-56 and 7-57).[29] The remaining segments of the skin of the foot contribute to the lymphatic channels through only very miniscule vessels.

Of the Toes

The lymphatics of the toes form a true plexus and envelop the toes completely. The lymphatic network is less developed on the dorsum of the toe and better defined on the lateral, medial, and plantar aspects. Lymphatic rootlets converge on the sides of the toe and form dorsal and plantar digital channels that may be converted into two main lateral and medial lymphatic channels coursing parallel and dorsal to the digital arteries. At the level of the metatarsophalangeal joints, the lymphatic trunks of two adjacent toes may unite or the four individual digital channels may form one common channel, which will then bifurcate and unite with the neighboring vessels. These multiple anastomoses result in a large lymphatic plexus covering the dorsum of the foot. At the level of the interdigital space the lymphatic plexus is

enriched by 3 to 4 lymphatic branches arising from the plantar aspect of the foot.[30] On the dorsum of the foot, Poirier and Charpy divide the superficial lymphatics into two collecting systems, medial and lateral.[30]

Medial System. The medial system is formed by the lymphatics of the big toe and the second toe and the skin of the inner third of the dorsum of the foot. This system is augmented by lymphatic branches arising from the sole of the foot. These medial marginal plantar branches, initially 14 to 15, are reduced to 4 to 5 branches as they reach the dorsum of the foot. All the collectors converge and form longitudinal lymphatic channels coursing along the greater saphenous vein. They terminate in the inguinal nodes.

Lateral System. The lateral system is formed by the lymphatics of the third, fourth, and fifth toes, of the lateral two thirds of the dorsal skin of the foot, and of the anterior half of the lateral foot margin. The collectors are oriented posteromedially and join the channels along the greater saphenous vein. The superficial lymphatics of the posterior half of the lateral border of the foot and of the corresponding segment of the heel form two to three channels, pass behind the lateral malleolus, and course along the lesser saphenous vein. They terminate in the most superficial popliteal node.

Of the Sole

As described by Sappey, the superficial lymphatics of the sole are divided into anterior, medial, and lateral groups.[29]

Anterior Group. The anterior group is formed by branches coursing toward the dorsum of the foot through the web space. There are 2 to 3 branches per web space.

Medial Group. The medial group is formed by 3 to 4 lymphatic branches. Of these, 3 cross the medial border of the foot obliquely to reach the dorsal system and are located anterior to the medial malleolus; the fourth branch is posterior to the medial malleolus.

Lateral Group. The lateral group is formed by 2 to 4 vessels. Of these, 1 passes behind the lateral malleolus and the others pass in front to reach the dorsal system.

DEEP LYMPHATICS OF THE FOOT

The deep lymphatics are satellites of the arterial trunks and are divided into three groups: dorsalis pedis and anterior tibial lymphatics, plantar and posterior tibial lymphatics, and peroneal lymphatics.

The dorsalis pedis and anterior tibial lymphatics originate in the planta pedis from the deep muscles. The lymphatic channels unite into one or two trunks, pass to the dorsum of the foot, and course along the dorsalis pedis and the tibialis anterior arteries. They also collect the deep lymphatics from the dorsum of the foot and terminate in the popliteal nodes.

The plantar and posterior tibial lymphatics originate in

Fig. 7-56. Superficial lymphatics of the foot and leg. (*A*) Lateral aspect. (1, Lymphatic network of lateral borders of foot; 2, lymphatic channels draining lateral border of foot and terminating in popliteal lymph nodes; 3, lymphatic vessels of dorsum of foot draining toes and anterior segment of plantar region; 4, lymphatic vessels crossing tibial crest.) (*B*) Medial aspect. (1, Lymphatic network of inner aspect of sole of foot; 2, lymphatic vessels that run from *1;* 3, other lymphatic trunks of dorsal surface of foot; 4, large lymphatic trunk passing in front of medial malleolus; 5, lymphatic vessels located anterior and posterior to *4;* 6, lymphatic vessels arising from lateral surface of leg; 7, lymphatic vessels located on medial aspect of leg.) (From Sappey PC: Traité d'Anatomie Descriptive, Vol II, Angiologie, p 791. Paris, Lecrosnier, 1888)

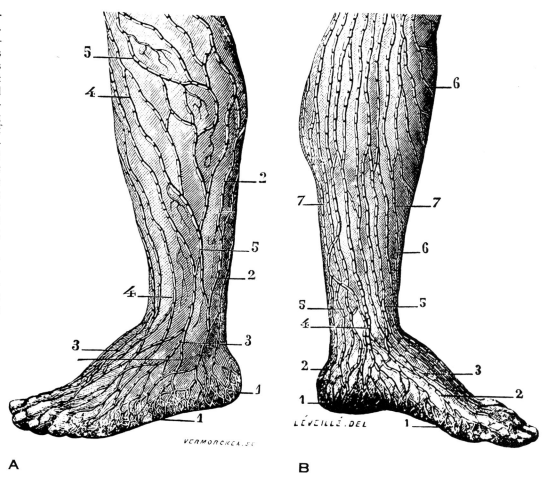

A   **B**

Fig. 7-57. Superficial lymphatics of the foot. (1, Lymphatic network of lateral border of foot; 2, lymphatic network of toe; 3, lymphatic network of skin of heel; 4, lymphatic vessels that accompany lateral saphenous vein and terminate in popliteal lymph nodes; 5, lymphatic trunks on dorsal surface of foot; 6, lymphatic trunks that run from lateral to medial aspect of leg; 7, lymphatic networks from which a single lymphatic vessel originates and connects with neighboring trunks.) (From Sappey PC: Traité d'Anatomie Descriptive, Vol II, Angiologie, p 789. Paris, Lecrosnier, 1888)

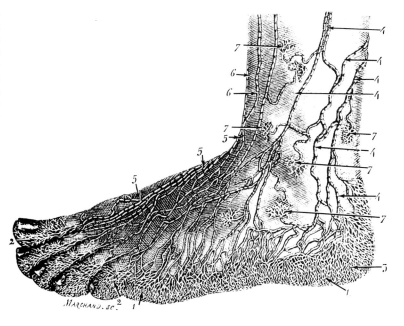

the sole and follow the plantar arteries and the posterior tibial artery. There are three or four collecting trunks around the latter; the trunks terminate in the popliteal nodes.[30]

The peroneal lymphatics have two collecting trunks accompanying the peroneal artery; they also terminate in the popliteal nodes.

LYMPHATICS OF THE JOINTS

The lymphatics of the interphalangeal joints drain into the collecting channels of the dorsum of the foot.[31]

Lymphatics of the metatarsophalangeal joints are divided into plantar and dorsal lymphatics.[31] The lymphatic channels drain into the plantar metatarsal channels coursing along the plantar metatarsal arteries. The plantar lymphatics of the metatarsophalangeal joint of the big toe reach the dorsum of the foot and unite with the superficial saphenous system or the deep system accompanying the dorsalis pedis artery. The dorsal lymphatics empty into the superficial lymphatics of the dorsum of the foot and occasionally into the deep dorsal collecting channels.

The lymphatics of the ankle are divided into superficial and deep channels.[31] The superficial lymphatics are anterior and posterior; they course along the saphenous veins and reach the inguinal and the popliteal node. The deep lymphatics are divided into three groups: anterior, posteromedial, and posterolateral.

The deep anterior lymphatics start on the anteromedial and anterolateral aspects of the articular capsule and their corresponding ligaments. Their lymphatic channels are directed transversely toward the anterior tibial artery, where they join the longitudinal lymphatic channels along the artery. The deep posteromedial lymphatics emerge from the deltoid ligament and the posteromedial articular capsule and drain into the posterior tibial lymphatic channel. The deep posterolateral lymphatics originate from the posterolateral capsule and ligaments and merge with the peroneal lymphatic channels.

REFERENCES

1. Dubreuil-Chambardel L: Variations des Artères du Pelvis et du Membre Inferieur, pp 191–271. Paris, Masson et Cie, 1925
2. Adachi B: Das Arteriensystem der Japaner, pp 215–291. Kyoto, Maruzen, 1928
3. Quain: Anatomy of the Arteries of the Human Body. London, 1844
4. Manno A: Arteriae plantares pedis mammalium. Int Monatsschr Anat Physiol 22, 1905
5. Huber JF: The arterial network supplying the dorsum of the foot. Anat Rec 80:373, 1941
6. Salvi, G: Sull' arteria dorsale pedis. Atti della Societa Toscana di Scienze Naturalli, Process Verbali, 12, 1898
7. Schwalbe G, Pfitzner W: Varietäten-Statistik und Anthropologie Dritte Mitteilung. Morphol Arb 3:459, 1894
8. Edwards EA: Anatomy of the small arteries of the foot and toes. Acta Anat 40:81, 1960
9. Gilbert A: Composite tissue transfers from the foot: Anatomic basis and surgical technique. Symposium on Microsurgery, 14, pp 230–241. St. Louis, CV Mosby, 1976
10. Man D, Acland RD: The microarterial anatomy of the dorsalis pedis flap and its clinical applications. Plast Reconstr Surg 65, No. 4:419, 1980
11. Poirier P, Charpy A: Traité d'Anatomie Humaine, Vol II, Angiologie, pp 839–847. Paris, Masson, 1902
12. Levame JH: Les artères des orteils: Etude anatomique et arteriographique: Conclusions chirurgicales. J Chir 86, No. 6:651, 1963
13. Murakami T: On the position and course of the deep plantar arteries, with special reference to the so-called plantar metatarsal arteries. Okajimas Folia Anat Jpn 48:295, 1971
14. Mulfinger GL, Trueta J: The blood supply of the talus. J Bone Joint Surg [Br] 52, No. 1:160, 1970
15. Wildenauer E: Die Blutvesorgung des Talus. Z Anat Entwicklungs 115:32, 1950
16. Aschner B: Zur Anatomie der Arterien der Fusssohle. Anat Hefte Beit Ref Anat Entwicklungs 27:345, 1905
17. Vann MH: A note on the formation of the plantar arterial arch of the human foot. Anat Rec 85:269, 1943
18. Pyka RA, Coventry MB: Avascular necrosis of the skin after operations on the foot. J Bone Joint Surg [Am] 43:955, 1961
19. Von Lanz R, Wachsmuth W: Praktische Anatomie, Bein und Statik Erster Band Vierter Teil, p 423. Berlin, Springer, 1972
20. Mathes SJ, Nahai F: Clinical Atlas of Muscle and Musculocutaneous Flaps, pp 263–307. St Louis, Mosby, 1979
21. Crock HV: The Blood Supply of the Lower Limb Bones in Man—Descriptive and Applied, pp 72–87. Edinburgh, Livingstone, 1967
22. Haliburton RA, Sullivan CR, Kelly PJ, Peterson LFA: The extraosseous and intraosseous blood supply of the talus. J Bone Joint Surg [Am] 40, No. 5:1115, 1958
23. Zchakaja MJ: Blutversorgung der Knochen des Fusses (ossa pedis). Fortschr Gebiete Röntgenol 45:160, 1932
24. Velluda C: Sur la vascularisation du scaphoid du tarse. Ann Anat Pathol 5:1016, 1928
25. Waugh W: The ossification and vascularisation of the tarsal navicular and their relation to Köhler's Disease. J Bone Joint Surg [Br] 40, No. 4:765, 1958
26. Kuster G, Lofgren EP, Hollinshead WH: Anatomy of the veins of the foot. Surg Gynecol Obstet 127:817, 1968
27. Winckler G: Les veines du pied. Arch Anat Histol Embryol 37:175, 1954–1955
28. Ascar O, Abdulah AS: The veins of the foot: Surgical anatomy and its relation to disorders of the venous return from the foot. J Cardiovasc Surg 16:53, 1975
29. Sappey PC: Traité d'Anatomie Descriptive, Vol II, Angiologie, pp 790–795. Paris, Lecrosnier, 1888
30. Poirier P, Charpy A: Traité d'Anatomie Humaine, Vol II, Fasc 4, The Lymphatics, pp 1158–1170. Paris, Masson, 1902
31. Rouvière H: Anatomy of the Human Lymphatic System: A compendium. Tobias MJ (trans): Ann Arbor, Edwards, 1938

8

Nerves

The nerve supply to the foot and ankle is provided by the branches of the sciatic nerve. The saphenous nerve, a branch of the femoral nerve, gives limited contribution. The branches of the sciatic nerve innervating the foot and ankle are the sural nerve, the superficial peroneal nerve and the accessory deep peroneal nerve, the deep peroneal nerve, and the posterior tibial nerve with its medial and lateral plantar nerves.

Sural Nerve

The sural nerve is formed by the medial sural nerve after receiving the anastomotic peroneal communicating nerve (Figs. 8-1–8-3). The medial sural nerve is a branch of the tibial nerve and the anastomotic peroneal communicating nerve a branch of the common peroneal nerve or of the lateral sural nerve.

When the anastomotic branch is absent, the medial sural nerve usually predominates and covers the territory of the sural nerve. Occasionally the lateral sural nerve or the peroneal communicating nerve takes over the same territory of innervation.

The medial sural nerve (median sural nerve, external saphenous nerve, tibial saphenous nerve) arises from the tibial nerve in the popliteal space. It courses between the two heads of the gastrocnemius muscle covered by the deep aponeurosis. It pierces the latter in the middle of the leg, receives the anastomotic peroneal communicating nerve, and forms the sural nerve. The sural nerve courses along the lateral border of the Achilles tendon and is anterolateral to the short saphenous veins. It turns around the posterior border of the lateral malleolus and passes 1 cm to 1.5 cm from the tip of the lateral malleolus from which it is sepa-

rated by the tendons of the peronei and their sheaths (Fig. 8-4). At the level of the tuberosity of the fifth metatarsal, the nerve divides into two terminal branches, lateral and medial (Fig. 8-5). The lateral branch is a direct continuation of the main nerve and terminates as the dorsolateral cutaneous nerve of the fifth toe. The larger medial branch obliquely crosses the dorsolateral aspect of the foot; it passes over the tendon of the long extensor of the fifth toe and divides over the anterior aspect of the fourth interosseous space into the dorsomedial cutaneous nerve of the fifth toe and the dorsolateral cutaneous nerve of the fourth toe.

The sural nerve provides the lateral calcaneal branches. One such branch originates 5 cm above the lateral malleolus and another 1.3 cm above and behind the tip of the lateral malleolus in 98% of the cases.[1] The sural nerve also supplies the lateral malleolar branch and an anastomotic branch that crosses the dorsum of the foot obliquely, passes under the dorsolateral vein, and unites with the lateral branch of the superficial peroneal nerve. Articular branches are provided by the sural nerve to the inferior tibiofibular joint, the ankle joint, and the talocalcaneal joint.

The formation of the sural nerve or the predominance of the medial sural nerve has been investigated by many authors and occurs with the frequency shown in Table 8-1.

The anastomosis between the medial sural nerve and the peroneal communicating branch usually takes place at mid leg but may occur as low as in the lower quarter of the leg or as high as above the level of the knee joint.[3]

A most common location of the sural nerve is at "10 cm above the tip of the lateral malleolus just at the lateral border of the Achilles tendon," and the diameter of the sural nerve is 2 mm average (1.25 mm–2.75 mm) according to Kosinski or 3 mm average according to Horwitz.[1,3]

(Text continues on p. 317.)

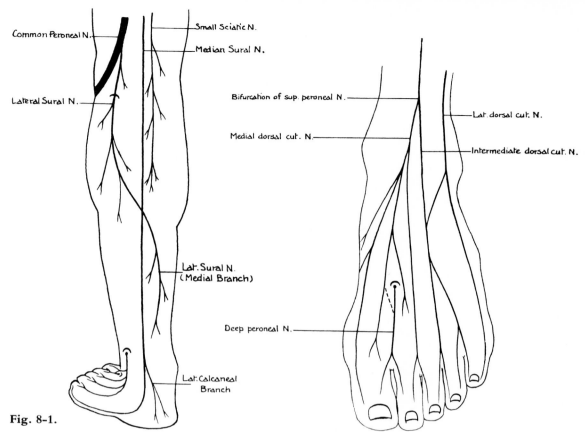

Fig. 8-1.

Common Peroneal N.

Small Sciatic N.

Median Sural N.

Lateral Sural N.

Bifurcation of sup. peroneal N.

Lat. dorsal cut. N.

Medial dorsal cut. N.

Intermediate dorsal cut. N.

Lat. Sural N. (Medial Branch)

Deep peroneal N.

Lat. Calcaneal Branch

Fig. 8-2.

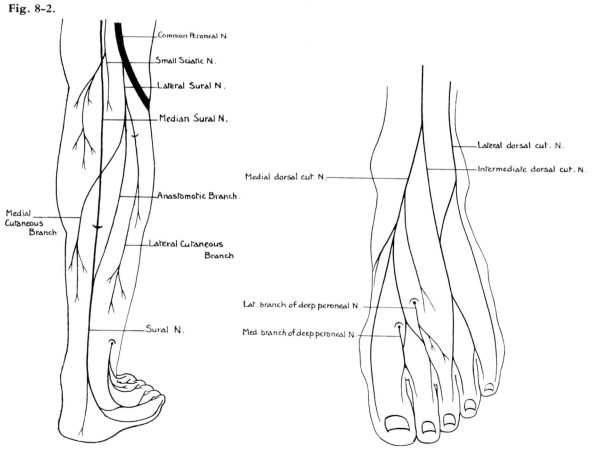

Common Peroneal N

Small Sciatic N.

Lateral Sural N.

Median Sural N.

Lateral dorsal cut. N.

Medial dorsal cut. N.

Intermediate dorsal cut. N.

Anastomotic Branch.

Medial Cutaneous Branch

Lateral Cutaneous Branch

Lat. branch of deep peroneal N.

Med. branch of deep peroneal N.

Sural N.

Fig. 8-1. Sural nerve type A (53%) formed by the medial sural nerve only. The lateral sural nerve terminates in the posterior aspect of the leg. The sural nerve forms the lateral dorsal cutaneous nerve of the dorsum of the foot and provides an anastomotic branch to the intemediate dorsal cutaneous nerve—a branch of the superficial peroneal nerve, which is increased. (From Kosinski C: The course, mutual relations and distribution of the cutaneous nerve of the metazonal region of the leg and foot. J Anat 60:274, 1926)

Fig. 8-2. Sural nerve type B (40%) formed by two roots: the medial and lateral sural nerves, connected by an anastomotic branch. The sural nerve forms the lateral dorsal cutaneous nerve of the foot united to the intermediate dorsal cutaneous nerve by an anastomotic branch. The deep peroneal nerve is increased, with a medial branch innervating the first web space and a lateral branch innervating the second web space. (From Kosinski C: The course, nutual relations and distribution of the cutaneous nerve of the metazonal region of the leg and foot. J Anat 60:274, 1926)

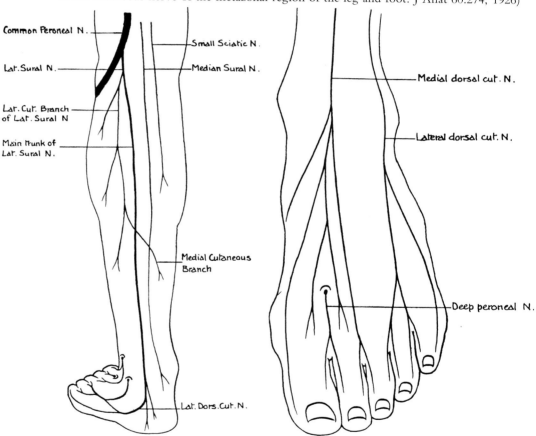

Fig. 8-3. Sural nerve type C (6%) formed by the lateral sural nerve only arising from the common peroneal nerve. The sural nerve forms the lateral dorsal cutaneous nerve, which is increased. (From Kosinski C: The course, mutual relations and distribution of the cutaneous nerve of the metazonal region of the leg and foot. J Anat 60:274, 1926)

TABLE 8-1   Frequency of Occurrence of Sural Nerve or Other Nerve Functioning as Such

			Functioning as Sural Nerve (%)	
Author	No. Legs	Sural Nerve With Two Roots (%)	Medial Sural Nerve	Lateral Sural Nerve or Peroneal Communicating Nerve
Catania[2]	94	51	35	14
Kosinski[3]	287	40.2 (type B)	53.8 (type A)	6 (type C)
Andreassi[4]	144	63.9	34.7	1.4
Soskolow[5]	500	52.2	43.8	3.6
Mogi[6]	180	83.3	16.7	0
P'an[7]	286	81.5	13.3	5.2
Williams[8]	257	83.7	15.9	0.4

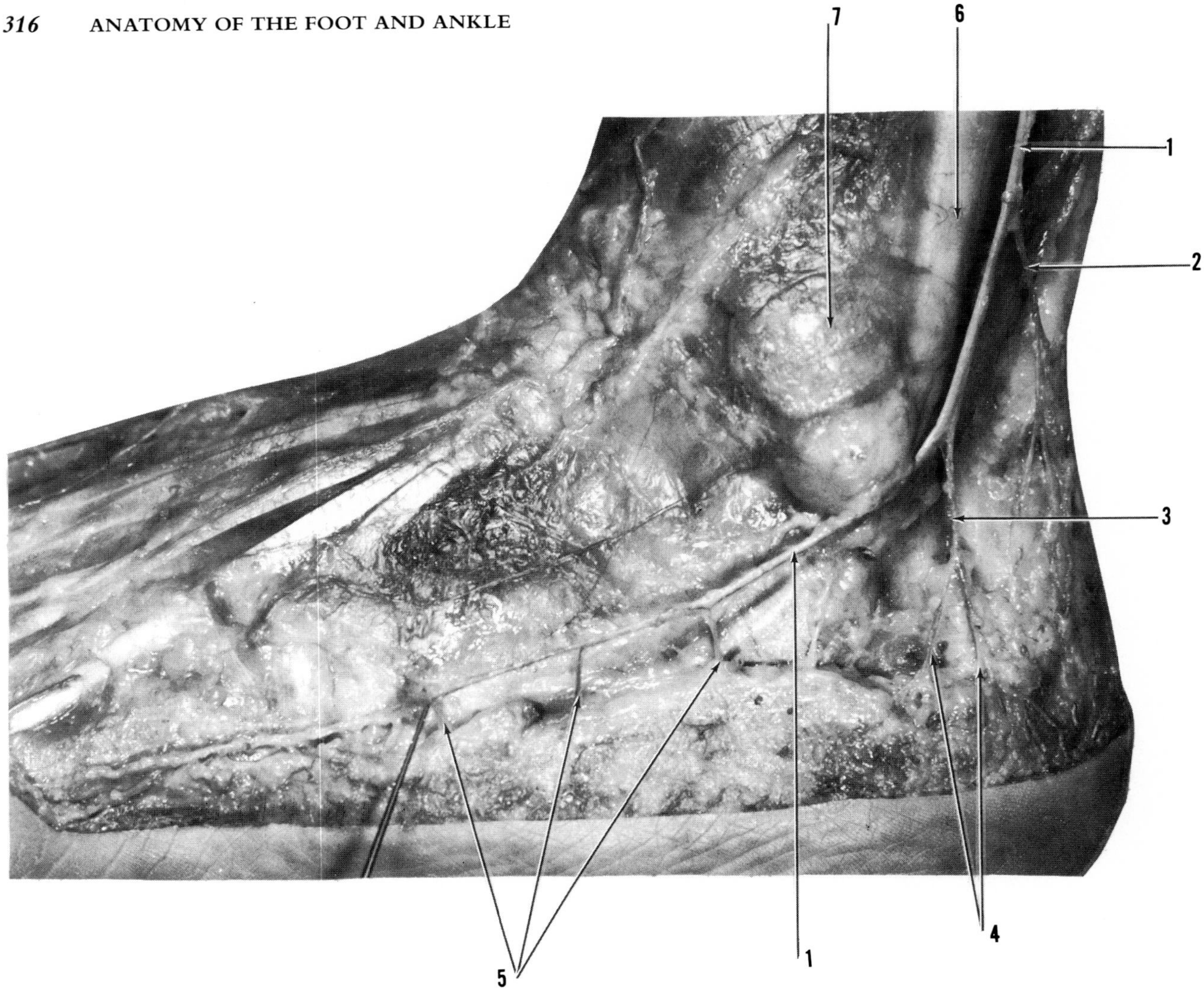

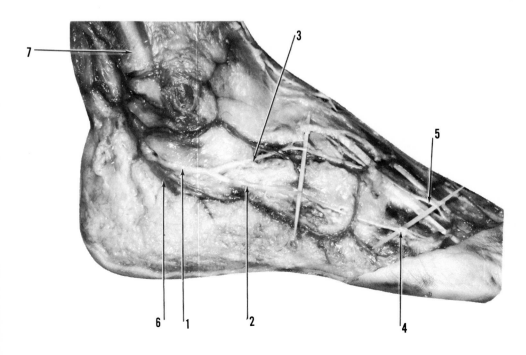

Fig. 8–4.   Sural nerve. (1, Sural nerve; 2, branch of sural nerve to posterolateral aspect of Achilles tendon area and calcaneal region; 3, lateral calcaneal branch of sural nerve with bifurcation branches [4]; 5, branches of sural nerve to lateral border of foot; 6, peronei tendons; 7, lateral malleolus [sural nerve passes 1 cm to 1.5 cm below tip of lateral malleolus].)

Fig. 8–5.   Lateral aspect of the right foot and ankle. (1, Sural nerve dividing into lateral branch [2] forming dorsolateral cutaneous nerve [4] and medial branch [3] uniting with intermediate dorsal cutaneous nerve [5] of superficial peroneal nerve; 6, shorter saphenous vein; 7, peronei tendons.)

Superficial Peroneal Nerve

The superficial peroneal nerve (musculocutaneous nerve), a branch of the common peroneal nerve, after coursing in the anterolateral compartment of the leg, pierces the deep fascia cruris in the lower third of the leg and divides into the medial and the intermediate dorsal cutaneous nerves of the dorsum of the foot. The piercing of the deep fascia of the leg by the superficial peroneal nerve occurs at different levels: In 100 legs, it occurred 12.5 cm above the tip of the lateral malleolus in 90%; 15 cm above the tip in 1%; 10 cm above the tip in 2%; 7.5 cm above the tip in 5%; and 5 cm above the tip in 2%.[1] In 118 legs, it occured 10.5 cm above the tip of the lateral malleolus in 74.7% and at a higher level in 23.4%.[3]

When the division of the superficial peroneal nerve into its cutaneous branches occurs at a higher level, the medial dorsal cutaneous branch pierces the fascia cruris at 12.7 cm and the intermediate dorsal cutaneous branch at 4.7 cm above the tip of the lateral malleolus.[3] After becoming subcutaneous, the cutaneous common trunk of the superficial peroneal nerve divides into its terminal branches, usually 6.4 cm above the lateral malleolus; this division occurs below this level in 3% and above the same level in 5% (12.5 cm).[1] Cutaneous branches are provided by the common trunk, and the largest of these, the lateral malleolar branch, may anastomose with the lateral sural nerve or with an accessory branch of the sural nerve.[9]

The most common site of the superficial peroneal nerve is "10.5 cm above the tip of the external malleolus just within the anterior border of the fibula in the groove between the peroneal group of muscles and the extensor digitorum longus."[1] In this location the nerve is subcutaneous in 91% and deep to the fascia in 9%.[1]

The *intermediate dorsal cutaneous nerve* (middle dorsal cutaneous nerve, external branch of the musculocutaneous nerve) is thinner than the medial branch and crosses the fifth and fourth extensor digitorum longus tendons obliquely and superficially. It courses over the third intermetatarsal space. At the anterior aspect of this space, the nerve provides the dorsolateral branch to the third toe and the dorsomedial branch to the fourth toe; it may also send an anastomotic branch to the sural nerve.

The *medial dorsal cutaneous nerve* is the largest bifurcation branch of the superficial peroneal nerve. It is directed medially toward the inner border of the foot. It crosses the inferior extensor retinaculum and takes a direction nearly parallel to the extensor hallucis longus tendon. The nerve divides into three branches: lateral, middle, and medial. The lateral branch takes off at the inferior border of the inferior extensor retinaculum, crosses the long extensor tendon of the second toe, and in the anterior aspect of the second intermetatarsal space divides into the dorsolateral branch of the second toe and the dorsomedial branch of the third toe. The middle branch courses in the interval corresponding to the first intermetatarsal space and, on the anterior aspect of the latter, divides into the dorsomedial branch of the second toe and the dorsolateral branch of the big toe. These two branches are very thin and receive reinforcement from the branches of the deep peroneal nerve. The medial branch is

directed medially, crosses the extensor hallucis longus tendon superficially and obliquely, and then runs parallel to the tendon, forming the dorsomedial cutaneous nerve of the big toe. This nerve branch is subcutaneous but is located within or immediately under the superficial fascia of the foot and yet is superficial to the extensor hallucis longus tendon and its investing fascia. The medial cutaneous branch anastomoses at the level of the metatarsophalangeal joint of the big toe with a terminal branch of the saphenous nerve.

The *accessory deep peroneal nerve,* a branch of the superficial peroneal nerve, was first recognized by Bryce and described in three cases.[10-12] The thin branch passed through the substance of the peroneus brevis muscle and terminated once in the ligament of the ankle joint and twice in the extensor digitorum brevis.

A comprehensive study of the same nerve is provided by Winckler, who described it in seven cases (five adults and two newborns).[13] The branch of the superficial peroneal nerve to the peroneus brevis muscle, after providing the motor branches to the latter, courses along the posterior border of the peroneus brevis tendon, remains in the compartment of the peronei, and reaches the posterior aspect of the lateral malleolus. At this level the nerve provides branches to the posterior talofibular ligament and to the calcaneofibular ligament and then turns around the lateral malleolus parallel to the tendon of the peroneus brevis, reaches the extensor digitorum brevis, and innervates its two lateral heads—to the fourth and third toes—and terminates in the dorsal capsule of the calcaneocuboid joint. Prior to entering the extensor digitorum brevis, the accessory deep peroneal nerve provides branches to the anterior talofibular ligament and to the capsule of the ankle joint.

As descrived by Winckler, the accessory deep peroneal nerve is associated with a strong development of the peroneus brevis muscle and with the presence of an accessory tendon extending from the peroneus brevis muscle to the fifth toe as the peroneal extensor of the fifth toe.[13] The nerve may be purely sensory, innervating the ankle joint or certain articulations of the tarsal and tarsometatarsal joints; however, it is usually mixed, and it is never pure motor, innervating only the extensor digitorum brevis.

Lambert, in an electromyographic investigation of 50 healthy persons, found evidence of the presence of this accessory deep peroneal nerve in 22% of the examined limbs.[14]

Deep Peroneal Nerve

The deep peroneal nerve, after piercing the extensor digitorum longus muscle, joins the anterior tibial artery. In the upper third of the leg the nerve is situated between the extensor digitorum longus and the tibialis anterior muscle. In the middle third the nerve is located between the extensor hallucis longus and the tibialis anterior muscle. In the distal third of the leg the deep peroneal nerve passes behind the obliquely directed extensor hallucis longus muscle–tendon, and at 2.5 cm to 5 cm above the ankle the nerve is located between the latter tendon and the extensor digitorum longus tendon.[1]

The deep peroneal nerve is lateral to the anterior tibial artery proximally and distally, but some variations are possible. Horwitz, in a study of 100 legs, mentions that in 90% of the cases the nerve is lateral to the artery in the upper and middle thirds of the leg and then at 10 cm above the ankle joint the nerve is anterolateral to the artery; at 5 cm above the joint the nerve is again lateral to the artery.[1] In 4% the nerve is lateral initially, crosses the artery posteriorly, and is medial farther down.[1] In 1% the nerve is lateral initially, crosses the artery anteriorly, and is medial to the latter distally.[1]

The deep peroneal nerve divides into a medial and a lateral terminal branch at 1.3 cm above the ankle joint in 98% of the cases.[1] In 2% the branching occurs at 6.4 cm above the ankle joint or at the level of the ankle joint.[1] At the level of the ankle the deep peroneal nerve is located under the reflected segment of the extensor pulley of the extensor hallucis longus tendon.

The medial branch usually is located medial to the dorsalis pedis artery. It is the larger branch and continues the direction of the nerve. Initially it is located between the extensor hallucis longus tendon and the medial border of the extensor hallucis brevis muscle. It is crossed superficially and obliquely by the latter and reaches the first intermetatarsal space, where it pierces the deep dorsal aponeurosis of the foot. It is now located between the extensor hallucis brevis tendon medially and the long extensor of the second toe laterally. The nerve divides into two branches and supplies the dorsolateral cutaneous branch to the big toe and the dorsomedial cutaneous branch to the second toe. Quite often the deep peroneal nerve joins the branches of the superficial peroneal nerve in going to the first web space.

The lateral branch of the deep peroneal nerve is directed anterolaterally, penetrates and innervates the extensor digitorum brevis muscle, and terminates into very thin branches that are applied against the tarsal skeleton and form the second, third, and fourth dorsal interosseous nerves. These branches provide the nerve supply to the tarsometatarsal, the metatarsophalangeal, and interphalangeal joints of the lesser toes.

The average diameter of the deep peroneal nerve is 1 mm to 3 mm, and the most constant site is 2.5 cm above the level of the ankle joint anteriorly, under the upper arm of the inferior extensor retinaculum between the extensor hallucis medially and the extensor digitorum longus laterally.[1]

The dorsal cutaneous nerve supply to the dorsum of the foot is very variable. Statistical information based on a collective study of 229 feet is presented in Figures 8-6–8-8. When the territory of the sural nerve increases that of the intermediate dorsal cutaneous branch decreases, and *vice versa*. In the same series, only in one case did the saphenous nerve supply the inner side of the big toe, and in another one it reached the inner side of the head of the first metatarsal bone.[15]

Posterior Tibial Nerve

The posterior tibial nerve (tibial nerve) extends from the arcade of the soleus muscle to the calcaneal canal (Fig. 8-9 and Fig. 8-10). It is in direct vertical continuity with the sciatic nerve and shifts slightly to the medial side to reach the tibiotalocalcaneal canal; within this canal the nerve divides into two terminal branches—medial and lateral plantar nerves.

In the upper two thirds of its course, the posterior tibial nerve is located in the deep posterior compartment of the leg in the interval between the tibialis posterior muscle and the flexor digitorum longus anteriorly. Farther down the nerve is located between the latter and the flexor hallucis longus.

In the inferior third of the leg, the posterior tibial nerve is more superficial as the soleus and the gastrocnemei are converted to the Achilles tendon, thus exposing the nerve. The posterior tibial nerve now runs along the medial border of the Achilles tendon; the flexor hallucis longus tendon is lateral to the posterior tibial nerve and the flexor digitorum longus is anteromedial. Posteriorly and medially the nerve is covered by the superficial and deep fascias of the leg. The posterior tibial nerve remains lateral and slightly posterior to the posterior tibial artery.

The most common site of the posterior tibial nerve is 7.5 cm above the tip of the medial malleolus, in line with the medial border of the Achilles tendon.[1] The posterior tibial nerve provides cutaneous, articular, and vascular branches.

The cutaneous branches are distributed to the skin of the medial malleolar area and to the inner aspect of the heel. The medial malleolar branch is very thin and perforates the aponeurosis of the ankle just proximal to the medial malleolus, supplies the skin covering the malleolus, and often anastomoses with a branch of the saphenous nerve.

The medial calcaneal nerve branches from the posterior tibial nerve in the distal third of the leg. Horwitz mentions that this nerve originates from the medial plantar nerve and in 4% takes off from the posterior tibial nerve 2.5 cm (3%) and 7.5 cm (1%) proximal to the bifurcation point.[1]

The medial calcaneal branch pierces the aponeurosis at a variable point and immediately divides into two branches, which could at times arise separately. The posterior branch or calcaneal branch proper is distributed to the skin covering the medial aspect of the Achilles tendon and the medial and posterior aspect of the heel. The anterior branch is a plantar branch; it courses along the inner border of the foot and passes through the very thick layer of adipose tissue, and its terminal branches are distributed to the skin of the posterior third of the region. Medially the terminal branches anastomose with the calcaneal branches of the saphenous nerve and the cutaneous branches of the medial plantar nerve. Laterally the terminal calcaneal branches anastomose with branches of the sural nerve and anteriorly with branches of the lateral plantar nerve.

The articular branches, one and occasionally two, arise from the posterior tibial nerve near its bifurcation. They are directed anteriorly, pass between the tibialis posterior tendon and the flexor digitorum longus tendon, and innervate the ankle joint. A few fibers penetrate between the deep and superficial layers of the deltoid ligament, whereas others remain on the surface of the superficial layer of the ligament.[16]

(Text continues on p. 322.)

Fig. 8-6. Variations in the distribution of the cutaneous nerves on the dorsum of the foot (229 feet examined). *Type I (55%): Most frequent distribution pattern, with the superficial peroneal nerve predominating. Type II (24%): Sural nerve is increased. Type III (8%): Sural nerve innervates the fourth web space and provides the lateral dorsal cutaneous branch of the little toe. Type IV (6 of 229): Similar to type I but the superficial peroneal nerve provides two anastomotic branches to the deep peroneal nerve. (SP, superficial peroneal nerve; IN, internal division branch of SP; EX, external division branch of SP; DP, deep peroneal nerve; S, sural nerve.) (Redrawn after Anatomical Society of Great Britain and Ireland: Report of Committee of Collective Investigation on the Distribution of Cutaneous Nerve on the Dorsum of the Foot. J Anat Physiol 26:89, 1891–1892)*

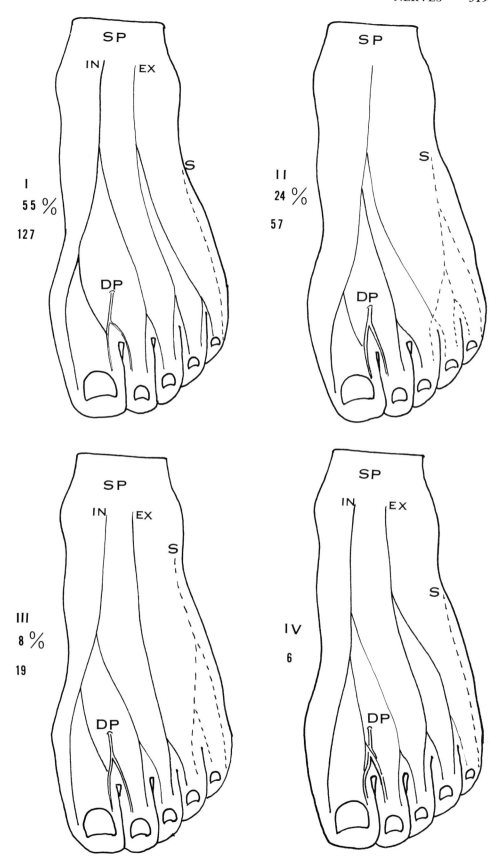

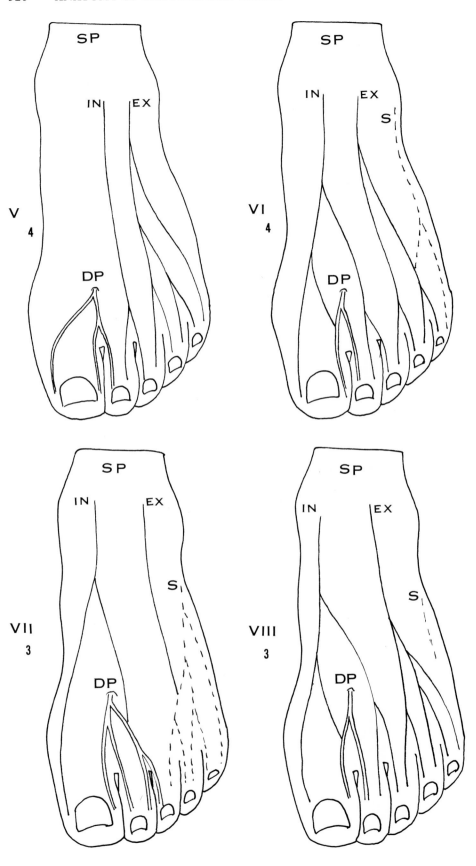

Fig. 8-7. Variations in the distribution of the cutaneous nerves on the dorsum of the foot (229 feet examined). *Type V* (4 of 229): The deep peroneal nerve predominates and the sural nerve is absent. *Type VI* (4 of 229): Similar to type I except for anastomotic branch from the sural nerve to the external division branch (intermediate cutaneous branch) of the superficial peroneal nerve. *Type VII* (3 of 229): The sural nerve and the deep peroneal nerve predominate. *Type VIII* (3 of 229): The sural nerve is nearly absent. (*SP*, superficial peroneal nerve; *IN*, internal division branch of *SP*; *EX*, external division branch of *SP*; *DP*, deep peroneal nerve; *S*, sural nerve.) (Redrawn after Anatomical Society of Great Britain and Ireland: Report of Committee of Collective Investigation on the Distribution of Cutaneous Nerve on the Dorsum of the Foot. J Anat Physiol 26:89, 1891–1892)

Fig. 8-8. Variations in the distribution of the cutaneous nerves on the dorsum of the foot (229 feet examined). *Type IX* (3 of 229): The deep peroneal predominates. The lateral peroneal nerve extends laterally. *Type X* (1 of 229): The deep peroneal nerve has minimal contribution. *Type XI* (1 of 229): The external division branch of the superficial peroneal nerve predominates. *Type XII* (1 of 229): The deep peroneal nerve has no contribution. The sural nerve predominates. (*SP*, superficial peroneal nerve; *IN*, internal division branch of *SP*; *EX*, external division branch of *SP*; *DP*, deep peroneal nerve; *S*, sural nerve.) (Redrawn after Anatomical Society of Great Britain and Ireland: Report of Committee of Collective Investigation on the Distribution of Cutaneous Nerve on the Dorsum of the Foot. J Anat Physiol 26:89, 1891–1892)

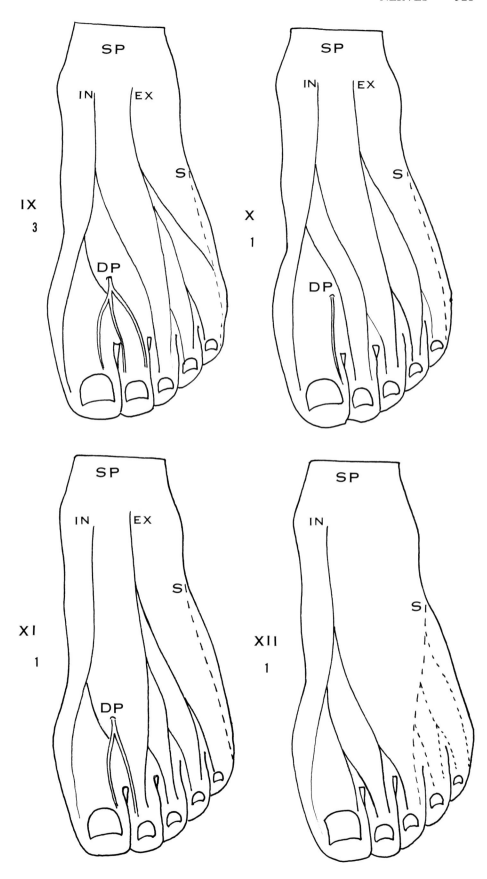

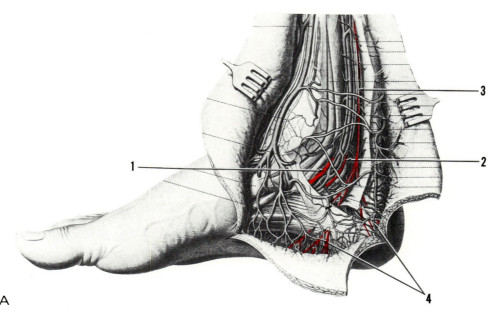

Fig. 8-9. Medial aspect of the foot and ankle. (*A*) (1, Medial plantar nerve; 2, lateral plantar nerve; 3, calcaneal branch of posterior tibial nerve; 4, division branches of *3*.) (*B*) Flexor retinaculum and abductor hallicus muscle reflected plantarward. (1, Posterior tibial nerve; 2, lateral plantar nerve; 3, medial plantar nerve; 4, calcaneal branch of posterior tibial nerve; 5, division branches of *4*; 6, 7, branches to abductor hallucis muscle; 8, hallucal medial plantar nerve.) (From Lanz T, Wachsmuth W: Praktische Anatomie Bein und Statik Erster Band, 4th ed, pp 339–340. Berlin, Springer-Verlag, 1972)

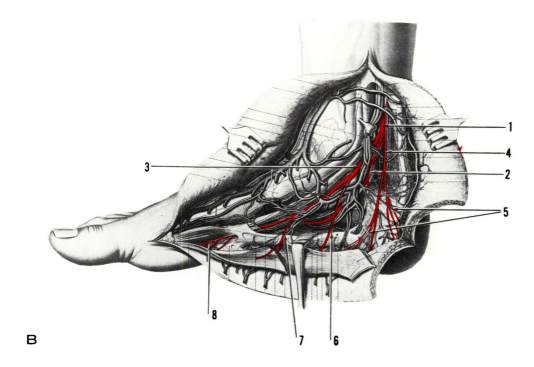

The vascular branches arise from the terminal portion of the posterior tibial nerve and form nerve loops around the posterior tibial artery; occasionally they form a plexus—the posterior tibial retromalleolar plexus of Lazorthe.[17] Among these vascular nerve branches there is usually one larger branch that bifurcates at the site of division of the posterior tibial artery, and each nerve branch accompanies the corresponding plantar medial and lateral arteries. This vascular branch anchors the bifurcation of the posterior tibial artery and nerve to each other.[18]

The terminal branches of the posterior tibial nerve are the medial and lateral plantar nerves. The division occurs in the talocalcaneal tunnel, 1.3 cm to 2.5 cm proximal to the division of the posterior tibial artery.[1] The bifurcation of the posterior tibial nerve into its terminal branches occurs proximal to the medial malleolus; according to Horwitz, the bifurcation occurs 1.3 cm proximal to the tip of medial malleolus, and according to Macaggi, it occurs 1.5 cm proximal to the tip of medial malleolus, with a higher bifurcation in 13.5%.[1, 19] Hovelacque mentions having observed one

Fig. 8-10.   Medial aspect of the left ankle and foot. (*A*) (1, Posterior tibial nerve; 2, calcaneal branch of *1*; 3, posterior tibial vessels.) (*B*) Posterior tibial vessels reflected plantarward. (1, Posterior tibial nerve; 2, medial planter nerve; 3, lateral plantar nerve; 4, 5, medial calcaneal cutaneous nerve branches.)

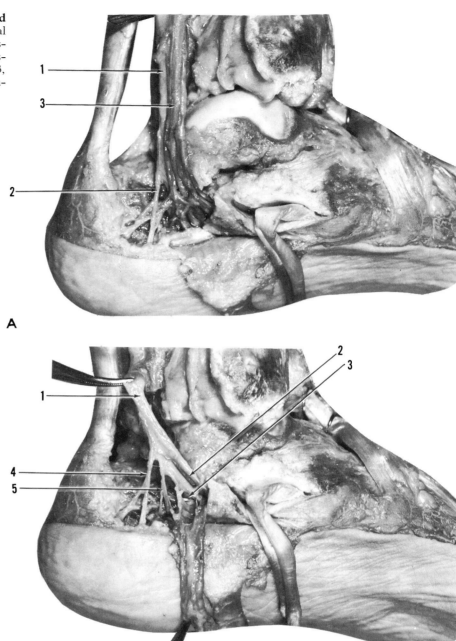

bifurcation at 6 cm and another one at 10 cm above the tip of the medial malleolus.[20]

MEDIAL PLANTAR NERVE

The medial plantar nerve is the anterior division branch of the posterior tibial nerve (Figs. 8-11–8-13). In general it is larger than the lateral plantar nerve. Directed obliquely downward and anteriorly, it crosses the lateral surface of the posterior tibial artery and locates itself anterior to the medial plantar artery. Proximally the posterior tibial neurovascular bundle is contained in a neurovascular compart-

ment limited posteriorly by the deep aponeurosis of the leg and located in the interval between the tunnel of the flexor hallucis longus laterally and the flexor digitorum longus anteromedially. In the lower segment the calcaneal canal is subdivided into two chambers, upper and lower, by the semitransverse interfascicular septum extending from the deep investing fascia of the abductor hallucis to the upper border of the flexor accessorius immediately below the tunnel of the flexor hallucis longus. The medial plantar nerve and the medial plantar artery pass through the upper chamber, the nerve remaining anterior to the artery. They are covered medially by the superior segment of the abductor hallucis muscle and the laciniate ligament. At this level the medial neurovascular bundle corresponds to the tunnel of the flexor hallucis longus tendon laterally. The medial plantar nerve leaves the calcaneal canal, penetrates the sole of the foot, and passes on the plantar aspect of intersection of the flexor hallucis longus and the flexor digitorum longus tendon. The nerve is located deep in the interval between the abductor hallucis and the flexor digitorum brevis and may be partially covered by the former. The medial plantar nerve now lies in the medial wall of the middle compartment of the sole of the foot, and at about the level of the base of the first metatarsal, the nerve divides into its terminal branches, medial and lateral.

During its course the medial plantar nerve provides cutaneous, muscular, articular, and vascular branches. The *cutaneous branches* arise as soon as the nerve enters the sole of the foot. They are directed downward in the interval between the abductor of the big toe and the flexor digitorum brevis, perforate the aponeurosis, and supply branches to the skin of the inner aspect of the sole of the foot. They anastomose with terminal branches of the medial calcaneal nerve. The *muscular branches* to the abductor hallucis, two or, occasionally, three in number, branch off from the medial aspect of the medial plantar nerve as separate branches or as a common trunk. They are directed anteriorly and medially, pass through small fibrous tunnels, and enter the muscle from the lateral side into the deep surface.[18] The muscular branch to the flexor digitorum brevis is often double and arises from the lateral border of the nerve, usually at the same level as the nerve of the abductor hallucis; it is directed anteriorly and laterally and penetrates the muscle from its deep surface near the inner border at the junction of the posterior third and anterior two thirds of the foot.[20] The *articular branches* arise from the medial border of the nerve, distal to the previous motor branches, and provide branches to the talonavicular and cuneonavicular joints. The *vascular branches* are very thin and variable in number (two or three) and reach the medial plantar artery and its branches.[18]

At the level of the base of the first metatarsal the medial plantar nerve divides into its terminal branches, medial and lateral. The medial branch is the thinner of the two; it courses anteromedially over the medial head of the flexor hallucis brevis between the flexor hallucis longus laterally and the abductor hallucis tendon medially. It terminates as the medial plantar cutaneous nerve of the big toe, which also provides a sensory branch reaching the dorsomedial aspect of the distal phalanx of the big toe. During its course the medial branch gives motor branches—one or two—to the medial head of the flexor hallucis brevis and often one branch to the lateral head of the same muscle. The lateral branch of the medial plantar nerve, the larger of the two, is located in the interval between the abductor hallucis brevis and the flexor digitorum brevis. This nerve now bulges into the middle compartment of the sole but still is separated from the latter by a layer of fascia.[21] It passes around the medial border of the flexor digitorum brevis, enters the superficial space (M_1) of the middle compartment of the sole, and divides into three common digital branches.[21]

The first common digital nerve is directed toward the first web space. It courses plantar to the lateral head of the short flexor of the big toe and is located between the flexor hallucis longus medially and the flexor digitorum longus to the second toe with its first lumbrical laterally. The nerve divides into the lateral plantar digital nerve of the big toe and the medial plantar digital nerve of the second toe. The bifurcation occurs proximal to or at the level of the deep transverse metatarsal ligament between the first and second toes. At this level the nerve is joined by the lateral bifurcation branch of the first plantar metatarsal artery. The nerve is more plantar than the artery, and both are embedded in a protective fat body.[22] Farther distally the nerves and the artery pass under the mooring ligament and the natatory ligament and reach the corresponding sides of the first and second toes. During its course the first common digital nerve provides a branch to the first lumbrical and one to the lateral head of the short flexor of the big toe. It also provides a cutaneous branch and an anastomotic branch with the medial plantar hallucal nerve. The latter passes obliquely over the plantar aspect of the flexor hallucis longus tunnel.[20]

The second common digital nerve turns around the medial border of the flexor digitorum brevis and is directed anteriorly and laterally. It crosses superficially the short flexor tendon to the second toe and passes between this tendon and the longitudinal tract of the plantar aponeurosis. During its course the nerve passes along the posterior border of the sagittal septa of the plantar aponeurosis to the second ray and divides into the lateral plantar nerve to the second toe and the medial plantar nerve to the third toe. Both are also embedded in a fat body at the level of the deep transverse metatarsal ligament and are joined by the digital artery merging from the space delineated by the proximal border of the same ligament and the transverse head of the adductor hallucis. The second common digital nerve provides, during its course, a branch to the second lumbrical muscle.

The third common digital nerve is directed anteriorly and laterally, crosses superficially the short flexor tendons corresponding to the second and third toes, and reaches the third interosseous space. The nerve courses under the plantar aponeurosis and makes a sharp turn against the free posterior border of the lateral sagittal septum of the aponeurosis of the third digit. The nerve divides into the lateral digital branch of the third toe and the medial digital branch of the fourth toe. Very often the third common digital nerve receives an anastomotic branch from the superficial branch of the lateral plantar nerve; the location and type of this anastomosis are very variable. As described by Hovelacque, most frequently the anastomotic branch arises from the lateral plantar nerve and is directed anteriorly and medially, coursing between the plantar aponeurosis and the short flexor of the toes and joining the third common digital nerve near its bifurcation. Sometimes the anastomotic branch passes deep to the short flexor tendons of the fifth and fourth toes and emerges between the tendons of the third and fourth toes. Rarely the anastomosis is double or Y-shaped, or it may extend obliquely outward and anteriorly from the medial plantar nerve to the lateral plantar nerve.

LATERAL PLANTAR NERVE

In the proximal segment of the talocalcaneal canal, the lateral plantar nerve is located initially behind the posterior tibial artery, crosses the latter near its bifurcation, and courses between the more anteriorly located medial plantar artery and the more posteriorly located lateral plantar artery (Figs. 8-11–8-13). At the level of the porta pedis the lateral plantar nerve passes in the lower chamber of the calcaneal canal and enters the medial plantar space M_2 sandwiched between the quadratus plantae and the flexor digitorum brevis. It runs obliquely, anteriorly and laterally, passing under the fascia of the quadratus plantae and anterior to the lateral plantar vessels. It now pierces the lateral intermuscular septum and extends forward. Opposite the base of the fifth metatarsal bone the nerve divides into terminal branches. During this segment of its course the lateral plantar nerve provides a motor branch to the abductor digiti quinti, which arises from the nerve at the level of the medial border of the flexor digitorum brevis as the nerve penetrates the middle compartment of the sole of the foot. This rather large motor branch is directed almost transversely laterally, passes anterior to the posterior tuberosities of the os calcis between the quadratus plantae and the flexor digitorum brevis, and penetrates the abductor digiti quinti on its deep surface near its origin.[20]

Fig. 8-11.   Plantar aspect of the right foot—superficial layer. (1, Medial division branch of medial plantar nerve; 2, first common digital nerve, branch of lateral division branch of medial plantar nerve; 3, second and third common digital nerve trunk, branch of lateral division branch of medial plantar nerve; 4, 5, motor branches to flexor hallucis brevis arising from medial division branch of medial plantar nerve; 6, motor branch to first lumbrical muscle; 7, medial plantar hallucal nerve, a continuation branch of medial division branch of medial plantar nerve; 8, plantar digital nerve to first web space; 9, plantar digital nerve to second web space; 10, plantar digital nerve to third web space; 11, cutaneous branches; 12, anastomotic branch between first common digital nerve and medial plantar hallucal nerve; 13, fourth common digital nerve, a division branch of superficial branch of lateral plantar nerve; 14, plantar digital nerves to fourth web space; 15, lateral plantar cutaneous nerve of little toe; 16, lateral plantar cutaneous nerve, a division branch of superficial branch of lateral plantar nerve; 17, anastomotic branch between common digital nerve to third web space and common digital nerve to fourth web space; 18, medial calcaneal nerve, branch of posterior tibial nerve.) (Redrawn after Hovelacque A: Anatomie des Nerfs Craniens et Rachidiens et du Système Grand Sympathique Chez l'Homme. Paris, Doin, 1927)

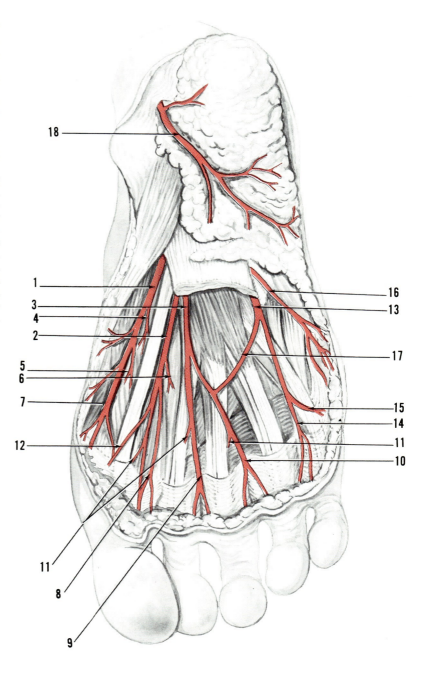

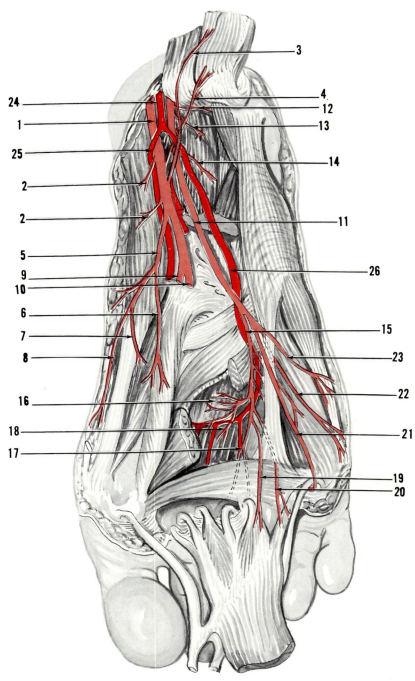

►

Fig. 8-12. Plantar aspect of the right foot—deep layer. (1, Medial plantar nerve; 2, anterior and posterior motor nerves to abductor hallucis muscle; 3, 4, motor branches to flexor digitorum brevis muscle; 5, medial division branch of medial plantar nerve; 6, motor branch to lateral head of flexor hallucis brevis, providing also a branch to medial head of same muscle; 7, motor branch to medial head of flexor hallucis brevis muscle; 8, medial plantar hallucal nerve; 9, 10, division branches of lateral division branch of medial plantar nerve; 11, lateral plantar nerve; 12, motor branch to abductor digiti quinti muscle; 13, posterior motor branch to quadratus plantae muscle; 14, anterior motor branch to quadratus plantae muscle; 15, deep branch of lateral plantar nerve; 16, motor branches to oblique head of adductor hallucis muscle; 17, motor branch to transverse head of adductor hallucis muscle, providing also an articular branch; 18, motor branch to interossei muscles of third interspace; 19, motor branch to third lumbrical muscle; 20, motor branch to fourth lumbrical muscle; 21, common digital nerve to fourth web space; 22, lateral collateral nerve to fifth toe; 23, lateral plantar cutaneous nerve; 24, posterior tibial artery; 25, medial plantar artery; 26, lateral plantar artery.) (Redrawn after Hovelacque A: Anatomie des Nerfs Craniens et Rachidiens et du Système Grand Sympathique Chez l'Homme. Paris, Doin, 1927)

Fig. 8-13.   Plantar aspect of the right foot—superficial and deep layers. (1, Medial plantar nerve; 2, motor branch to flexor digitorum brevis muscle; 3, motor branch to abductor hallucis; 4, medial division branch of medial plantar nerve; 5, lateral division branch of medial plantar nerve; 6, medial plantar hallucal nerve; 7, motor branches to medial head of flexor hallucis muscle; 8, first common digital nerve; 9, common trunk of second and third common digital nerves; 10, motor branch to first lumbrical muscle; 11, motor branch to second lumbrical muscle; 12, motor branch to lateral head of flexor hallucis brevis muscle; 13, interfascicular septum; 14, plantar digital nerve to first web space; 15, plantar digital nerve to second web space; 16, plantar digital nerve to third web space; 17, lateral plantar nerve; 18, motor branch to abductor digiti quinti muscle; 19, posterior motor branch to quadratus plantae muscle; 20, anterior motor branch to quadratus plantae muscle; 21, motor branch to opponens of fifth toe; 22, deep branch of lateral plantar nerve; 23, motor branch to short flexor of fifth toe; 24, motor branch to interossei of third interspace; 25, lateral plantar cutaneous nerve of fifth toe; 26, anastomotic branch between trunk of second–third common digital nerve and fourth common digital nerve; 27, fourth common digital nerve; 28, motor branches to adductor hallucis oblique head, interossei of second space, and transverse head of adductor hallucis; 29, motor branches to interossei muscles of second and third interspaces; 30, motor branch to transverse head of adductor hallucis muscle; 31, motor branch to opponens of fifth toe; 32, motor branch to third lumbrical muscle; 33, motor branch to calcaneocuboid ligament.) (From Dujarier CH: Anatomie des Membres: Dissection-Anatomie Topographique, 2nd ed. Paris, Masson, 1924)

The lateral plantar nerve also provides motor branches to the quadratus plantae. Generally two in number, these are more anterior than the preceding motor branch. They penetrate each head of the muscle from the plantar aspect. Quite often the nerve enters between the two muscular heads and then divides into muscular branches for each and also provides a branch to the calcaneocuboid ligament.[17, 20]

There are two terminal branches of the lateral plantar nerve, superficial and deep.

Superficial Branch

The superficial branch is located in the interval between the flexor digitorum brevis and the abductor digiti quinti; from its inferior surface, it provides for the outer aspect of the sole, several cutaneous branches, which pass through the plantar aponeurosis. It also provides from its lateral border a branch for the short flexor and another branch for the opponens of the fifth toe. These motor branches may arise more anteriorly from the lateral plantar cutaneous branch of the fifth toe or even from the deep branch.[20] The superficial branch now divides into the fourth common digital nerve and the lateral plantar cutaneous nerve to the fifth toe. The lateral plantar cutaneous nerve to the fifth toe is directed obliquely anteriorly and laterally, crosses the short muscles of the fifth toe, and runs alongs its lateral border. The fourth common digital nerve turns around the lateral border of the flexor digitorum brevis, enters the middle plantar space M_1, and divides into the lateral plantar nerve of the fourth toe and the medial plantar nerve of the fifth toe. As described above, it is this nerve to the fourth space that provides the anastomotic branch with the third common digital nerve.

Deep Branch

The deep branch of the lateral plantar nerve follows the direction of the lateral plantar artery, perforates the lateral intermuscular septum 2.5 cm distal to the tuberosity of the fifth metatarsal, and enters the middle plantar space M_3 and subsequently M_4 dorsal to the oblique head of the adductor hallucis. The nerve, posterior to the artery, now courses between the adductor hallucis muscle and the plantar interossei. It passes across the metatarsals 4, 3, and 2 near their base and traces a curve with a posteromedial concavity.

During its course the deep branch of the lateral plantar nerve provides, from its concavity, articular branches to the tarsal and the tarsometatarsal joints. From its convexity the nerve gives off motor branches to the lateral two or three lumbricals, to the interossei of the second, third, fourth space, and to the transverse head of the adductor hallucis; the branches of the latter penetrate the muscle from the posterior border of the dorsal surface.

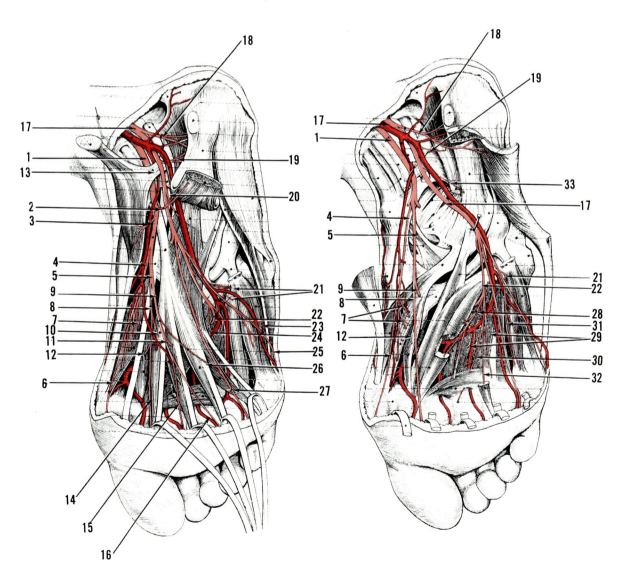

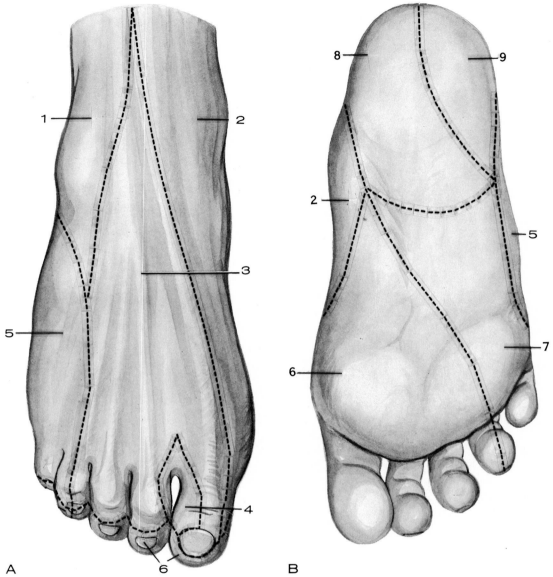

Fig. 8-14.   Cutaneous innervation of the foot. (*A*) Dorsum of the foot. (*B*) Sole of the foot. (1, Peroneal cutaneous nerve; 2, saphenous nerve; 3, superficial peroneal nerve; 4, deep peroneal nerve; 5, sural nerve; 6, medial plantar nerve; 7, lateral plantar nerve; 8, medial calcaneal nerve; 9, lateral calcaneal nerve.)

The deep branch of the lateral plantar nerve terminates by providing branches to the oblique head of the adductor hallucis and the muscles of the first interosseous space. One of the most posterior branches to the adductor hallucis perforates the muscle from the depth to the surface and, before reaching the lateral head of the flexor hallucis, anastomoses with a similar branch provided by the medial plantar nerve. This motor anastomosis, described by Hallopeau, is the equivalent of the Riche and Cannieu motor anastomosis seen in the hand.[20, 23] The very thin anastomosis occurs in the substance of the flexor hallucis brevis or on the plantar aspect of the latter, dorsal to the flexor hallucis longus tendon.[23]

Saphenous Nerve

The saphenous nerve is the terminal branch of the femoral nerve. It courses with the femoral artery, and at the tendinous arch of the adductor magnus, it perforates the fascial covering of the adductor canal. It passes to the medial aspect of the knee deep to the sartorius, pierces the fascia lata between the sartorius and the gracilis, and becomes subcutaneous. It now runs distally in the leg behind the medial border of the tibia, just posterior to the greater saphenous vein. It divides into two branches: one branch, smaller, terminates at the level of the ankle, whereas the second branch passes in front of the medial malleolus and provides

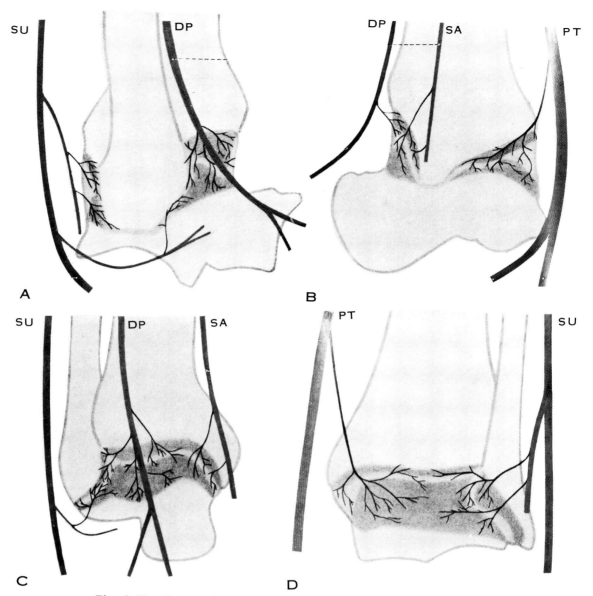

Fig. 8-15. Innervation of the ankle joint. (*A*) Lateral aspect. (*B*) Medial aspect. (*C*) Anterior aspect. (*D*) Posterior aspect. (*SU,* sural nerve; *DP,* deep peroneal nerve; *PT,* posterior tibial nerve; *SA,* saphenous nerve.) (From Lippert J: Zur Innervation der menschlichen Fussgelenke. Anat Entwgesh 123:299, 1962)

branches to the medial side of the foot, extending up to the medial side of the big toe. This branch anastomoses with the medial branch of the superficial peroneal nerve.

Horwitz provides the following data concerning the level of the terminal division of the saphenous nerve: 15 cm from the medial malleolus in 89%, 12.5 cm from the medial malleolus in 5%, 7.5 cm from the medial malleolus in 3%, and 5 cm from the medial malleolus in 3%.[1]

The most constant site of the saphenous nerve is 18 cm above the medial malleolus at the medial border of the tibia, superficial to the deep fascia and posterior or posteromedial

to the saphenous vein.[1] The average diameter of the nerve is 3 mm.[1]

The cutaneous innervation of the foot is shown in Figure 8-14.

Nerves of the Joints of the Foot and Ankle

The first comprehensive study of the innervation of the joints of the foot and ankle was provided by Rudinger.[16]

The more recent studies include those of Morin and Roasenda, Lippert, Gardner and Gray, and Champetier.[24–27] The contribution to the innervation of the joints by the accessory deep peroneal nerve has been described by Bryce and Winckler, as presented previously.[10–13]

The *ankle joint* is innervated by all the nerves crossing the joint, but the more important contribution is from the deep nerves (Fig. 8-15). This innervation is extremely variable.[27] The articular branches from the deep peroneal nerve, three to five in number, arise at the level of the articular interline.[25, 27] A branch may arise proximally in the distal third of the leg, covered by the tibialis anterior tendon. Some branches may have a low origin below the ankle joint interline and they have then a recurrent course to reach the joint. The articular branches from the deep peroneal nerve

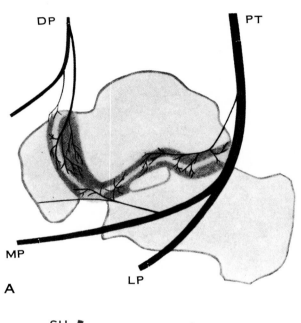

are located behind the tendons and may pass anterior or posterior to the anterior tibial artery. They innervate the anterior aspect of the capsule of the ankle joint, the anterior and inferior tibiofibular ligament, and the anterior talofibular ligament. The posterior tibial nerve provides three to five articular branches and innervates the entire medial aspect of the articulation and the posterior and anterior aspect of the medial malleolus.[25, 27] It extends its innervation to the anterior and posterior aspects of the ankle joint. The articular branches originate from the posterior tibial nerve when the latter divides below the medial malleolus; they may, however, originate from the medial plantar nerve or even the lateral plantar nerve when the division of the posterior tibial nerve is proximal to the level of the medial malleolus. There are also quite often articular branches arising proximally at the junction of the middle third and the distal third of the leg.[27] The nerve to the abductor hallucis from the medial plantar nerve may give articular branches to the ankle joint.

To reach the joint, the articular branches pass lateral or medial to the flexor digitorum longus and always lateral to the tibialis posterior tendon between the deep surface of the sheath and the capsuloligamentous plane.[27]

The saphenous nerve has a modest contribution, with two short branches to the anterior aspect of the medial malleolus and the corresponding capsuloligamentous plane at the same location. These articular branches originate at the level of the medial malleolus and pass behind the tendon of the tibialis anterior before entering the capsule of the joint.

The sural nerve provides articular branches to the perilateral malleolar capsule and ligament. Anterior branches arise sometimes from a long premalleolar branch at the level of the distal third of the leg. Inferior branches take off from the submalleolar arcade of the nerve; these branches pass over the peronei tendons and reach the joint. Posterior branches take off directly from the trunk of the sural nerve and pass deep to the peronei tendons or may originate from a long posterior branch of the sural nerve. The articular branches cross the adipose tissue between the Achilles tendon and the flexors and reach the ankle joint posteriorly.

Champetier describes an inconstant contribution to the innervation of the ankle joint from the superficial peroneal

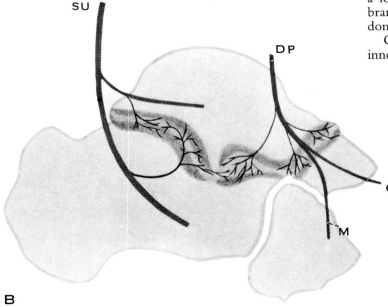

Fig. 8-16. **Innervation of the talocalcaneonavicular joint.** (*A*) Medial aspect. (*B*) Lateral aspect. (*PT,* posterior tibial nerve; *DP,* deep peroneal nerve; *SU,* sural nerve; MP, medial plantar nerve; LP, lateral plantar nerve; M, muscular branch of deep peroneal nerve; C, cutaneous branch of deep peroneal nerve.) (From Lippert J: Zur Innervation der menschlichen Fussgelenke. Z Anat Entwgesh 123:299, 1962)

nerve; anterolateral and anteromedial branches may be provided by the superficial peroneal nerve to the ankle joint.[27] This nerve may also supply an articular branch through the accessory deep peroneal nerve.

The *talotarsal joint* receives its nerve supply from the posterior tibial nerve, the medial plantar nerve, the deep peroneal nerve, the sural nerve, and, when present, the accessory deep peroneal nerve (Fig. 8-16).[25, 26] The *posterior talocalcaneal joint* is innervated medially by a branch from the posterior tibial nerve and laterally by two branches from the sural nerve. The sinus tarsi receives nerve twigs from a branch of the deep peroneal nerve and the canalis tarsi from the posterior tibial nerve. The *talocalcaneonavicular joint* is supplied on the inferomedial aspect by the medial plantar nerve and on the dorsomedial, dorsal, and lateral aspects by the branches from the deep peroneal nerve; the lateral aspect of the joint may receive a branch from the accessory deep peroneal nerve.

On the plantar aspect, all the *articular connections of the cuboid* with the surrounding bones are innervated by the lateral plantar nerve before it gives off its deep branch (Fig. 8-17).[25, 26] On the dorsal aspect, the calcaneocuboid joint is supplied by branches from the sural nerve, the deep peroneal nerve, and the accessory deep peroneal nerve. Dorsally, the cuboid–lateral cuneiform joint is supplied by the deep peroneal nerve, and the cuboid–metatarsals 4 and 5 are innervated by branches from the sural nerve and the lateral branch of the superficial peroneal nerve.

The *cuneonavicular joints,* the *intercuneiform joints,* and the *cuneometatarsal$_{1-3}$ joints* are all innervated on the dorsum by the deep peroneal nerve. On the plantar side the medial plantar nerve innervates the same joints except for the joints of the lateral cuneiform, which are supplied by the lateral plantar nerve.[25, 26]

The *intermetatarsal joints* between metatarsal bases 1, 2, 3, and 4 are innervated on the dorsum by the deep peroneal nerve.[25, 26] On the plantar aspect the intermetatarsal joint 1–2 is supplied by the medial plantar nerve and the intermetatarsal joints 2–3, 3–4 by the deep branch of the lateral plantar nerve. The intermetatarsal joint 4–5 is supplied on the plantar side by the lateral plantar nerve before giving off its deep branch and on the dorsal aspect by branches from the sural nerve and the lateral branch of the superficial peroneal nerve.

The *metatarsophalangeal joints* and the *interphalangeal joints* of the toes receive their main supply from the plantar interdigital nerves (Fig. 8-18).[25, 26]

The digital branches of the medial plantar nerve give articular branches to the plantar aspects of the metatarsophalangeal joints of the first, second, and third toes and the medial aspect of the fourth toe. The digital branches of the lateral plantar nerve provide articular branches to the plantar aspect of the metatarsophalangeal joint of the fifth toe and the lateral aspect of the fourth toe. The plantar aspects of the metatarsophalangeal joints of the second, third, and fourth toes also receive long filaments arising from the deep branch of the lateral plantar nerve.

The medial dorsal cutaneous branch of the superficial peroneal nerve supplies sensory branches to the dorsomedial aspect of the metatarsophalangeal joint and to the inter-

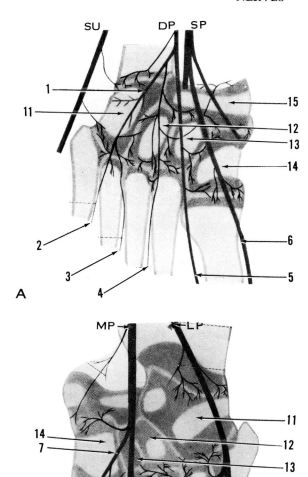

Fig. 8-17.   Innervation of the tarsus and the tarsometatarsal joint. (*A*) Dorsal aspect. (*B*) Plantar aspect. (*SU,* sural nerve; *DP,* deep peroneal nerve; *SP,* superficial peroneal nerve; *MP,* medial plantar nerve; *LP,* lateral plantar nerve; 1, muscular branch of deep peroneal nerve; 2, nerve to dorsal interosseous space 4; 3, nerve to dorsal interosseous space 3; 4, nerve to dorsal interosseous space 2; 5, cutaneous branch of deep peroneal nerve; 6, dorsaltibial cutaneous hallucal nerve; 7, plantartibial cutaneous hallucal nerve; 8, commn digital plantar nerves; 9, deep branch of lateral plantar nerve; 10, plantar lateral cutaneous branch to fifth toe; 11, cuboid; 12, third cuneiform; 13 second cuneiform; 14, first cuneiform; 15, navicular.) (From Lippert J: Zur Innervation der menschlichen Fussgelenke. Z Anat Entwgesh 123:299, 1962)

phalangeal joint of the big toe, whereas the deep peroneal nerve supplies the same joints on the dorsolateral aspect and the digital joints of the second toe medially. The digital branches of the intermediate dorsal cutaneous nerve can be traced up to the tip of the third toe, the lateral aspect of the

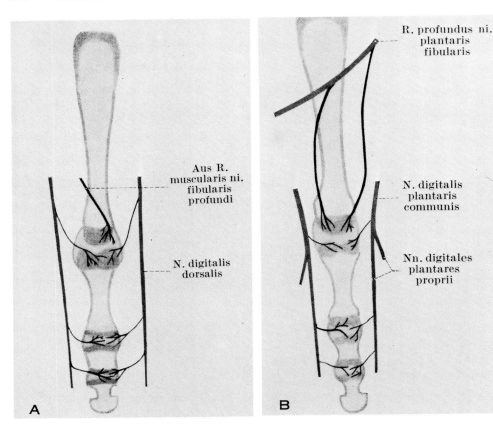

Aus R.
muscularis ni.
fibularis
profundi

N. digitalis
dorsalis

A

R. profundus ni.
plantaris
fibularis

N. digitalis
plantaris
communis

Nn. digitales
plantares
proprii

B

Fig. 8-18. Innervation of the lesser toes. (*A*) Dorsal aspect. (*B*) Plantar aspect. (From Lippert J: Zur Innervation der menschlichen Fussgelenke. Z Anat Entwgesh 123:299, 1962)

second toe, and the medial aspect of the fourth toe, but "in most cases branches of these nerves could not be traced to the metatarso-phalangeal and inter-phalangeal joints."[26] The lateral dorsal cutaneous nerve, a branch of the sural nerve, provides articular filaments to the metatarsophalangeal joint of the fifth and the fourth toe, "but branches to the inter-phalangeal joints of these toes were inconstant."[26]

REFERENCES

1. Horwitz MT: Normal anatomy and variations of the peripheral nerves of the leg and foot. Arch Surg 36:626, 1938
2. Catania V: Il comportamento dei nerve cutanei dorsali del piede (ricerche statistiche nei Siciliani). Arch Ital Anat Embriol 21:295, 1924
3. Kosinski C: The course, mutual relations and distribution of the cutaneous nerve of the metazonal region of the leg and foot. J Anat 60:274, 1926
4. Andreassi G: Osservazioni intorno all'origine, comportamenta e distribuzione dei nervi cutaneo mediale della sura, ramo anastomotico peoniero e cutaneo laterale della sura nell'uoma. Ric Mofologia 2:83, 1931
5. Soskolow PA: Zur anatomie des N. Suralis beim Menschen und Affen. Z Anat Entwgesh 100:194, 1933
6. Mogi E: Über die sensiblen Wadennerven bei den Japanischen Zwillingen. Okajimas Folia Anat Jap 16:229, 1938
7. P'an MT: Formation of sural nerve in the Chinese. Am J Physiol Anthropol 25:311, 1939
8. Williams DD: A study of the human fibular communicating nerve. Anat Rec 120:533, 1954
9. Cruveilhier J: Anatomie Descriptive, Vol IV, p 868. Paris, Bechet Jeune, 1836
10. Bryce TH: Note of a case in which the deep accessory peroneal nerve supplied the extensor brevis digitorum pedis on both sides in the same subject. J Anat Physiol 38:79, 1903–1904
11. Bryce TH: Long muscular branch of the musculocutaneous nerve of the leg. J Anat 31:5, 1896–1897
12. Bryce TH: Deep accessory peroneal nerve. J Anat 35:69, 1900–1901
13. Winckler G: Le nerf péronier accessoire profond: Etude d'anatomie comparée. Arch Anat Histol Embryol 18:186, 1934
14. Lambert EH: The accessory deep peroneal nerve: A common variation in innervation of extensor digitorum brevis. Neurology 19:1169, 1969
15. Anatomical Society of Great Britain and Ireland: Report of Committee of Collective Investigation on the Distribution of Cutaneous Nerve on the Dorsum of the Foot. J Anat Physiol 26:89, 1891–1892
16. Rudinger N: Die Glenknerven des Menschlichen Körpers. Enke Erlangen, 1857
17. Paturet G: Traité d'Anatomie Humaine, Vol II, pp 1067–1069. Paris, Masson, 1951
18. Dujarier CH: Anatomie de Membres: Dissection-Anatomie Topographique, 2nd ed, p 323. Paris, Masson, 1924
19. Macaggi: Sul livetto di biforcazione del nervo tibiale posteriore. Arch Ital Chirurg 3:507, 1921
20. Hovelacque A: Anatomie des Nerfs Craniens et Rachidiens et du Système Grand Sympathique Chez l'Homme, pp 627–635. Paris, Doin, 1927
21. Grodinsky M: A study of the fascial spaces of the foot and their bearing on infections. Surg Obstet Gynecol 49, No. 6:737, 1929
22. Bosjen-Møller F, Flagstad KE: Plantar aponeurosis and internal architecture of the ball of the foot. J Anat 121:599, 1976
23. Hallopeau P: Note sur le nerf de l'adducteur oblique du gros orteil. Bull Mem Soc Anat Paris 2:1078, 1900
24. Morin F, Roasenda F: Le Enervazioni Articolari. Minerva Medica, Torino, 1948
25. Lippert J: Zur Innervation der menschlichen Fussgelenke. Z Anat Entwgesh 123:299, 1962
26. Gardner E, Gray DJ: The innervation of the joints of the foot. Anat Rec 161:141, 1968
27. Champetier J: Innervation de l'articulation tibio-tarsienne (articulatio talo-cruralis). Acta Anat 77:398, 1970

9

Topographic Anatomy

Anterior Aspect of the Ankle and Dorsum of the Foot

The anterior aspect of the ankle is a passage zone from the anterior compartment of the leg to the dorsum of the foot. Morphologically, the distal narrow leg gradually enlarges at the bimalleolar level and is in continuity with the foot plate. The latter is convex dorsally in the proximal and mid segments. Distally, at the level of the metatarsal heads, the foot plate is larger and horizontal.

SURFACE ANATOMY

The lateral and medial malleoli are easily palpated. The lateral malleolus is more distal—about 1 cm—and more posterior than the medial malleolus. The bimalleolar axis is thus turned posterolaterally, with an average angle of rotation of 20° to 30°. A line, nearly horizontal, drawn 2 cm proximal to the tip of the lateral malleolus and 1 cm proximal to the tip of the medial malleolus closely delineates the talotibial joint anterior interline (Fig. 9-1).

On the anterior aspect of the ankle, the tendons of the tibialis anterior medially and of the extensor digitorum longus laterally are easily palpated. Lateral to the latter and medial to the former are the medial and lateral premalleolar depressions where the synovium of the ankle joint may bulge in the presence of effusion. Between these two tendons but deeper is the tendon of the extensor hallucis longus; the tibialis anterior pulse may be taken just lateral to this tendon. A line drawn from the midpoint of the bimalleolar axis to the tip of the first intermetatarsal space traces the direction of the dorsalis pedis artery when the latter is present in its typical location (Fig. 9-1). The dorsalis pedis pulse is felt for along this line, lateral to the extensor hallucis longus tendon and distal to the inferior extensor retinaculum. In young individuals the pulse of the first dorsal metatarsal artery may be found in the first intermetatarsal space and felt up to the level of the head of the first metatarsal. A lateral premalleolar fat pad may be seen and palpated. At the level of the sinus tarsi, a second soft tissue bulge is frequently found, representing the well-developed origin of the extensor digitorum brevis muscle.

On the lateral borders of the foot, the tuberosity of the fifth metatarsal is easily found. The calcaneocuboid joint line is one fingerbreadth proximal to this tuberosity. On the medial border of the foot the tuberosity of the navicular is palpated and, farther distally, the tubercle of the first metatarsal base; the latter is located at the midpoint of the medial border of the foot. The talar head is located medially at the midpoint of a line joining the tuberosity of the navicular to the tip of the medial malleolus. A line drawn across the foot from the calcaneocuboid interline to the middle of a line connecting the head of the talus with the tuberosity of the navicular closely locates Chopart's joint line.[1] A line, slightly convex anteriorly, drawn across the foot from the tuberosity of the fifth metatarsal to the tubercle of the first metatarsal base closely corresponds to Lisfranc's joint interline.[1]

On the dorsum of the foot, in addition to the digital extensor tendons and the tibialis anterior tendon, the examining hand may palpate the intermediate cutaneous branch of the superficial peroneal nerve, which in certain individuals stands up like a thin, tense cable when the foot is inverted and plantar flexed. This nerve courses in the direction of the third web space.

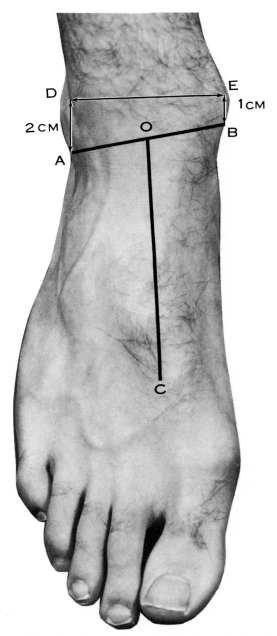

Fig. 9-1.   The dorsal vascular axis. The bimalleolar axis of the ankle is indicated by the line *AB*. Point *O* is the middle of line *AB*. Point *C* is the proximal end of the first intermetatarsal space. Line *OC* indicates the direction and location of the dorsalis pedis artery. Line *DE* indicates the location of the talotibial articular interline. It is 2 cm proximal to the tip of the lateral malleolus and 1 cm proximal to the tip of the medial malleolus.

SKIN AND SUBCUTANEOUS LAYER AND SUPERFICIAL VEINS AND NERVES

Skin and Subcutaneous Layer

The skin on the anterior aspect of the ankle and the dorsum of the foot is thin and supple and may be easily moved over the underlying structures. At the level of the lateral border of the foot it is more intimately connected to the subcutaneous tissue and appreciably loses its mobility.

The cleavage lines of the dorsal skin are shown in Figure 9-2. Along the tibial aspect of the leg and across the anterior aspect of the ankle and the dorsum of the big toe, the lines run parallel to the long axis of the foot. In the remaining segment of the dorsum of the foot, the cleavage lines veer laterally, and at the level of the fifth ray, the obliquity of the lines may reach 45°. Around the lateral aspect of the ankle, the cleavage lines follow more or less the contour of the lateral malleolus. Over the lateral and the medial borders of the foot, the lines are longitudinally oriented. Surgical incisions parallel to the cleavage lines leave finer linear scars, whereas incisions at right angles to these lines are subjected to increased tension and may leave wider scars.

The subcutaneous tissue is formed by a loose-meshed connective tissue, lamellar in structure and mobile relative to the underlying structures. It contains a variable amount of adipose tissue. This layer may form a thin transparent fascia covering or carrying the superficial nerves and veins and may be reflected with ease, exposing the superficial dorsal aponeurosis.

Superficial Veins

The superficial veins of the dorsum of the foot and the anterior ankle are usually superficial to the sensory nerves (Col. Fig. 9-3).[2] The venous network is formed centrally by longitudinally and obliquely oriented veins and distally by the dorsal venous arcade, which receives the superficial dorsal metatarsal veins.

The dorsomedial vein of the big toe, a set of parallel superficial veins crossing the medial border of the foot, and the medial deep perforating veins join the proximal medial extension of the dorsal venous arcade to form the greater saphenous vein. The greater saphenous vein courses anterior to the medial malleolus and receives from its lateral border most of the longitudinally oriented dorsal veins. A medial malleolar vein crosses the medial malleolus inferiorly and transversely and unites the greater saphenous vein with the posterior tibial vein.

The medial perforating veins surface between the superior border of the abductor hallucis and the tarsus. They are usually four in number, one located at the level of the cuneo$_1$ metatarsal$_1$ joint, two periscaphoid, and one more proximal, arising from the medial plantar vein.

On the dorsum of the first web space a perforating vein connects the dorsal venous arcade with the medial end of the deep plantar venous arch. The proximal lateral extension of the dorsal venous arcade receives a set of parallel veins (average number 15) crossing the lateral border of the foot; this forms the lesser saphenous vein, which courses along the posterior aspect of the lateral malleolus.

Fig. 9-2. The cleavage lines of the dorsal and plantar skin of the foot. (*A*) On the dorsal and medial aspect, the cleavage lines are parallel to the medial border of the foot. In the remaining surface the lines are oblique, making about a 45° angle with the long axis of the foot. (*B*) On the plantar aspect, the lines are longitudinally oriented with a slight curvature, convex to the fibular side. At the level of the heel the lines are arciform and parallel to the plantar border of the heel. Incisions placed in the cleavage lines leave fine linear scars, whereas incisions at right angles to these lines may leave wide scars. (Direction of cleavage lines adapted from Cox HT: The cleavage lines of the skin. Br J Surg 29:234, 1941)

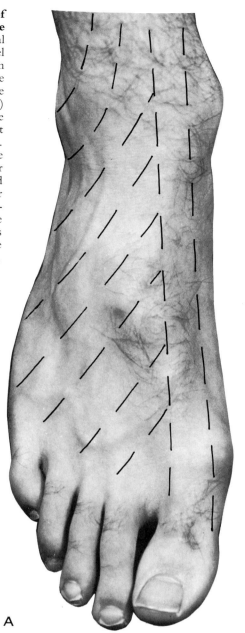

A

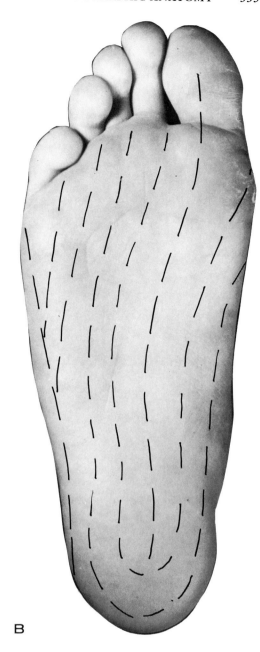

B

The lateral perforating veins join the lesser saphenous vein. They are the peroneal perforating veins, distal and proximal. The distal peroneal perforating vein emerges on the lateral border of the peroneus brevis tendon near its insertion and arises from the dorsal aspect of the calcaneo-cuboid joint. The proximal peroneal perforating vein originates from the plantar aspect of the calcaneocuboid joint, emerges deep to the peroneus longus tendon, and unites with the lesser saphenous vein. The lesser saphenous vein also receives, from its medial border, the deep lateral malleolar veins that pass under the extensor digitorum longus tendons and unite with the dorsalis pedis vein.

The venous flow in the foot is bidirectional, but when valves are present, the flow is from the depth of the planta pedis to the superficial dorsal system.

Superficial Nerves

The superficial nerves of the dorsum of the foot are provided by the superficial peroneal nerve, the terminal branch of the deep peroneal nerve, the lateral sural nerve, and the saphenous nerve (Fig. 9-3).

The superficial peroneal nerve trunk is usually found subcutaneously along the anterior border of the fibula, 10.5 cm above the tip of the lateral malleolus, in the groove between the peroneal group of muscles and the extensor digitorum longus.[3] The nerve divides into its terminal branches—intermediate and medial dorsal cutaneous nerves—at an average 6.5 cm proximal to the tip of the lateral malleolus.[3] The intermediate dorsal cutaneous nerve courses along the tibiofibular syndesmosis, passes over the

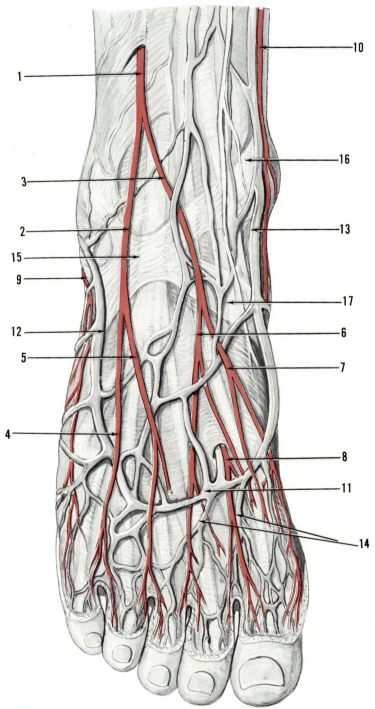

Fig. 9-3. Superficial layer of the dorsum of the foot and ankle. (1, Superficial peroneal nerve; 2, intermediate dorsal cutaneous nerve; 3, medial dorsal cutaneous nerve; 4, dorsal cutaneous nerve to fourth web space; 5, dorsal cutaneous nerve to third web space; 6, dorsal cutaneous nerve to second web space with branch to dorsum of big toe; 7, dorsomedial cutaneous nerve to big toe; 8, nerve branch from deep peroneal nerve to first interspace; 9, sural nerve; 10, saphenous nerve; 11, dorsal venous arcade; 12, lesser saphenous vein; 13, greater saphenous vein; 14, dorsal metatarsal veins; 15, stem of inferior extensor retinaculum; 16, superomedial band of inferior extensor retinaculum; 17, inferomedial band of inferior extensor retinaculum.)

root of the inferior extensor retinaculum, crosses obliquely the fifth and fourth extensor digitorum longus tendons, and courses over the third intermetatarsal space. This nerve can be palpated through the skin. Distally the nerve divides into the dorsolateral branch of the third toe and the dorsomedial branch of the fourth toe. An anastomic branch to the sural nerve may be present. The variations of the distributions of the sensory nerves are dealt with in Chapter 8.

The medial dorsal cutaneous branch is located laterally over the anterior aspect of the ankle and overlies the extensor digitorum longus tendons. It runs parallel to the extensor hallucis longus tendon, crosses the inferior extensor retinaculum, and, distal to the latter, divides into three branches: lateral, middle, and medial.

The lateral branch obliquely crosses the long extensor tendon of the second toe and bifurcates in the anterior segment of the second intermetatarsal space into the dorsomedial branch of the third toe and the dorsolateral branch of the second toe.

The middle branch courses superficially over the first intermetatarsal space and divides into two thin branches supplying the dorsomedial aspect of the second toe and the dorsolateral aspect of the big toe. These two branches are reinforced by the deep peroneal nerve.

The medial branch is directed medially; it crosses the extensor hallucis longus tendon and forms the dorsomedial cutaneous nerve of the big toe. This is the superficial nerve branch that is to be looked for and reflected laterally during the bunionectomy of the big toe through a medial approach.

The intermediate and medial dorsal cutaneous nerves are to be dealt with in the anterolateral approach to the lateral malleolus and the ankle joint, in the lateral approach for a triple arthrodesis, in the transverse or longitudinal approach for a tarsometatarsal mobilization, in the midtarsal osteotomy, or in the central metatarsal osteotomies. The longitudinally oriented superficial nerves are most vulnerable in the transverse dorsal incisions.

The saphenous nerve is located on the anterior aspect of the medial malleolus, posteromedial to the greater saphenous vein, and may extend along the medial border of the foot and reach the medial aspect of the big toe.

The sural nerve, after turning around the lateral malleolus, divides into two branches—lateral and medial—at the base of the fifth metatarsal bone. The lateral branch terminates as the dorsolateral nerve of the fifth toe. The medial branch obliquely crosses the long extensor tendon of the fifth toe and forms the dorsomedial branch to the fifth toe. As mentioned above, an anastomotic branch may be present between the sural nerve and the lateral division branch of the intermediate dorsal cutaneous nerve.

DORSAL APONEUROSIS AND DORSAL FASCIAL SPACES AND CONTENTS

Dorsal Aponeurosis

The superficial dorsal aponeurosis of the foot is encountered after reflection of the skin and the subcutaneous layer carrying the fascia superficialis and the incorporated superficial veins and nerves. This thin, semitransparent layer invests the musculotendinous units, the arteries, and their accom-

Fig. 9-4.   Second layer of the dorsum of the foot and ankle. (1, Anterior tibial artery; 2, anterior medial malleolar artery; 3, anterior lateral malleolar artery; 4, dorsalis pedis artery; 5, first dorsal metatarsal artery; 6, arcuate artery; 7, dorsal metatarsal arteries 2, 3, 4; 8, medial tarsal artery; 9, 10, deep peroneal nerve; 11, motor nerve branch to extensor digitorum brevis; 12, inferior extensor retinaculum; 13, superomedial band of inferior extensor retinaculum; 14, inferomedial band of inferior extensor retinaculum; 15, superolateral band of inferior extensor retinaculum; 16, superior extensor retinaculum; 17, tibialis anterior tendon; 18, extensor hallucis longus tendon; 19, extensor digitorum longus tendon; 20, extensor digitorum brevis muscle to toes 2, 3, 4; 21, extensor hallucis brevis muscle.)

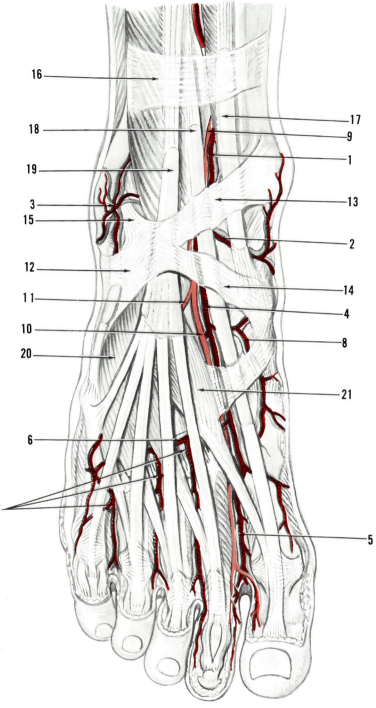

panying deep veins. It is attached to the dorsal skeletal frame medially and laterally and creates a true osteofascial space: spatium dorsalis pedis.[4] Laterally the aponeurosis attaches on the os calcis, the cuboid, and the tuberosity and the lateral border of the fifth metatarsal bone. The medial marginal insertion extends from the sustentaculum tali to the tuberosity of the scaphoid and the medial border of the first metatarsal bone.

The superficial dorsal aponeurosis extends vertical fibers to the skin and closes the dorsal subcutaneous space along its margins. Distally the thin aponeurosis attaches to the fibrous sheath of the extensor tendons, and proximally it is in continuity with the inferior extensor retinaculum.

The inferior extensor retinaculum is a retention system acting as multiple pulleys for the tendons crossing the anterior aspect of the ankle and of the foot, preventing their bowstringing (Figs. 9-4 and 9-5). Their surgical preservation or reconstruction is essential.

At first sight the delineation of the borders of this retinaculum might not be very clear, as distally it is in conti-

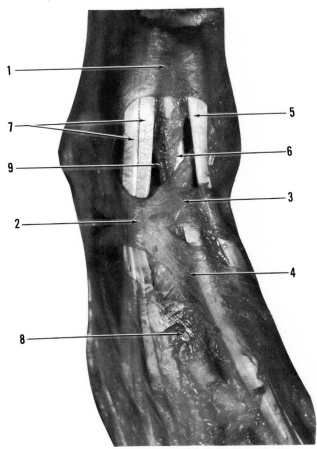

Fig. 9-5. Dorsum of the ankle and foot. (1, Superior extensor retinaculum; 2, stem of inferior extensor retinaculum; 3, superomedial band of inferior extensor retinaculum; 4, inferomedial band of inferior extensor retinaculum; 5, tibialis anterior tendon; 6, extensor hallucis longus tendon; 7, extensor digitorum longus tendons; 8, extensor digitorum brevis muscle; 9, neurovascular bundle—deep peroneal nerve and dorsalis pedis artery.)

nuity with the dorsal aponeurosis and proximally with the distal segment of the aponeurosis cruris and the superior extensor retinaculum. The inferior extensor retinaculum originates from the sinus tarsi and sinus canal with three roots: lateral, intermediate, and medial (Fig. 9-6). The lateral root inserts on the lateral border of the sinus tarsi and over the inferior peroneal retinaculum; it is lateral to the origin of the extensor digitorum brevis muscle. The intermediate root originates in the center of the sinus tarsi, me-·dial to the extensor digitorum brevis muscle and posterior to the cervical ligament. The medial root inserts in the sinus tarsi, next to the intermediate root; in the canalis tarsi it is anterior to the interosseous ligament and sends an arm to the talar roof of the tarsal canal. The lateral and intermediate roots envelop the origin of the extensor digitorum brevis, unite, and form the stem of the inferior extensor retinaculum. The medial root courses superomedially and attaches to the deep surface of the stem immediately medial to the extensor digitorum longus tendons, contributing to the formation of the powerful lateral retention sling for these ten-

dons. Anteriorly the retinacular stem divides into two arms, superomedial and inferomedial. The superomedial arm passes over the tendon of the extensor hallucis longus, covers the tendon of the tibialis anterior, and inserts on the anterior aspect of the medial malleolus. On the medial border of the extensor hallucis longus tendon, deep retinacular fibers loop around the tendon posteriorly and insert either on the talar neck or on the deep surface of the lateral sling. These recurrent fibers form a retention tunnel for the extensor hallucis longus tendon. Farther medially the superomedial arm of the retinaculum reaches the tibialis anterior tendon and forms two retention systems: superior and inferior. The superior tunnel has a very thin or absent superficial cover, whereas the deep layer is thick and inserts on the medial malleolus. The inferior tunnel is well structured. The anterior and posterior walls of the tunnel unite on the medial border of the tendon and insert on the anterior aspect of the medial malleolus.

The inferomedial arm of the retinaculum courses anteromedially and reaches the medial border of the foot at the level of the cuneonavicular joint. The fibers pass over the dorsalis pedis vessels, the deep peroneal nerve, and the extensor hallucis longus tendon, and as they reach the tibialis anterior tendon, they form a terminal tunnel for the latter. This segment of the retinaculum splits into deep fibers, which insert on the navicular and medial cuneiform, and superficial fibers, which are in continuity with the investing fascia of the abductor hallucis muscle.

In 25% of the cases the inferior extensor retinaculum has an oblique superolateral extension band that gives to the retinaculum a cruciate configuration. This band originates from the lateral sling, from the superomedial band, or from both. It courses upward and laterally and inserts on the lateral surface of the lateral malleolus and the lateral crest of the lower segment of the fibula.

Dorsal Fascial Spaces and Contents

The dorsal osteoaponeurotic space of the foot is subdivided into four fascial gliding spaces by three layers of tissue.[4]

The first layer is formed by the tendons of the tibialis anterior, extensor hallucis longus, extensor digitorum longus, and peroneus tertius, surrounded by their synovial sheaths or peritenon. The tendons are united to each other with loose connective tissue. Laterally and medially this loose connective tissue blends with the superficial dorsal aponeurosis.

The second layer is muscular and is formed by the extensor digitorum brevis and its investing fascia. This fascia, attached to the deep surface of the extensor hallucis longus synovial sheath, passes over the dorsalis pedis vessels and the deep peroneal nerve. It encounters the medial border of the extensor digitorum brevis, where it splits into two investing layers, superficial and deep. On the lateral margin of the muscle the two layers unite, and the aponeurosis inserts on the deep surface of the superficial dorsal aponeurosis and on the tarsal skeleton.

The third layer, neurovascular, is formed by an adipoconnective lamina carrying the dorsalis pedis vessels with their tributaries and the deep peroneal nerve with its branches.

At the level of the metatarsals the dorsal interosseous aponeurosis is the last investing layer.

The four gliding fascial spaces are the potential spaces located between the dorsal aponeurosis, the three soft tissue layers, and the dorsal osteoligamentous frame.

First Layer.   On the anterior aspect of the ankle, the crossing tendons are grouped over the distal tibia and do not cover the anterior aspect of the malleoli (Fig. 9-4). The tibialis anterior tendon on the medial side and the extensor digitorum longus tendon with the peroneus tertius tendon laterally are more superficial than the centrally located extensor hallucis longus tendon.

The reflection of the superficial dorsal aponeurosis reveals the same tendons on the dorsum of the foot but in a diverging pattern. On the medial aspect, the tendon of the tibialis anterior is directed obliquely anteromedially and plantarward, winds around the medial border of the foot, and inserts on the base of the first metatarsal inferomedially and on the medial aspect of the first cuneiform. The synovial tendon sheath of the tibialis anterior tendon extends from above the superior arm of the inferior extensor retinaculum to the level of the talonavicular joint.

The extensor hallucis longus tendon is located lateral to the tibialis anterior tendon. It is directed anteromedially, diverging slightly from the tibialis anterior tendon. The tendon approaches the first metatarsal bone at an acute angle; it courses on the dorsolateral aspect of the bone and remains centralized on the dorsum of the metatarsophalangeal joint of the big toe. The lateral border of the extensor hallucis longus is an important guideline, as it parallels the direction of the vascular axis of the dorsum of the foot. The synovial sheath of the extensor hallucis tendon extends from just above the upper arm of the inferior extensor retinaculum to the level of the $cuneo_1$-$metatarsal_1$ joint.

The extensor digitorum longus tendons, usually two in number, are located under the stem of the inferior extensor retinaculum and divide into four tendons as they exit from their retinacular tunnel. On the dorsum of the foot these tendons fan out, cross the extensor digitorum brevis muscle, may exchange thin connecting fibers, and reach their respective toes 2 to 5. The long extensor tendons to the fourth and fifth toes are oriented anterolaterally.

The peroneus tertius tendon is lateral to the tendons of the extensor digitorum longus. The tendon diverges anterolaterally, obliquely crosses the underlying extensor digitorum brevis muscle, fans out, and inserts on the superior surface of the fifth metatarsal base; this tendon is absent in 8.5% of the cases.

The common synovial tendon sheath of the extensor digitorum longus and the peroneus tertius starts about 1 cm proximal to the tendon sheath of the extensor hallucis longus. It enlarges distally and forms a triangular sac that terminates at the level of the cuneonavicular joint. Four small synovial projections may extend farther distally over the four toe extensors. The tenosynovial compartments described above are normally flat, unimpressive structures, but they have great relevance when involved by an inflammatory or infectious process.

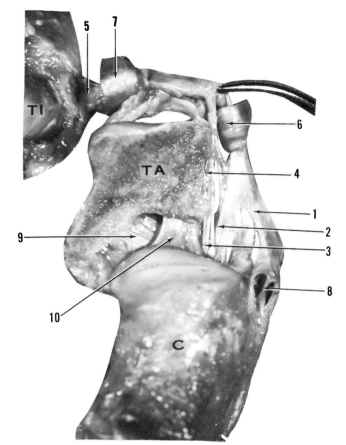

Fig. 9-6.   The roots of the inferior extensor retinaculum on the right foot. The posterior aspect of the talus is removed, exposing the canalis tarsi. (*C,* calcaneum; *TA,* talus; *TI,* tibia; 1, lateral root of inferior extensor retinaculum; 2, intermediary root of inferior extensor retinaculum; 3, medial root of inferior extensor retinaculum; 4, talar attachment of 3; 5, superomedial attachment of inferior extensor retinaculum on tibia; 6, tendon of extensor digitorum longus; 7, tibialis anterior tendon; 8, inferior peroneal retinaculum; 9, interosseous ligament of canalis tarsi; 10, anterior capsular ligament of posterior talocalcaneal joint.)

Second Layer.   The extensor digitorum brevis muscle originates in the sinus tarsi between the superficial and intermediate roots of the inferior extensor retinaculum. Initially the muscle covers the lateral half of the tarsus, is directed anteromedially, and divides into four small muscles followed by their corresponding tendons. The extensor hallucis brevis component is the largest of the four, and it obliquely crosses the distal segment of the dorsalis pedis artery. When the muscle is well developed, the medial border covers the mid segment of the same artery. The tendon of the extensor hallucis brevis joins the extensor hallucis longus from the peroneal side and is deep to the latter and its extensor lamina.

The extensor digitorum brevis tendons to the second, third, and fourth toes join the long extensor tendinous complex from the peroneal side. Proximally they are deeper relative to the long extensor tendon. The fifth toe does not

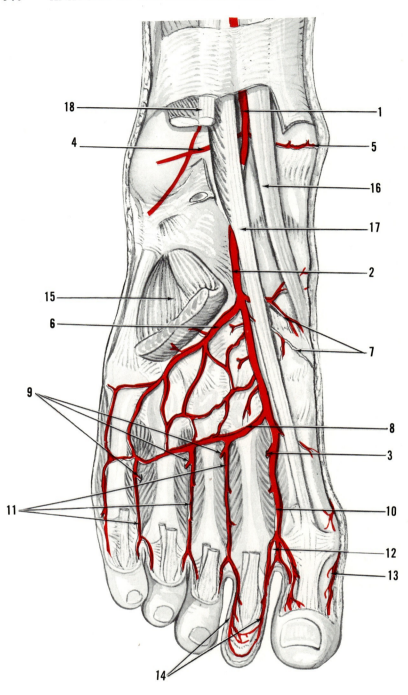

Fig. 9-7. Deep layer of the dorsal aspect of the foot and ankle. (1, Anterior tibial artery; 2, dorsalis pedis artery; 3, first proximal perforating artery; 4, anterior lateral malleolar artery; 5, anterior medial malleolar artery; 6, lateral tarsal artery; 7, medial tarsal arteries; 8, arcuate artery; 9, proximal perforating arteries 2, 3, 4; 10, first dorsal metatarsal artery; 11, dorsal metatarsal arteries 2, 3, 4; 12, first distal perforating artery; 13, dorsomedial hallucal artery; 14, dorsal digital collateral arteries; 15, extensor digitorum brevis muscle; 16, tibialis anterior tendon; 17, extensor hallucis longus tendon; 18, extensor digitorum longus tendon.)

have an extensor brevis muscle and cannot be a donor of long extensor tendon as a graft.

Reflection of the extensor digitorum brevis and its aponeurosis reveals the connective tissue layer carrying the dorsal pedis vessels and the deep peroneal nerve, with their divisions (Fig. 9-7).

Third Layer. As mentioned previously, the dorsalis pedis vascular axis is delineated by a line joining the midpoint of the bimalleolar axis to the proximal end of the first interosseous space.

At the level of the ankle joint interline, the tibialis anterior artery becomes the dorsalis pedis artery. Above the ankle joint the artery is covered by the extensor hallucis longus tendon. At the ankle the extensor hallucis longus tendon crosses the dorsalis pedis artery, and is then medial to the artery. Under the inferior extensor retinaculum the artery is deep and located posterolateral to the tunnel of the extensor hallucis longus tendon.

The two accompanying veins and the deep branch of the peroneal nerve located on the lateral side of the vessels are all applied against the osteoarticular layer. Lateral detachment of the roots of the inferior extensor retinaculum and of the origin of the extensor digitorum brevis followed by medial reflection of this entire unit will carry all the tendons but leave the neurovascular structures against the joint.

Distal to the inferior extensor retinaculum, the dorsalis pedis artery is located lateral to the extensor hallucis longus tendon and medial to the medial border of the extensor hallucis brevis muscle. In the mid segment of the foot the artery is covered by the medial border of the same muscle, and distally it is lateral to the tendon of the same muscle.

To expose the dorsalis pedis artery, a skin incision is made on the dorsum of the foot along a line extending from the midpoint of the bimalleolar axis to the base of the first interosseous space. The superficial aponeurosis is incised, followed by incision of the second aponeurosis along the medial border of the extensor digitorum brevis, which is retracted laterally, providing access to the artery.

The above description of the dorsalis pedis artery applies to the majority of the cases. However, the artery may be absent in 12% of the cases or may have a lateral deviation in 5.5% and a medial deviation in 3.5%.[5]

The dorsalis pedis artery plunges plantarward at a 90° angle through the space limited by the arch of the first dorsal interosseous muscle and the bases of the first and second metatarsals. After making another 90° lateral turn, it inosculates with the deep branch of the lateral plantar artery. At the level of the ankle the dorsalis pedis artery provides the transversely oriented anterior lateral and medial malleolar arteries; these two arteries are deep to the tendons crossing the ankle.

At the level of the talar neck a few talar branches take off, including the artery of the sinus tarsi. The lateral tarsal artery originates at the level of the talar head and courses obliquely over the dorsum of the cuboid under the extensor digitorum brevis. It provides the arterial branches to the extensor digitorum brevis, contributes to the vascularization of the talus, and divides over the cuboid into two or three longitudinal arterial branches, which join the arcuate artery. The latter originates from the dorsalis pedis artery at the level of the cuneo$_1$-metatarsal$_1$ joint, crosses transversely the bases of the second, third, and fourth metatarsals, and provides the dorsal metatarsal arteries 2 to 4.

The first dorsal metatarsal artery takes off from the terminal segment of the dorsalis pedis artery and courses over the first dorsal interosseous muscle. It provides the dorsal arteries to the big toe and the dorsotibial artery to the second toe. It plunges plantarward at the first web space and becomes the first distal perforating artery.

The dorsal metatarsal arteries 2 to 4 course in their respective intermetatarsal spaces. Each provides the proximal perforating artery in the proximal segment of the interspace, supplies the dorsal arteries to the adjacent toes, and terminates as the distal perforating artery in the web space. At the level of the metatarsal necks the dorsal metatarsal artery also provides two transverse plantar anastomotic branches. The medial tarsal arteries take off from the medial aspect of the dorsalis pedis artery at the level of the navicular and the cuneonavicular joint and course transversely under the tibialis anterior tendon. The transversely crossing arcuate artery and the longitudinal tributaries of the lateral tarsal ar-

tery are dealt with during tarsometatarsal surgical mobilization.

The deep branch of the peroneal nerve is lateral to the anterior tibial vessels. Just proximal to the ankle joint interline the nerve divides into medial and lateral branches. Under the inferior extensor retinaculum the nerves remain lateral to the dorsalis pedis vessels. The larger medial branch continues the direction of the nerve trunk and courses along the medial side of the dorsalis pedis artery. At the base of the first intermetatarsal space the nerve divides into two branches: the dorsolateral branch of the big toe and the dorsomedial branch of the second toe.

The lateral branch of the deep peroneal nerve is directed anterolaterally and innervates the extensor digitorum brevis muscle. Both medial and lateral branches provide articular filaments to the tarsal skeleton, the tarsometatarsal joints, and the digital joints.

Posterolateral Aspect of the Ankle and Foot

The posterolateral aspect of the ankle and foot comprises the concave region located between the lateral border of the Achilles tendon and the peronei tendons. It extends distally over the convex lateral aspect of the heel and the lateral border of the foot up to the tuberosity of the fifth metatarsal.

SKIN, SUBCUTANEOUS LAYER, AND SUPERFICIAL VEINS AND NERVES

The skin is mobile proximally but relatively fixed over the heel and the lateral border of the foot (Fig 9-8). The skin cleavage lines are oblique, oriented downward and anteriorly except on the lateral border, where they are longitudinal.

The subcutaneous layer is thicker and more adipose than that of the anterior aspect of the ankle. The connective tissue is organized in lamellae and forms a superficial fascia that carries the superficial nerves and vessels.

The short saphenous vein courses along the lateral border of the Achilles tendon, turns around the lateral malleolus, and reaches the lateral aspect of the foot. It receives from its inferior border an average of three lateral calcaneal veins, and from its anterior border, it receives the anterolateral malleolar vein arising from the dorsalis pedis vein. Farther distally, two peroneal communicating veins—proximal and distal—are tributaries of the short saphenous vein. The proximal peroneal vein arises from the plantar aspect of the calcaneocuboid joint and passes deep to the peroneus longus tendon. The distal peroneal vein arises from the dorsum of the calcaneocuboid joint and passes between the peroneus brevis and the peroneus longus tendon to join the lesser saphenous vein.

The retromalleolar branch of the posterior peroneal artery, after piercing the deep and superficial aponeuroses, accompanies the short saphenous vein and provides the lateral arterial calcaneal branches.

Proximal to the ankle joint, the sural nerve is lateral to

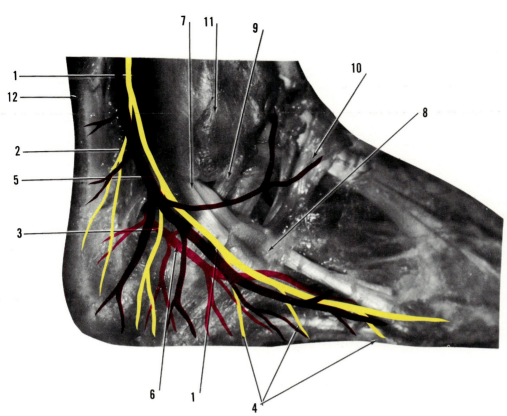

the lesser saphenous vein. With the latter, the nerve courses behind the posterior border of the lateral malleolus and the retained peronei tendons. The nerve passes 1 cm to 1.5 cm distal to the tip of the lateral malleolus. It is anterior to the vein and remains posterior to the peronei tendons. At times the peronei tendons are crossed by the nerve. At the level of the tuberosity of the fifth metatarsal base, the sural nerve divides into its two terminal branches. From its posterior border the nerve provides two lateral calcaneal branches originating about three fingerbreadths and one fingerbreadth proximal to the tip of the lateral malleolus. Farther distally the nerve provides from its lower border a set of three to four, vertical or slightly oblique lateral marginal branches. In a transverse surgical incision across the sheath of the peronei tendons, the sural nerve is to be dealt with.

SUPERFICIAL APONEUROSIS AND SUPERFICIAL POSTEROLATERAL COMPARTMENT

The superficial aponeurosis, after investing the Achilles tendon, covers the space between the latter and the fibrous proximal tunnel of the peronei tendons formed by the lateral expansion of the deep crural aponeurosis. Inferiorly the superficial aponeurosis is reinforced and forms the superior peroneal retinaculum or lateral annular ligament, a quadrilateral lamina that originates from the tip and posterior border of the lateral malleolus. This lamina is oriented pos-

teroinferiorly and inserts over the lateral aspect of the os calcis. The short saphenous vein and the sural nerve cross this lamina superficially and obliquely.

Farther distally a second reinforcement of the superficial aponeurosis contributes to the formation of the inferior peroneal retinaculum. The latter originates from the posterior segment of the lateral rim of the sinus tarsi in common with the lateral root of the inferior extensor retinaculum. It is directed posteroinferiorly, crosses the trochlear process (to which it provides fibers of attachment), and terminates on the lateral tuberosity of the os calcis. The inferior peroneal retinaculum forms two tunnels at the level of the trochlear process. The upper tunnel lodges the peroneus brevis tendon and the lower tunnel the peroneus longus tendon.

The common synovial sheath of the peronei tendons extends proximally about two fingerbreadths from the tip of the lateral malleolus. Distally the synovial sheath bifurcates at the level of the trochlear process. The sheath of the peroneus brevis tendon terminates about one fingerbreadth short of the insertion of the tendon. The synovial sheath of the peroneus longus reaches the plantar groove of the cuboid.

Below the free tip of the lateral malleolus, the peronei tendons cross the calcaneofibular ligament in an X (see Fig. 9-8). An incision of the superficial aponeurosis along the lateral border of the Achilles tendon provides safe entrance to the pre-Achilles space (filled centrally by the pre-Achilles fat pad) and leads to the deep aponeurosis.

TOPOGRAPHIC ANATOMY 343

DEEP APONEUROSIS AND DEEP POSTEROLATERAL COMPARTMENT

The deep aponeurosis forms the retromalleolar fibrous tunnel of the peronei tendons, covers the flexor hallucis muscle–tendon unit, and sends a septum on the medial border of the latter, forming a wide tunnel that corresponds to the posterolateral corner of the tibia. This second tunnel also contains the posterior peroneal vessels coursing along the posterior aspect of the tibiofibular syndesmosis.

The distal extension of the deep aponeurosis toward the dorsum of the os calcis and the talus may acquire thick fibers and form the fibulotalocalcaneal ligament of Rouvière and Canela Lazaro.[6] This ligament originates from the medial lip of the fibular canal for the peronei tendons and from the lower segment of the posterior tibiofibular ligament. It is flat anteroposteriorly, enlarges as it courses inferomedially, and divides into two bands—inferolateral or fibulocalcaneal and superomedial or talofibular. The fibulocalcaneal

component is the larger and inserts transversely over the dorsum of the os calcis. The talofibular component is oriented transversely and terminates over the posterolateral tubercle of the talus and the fibrous tunnel of the flexor hallucis longus tendon.

The fibulotalocalcaneal ligament is present in 60% of the cases; it covers the posterior talofibular ligament and is separated from the latter by adipose tissue.[6] This ligament is tight with dorsiflexion of the foot, and in clubfeet it contributes to the equinus deformity.

Incision of the deep aponeurosis in the posterolateral compartment above the ankle joint line gives access to a triangular interval with a proximal apex and a distal base. The lateral border of the space is formed by the peroneus brevis muscle, the medial border by the flexor hallucis. Enlargment of the triangular space provides access to the posterolateral end of the tibia and to the posterior tibiofibular joint.[7] The posterior peroneal vessels longitudinally cross the space and are to be dealt with in the surgical exposure (Fig. 9-9).

Fig. 9-9. Posterior aspect of the ankle. (A) Superficial aspect. (B) Deep aspect. (1, Sural nerve; 2, lateral calcaneal nerve, posterior branch; 3, medial calcaneal and posteromedial nerve branches of posterior tibial nerve; 4, posteromedial and medial calcaneal arteries, branch of posterior tibial artery; 5, lateral calcaneal artery, branch of posterior peroneal artery; 6, lesser saphenous vein; 7, posterior medial malleolar vein; 8, superficial aponeurosis cruris, which splits and invests Achilles tendon [10] and plantaris tendon [11]; 9, deep aponeurosis cruris; 12, posterior tibial nerve; 13, posterior tibial artery; 14, posterior tibial vein; 15, posterior peroneal artery and veins; 16, tibialis posterior tendon; 17, flexor digitorum longus tendon; 18, peroneus brevis muscle–tendon; 19, peroneus longus tendon; 20, pre-Achilles tendon fat pad located in "safe zone" between superficial and deep aponeuroses cruris.) (After Testut L, Jacob O: Traité d'Anatomie Topographique avec Applications Médico-Chirurgicales, 2nd ed, Vol II: pp 1036, 1045. Paris, Doin, 1909)

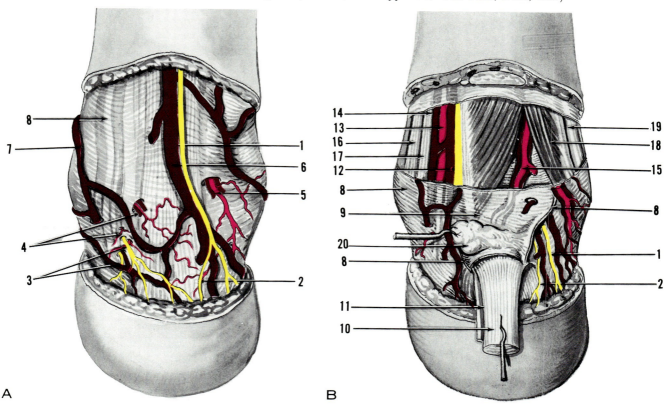

A
B

Posteromedial Aspect of the Ankle and the Tibiotalocalcaneal Tunnel

The posteromedial aspect of the ankle and the tarsal tunnel or calcaneal canal constitute the major passageway from the posterior compartment of the leg to the sole of the foot.

SURFACE ANATOMY

The medial malleolus is felt with ease. The sustentaculum tali is found about 2.5 cm below the tip of the medial malleolus. At the midpoint of the line uniting the tuberosity of the scaphoid to the tip of the medial malleolus is located the head of the talus. The tendon of the tibialis posterior may be palpated prior to its scaphoid insertion. The posterior tibial pulse is found one fingerbreadth behind the medial malleolus.

SKIN, SUBCUTANEOUS LAYER, AND SUPERFICIAL VEINS AND NERVES

The skin is mobile over the medial malleolus but semifixed over the medial aspect of the heel. The skin cleavage lines are oriented as indicated in Figure 9-10. The subcutaneous tissue has a lamellar constitution and may form a thin fascia superficialis carrying the superficial veins and nerves. Longitudinally oriented veins course over the superficial fascia, which bridges the interval between the posterior tibia and the medial border of the Achilles tendon. The superficial veins collect the medial calcaneal veins. A transverse vein crosses the lower border of the medial malleolus and unites the greater saphenous vein to the posterior tibial vein and contributes to the formation of the medial malleolar venous rete.

Two perforating veins are located around the scaphoid and surface at the upper border of the abductor hallucis muscle. These veins arrive from the plantar aspect of the scaphocuneiform and calcaneocuboid joints. A third perforating vein unites the greater saphenous vein with the medial plantar vein.

Sensory, longitudinally oriented nerve filaments are provided by the saphenous nerve. A medial calcaneal sensory nerve trunk, a branch of the posterior tibial nerve, perforates the superficial aponeurosis just proximal to the superior border of the abductor hallucis muscle. It courses superficially and divides into two groups, posterior and anterior. The posterior group is formed by two or three filaments and terminates in the skin of the heel. The anterior set, formed also by two or three filaments, terminates on the medial border of the foot.

SUPERFICIAL AND DEEP APONEUROSIS AND TIBIOTALOCALCANEAL TUNNEL

At the level of the distal leg posteriorly, the superficial aponeurosis splits and incorporates the triceps surae. The deep aponeurosis covers the tibialis posterior, the flexor digitorum longus, and the flexor hallucis longus muscles and the posterior tibial neurovascular bundle. It forms the deep compartment of the leg separated from the triceps surae and its investing superficial aponeurosis. Distally, a new fascial layer covers the tibialis posterior and the flexor digitorum longus muscles. Beyond the point where the two muscles cross, the corresponding tendons pass through individual fibrous tunnels covered by the deep aponeurosis. The flexor hallucis longus muscle and the posterior tibial neurovascular bundle are in a common compartment under the deep aponeurosis. At the level of the talotibial joint line

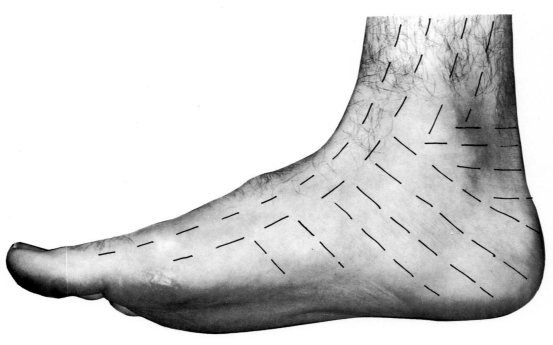

Fig. 9-10. The cleavage lines of the skin on the medial aspect of the ankle and foot. The cleavage lines are longitudinally oriented on the dorsomedial aspect. The lines are transverse and parallel on the posterior aspect of the ankle and are oblique in the remaining segment of the foot. (Direction of the cleavage lines adapted from Cox HT: The cleavage lines of the skin. Br J Surg 29:234, 1941)

Fig. 9-11.   Posteromedial aspect of the ankle and foot—tarsal tunnel. (1, Superficial aponeurosis, reflected off the deep aponeurosis [2]; 3, posterior tibial nerve; 4, posterior tibial artery and veins; 5, tibialis posterior tendon; 6, flexor digitorum longus tendon; 7, flexor hallucis longus tendon; 8, Achilles tendon; 9, peronei tendons.)

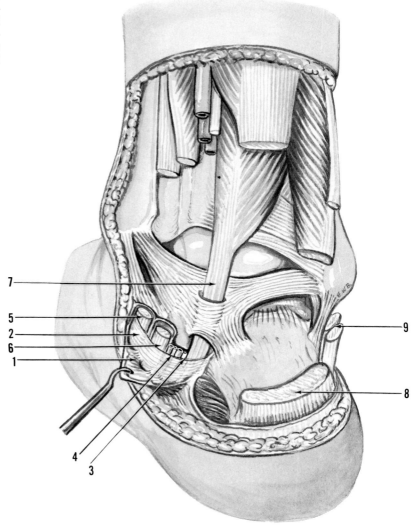

or just proximal to it, a fascial plane appears, forming a tunnel to the flexor hallucis longus muscle–tendon unit and separating the latter from the posterior tibial neurovascular bundle (Fig. 9-11). This fascial plane covers the free interval between the flexor hallucis longus tunnel and the tunnel of the flexor digitorum longus. All four tunnels, three tendinous and one neurovascular, are covered by the deep aponeurosis and retained in the deep compartment. The superficial compartment is now reduced to the Achilles tendon and the plantaris tendon. The space between these two compartments has enlarged and is filled with the pre-Achilles adipose tissue; it is considered a posteromedial "safe" zone. The superficial and the deep fascias are adherent at the level of the fibrous sheath of the tibialis posterior and the flexor digitorum longus tendon in the retromedial malleolar position, and farther down, they form the flexor retinaculum. The segment of the deep investing fascia that formed the tunnel of the flexor hallucis longus and separated the latter from the neurovascular bundle continues distally as the investing fascia of the quadratus plantae muscle.

Flexor Retinaculum

The flexor retinaculum or laciniate ligament formed by the fusion of the superficial and deep aponeuroses of the leg is triangular in shape with malleolar apex, inferior base, and anterior and posterior borders (Fig. 9-12).[8] The delineation of the last two borders is difficult, as they are in continuity: the posterior with the superficial aponeurosis of the leg and the anterior with the dorsal aponeurosis of the foot. A vertical line extended from the anterior border of the medial malleolus to the medial border of the foot marks approximately the anterior border of the flexor retinaculum. The posterior border follows more or less an oblique line drawn from the anterior border of the medial malleolus to the posterosuperior corner of the os calcis. The descending fibers of the retinaculum reach the superior border of the abductor hallucis muscle, split, and incorporate the muscle; they are in continuity with the plantar fascia. The superficial apical fibers of the flexor retinaculum insert on the subcutaneous anterior and medial surfaces of the medial malleo-

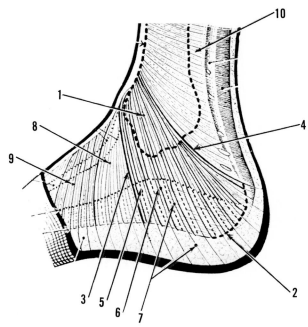

Fig. 9-12. Flexor retinaculum. (1, Apex of flexor retinaculum; 2, posteromedial border of calcaneum; 3, anterior border of flexor retinaculum; 4, posterosuperior border flexor retinaculum; 5, deep layer of flexor retinaculum investing abductor hallucis muscle; 6, superficial layer of flexor retinaculum investing abductor hallucis muscle; 7, superficial fibers of flexor retinaculum continued by retinaculum cutis; 8, superficial dorsal aponeurosis of foot; 9, inferomedial band of inferior extensor retinaculum; 10, adherent superficial and deep aponeuroses of leg.) (From Bellocq P, Meyer P: Le ligament annulaire interne du cou- de- pied. Arch Anat Histol Embryol 37:23, 1954)

lus. The deep apical fibers contribute to the formation of the tibialis anterior tunnel, insert on the deep surface of the superior extensor retinaculum, and exchange fibers with the superomedial band of the inferior extensor retinaculum.

Tibiotalocalcaneal Tunnel

The tibiotalocalcaneal tunnel extends from the posteromedial aspect of the ankle to the plantar aspect of the navicular to the crossing point of the flexor digitorum longus and flexor hallucis longus tendons (Figs. 9-13 and 9-14).[9, 10] This passageway is concave anteriorly and may be divided into two compartments: upper or tibiotalar and lower or talocalcaneal or tarsal tunnel.

Tibiotalar Compartment. The osseous canal of the tibiotalar compartment is formed by the posterior aspect of the distal tibia, the retromedial malleolar surface, the posterior border of the talus with its central sulcus flanked by the posterior talar tubercles, and the posterior segment of the medial talar surface. The canal is converted into a large compartment by the deep aponeurosis of the leg. The latter is attached medially to the posteromedial border of the tibia and the posterior border of the medial malleolus and laterally to the fibrous sheath of the peronei tendons. Anteriorly

the deep aponeurosis is covered by or adherent to the superficial aponeurosis. Posteriorly the two aponeurosis part; the superficial aponeurosis courses toward the medial border of the Achilles tendon and the deep aponeurosis is directed laterally toward the fibrous tunnel of the peronei tendons. Distally, the deep aponeurosis is attached to the superomedial surface of the os calcis. In the proximal tibial segment of the tunnel are located, from a medial to a lateral direction, the following structures:

The fibrous tunnel of the tibialis posterior tendon
The fibrous tunnel of the flexor digitorum longus adherent to the former
The superficial compartment for the posterior tibial neurovascular bundle
The large loose compartment for the flexor hallucis longus muscle–tendon unit and the peroneal vessels laterally (Fig. 9-15)

In the distal malleolar–talar segment of the tunnel, the same relationship is present with some modifications. The flexor hallucis longus is all tendinous and passes through a strong fibrous tunnel on the posterior border of the talus. The peronei vessels have parted. The posterior tibial neurovascular compartment is superficial and overlies the tunnel of the flexor hallucis longus and the intertendinous interval between the latter and the flexor digitorum longus tunnel.

Within the tibiotalar compartment the tunnel of the tibialis posterior tendon attaches to the posterior tibia, the medial and lateral crests of the retromalleolar canal, and the posterior talotibial fibers of the deltoid ligament. The tunnel of the flexor digitorum longus is usually lateral and occasionally posterolateral to the tunnel of the tibialis posterior tendon and attaches to the posterior tibia, the posterior capsule of the talotibial joint and the posterior bimalleolar ligament, and the posteromedial talar tubercle with the reaching posterior talotibial fibers of the deltoid ligament.

The neurovascular tunnel is more superficial, covering the tunnel of the flexor hallucis longus and the interval between the latter and the flexor digitorum longus tunnel. Within this compartment are located, medially to laterally, the posterior tibial veins (three), artery, and nerve (Fig. 9-16). Proximal to the tip of the medial malleolus (1.3 cm–1.5 cm), the posterior tibial nerve divides into its terminal medial and lateral plantar branches.[3] The posterior tibial artery is still undivided.

The tunnel of the flexor hallucis longus tendon is the most lateral in the deep compartment and attaches to the posterior tibia, the posterior tibiotalar capsule and laterally to the fibrous sheath of the peronei tendons, the posterior talofibular ligament, the talar component of the fibulotalocalcaneal ligament of Rouvière and Canela Lazaro, the posterior talar sulcus and lateral and medial posterior talar tubercles, and the posteromedial corner of the posterior talocalcaneal joint capsule.[6]

Talocalcaneal Tunnel. The osseous canal of the talocalcaneal or tarsal tunnel is formed from above downward by the medial surface of the talus and the inferomedial segment of the navicular, the sustentaculum tali, and the

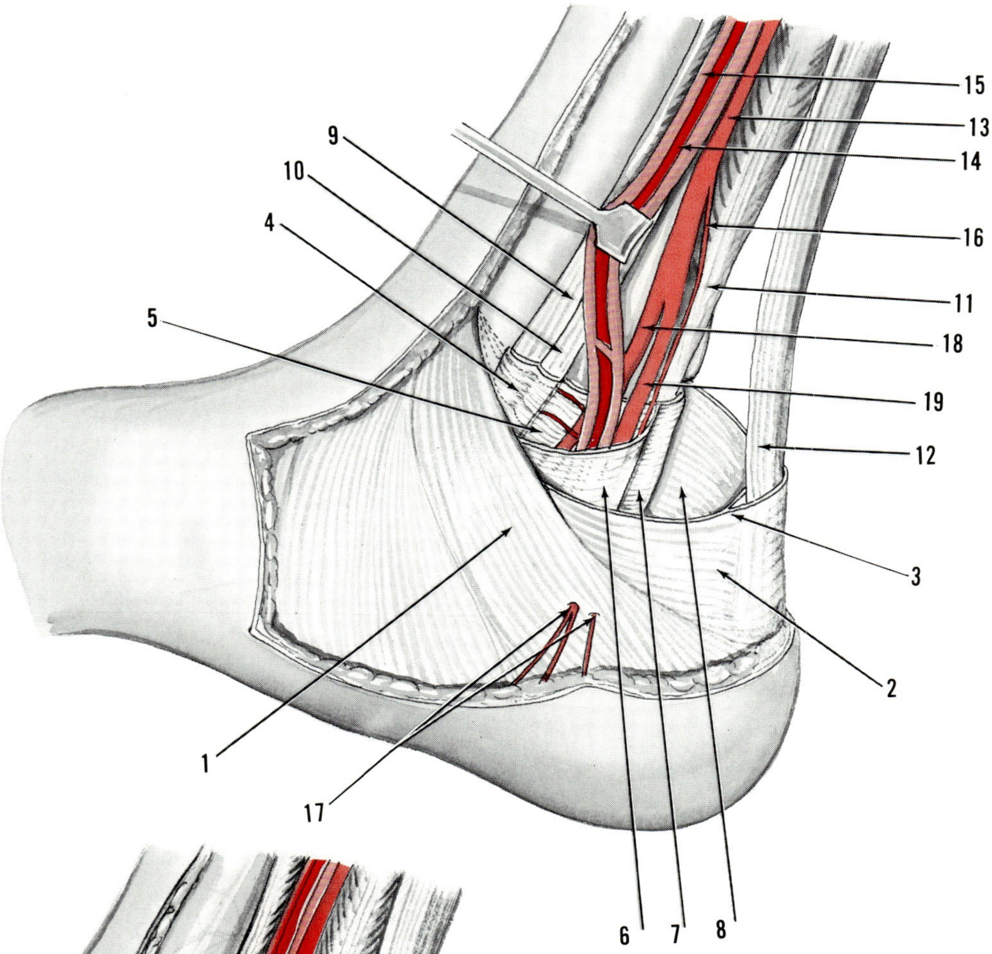

Fig. 9-13. Proximal aspect of the tibiotalocalcaneal canal. The posterior tibial arteriovenous bundle is retracted anteriorly to expose the posterior tibial nerve and its division branches. (1, Flexor retinaculum; 2, superficial aponeurosis splitting [3] to incorporate Achilles tendon [12]; 4, deep aponeurosis covering fibrous tunnels to tibialis posterior tendon [9] and flexor digitorum longus tendon [10]; 5, intermediary intertendinous aponeurosis forming floor of neurovascular compartment; 6, deep aponeurosis forming roof of neurovascular compartment and continuing over tunnel of flexor hallucis longus tendon [7]; 8, "safe zone," in front of Achilles tendon and behind neurovascular tunnel; 11, flexor hallucis longus tendon; 13, posterior tibial nerve; 14, posterior tibial artery; 15, posterior tibial vein; 16, posteromedial calcaneal nerve piercing aponeurosis at 17; 18, medial plantar nerve; 19, lateral plantar nerve.)

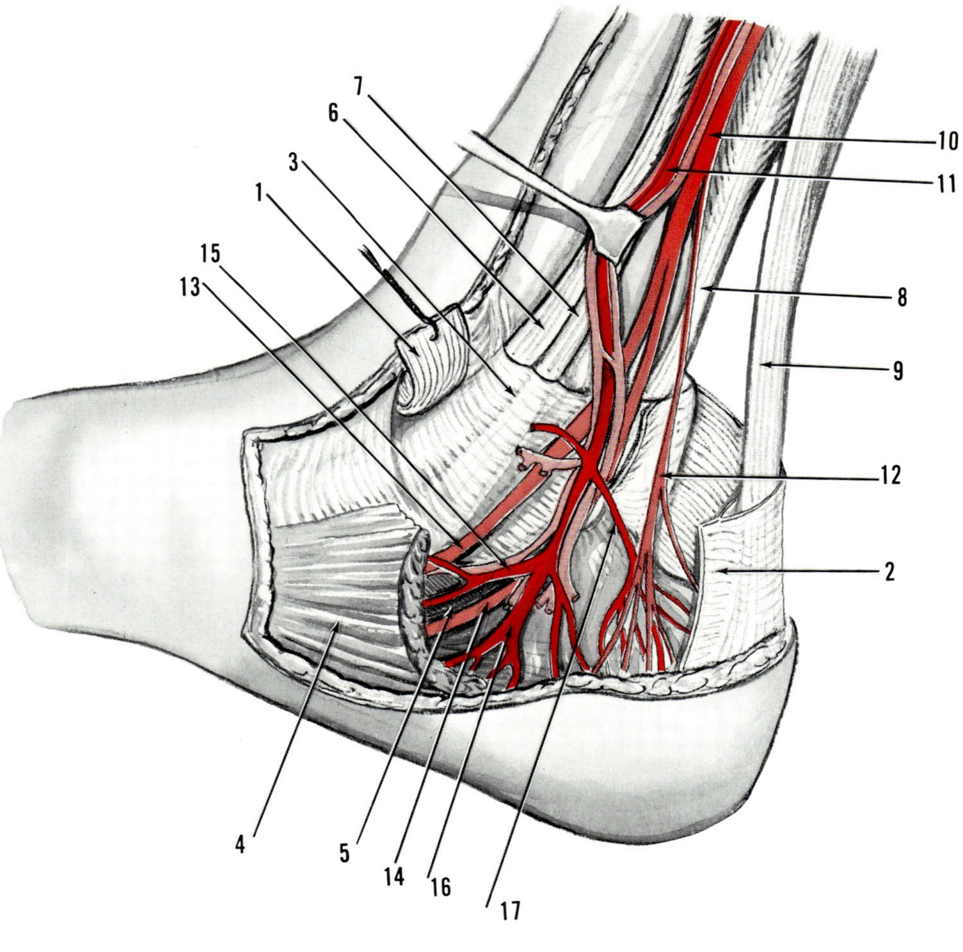

Fig. 9-14. Deep aspect of the tibiotalocalcaneal canal. (1, Reflected apex of flexor retinaculum; 2, superficial aponeurosis investing Achilles tendon [9]; 3, deep aponeurosis contributing to formation of fibrous tunnel of tibialis posterior tendon [6] and flexor digitorum longus tendon [7]; 4, abductor hallucis muscle; 5, interfascicular septum dividing calcaneal canal into upper and lower chambers; 8, flexor hallucis longus tendon; 10, posterior tibial nerve; 11, posterior tibial artery and veins; 12, posteromedial calcaneal nerve; 13, medial plantar nerve passing through upper chamber of calcaneal canal; 14, lateral plantar nerve passing through lower chamber of calcaneal canal; 15, medial plantar artery; 16, lateral plantar artery; 17, medial calcaneal artery.) (Modified after Dujarier C: Anatomie des Membres Dissection—Anatomie Topographique, 2nd ed. Paris, Masson, 1924)

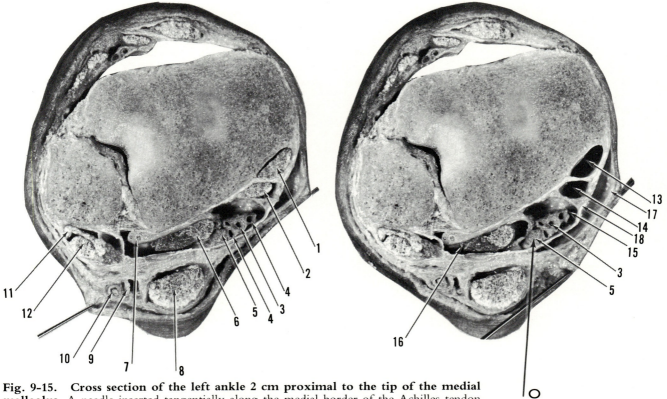

Fig. 9-15. Cross section of the left ankle 2 cm proximal to the tip of the medial malleolus. A needle inserted tangentially along the medial border of the Achilles tendon reaches the posterior tibial nerve, avoiding the vascular bundle (direction indicated by the *arrow O.*) This is a safe guide for anesthetic block of the posterior tibial nerve. (1, Tibialis posterior tendon; 2, flexor digitorum longus tendon; 3, posterior tibial artery; 4, posterior tibial veins; 5, posterior tibial nerve; 6, flexor hallucis longus tendon and muscle; 7, posterior peroneal vessels; 8, Achilles tendon; 9, sural nerve, 10, saphenous vein; 11, peroneus brevis tendon; 12, peroneus longus tendon; 13, tunnel of tibialis posterior tendon; 14, tunnel of flexor digitorum longus tendon; 15, tunnel of posterior tibial neurovascular bundle; 16, tunnel of flexor hallucis longus tendon and muscle; 17, superficial aponeurosis; 18, deep aponeurosis.)

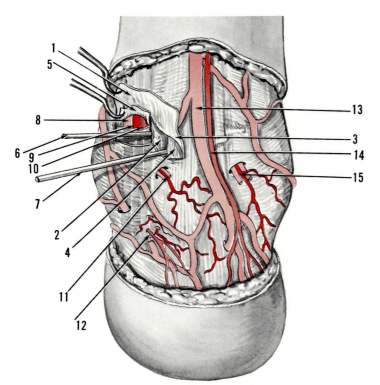

Fig. 9-16. Posterior aspect of the ankle. (1, Superficial aponeurosis, reflected upward; 2, anterior split layer of *1* investing Achilles tendon [4]; 3, posterior split layer of *1* investing Achilles tendon; 5, deep aponeurosis reflected upward exposing posterior tibial neurovascular bundle in VAN sequence [*8,* posterior tibial *v*ein; *9,* posterior tibial *a*rtery; *10,* posterior tibial *n*erve]; 6, probe passing between deep and superficial aponeuroses; 7, probe passing on anterior aspect of Achilles tendon but deep to anterior split layer of superficial aponeurosis; 11, posterior calcaneal artery; 12, posteromedial cutaneous nerve; 13, lesser saphenous vein; 14, sural nerve; 15, lateral calcaneal artery, branch of posterior peroneal artery.) (After Testut L, Jacob O: Traité d'Anatomie Topographique avec Applications Médico-Chirurgicales, 3nd ed, Vol II, p 1036. Paris, Doin, 1909)

curved, excavated medial surface of the os calcis. The surface is buttressed above by the superficial deltoid ligament and below by the quadratus plantae muscle. The talocalcaneal canal is converted to a tunnel by the covering flexor retinaculum above and the abductor hallucis muscle with its investing fascia below. Anterior to the flexor retinaculum the aponeurotic coverage is provided by the superficial dorsal aponeurosis of the foot and the inferomedial band of the inferior extensor retinaculum. Within the talocancaneal compartment, the tunnel of the tibialis posterior tendon attaches to the posterior talotibial segment of the deltoid ligament, the calcaneotibial component of the deltoid ligament over the medial surface of the talus, the superomedial calcaneonavicular ligament crossing the anterior talocalcaneal joint, and the inferior calcaneonavicular ligament.

Subsequently the tibialis posterior tendon divides into three parts: navicular, plantar, and recurrent. The recurrent part inserts on the sustentaculum tali and contributes to the roof of the distal segment of the tunnel.

The tunnel of the flexor digitorum longus attaches to the posteromedial talar tubercle, the posterior talotibial fibers of the deltoid ligament, and the medial border of the sustentaculum tali and the tibiocalcaneal component of the deltoid ligament. It shares distally a common tunnel with the flexor hallucis longus tendon.

The tunnel of the flexor digitorum longus crosses the medial opening of the tarsal canal. It is a useful guideline for the surgical location of the midsegment of the medial talocalcaneal joint interline. Occasioally the tunnel may shift downward and partially cover the tunnel of the flexor hallucis longus, which is attached to the lateral and medial borders of the osseous canal formed on the inferior surface of the sustentaculum tali. The bony canal disappears at the anterior border of the os calcis, and the tunnels of the flexor hallucis longus and the flexor digitorum longus lose their intermediary septum and share a common tunnel.[10] This segment of the tunnel corresponds to the master knot of Henry.[7] It is located on the inner aspect of the anterior segment of the os calcis, "a thumb's width lateral to the navicular tubercle."[7] The roof of the tunnel corresponds to the inferior calcaneonavicular ligament reinforced by a thick fibrous plate and by the recurrent segment of the tibialis posterior tendon. Medially the tunnel is attached to the deep aponeurosis of the abductor hallucis muscle and laterally to the os calcis. The floor of the common tunnel is thin and corresponds to the compartment of the medial plantar neurovascular bundle.

The neurovascular tunnel is initially superficial and corresponds to the interval between the tunnel of the flexor digitorum longus and the tunnel of the flexor hallucis longus (Fig. 9-17). Gradually, as the latter approaches the former, the intertendinous space disappears and the neurovascular tunnel is located on the medial aspect of the os calcis, posterior to the flexor hallucis longus tunnel.

In the lower segment of the calcaneal tunnel the neurovascular compartment is divided into an upper and a lower chamber by the transversely oriented interfascicular septum (Figs. 9-17 and 9-18). The lower neurovascular chamber is limited laterally by the quadratus plantae muscle covering the medial calcaneal surface, medially by the abductor hallucis muscle covered by the deep aponeurosis, above by the interfascicular septum, and below by the interspace between the inferior borders of the abductor hallucis and of the quadratus plantae. The upper neurovascular chamber is limited laterally by the tunnel of the flexor hallucis longus, medially by the flexor retinaculum, above by the tunnel of the flexor digitorum longus, and below by the interfascicular septum.

The posterior tibial artery divides into the medial and lateral plantar arteries proximal to the free concave border of the interfascicular septum. The medial plantar nerve and vessels penetrate the upper chamber of the calcaneal canal, whereas the lateral plantar nerve and vessels penetrate the lower chamber and reach the middle plantar compartment of the planta pedis. In both chambers the nerve is anterior to the corresponding artery.

The posterior tibial nerve bifurcates into the medial and lateral plantar nerves at 1.3 cm to 1.5 cm proximal to the tip of the medial malleolus.[3] Higher bifurcation occurs in 13.5%.[3] Hovelacque has observed one bifurcation at 6 cm and another at 10 cm proximal to the tip of the medial malleolus.[11] The bifurcation of the posterior tibial artery into the medial and the lateral plantar artery occurs 1.3 cm to 2.5 cm distal to the bifurcation of the posterior tibial nerve; this occurs in the majority of cases (86.5%).[3, 12] Occasionally the bifurcation of both is at the same level (11.5%) or, rarely, that of the artery is proximal to that of the nerve (2%).[12] The posterior tibial nerve has the most common site of location at 7.5 cm proximal to the tip of the medial malleolus, in line with the medial border of the Achilles tendon but located in the neurovascular compartment.[3] The medial calcaneal nerve branches from the posterotibial nerve proximal to the bifurcation or may originate from the medial plantar nerve. It pierces the aponeurosis at a variable level, and as described previously, it divides into two main calcaneal branches. The long motor branch of the abductor digiti minimi takes off from the lateral plantar nerve in the canal.

The posterior tibial artery provides proximally two transverse anatomotic branches—lateral and medial. The lateral branch passes under the flexor hallucis longus tendon and unites with a similar branch of the posterior peroneal artery. The medial branch courses over the tunnels of the flexor digitorum longus and tibialis posterior tendons and anastomoses with the anterior medial malleolar artery. This branch supplies the skin overlying the medial malleolus. At about 1 cm proximal to the bifurcation of the posterior tibial artery originates the artery of the tarsal canal.[13] It passes between the tunnels of the flexor digitorum longus and flexor hallucis longus tendons and enters the tarsal canal. The artery of the tarsal canal occasionally originates from the medial plantar artery (16.6%) or may be double (3.3%) or absent (3.3%).[13]

A deltoid arterial branch takes off from the artery of the tarsal canal at 5 mm from its origin. It passes between the tibiocalcaneal and the talotibial components of the deltoid ligament. Occasionally the deltoid branch originates from the posterior tibial artery (30%), or it may be double (6.6%).[13]

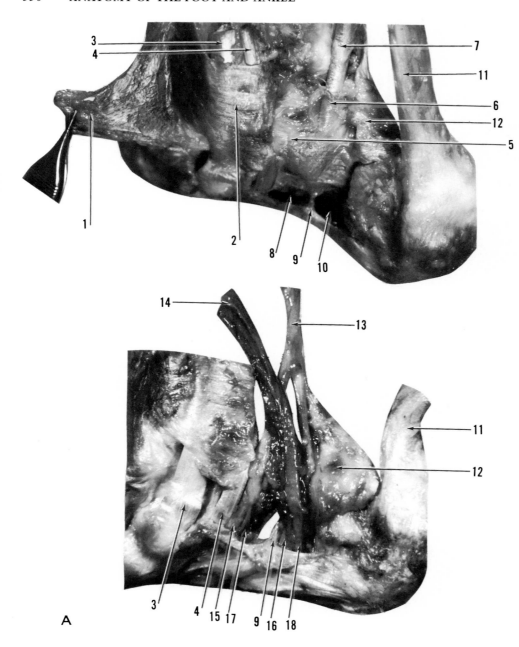

Fig. 9-17. (*A*) **Talocalcaneal canal.** The medial plantar nerve and artery pass in the upper calcaneal chamber; the lateral plantar nerve and artery pass in the lower calcaneal chamber. (1, Reflected flexor retinaculum, superficial aponeurosis; 2, deep aponeurosis covering tunnel of tibialis posterior [3] and flexor digitorum longus tendons [4]; 5, intermediary aponeurosis interposed between tunnels of the flexor digitorum longus [4] and flexor hallucis longus [6] tendons; 7, flexor hallucis longus muscle–tendon; 8, upper chamber of calcaneal canal; 9, interfascicular septum; 10, lower chamber of calcaneal canal; 11, Achilles tendon; 12, pre-Achilles fat pad; 13, posterior tibial nerve with proximal division; 14, posterior tibial artery and veins reflected anteriorly; 15, medial plantar nerve; 16, lateral plantar nerve; 17, medial plantar artery; 18, lateral plantar artery.) (continued)

A

Sole of the Foot

SURFACE ANATOMY

The sustentaculum tali located 2.5 cm below the medial malleolus, the tubercle of the navicular, and the tuberosity of the base of the fifth metatarsal are important points of reference. Delorme has provided guidelines for the location of the plantar neurovascular bundles and the intermuscular septa.[14]

A vertical line is drawn along the posterior border of the medial malleolus and continues transversely across the heel. A line is drawn from the tubercle of the navicular to the sustentaculum tali. With the foot held at 90°, the intersection of these two lines indicates the point of division of the posterior tibial artery (Fig. 9-19).

A line is drawn from the tuberosity of the fifth metatarsal to the bifurcation point of the posterior tibial artery and to the medial end of the plantar fold of the big toe. These lines determine, with the medial border of the foot, a triangle that encompasses the plantar arteries.

A line drawn from the midpoint of the transverse heel line to the third web space indicates the direction of the lateral intermuscular septum. The portion of this line located within the above-traced triangle represents the direction of the posteroanterior portion of the lateral plantar artery.

A line drawn transversely from the tubercle of the first

Fig. 9-17 (continued)

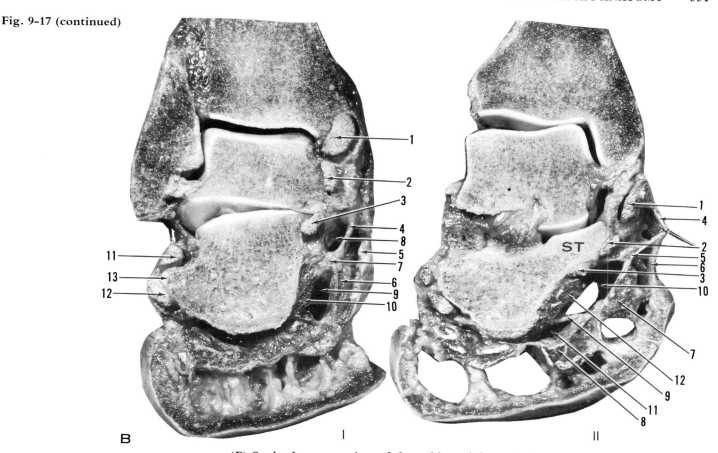

(B) Sagittal cross section of the ankle and foot. (*I*) Cross section passing through the posterior talocalcaneal joint. (1, Tibialis posterior tendon; 2, flexor digitorum longus tendon; 3, flexor hallucis longus tendon; 4, deep investing layer of flexor retinaculum; 5, superficial investing layer of flexor retinaculum; 6, abductor hallucis muscle being invested by *4* and *5*; 7, interfascicular septum; 8, upper calcaneal chamber; 9, lower calcaneal chamber; 10, quadratus plantae muscle; 11, peroneus brevis tendon; 12, peroneus longus tendon; 13, peroneal trochlea.) (*II*) Cross section passing at the level of the sustentaculum tali (*ST*). (1, Tibialis posterior tendon applied against tibiocalcaneal component of deltoid ligament; 2, flexor digitorum longus tendon applied against medial border of sustentaculum tali; 3, flexor hallucis longus tendon applied against inferior surface of sustentaculum tali; 4, flexor retinaculum with its deep [5] and superficial [6] layers investing abductor hallucis muscle [7]; 8, flexor digitorum brevis muscle; 9, interfascicular septum; 10, upper calcaneal chamber; 11, lower calcaneal chamber; 12, quadratus plantae muscle.)

metatarsal intersects the anterior border of the previously traced triangle and indicates the position of the deep lateral plantar arch.

The midpoint of the inner half of the transverse heel line is marked and connected to the first web space; this line indicates the medial intermuscular septum. The portion of this line located within the above-described triangle locates the posteroanterior portion of the medial plantar artery.

SKIN

The skin of the sole of the foot is tight and fixed. It is thick at the level of the heel and the lateral margin and the ball of the foot; it is thinner along the medial longitudinal arch.

The cleavage lines run longitudinally and have a lateral convexity. These lines are arcuate at the heel (Fig. 9-2).

SUBCUTANEOUS TISSUE AND SUPERFICIAL VESSELS AND NERVES

The subcutaneous tissue is fit to bear weight and to act as a cushion (Fig. 9-20).

At the level of the heel, the thickness is close to 2 cm. Fibrous lamellae are arranged in a complex spiral fashion around the os calcis and form multiple chambers retaining the adipose tissue (Figs. 9-21 and 9-22). Similarly, farther anteriorly, especially in the ball of the foot, vertical fibers
(Text continues on p. 355.)

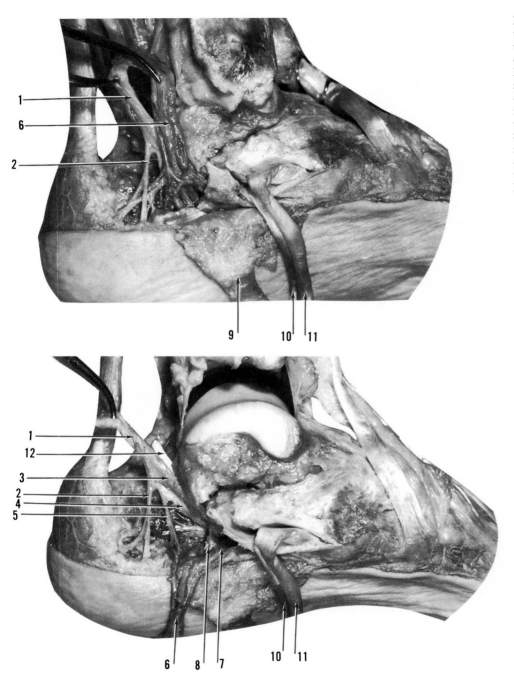

Fig. 9-18.   Neurovascular bundle in the tibiotalocalcaneal canal. (1, Posterior tibial nerve; 2, posteromedial calcaneal nerve; 3, medial plantar nerve; 4, lateral plantar nerve; 5, medial calcaneal nerve; 6, posterior tibial artery veins covering posterior tibial nerve in top figure and reflected downward in bottom figure; 7, upper calcaneal chamber; 8, interfascicular septum; 9, reflected flexor retinaculum; 10, reflected flexor digitorum longus tendon; 11, reflected tibialis posterior tendon; 12, flexor hallucis longus tendon.)

Fig. 9-19.   Guidelines to the posterior tibial artery and the plantar arteries. Both plantar arteries are incorporated in the *V* formed by the line *OFG*. Each plantar artery has an oblique and a posteroanterior longitudinal portion. The oblique portion of the medial plantar artery is situated along the line *OH*. *H* is located on the line *DD′* at a point equidistant from points *B* and *C*. The longitudinal section of the medial plantar artery is along the medial intermuscular septum line, within the previously determined *V*. The oblique portion of the lateral plantar artery is along the line *OF*, extending from *O* up to its intersection with *EE′*. The longitudinal portion of the lateral plantar artery is located along the *EE′* line within the vascular *V*. The transverse portion of the lateral plantar artery is located along a transverse line *YY′* drawn across the sole. (1, Posterior tibial artery; 2, medial plantar artery; 3, lateral plantar artery; *AX*, line tangential to posterior border of tibia; *B*, tuberosity of navicular; *C*, sustentaculum tali; *BC*, line that extended posteriorly intersects line *AX* at *O*, which represents bifurcation point of posterior tibial artery into medial and lateral plantar arteries; *AX*, line extended transversely across heel and forms line *XX′*; *E*, midpoint of *XX′*; *D*, midpoint of *XE*; *D′*, first web space; *E′*, third web space; *F*, tuberosity of fifth metatarsal; *G*, medial border of flexion crease of big toe; *Y*, tuberosity of first metatarsal; *DD′*, line indicating direction of medial intermuscular suptum; *EE′*, line indicating direction of lateral intermuscular septum.) (After Delorme: Ligature des artères de la paume de la main et de la plante du pied. Mem Acad Med 1882. Cited in Testut L, Jacob O: Traité d'Anatomie Topographique avec Applications Médico-Chirurgicales, 2nd ed, Vol II, p 1084. Paris, Doin, 1909)

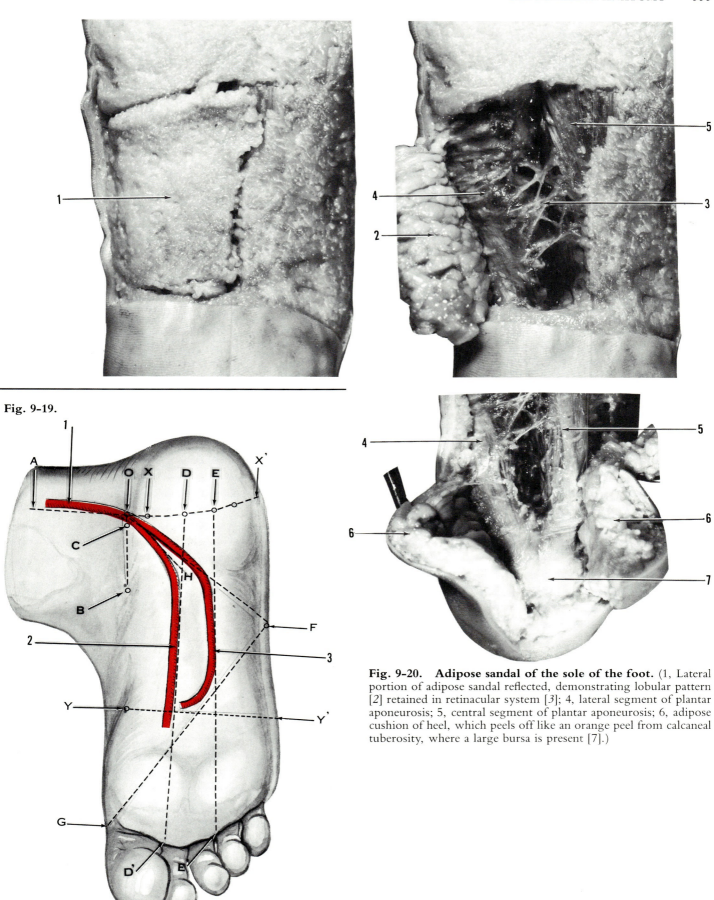

Fig. 9-19.

Fig. 9-20. Adipose sandal of the sole of the foot. (1, Lateral portion of adipose sandal reflected, demonstrating lobular pattern [2] retained in retinacular system [3]; 4, lateral segment of plantar aponeurosis; 5, central segment of plantar aponeurosis; 6, adipose cushion of heel, which peels off like an orange peel from calcaneal tuberosity, where a large bursa is present [7].)

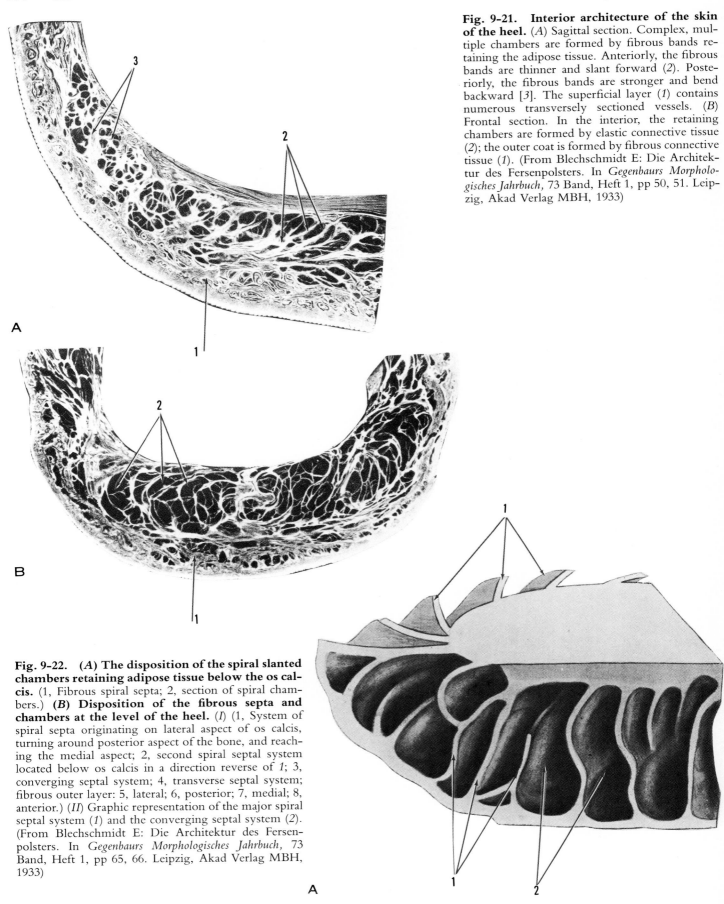

A

B

Fig. 9-21. Interior architecture of the skin of the heel. (*A*) Sagittal section. Complex, multiple chambers are formed by fibrous bands retaining the adipose tissue. Anteriorly, the fibrous bands are thinner and slant forward (*2*). Posteriorly, the fibrous bands are stronger and bend backward [*3*]. The superficial layer (*1*) contains numerous transversely sectioned vessels. (*B*) Frontal section. In the interior, the retaining chambers are formed by elastic connective tissue (*2*); the outer coat is formed by fibrous connective tissue (*1*). (From Blechschmidt E: Die Architektur des Fersenpolsters. In *Gegenbaurs Morphologisches Jahrbuch,* 73 Band, Heft 1, pp 50, 51. Leipzig, Akad Verlag MBH, 1933)

Fig. 9-22. (*A*) **The disposition of the spiral slanted chambers retaining adipose tissue below the os calcis.** (1, Fibrous spiral septa; 2, section of spiral chambers.) (*B*) **Disposition of the fibrous septa and chambers at the level of the heel.** (*I*) (1, System of spiral septa originating on lateral aspect of os calcis, turning around posterior aspect of the bone, and reaching the medial aspect; 2, second spiral septal system located below os calcis in a direction reverse of *1*; 3, converging septal system; 4, transverse septal system; fibrous outer layer: 5, lateral; 6, posterior; 7, medial; 8, anterior.) (*II*) Graphic representation of the major spiral septal system (*1*) and the converging septal system (*2*). (From Blechschmidt E: Die Architektur des Fersenpolsters. In *Gegenbaurs Morphologisches Jahrbuch,* 73 Band, Heft 1, pp 65, 66. Leipzig, Akad Verlag MBH, 1933)

A

connect the dermis to the plantar aponeurosis. These connections fix the skin and retain the adipose tissue. A large subcutaneous, subcalcaneal bursa is present at the heel.

A very superficial intradermal and subdermal venous network covers the sole of the foot and forms, at the foot margins, the medial and lateral marginal veins that drain into the dorsal veins. The superficial mid plantar region drains into a distal superficial venous arcade joining at each end the dorsomedial and dorsolateral marginal veins of the first and fifth toes.

The arterial blood supply of the sole of the foot is rich. In the mid segment, multiple small perforating vessels pass through the medial and lateral sulci of the sole and supply the skin. They are provided by the lateral and medial plantar arteries. The ball of the foot is vascularized by perforating cutaneous branches arising from the common plantar digital arteries. The medial aspect of the heel is supplied by the medial calcaneal arteries provided by the lateral plantar artery. The first medial calcaneal branch may emanate from

the end of the posterior tibial artery. The lateral aspect of the heel is supplied by the posterior peroneal or the posterior tibial artery. The anterior calcaneal branches may be supplemented by the lateral plantar artery, the anterior peroneal artery, or the lateral tarsal artery.

The sural nerve provides two calcaneal branches to the lateral aspect of the heel. The medial calcaneal nerves are branches of the posterior tibial nerve. The most posterior branch supplies the medial aspect of the heel. The anterior medial calcaneal nerve courses anterolaterally through the thick adipose tissue accompanying the medial calcaneal artery and supplies the skin to the posterior third of the sole. The remaining segment of the sole is innervated by the medial plantar nerve in its inner two thirds and by the lateral plantar nerve in the outer one third.

The cutaneous branches surface at the level of the medial and lateral sulci. The superficial neurovascular branches at the level of the heel and the sole of the foot are difficult to dissect.

Fig. 9-22 (continued)

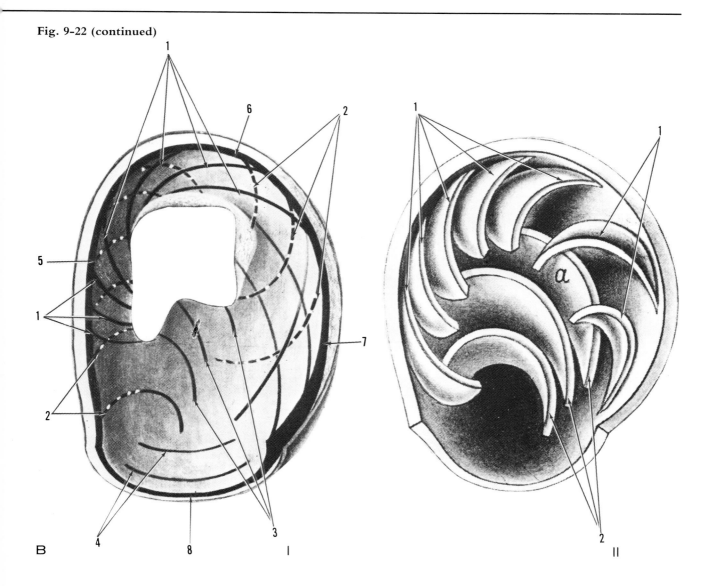

B

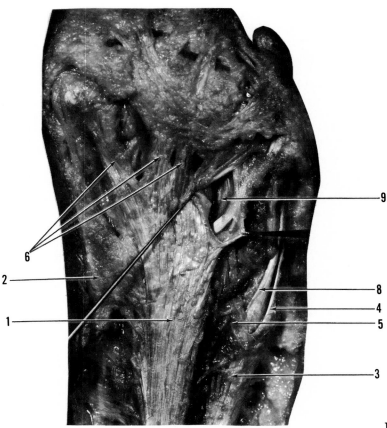

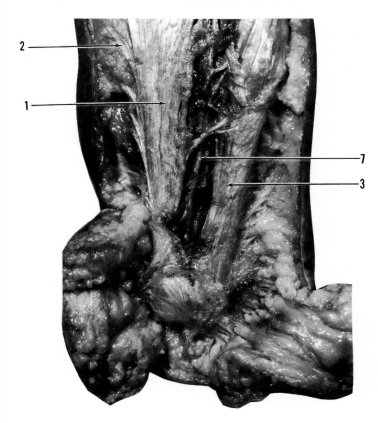

Fig. 9-23. Plantar aponeurosis. (1, Central segment; 2, medial segment; 3, lateral segment; 4, lateral crus of lateral segment; 5, medial crus of lateral segment; 6, longitudinal bands of central segment; 7, lateral intermuscular septum; 8, tendon of abductor digiti quinti passing through crura of lateral component; 9, lateral intermuscular septum pierced by long flexor tendon of fifth toe.)

PLANTAR APONEUROSIS, INTERMUSCULAR SEPTA, AND COMPARTMENTS

Plantar Aponeurosis

The plantar aponeurosis is a strong fibrous structure with three components: central, lateral, and tibial (Fig. 9-23).

The central component is the strongest and the thickest and has a glistening appearance. It is triangular in contour, with a proximal apex originating from the posteromedial calcaneal tubercle and a distal base. At the origin the aponeurosis measures 1.5 cm to 2 cm in width; it narrows slightly and then gradually enlarges as it progresses anteriorly. At mid metatarsal level, the fibers group into five longitudinally oriented bands that diverge. Just proximal to the level of the metatarsal heads, each band divides into three components, one superficial and two deep.

The superficial fibers insert subcutaneously in the distal segment of the ball of the foot. The deep fibers reach the depth in the form of two sagittal septa around each flexor tendon.

The lateral component of the plantar aponeurosis is thick posteriorly and thin anteriorly. It originates from the lateral margin of the medial calcaneal tubercle, extends in the direction of the cuboid, and divides into a lateral component, which inserts on the base of the fifth metatarsal, and a medial deep component, which extends to the plantar plate of the fourth toe. Through the bifurcation of this aponeurosis passes the tendon of the abductor digiti quinti.

The medial component of the plantar aponeurosis is thin posteriorly and thicker anteriorly. It forms the covering fascia of the abductor hallucis and is in continuity medially with the dorsal aponeurosis of the foot, the inferior arm of the inferior extensor retinaculum, and the flexor retinaculum.

Two longitudinal grooves, lateral and medial, are present on each side of the central component of the plantar aponeurosis. The lateral groove is better defined and larger than the medial and extends from the level of the calcaneal tubercle to the level of the fifth metatarsal tuberosity. This interval is bridged by a complex retinacular network uniting the central and the lateral components of the plantar aponeurosis. The retinacular fibers form a retaining system for the adipose lobules. Through this interval emerge the cutaneous branches arising from the lateral neurovascular bundle.

The medial groove located between the central and medial components is better defined in its proximal half and gives passage to the cutaneous branches arising from the medial plantar neurovascular bundle.

From the mid segment of the sulci surfaces, on the medial side, the medial plantar neurovascular bundle of the big toe and, on the lateral side, the lateral plantar neurovascular bundle of the fifth toe.

Intermuscular Septa

From the borders of the central component of the plantar aponeurosis, two intermuscular septa extend into the planta pedis—the lateral and the medial septum.

The lateral intermuscular septum is attached to the medial calcaneal tubercle, the calcaneocuboid ligament, and the sheath of the peroneus longus. Distally the septum splits, encloses the third plantar interosseous muscle, and inserts on the medial border of the fifth metatarsal shaft and the medial aspect of the base of the proximal phalanx of the little toe.

The medial intermuscular septum is less defined and forms a set of vertical fascicles arranged like the teeth of a comb and giving passage to the tendons and neurovascular structures.[1]

The posterior segment of the medial intermuscular septum is formed by the interfascicular lamina of the calcaneal tunnel and is attached to the medial surface of the os calcis under the sustentaculum tali. Farther distally the septum is attached to the navicular, the medial cuneiform, and the lateral aspect of the first metatarsal shaft after passing between the adductor hallucis and the flexor hallucis brevis and contributes to the formation of their sheaths.

Compartments

The plantar aponeurosis and the intermuscular septa divide the planta pedis into three compartments: central, lateral, and medial.

Central Compartment.   The central compartment is formed superficially by the central segment of the plantar

aponeurosis, laterally by the lateral intermuscular septum, and medially by the medial intermuscular septum. The floor or deep surface corresponds proximally to the tarsal bones, their plantar ligamentous structures, the tendon of the tibialis posterior with its ramifications, and the covering peroneus longus tendon with its sheath. Distally the floor is formed by the central metatarsals 2, 3, and 4 and the interossei muscles covered by the interossei fascia.

The central compartment contains three muscular layers—the flexor digitorum brevis, the quadratus plantae with the flexor digitorum longus tendons, and the adductor hallucis, oblique head—separated by four fascial spaces (Figs. 9-24 and 9-25):[15]

Space 1: between the deep surface of the plantar aponeurosis and the flexor digitorum brevis

Space 2: between the deep surface of the flexor digitorum brevis and the quadratus plantae–flexor digitorum longus unit

Space 3: between the deep surface of the quadratus plantae–flexor digitorum longus and the tarsus with its ligaments posteriorly (posterior to the tendon of the peroneus longus), the adductor hallucis obliquis, and

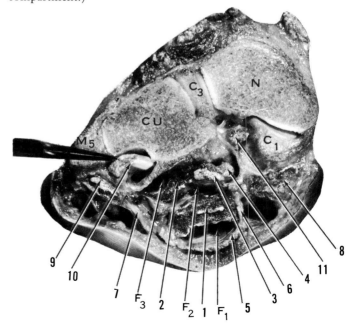

Fig. 9-24.   Cross section of the left midfoot, passing transversely through the navicular and cuboid. (*CU,* cuboid; *N,* navicular; *C₃,* lateral or third cuneiform; *C₁,* first cuneiform; *M₅,* base of fifth metatarsal bone; 1, flexor digitorum brevis; 2, quadratus plantae united with flexor digitorum longus [*3*]; 4, flexor hallucis longus; 5, central segment of plantar aponeurosis; 6, medial intermuscular septum; 7, lateral intermuscular septum; 8, abductor hallucis muscle; 9, abductor digiti quinti muscle; 10, peroneus longus tendon in cuboid tunnel; 11, tibialis posterior tendon, plantar component; *F₁,* fascial space 1 of middle compartment; *F₂,* fascial space 2 of middle compartment; *F₃,* fascial space 3 of middle compartment.)

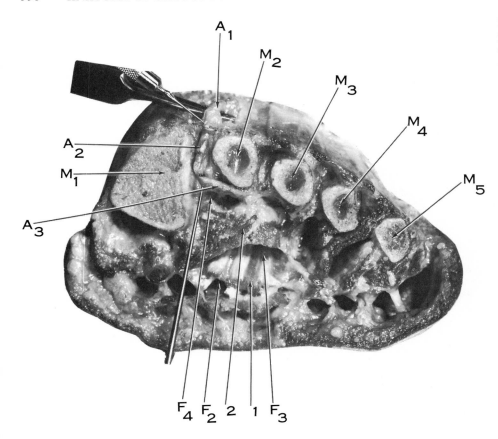

Fig. 9-25. Cross section of the left foot, passing through the base of the first metatarsal and the bases of metatarsals 2 to 5. (M_1–M_5; metatarsals 1 to 5; A_1, dorsalis pedis artery on dorsum of first intermetatarsal space; A_2, vertical, plunging portion of dorsalis pedis artery; A_3, transverse plantar portion of dorsalis pedis artery [dorsalis pedis artery makes two 90° turns before uniting by inosculation with transverse portion of lateral plantar artery]; 1, flexors digitorum longus with their lumbricals; 2, adductor hallucis muscle, oblique portion; F_2, fascial space 2 of middle compartment; F_3, fascial space 3 of middle compartment; F_4, fascial space 4 of middle compartment.)

the plantar and dorsal interossei muscles of the fourth and partially the third interspace anteriorly

Space 4: between the deep surface of the oblique head of the adductor hallucis and the underlying second and third intermetatarsal spaces covered by their interossei

Fascial space 1 extends anteriorly to the mid metatarsal level, and in the space are found the superficial common plantar digital arteries arising from the lateral superficial branch of the medial plantar artery (Fig. 9-26). The superficial arteries connect distally with the corresponding plantar metatarsal arteries 1 to 3. Occasionally a similar superficial arterial branch is given off by the lateral plantar artery and joins the medial superficial group to form the superficial arterial arcade. The details concerning the frequency of occurrence are provided in Chapter 7.

The first, second, and third common digital branches of the medial plantar nerve enter the space from the medial side and course with their corresponding superficial common plantar digital arteries. The space is penetrated from the lateral side by the anastomotic branch between the third common digital nerve and the fourth common digital nerve, a branch of the lateral plantar nerve. This anastomotic branch sometimes passes deep to the short flexor tendons of the fifth and fourth toes and emerges between the tendons of the third and fourth toes. It may also be double or Y-shaped.[11]

Space 1 does not exist under the posterior third of the plantar aponeurosis as the latter gives insertion to the flexor digitorum brevis muscle. This muscle divides into four tendons for the lesser toes. The tendons of the inner three toes continue in the direction of the muscle, whereas the tendon of the little toe diverges clearly outward and is, at times, absent.

During the surgical mobilization of the inner border of the flexor hallucis brevis muscle, one not only is to mobilize the superficial neurovascular branches but also is to protect the motor branch of the muscle arising from the medial plantar nerve and penetrating the muscle from the deep surface of the medial border. The mobilization of the lateral border of the muscle requires the protection of the sensory branch to the fourth interspace that, coming from the depths, contours the border of the muscle.

Fascial space 2 extends anteriorly to the level of a transverse line drawn from the base of the fifth metatarsal. At this level the two layers forming the floor and the ceiling are joined by loose areolar tissue (Fig. 9-27).

Under pressure, the connecting layer may yield, and the area communicates with the interseptal spaces determined by the deep extensions of the plantar aponeurosis. Posteriorly, fascial space 2 leads to the lower chamber of the calcaneal canal. The lateral plantar neurovascular bundle enters the mid plantar space obliquely—anterolaterally—and courses over the quadratus plantae muscle under its invest-

Fig. 9-26. Central compartment of the sole of the foot. (F_1, fascial space 1 between central segment of plantar aponeurosis [1] and flexor digitorum brevis [2], which is adherent to 1 in the posterior third [3], where the space obliterates; F_2, fascial space 2 between flexor digitorum brevis and quadratus plantae–flexor digitorum longus [this space is crossed posteriorly by lateral plantar nerve (4) passing anterior to lateral plantar artery (5) and veins; lateral neurovascular bundle pierces lateral intermuscular septum twice; to leave the central compartment (6) and to reenter the latter (6′)]; 7, superficial branch of lateral plantar nerve; 8, superficial division branch of medial plantar nerve passing around medial border of flexor digitorum brevis and dividing into common digital plantar nerve to the third web space [9], the second web space [10], and the first web space [11]; 12, anastomotic branch between third [9] and fourth [13] common digital plantar nerves.) (After Testut L, Jacob O: Traité d'Anatomie Topographique avec Applications Médico-Chirurgicales, 2nd ed, Vol II, p 1080. Paris, Doin, 1909)

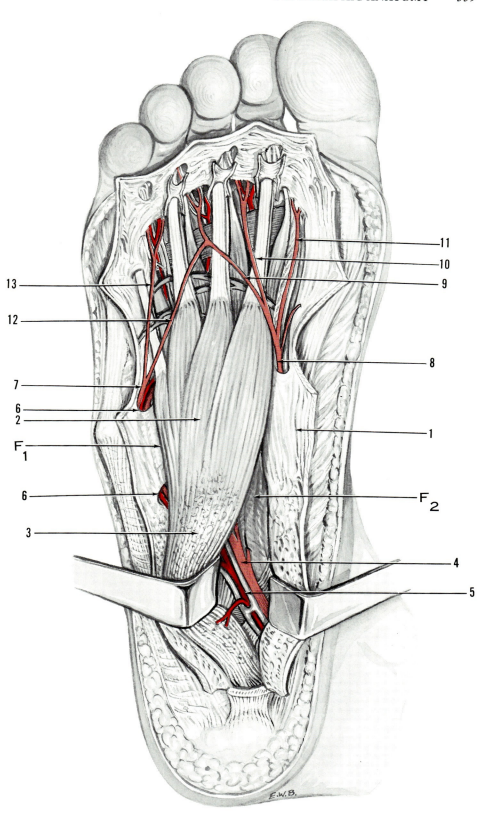

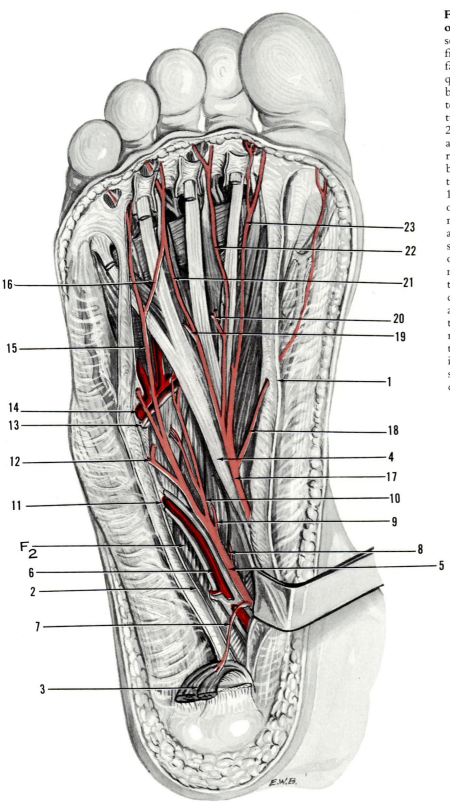

16
15
14
13
12
11
F
2
6
2
7
3

23
22
21
20
19
1
18
4
17
10
9
8
5

E.W.B.

Fig. 9-27. Central compartment of the sole of the foot. The superficial nerve branches preserved in this illustration are passing through the first fascial space in the central compartment. (F_2, fascial space 2 between flexor digitorum longus–quadratus plantae layer [4] and flexor digitorum brevis [3; here reflected backward]; 1, Medial intermuscular septum; 2, lateral intermuscular septum; 5, lateral plantar nerve crossing fascial space 2 and passing anterior to lateral plantar artery [6] and vein; 7, motor nerve branch to flexor digitorum brevis muscle; 8, motor posterior nerve branch to quadratus plantae muscle; 9, motor anterior nerve branch to quadratus plantae muscle; 10, motor nerve branch to adductor hallucis oblique segment; 11, perforation of lateral intermuscular septum by exiting lateral plantar artery and vein; 12, perforation of lateral intermuscular septum by exiting lateral plantar nerve; 13, reentry of lateral plantar nerve into central compartment; nerve is now posterior to lateral plantar artery, transverse segment [14]; 15, superficial plantar common digital nerve to fourth web space; 16, anastomotic branch between third and fourth plantar digital nerves; 17, medial plantar nerve; 18, medial plantar hallucal nerve; 19, sensory branch to plantar skin; 20, motor branch to second lumbrical muscle and sensory branch to plantar skin; 22, second common superficial plantar nerve; 23, first common superficial plantar nerve.)

ing fascia. It pierces the lateral intermuscular septum and enters the lateral compartment. The lateral plantar nerve remains anterior to the lateral plantar artery and its accompanying two veins. The nerve to the abductor of the fifth toe, which has taken off near the origin of the lateral plantar nerve, crosses the space in its most posterior aspect and penetrates the abductor of the fifth toe from its deep surface. Two small branches of the lateral plantar nerve pass under the lateral plantar vessels and supply the quadratus plantae and the calcaneocuboid ligament. The lateral plantar artery provides muscular branches to the flexor digitorum brevis and to the abductor digiti minimi. The flexor digitorum longus tendon passes through the medial intermuscular septum, anterior to the lateral neurovascular bundle. The margins of the septum are closely adherent to the tendon; however, the seal may yield to pressure. The flexor digitorum longus tendon receives an extension from the flexor hallucis longus and fans out into four long tendons for the corresponding lesser toes. The long flexor of the fifth toe passes through the distal end of the lateral intermuscular septum to reach its destination. The lumbricals are located on the tibial aspect of the long flexor tendons. The first lumbrical originates from the tibial border of the tendon to the second toe; the other three lumbricals take off from the corresponding intertendinous spaces 2 to 4.

The quadratus plantae is a flat, quadrilateral muscle with a large medial component arising from the medial surface of the os calcis and a smaller lateral component originating from the inferior surface of the os calcis near the lateral tuberosity. The two muscular heads unite and insert on the common tendon of the long flexor or, mainly, on the long flexors of the third and fourth toes.

Fascial space 3 is limited anteriorly by a connective tissue septum that inserts along a line extending from the middle of the fifth metatarsal shaft to the head of the third metatarsal (Fig. 9-28). This connection is loose and areolar and could be followed farther distally in the form of four extensions that are located under the lumbrical muscle grooves but do not extend beyond the level of the metatarsal heads unless disrupting the bond.

The lateral plantar artery and nerve reenter the mid plantar compartment and the fascial space 3 by piercing the lateral intermuscular septum just distal to the base of the fifth metatarsal bone. The lateral plantar nerve is now posterior to the artery. The fourth superficial metatarsal and intermetatarsal arteries and the distal segment of the third superficial metatarsal artery are, in this space, covered by the interossei fascia. The deep branch of the lateral plantar nerve provides, at this point, motor branches to the oblique and transverse heads of the adductor hallucis, the two lateral lumbricals, and the interossei muscles of the second and third interspaces.

Fascial space 4 is very deep and located on the dorsal surface of the oblique head of the adductor hallucis (Fig. 9-29). The entrance to the space is located on the lateral border of the muscle. It is delineated by a line extending from the base of the fourth metatarsal bone to the lateral side of the base of the proximal phalanx of the big toe. This deep fascial space covers completely the first interosseous space, the

proximal half of the second interosseous space, and the proximal end of the third interosseous space.

The fourth interosseous space then corresponds only to fascial space 3 and the first interosseous space to fascial space 4. The second interosseous space shares distally the third fascial space and proximally the fourth. The lateral plantar artery and nerve course transversely in fascial space 4. The lateral plantar artery crosses the bases of the metatarsals 4, 3, and 2 and terminates by inosculation in the perforating deep branch of the dorsalis pedis artery at the base of the first metatarsal. It forms the plantar arterial arcade that provides the metatarsal arteries 1 to 4 and the proximal intermetatarsal perforating arteries 2, 3, and 4.

The common course of the plantar metatarsal arteries is along the shaft of metatarsals 2 to 4. The potential division of the metatarsal arteries into deep and superficial metatarsal arteries and deep and superficial intermetatarsal arteries is presented in Chapter 7.

The deep branch of the lateral plantar nerve provides motor branches to the oblique head of the adductor hallucis and the interossei of the first intermetatarsal space; a branch may extend into the lateral head of the short flexor of the big toe. This last branch may send an anastomotic branch to a similar motor branch arising from the medial plantar nerve and form the anastomotic motor branch of Hallopeau, the equivalent of Riche and Cannieu motor anastomosis as seen in the hand.[16]

The oblique head of the adductor hallucis muscle arises from the mid segment of the peroneus longus tendon sheath, the calcaneocuboid ligament, the crest of the cuboid, the base of metatarsals 4, 3, and 2, and the lateral cuneiform. The strong muscle courses anteromedially. It is joined by the transverse head of the adductor hallucis and shares insertion with the lateral head of the flexor hallucis brevis; this insertion takes place on the lateral sesamoid and the lateral aspect of the base of the proximal phalanx of the big toe.

A pyogenic collection in fascial spaces 2, 3, and 4 of the central compartment of the sole of the foot may extend into the calcaneal canal and reach the deep compartment of the leg. Further details concerning these possible extensions are provided in Chapter 3.

Lateral Compartment. The lateral compartment is formed by the lateral intermuscular septum medially and the lateral component of the plantar aponeurosis on the plantar and lateral aspects. The lateral aponeurosis provides dorsolateral fibers that insert over the os calcis, the sheath of the peronei, and subsequently the base and shaft of the fifth metatarsal. Three muscles are present in this compartment: the abductor digiti quinti and the short flexor and the opponens of the fifth toe.

The abductor digiti quinti originates from the posterolateral and posteromedial tuberosities of the os calcis, the deep surface of the plantar aponeurosis, and the lateral intermuscular septum. The muscle is directed anterolaterally, and at the level of the base of the fifth metatarsal, it may glide over a bursa or receive supplementary fibers of attachment. The shiny, flat tendon passes through the bifur-

(Text continues on p. 364.)

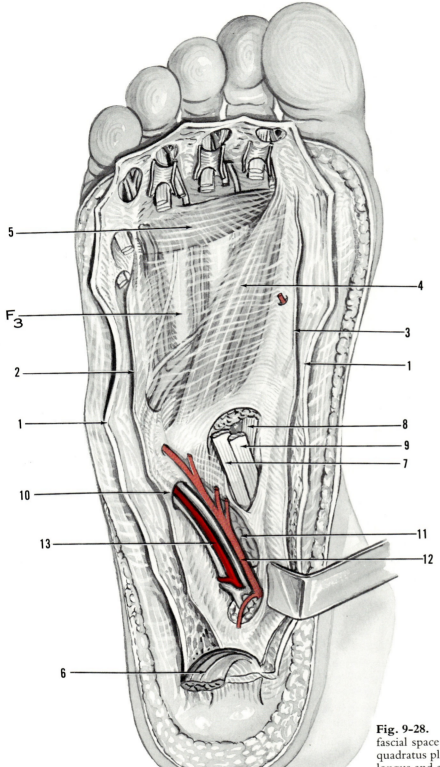

Fig. 9-28. Central compartment of the sole of the foot. (F_3, fascial space 3, proximally between the flexor digitorum longus–quadratus plantae and the tarsus, distally between flexor digitorum longus and adductor hallucis oblique head, including a segment of plane of the interossei muscles; 1, Plantar aponeurosis; 2, lateral intermuscular septum; 3, medial intermuscular septum; 4, adductor hallucis muscle, oblique head; 5, adductor hallucis muscle, transverse head; 6, flexor digitorum brevis reflected posteriorly; 7, flexor digitorum longus tendon; 8, flexor hallucis longus tendon; 9, expansion band of flexor hallucis longus; 10, foramen of exit of lateral plantar vessels; 11, quadratus plantae muscle; 12, lateral plantar nerve; 13, lateral plantar artery and veins.) (After Testut L, Jacob O: Traité d'Anatomie Topographique avec Applications Médico-Chirurgicales, 2nd ed, Vol II, p 1078. Paris, Doin, 1909)

Fig. 9-29.   Central compartment of the sole of the foot. (F_4, fascial space 4 between oblique head of adductor hallucis muscle and plane of interossei; F_3, fascial space 3, posterior segment, between quadratus plantae muscle and osteoligamentous plane of tarsus; F_2, fascial space 2 between quadratus plantar muscle and reflected flexor digitorum brevis; 1, flexor digitorum brevis muscle, reflected posteriorly; 2, abductor hallucis muscle; 3, abductor digiti quinti muscle; 4, quadratus plantae muscle; 5, adductor hallucis muscle, oblique head; 6, adductor hallucis muscle, transverse head; 7, medial intermuscular septum; 8, lateral intermuscular septum; 9, flexor digitorum longus tendon; 10, peroneus longus tendon; 11, lateral plantar nerve, exiting at *14*; 12 lateral plantar artery, exiting at *13*; 15, lateral plantar nerve, deep branch, passing posterior to deep branch of lateral plantar artery [16]; 17, motor nerve branch to transverse head of adductor hallucis; 18, motor nerve branch to second plantar interosseous muscle; 19, motor nerve branch to first plantar interosseous muscle; 20, motor branch to oblique head of adductor hallucis; 21, motor branch to second dorsal interosseous muscle; 22, motor branch to lateral head flexor hallucis brevis; 23, medial plantar nerve; 24, medial plantar artery; 25, superficial tibial plantar artery; 26, first plantar metatarsal artery; 27, medial plantar hallucal artery; 28, 29, plantar metatarsal arteries.)

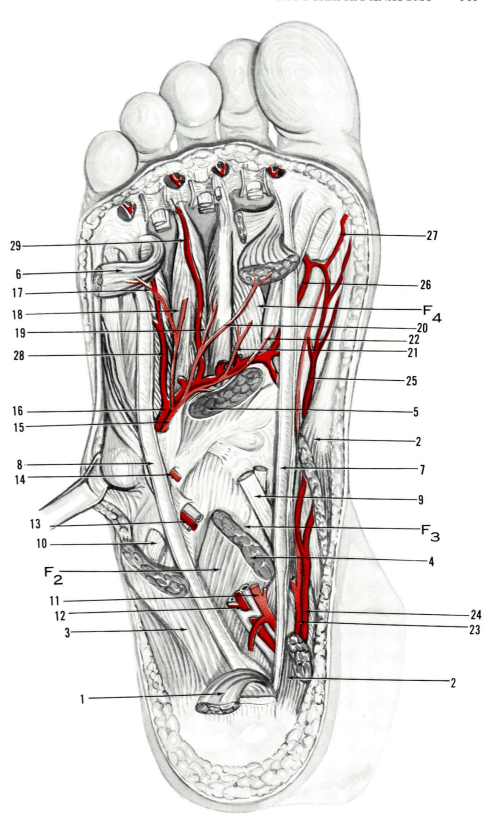

cation of the lateral plantar aponeurosis and inserts on the lateral aspect of the proximal phalanx of the fifth toe and in the plantar plate of the metatarsophalangeal joint of the same toe. The deep covering fascia of the muscle is attached to the long calcaneocuboid ligament, the peroneus longus tendon sheath, and, more anteriorly, the flexor digiti quinti brevis fascia. A space is present between the deep investing fascia and the muscle. With increased pressure, the space yields into the peroneus longus tunnel or into the mid compartment.

The short flexor of the fifth toe is covered almost completely by the abductor muscle of the same toe. This small and thin muscle originates from the sheath of the peroneus longus tendon and the base of the fifth metatarsal. It inserts through a flat tendon on the base of the proximal phalanx of the toe laterally.

The opponens of the fifth toe is located on the inner aspect of the short flexor of the toe and has a common origin with the latter. The muscle inserts on the anterior two thirds of the fifth metatarsal shaft. Quite often, this muscle is absent or fused to the short flexor.

The lateral plantar artery and nerve, after emerging from the midplantar space, extend forward and are located between the lateral intermuscular septum and the deep sheath of the abductor digiti quinti muscle. About 2.5 cm distal to the base of the fifth metatarsal bone, the artery goes deep to the medial aspect of the short flexor of the fifth toe and pierces again the lateral intermuscular septum to reenter the mid plantar space. Just distal to the fifth metatarsal base, the lateral plantar artery gives off the superficial fibular plantar artery of the little toe and may provide the fourth superficial plantar common digital plantar artery, which contributes to the formation of the superficial plantar arterial arcade.

The lateral plantar nerve is initially anterior and then medial to the artery. Opposite the base of the fifth metatarsal, the nerve divides into one deep and two superficial branches (lateral and medial). The deep lateral neurovascular bundle makes a medial turn, perforates the lateral intermuscular septum, and penetrates the middle compartment. The lateral superficial nerve is located in the interval between the flexor digitorum brevis and the abductor digiti quinti. It provides motor branches to the short flexor, opponens, and abductor of the fifth toe and continues as the lateral plantar cutaneous nerve of the latter. The medial superficial nerve branch obliquely and superficially crosses the short flexor tendon to the fifth toe. It provides the common digital nerve to the fourth interosseous space and an anastomotic branch to the nerve of the third web space. Variations of the pattern of division of the lateral plantar nerve are possible, and the superficial branch may initially have a common stem that subsequently bifurcates.

Medial Compartment. The medial compartment of the foot is limited laterally by the medial intermuscular septum and on the plantar and medial sides by the medial component of the plantar aponeurosis. The latter inserts along the first metatarsal shaft, medial cuneiform, and navicular. Within the compartment are located the abductor

hallucis muscle, the flexor hallucis brevis muscle, and the flexor hallucis longus tendon.

The abductor hallucis muscle originates from the medial calcaneal tuberosity, the deep surface of the plantar aponeurosis, the posterior end of the medial intermuscular septum, and the flexor retinaculum. It establishes fascial connections with the medial surface of the os calcis through the interfascicular septum of the calcaneal canal and with the common sheath of the flexor digitorum longus and the flexor hallucis longus tendon. Further connections are established at the level of the tuberosity of the navicular. The lateral border of the muscle is quite adherent to the plantar aponeurosis. The tendon of insertion appears on the medial aspect of the muscle; it is flat and slightly plantar in location. The inferolateral fibers insert on the medial sesamoid of the big toe in conjunction with the medial head of the flexor hallucis brevis. The superomedial fibers contribute to the transverse lamina of the extensor aponeurosis.

The flexor hallucis brevis muscle arises from the medial intermuscular septum and has a Y-shaped tendinous origin. The medial limb of the Y is in continuity with the tibialis posterior tendon, and the lateral limb is anchored to the cuboid and the lateral cuneiform.

The muscle is oriented anteromedially, crosses obliquely the first interosseous space, and, before reaching the metatarsophalangeal joint of the big toe, divides into two heads, lateral and medial. The lateral head, which is crossed by the flexor hallucis longus tendon, has a spiral twist to its fibers and inserts on the lateral aspect of the plantar plate, the lateral sesamoid, and the base of the proximal phalanx of the big toe in conjunction with the tendon of the adductor hallucis. As mentioned above, the medial head of the short flexor has a common insertion with the tendon of the abductor hallucis.

The tendon of the flexor hallucis longus, after being crossed on its plantar aspect by the flexor digitorum longus tendon, provides a tendinous slip to the latter but remains in the medial compartment and courses initially between the medial intermuscular septum and the abductor hallucis. It obliquely crosses the lateral head of the flexor hallucis brevis and enters the fibrous tunnel at the level of the plantar plate of the big toe.

The medial plantar neurovascular bundle reaches the medial compartment through the upper chamber of the calcaneal canal (Fig. 9-30). The nerve is anterior to the artery. As the flexor digitorum longus tendon becomes oblique to enter the middle compartment, the neurovascular bundle passes over the same tendon superficially. The artery crosses the nerve superficially and locates on the medial side of the nerve. From there until their branching, the medial plantar nerve and artery remain on the medial side of the flexor hallucis longus tendon and nearly within the substance of the medial intermuscular septum. The nerve provides two motor branches to the abductor hallucis muscle; they are located two and three finger-breadths behind the tuberosity of the navicular and enter the muscle from the deep lateral border.[7] These branches pass through fibrous tunnels and superficially cross the vessels. A third motor branch is provided by the median plantar nerve to the flexor hallucis brevis and penetrates the muscle from the medial border.

Fig. 9-30.   Plantar aspect of the foot. (1, Abductor hallucis muscle detached from its origin [2]; 3, interfascicular septum; 4, flexor digitorum brevis; 5, abductor digiti quinti; 6, quadratus plantae; 7, flexor digitorum longus; 8, flexor hallucis longus; 9, lateral plantar nerve; 10, medial plantar nerve; 11, posterior tibial artery; 12, motor nerve branch to abductor digiti quinti; 13, medial calcaneal artery; 14, lateral plantar artery; 15, medial plantar artery; 16, posterior motor nerve branch to quadratus plantae; 17, motor nerve branch to flexor digitorum brevis; 18, motor nerve branch to abductor hallucis muscle; 19, medial division branch of medial plantar nerve providing motor branches to medial head of flexor hallucis brevis and forming medial plantar hallucal nerve [22]; 20, lateral division branch of medial plantar nerve providing motor branch to first lumbrical muscle [21] and then branch to lateral head of flexor hallucis brevis and forming first common superficial digital nerve [23]; the nerve courses laterally and provides second and third common superficial digital nerves [24] and anastomotic branch [25] to fourth common superficial nerve [31]; 26, anterior motor nerve branch to quadratus plantae muscle; 27, motor nerve branch to opponens digiti quinti; 28, motor nerve branches to flexor digiti quinti; 29, deep motor branch of lateral plantar nerve; 30, motor nerve branch to adductor hallucis, transverse head; 32, first plantar metatarsal artery; 33, superficial plantar lateral artery to fifth toe; 34, fourth plantar metatarsal artery.) (Redrawn after Dujarier C: Anatomie des Membres Dissection—Anatomie Topographique, 2nd ed, p 322. Paris, Masson, 1924)

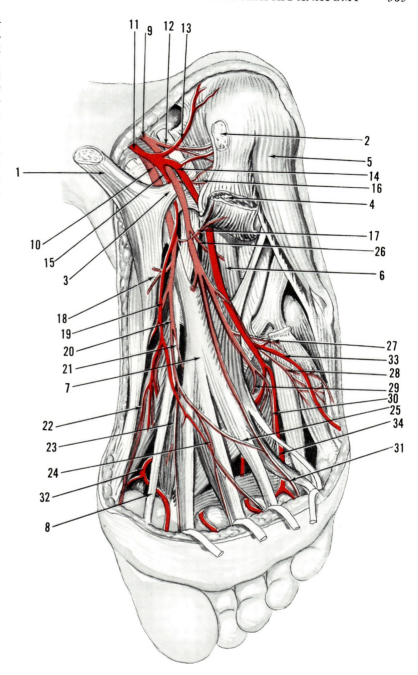

Slightly distal to the level of the tuberosity of the fifth metatarsal, the medial plantar nerve divides into two branches: medial and lateral. The medial branch courses along the lateral side of the abductor hallucis tendon, provides multiple motor branches to the medial head of the flexor hallucis brevis, and terminates as the medial plantar digital nerve of the big toe. The lateral branch bifurcates, and its medial branch innervates the lateral head of the flexor hallucis brevis and the first lumbrical and terminates as the common plantar digital nerve to the first web space. The lateral branch of the bifurcation turns around the medial border of the flexor digitorum brevis and divides within fascial space 1 into the motor branches to the second lum-

brical and the sensory common plantar digital nerves to the second and third web spaces. The nerve to the last space may receive an anastomotic branch from the common digital nerve of the fourth space.

The medial plantar artery, located on the medial side of the nerve, has variable divisions. In general the artery divides into two branches, superficial and deep. The superficial branch emerges between the abductor hallucis and the flexor digitorum brevis and divides into the superficial tibial plantar artery of the big toe and the common plantar digital artery. The former courses over the flexor hallucis brevis muscle on the tibial side of the flexor hallucis longus tendon. On the medial border of the first metatarsal neck, the su-

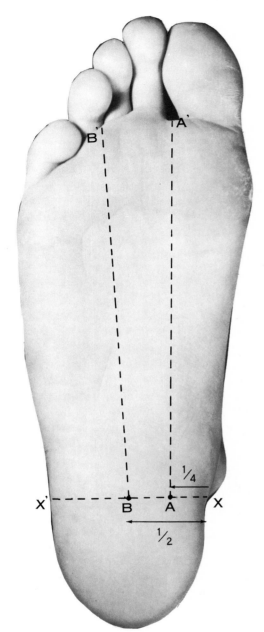

Fig. 9-31.   Guidelines for the locations of the intermuscular septa. *XX'*, plantar continuation of line drawn tangentially to posterior border of tibia; *B*, midpoint of *XX'*; *A*, midpoint of *BX*; *AA'*, line drawn from *A* to first web space indicates location of medial intermuscular septum; *BB'*, line drawn from *B* to third web space indicates location of lateral intermuscular septum.) (Guidelines redrawn after Testut L, Jacob O: Traité d'Anatomie Topographique avec Applications Médico-Chirurgicales, 2nd ed, Vol II, p 1077. Paris, Doin, 1909)

perficial tibial plantar artery passes between the medial head of the flexor hallucis brevis and the bone and anastomoses with the first plantar metatarsal artery.

The common plantar digital artery crosses obliquely the flexor hallucis longus tendon, passes between the plantar aponeurosis and the flexor digitorum brevis, and provides the common digital plantar arteries 1 to 3, which will join the corresponding plantar metatarsal arteries. As mentioned previously, a superficial plantar arterial arcade is formed when the third common digital plantar artery receives a similar superficial branch from the lateral plantar artery.

The deep branch of the medial plantar artery is divided into a tibial and a peroneal branch. The deep tibial branch courses along the skeletal margin of the foot and may anastomose with the first plantar metatarsal artery or continue into the dorsal tibial hallucal artery. The deep peroneal branch passes dorsal to the peroneus longus tendon near its insertion and terminates in the deep plantar arterial arch.

A fascial space is present between the deep surface of the abductor hallucis muscle and its investing fascia. This is a closed space and may yield only into the subcutaneous space.

The middle compartment of the sole of the foot may be approached surgically directly on either side of the flexor digitorum brevis. The incision is placed along the line delineating either the medial or the lateral plantar groove, which will lead to the major neurovascular bundles or to the central compartment. The guidelines for the placement of these incisions have been presented in the surface anatomy (Fig. 9-31).

The incision is extended as needed to the medial retromalleolar area in a curvilinear manner, passing over the abductor hallucis muscle and centered over the neurovascular tunnel located about one fingerbreadth behind the medial malleolus. The control of the neurovascular bundle permits the safe exposure of the tendinous or osteoligamentous layer.

Henry advocates a medial approach to the planta pedis.[7] A curvilinear incision on the medial border of the foot from the ball of the great toe to the heel is followed by the mobilization of the upper border of the abductor hallucis muscle, allowing the downward hinging of the muscle. The two motor branches of the muscle are to be protected; they are located two and three fingerbreadths behind the tuberosity of the navicular. The medial intermuscular septum, presenting itself as a "defective fascia," is dissected, and the bifurcation of the medial and lateral plantar neurovascular bundles is located. A thumbwidth lateral to the tuberosity of the navicular is the common sheath of the flexor digitorum longus and flexor hallucis longus tendons; this "master knot" is detached. The origin of the flexor hallucis brevis is released. The musculotendinous units of the medial and central compartments, including the plantar neurovascular bundles, are retracted plantarward, thus providing access to the osteoligamentous plantar plane, including the long and short plantar calcaneocuboid ligaments. The short plantar calcaneocuboid ligament is recognized by its obliquity toward the big toe. The inferior calcaneonavicular ligament crossed by the plantar component of the tibialis posterior tendon is well in view.

Ball of the Foot and Big Toe

SURFACE ANATOMY

The ball of the foot extends from the level of the metatarsal necks to the distal plantar digital flexion crease. The skin is convex in the sagittal plane as it curves dorsally. The flexion crease is convex distally, with the apex centered on the second toe. It crosses the toes at the level of the proximal phalanges, and in the little toe, it may reach the proximal interphalangeal joint. The five metatarsal heads and the medial and the lateral sesamoids of the big toe are easily felt through the skin.

SKIN

The skin of the ball of the foot is thick and semimobile. It tenses and acquires fixation with the extension of the toes. The subcutaneous adipose layer is thin at the level of the dermal insertion of the longitudinal bands of the plantar aponeurosis. The cushioning of the ball of the foot is provided by the pretendinous submetatarsal adipose cushions and the intermetatarsal fat bodies.[17]

Subcutaneous bursae may be present under the heads of the first and fifth metatarsals. Venous longitudinal branches arising from the distal venous arcade course distally toward the corresponding web spaces to drain in the dorsal venous system.

PLANTAR APONEUROSIS AND SUBCOMPARTMENTS AND CONTENTS

The plantar aponeurosis, proximal to the metatarsal heads, is structured into five bands—one medial, three central, and one lateral. The medial and the lateral bands course obliquely over the metatarsophalangeal joint area of the big and little toes. The central bands diverge and proceed individually toward the first interdigital space, the third toe, and the fourth interdigital space. They insert into the dermis distal to the metatarsophalangeal joint and segmentally close the subcutaneous space. The distal fibers pass over the natatory ligaments and contribute to their formation. No fibers reach or insert on the skin at the level of the plantar digital crease, where a transverse band of adipose tissue is interposed between the skin and the most frontal part of the natatory ligament.

Proximal to the metatarsal heads, transversely oriented aponeurotic thin bands cross the plantar aponeurosis and extend into the dermis. Adipose tissue is retained between the layers. The medial and lateral ends of these transverse bands turn anteriorly and contribute to the formation of the natatory ligaments.

The longitudinally oriented aponeurotic bands, the transverse fasciculi proximally and the transversely oriented natatory ligaments distally, delineate spaces that are oval to quadrilateral in shape. Adipose tissue corresponding to the fat bodies protrudes in these spaces and forms the monticuli of the skin. Within these windows course superficially the superficial common plantar digital arteries 1 to 4 and the common digital plantar nerves to spaces 1 to 4. The common plantar digital arteries are deeper and well covered with the fat body.

The medial plantar nerve of the big toe courses under the medial prong of the plantar aponeurosis. The lateral plantar nerve of the fifth toe and the accompanying plantar arterial branch pass under the lateral prong of the plantar aponeurosis.

Proximal to the metatarsal heads, each longitudinal band of the plantar aponeurosis extends, on each side of the corresponding long flexor tendon, two aponeurotic septa (Fig. 9-32). These septa insert on the interosseous fascia, the fascia of the transverse head of the adductor hallucis, the deep transverse metatarsal ligament, and the plantar plate and its junction with the accessory collateral ligament of the metatarsophalangeal joint. The two septa of a given band may interchange fibers proximally and form a foramina through which pass the long flexor tendons and may also extend insertional fibers to the adjacent septa.

The longitudinal septa separate the long flexor tendon from the lumbrical muscle, and the origin of the latter limits the proximal extension of the sagittal septum.

At the level of the metatarsal heads, the septa are in continuity with vertical fibers (Figs. 9-33 and 9-34). These fibers arise from the sides of the fibrous flexor tendon sheath and from the plantar plate. They course plantarward, connect with the longitudinal aponeurotic band, and insert with the latter on the skin. Some of the vertical fibers arch over the flexor tendon sheath and form a compartment filled with adipose tissue, called the "submetatarsal cushion."[17] Both sesamoids of the big toe are covered by such a common cushion.

At the level of the metatarsophalangeal joint on the tibial side, a fascia splits off the longitudinal septum and forms a compartment for the lumbrical tendon. The intermetatarsal capitular space, over the plantar aspect of the transverse metatarsal ligament, is occupied by an encapsulated fat body that covers the common plantar digital neurovascular bundle.[17]

Distal to the level of the metatarsal heads, the fibrous sheaths of the flexor hallucis longus and of the flexor digitorum longus–brevis are joined by a transversely directed retinacular ligament, arching from sheath to sheath, called the "mooring ligament."

The distal segment of the ball of the foot and web space is crossed transversely by the natatory or interdigital ligament. This ligament has a multilamellar (six to eight transverse layers) or retinacular weblike structure.[17] It is deep to the insertional fibers of the longitudinal bands of the plantar aponeurosis. It attaches to the flexor tendon sheath and the mooring ligament and covers the intertendinous space on the plantar aspect of the web space. The plantar digital neurovascular bundle passes dorsal to this ligament. Superficially, the natatory ligament attaches to the dermis and retains within its layer a substantial amount of adipose tissue.

Proximal transection of the plantar aponeurosis and detachment of the longitudinal septa allows reflection of the aponeurosis. The superficial common plantar digital nerves and arteries now are crossing the plantar aspect of the flexor digitorum brevis tendons. These structures with the flexor

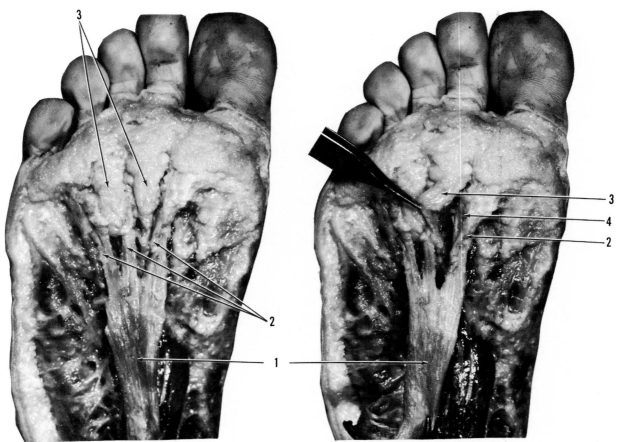

Fig. 9–32.   Longitudinal bands of the plantar aponeurosis. (1, Plantar aponeurosis; 2, longitudinal superficial tracts 2, 3, 4 of plantar aponeurosis; 3, fat bodies; 4, septum of deep component of longitudinal tract of plantar aponeurosis.)

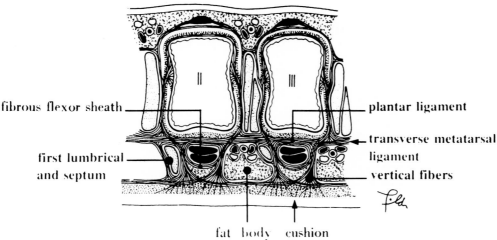

Fig. 9–33.   Cross section through metatarsal heads 2 and 3. (From Bojsen-Møller F: Anatomy of the forefoot, normal and pathologic. Clin Orthop 142:17, 1979)

Fig. 9-34.   Cross section passing through metatarsal heads 2, 3, 4. (1, Chamber retaining fat body; 2, vertical fibers arising from flexor tendon sheath; 3, arciform fibers forming chamber of fatty, preflexor cushion [*4*]; 5, plantae plate; 6, flexors digitorum longus and brevis in their fibrous tunnel; 7, lumbrical tendon; 8, metatarsal head.)

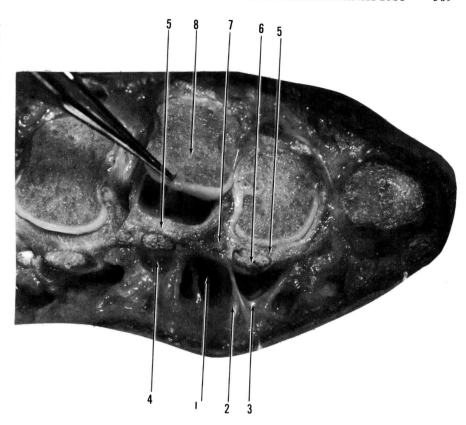

digitorum longus are retracted to bring into view the transverse head of the adductor hallucis and a segment of the interossei covered by their fascia.

The transverse head of the adductor hallucis arises from the proximal border of the plantar plate of the third, fourth, and fifth metatarsophalangeal joints; the proximal border of the deep transverse metatarsal ligament of the second, third, and fourth spaces; and the lateral crux of the lateral segment of the plantar aponeurosis.

The covering fascia gives attachment to the longitudinal septa of the plantar aponeurosis. The transversely oriented muscle fibers overlap, and the longest fibers are the most posterior and have a lateral origin. The transverse head of the adductor hallucis joins the oblique head for a common insertion on the lateral aspect of the proximal phalanx of the big toe and the lateral sesamoid.

Opposite the proximal border of the second, third, and fourth deep transverse metatarsal ligaments and the transverse head of the adductor hallucis, small apertures for the passage of the common plantar digital arteries are present. These openings are seen at times as a foramina through the substance of the deep transverse metatarsal ligament. Reflection of the transverse head of the adductor hallucis brings into view the origins of the common plantar digital arteries and of the premetatarsal vascular triangle.

Over the central metatarsal 2, 3, and 4, the vascular triangle is located on the plantar aspect of the corresponding metatarsal neck (Fig. 9-35). The base is distal and formed by the proximal border of the plantar plate, the apex is proximal, and the sides are formed by the parting interossei muscles. The plantar metatarsal artery bifurcates in this space into lateral and medial branches. Each branch passes between the distal border of the transverse head of the adductor of the big toe and the proximal border of the deep transverse metatarsal ligament and courses on the plantar aspect of the latter as the common digital plantar artery. Quite often only the lateral limb of the bifurcation is substantial or present, and this continues as the common digital plantar artery and joins distally, in the web space, the distal perforating branch of the corresponding dorsal metatarsal artery, which in turn divides into the plantar digital arteries of the adjacent toes.

Further details concerning the contribution of the metatarsal arteries to the digital arteries are provided in Chapter 7.

BIG TOE

The prominent head of the first metatarsal is covered on the plantar and the dorsomedial aspect by two subcutaneous bursae.

On the plantar aspect, a thin layer of subcutaneous fat is present, which covers the oblique superficial aponeurotic tract of the plantar fascia. Two deep aponeurotic septa extend from the superficial tract on each side of the flexor hallucis longus tendon (Fig. 9-36). The medial septum inserts on the medial sesamoid, the medial border of the plantar plate, and the medial head of the flexor hallucis brevis. The lateral septum inserts on the lateral sesamoid, the lateral border of the plantar plate, the lateral head of the flexor hallucis brevis, and the distal end of the medial intermuscular septum.

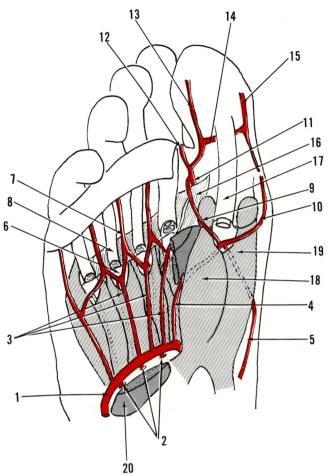

Fig. 9-35.   Disposition of the plantar arteries in the forefoot.
(1, Plantar arterial arcade; 2, proximal perforating arteries; 3, metatarsal arteries 2, 3, 4; 4, first plantar metatarsal artery; 5, medial branch of medial plantar artery; 6, vascular triangle formed by interossei and proximal border of plantar plate; 7, common plantar digital artery; 8, flexor tunnel; 9, lateral division branch of first plantar metatarsal artery; 10, medial division branch of first metatarsal artery; 11, vertical segment of first dorsal metatarsal artery; 12, medial plantar artery of second toe; 13, lateral plantar hallucal artery; 14, transverse anastomotic branch of plantar hallucal arteries; 15, medial plantar hallucal artery; 16, deep transverse metatarsal ligament; 17, flexor hallucis longus tunnel; 18, flexor hallucis brevis, lateral head; 19 flexor hallucis brevis, medial head; 20, adductor hallucis muscle, oblique head.)

Anterior to the aponeurotic septa, the metatarsophalangeal joint is covered by the pretendinous, premetatarsal fat or cushion. The cushion is retained in the compartment by vertical fibers extending from each side of the joint and arching at a distance over the fibrous tunnel of the flexor hallucis longus tendon. This adipose cushion covers both sesamoids.

Distally, the medial ends of the mooring arms of the natatory ligaments insert on the long flexor tunnel. Proximally the lateral septum may send a strong connecting band to the medial septum of the second toe, and it is also a termination point for the medial intermuscular septum.

The deep transverse metatarsal ligament joins the lateral border of the plantar plate of the big toe to the medial border of the plantar plate of the second toe. The adductor tendons reach the big toe dorsal to the deep transverse metatarsal ligament. The tendon of the transverse head of the adductor inserts on the extensor aponeurosis, and the remaining fibers pass over the insertional fibers of the oblique head of the adductor hallucis, share their insertion on the lateral sesamoid, and terminate on the fibrous sheath of the flexor hallucis longus.

The oblique head of the adductor hallucis has three components: medial, central, and lateral. The medial component with fleshy fibers, inserts directly on the lateral sesamoid. The central deep component is tendinous and takes a firm grip on the plantar aspect of the lateral sesamoid. The lateral component has a broader tendon that inserts on the lateral sesamoid and the plantar lateral aspect of the proximal phalanx, with minor contribution to the extensor aponeurosis (Fig. 9-37).

The lateral head of the flexor hallucis penetrates the plantar plate through a flat tunnel laterally at a distance from the tendons of the adductor hallucis. The fibers insert on the lateral aspect of the plantar plate, the central and medial aspects of the lateral sesamoid, and the lateral aspect of the proximal phalanx. The tendons of the adductor hallucis and of the lateral head of the short flexor of the big toe are conjoint only at the distal insertional point.

The medial head of the flexor hallucis brevis inserts on the medial aspect of the plantar plate, the lateral and central aspect of the medial sesamoid, and the medial aspect of the base of the proximal phalanx in conjunction with the abductor hallucis tendon (Fig. 9-38). The inferolateral tendinous fibers of the latter insert on the medial sesamoid and on the medial plantar tubercle of the proximal phalanx of the big toe. The superomedial tendinous fibers connect with the medial aspect of the transverse lamina of the hallucal extensor aponeurosis. A triangle is formed on the plantar aspect of the first metatarsal neck and is similar to the ones found in the lesser toes (see Fig. 9-35). This triangle has a distal base that corresponds to the proximal border of the plantar plate. The apex and the sides are formed by the parting of the two heads of the flexor hallucis brevis muscle. The first plantar metatarsal artery, after coursing proximally on the plantar aspect of the first dorsal interosseous muscle, passes from the lateral side under the flexor hallucis brevis muscle and the first metatarsal shaft. It appears in the depths of the described triangle and bifurcates into lateral and medial branches. The deep medial branch of the medial plantar artery passes between the medial head of the flexor hallucis brevis and the first metatarsal shaft from the medial side and joins the bifurcation point of the first plantar metatarsal artery (see Fig. 9-35). The anastomosis and the branching form a cruciform arterial pattern. The medial division branch of the first plantar metatarsal artery passes under the flexor hallucis longus tendon, turns over or around the medial sesamoid, and joins the tibial plantar hallucal artery, which is a branch of the perforating branch of the first dorsal metatarsal artery. The medial division branch of the first plantar metatarsal artery is joined on the medial aspect of the big toe by the medial or tibial marginal artery, which is

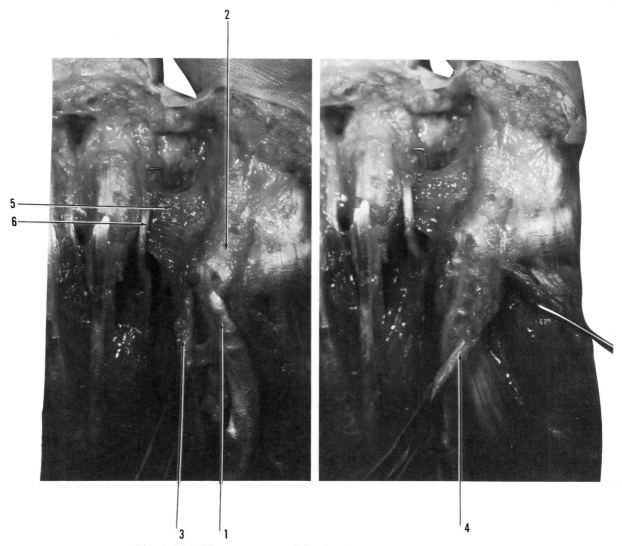

Fig. 9-36. Plantar aspect of the first intercapitular space. (1, Flexor hallucis longus; 2, tunnel of *1*; 3, lateral vertical septum of first longitudinal band of plantar aponeurosis; 4, medial vertical septum of first longitudinal band of plantar aponeurosis; 5, intermetatarsal ligament; 6, lumbrical tendon.)

a lateral division of the superficial branch of the medial plantar artery. The lateral division branch of the first plantar metatarsal artery exits from the vascular triangle and crosses the lateral head of the flexor hallucis brevis and the adductor hallucis. It passes around the lateral sesamoid on the plantar aspect of the deep transverse metatarsal ligament and joins the perforating branch of the first dorsal metatarsal artery in the first web space. Subsequent to this anastomosis, the first dorsal metatarsal artery divides into the plantar lateral artery of the big toe and the medial plantar artery of the second toe.

The lateral plantar hallucal artery sends a transverse branch across the mid segment of the proximal phalanx between the bone and the flexor hallucis longus tendon and forms the medial plantar hallucal artery, which is joined by the medial division branch of the first plantar metatarsal artery. The lateral plantar hallucal artery is the major artery

of the big toe, and the variations of the arterial supply are presented in Chapter 7.

The first common plantar digital nerve provides the lateral plantar nerve to the big toe which passes plantar to the deep transverse metatarsal ligament.

The medial plantar digital nerve of the big toe courses along the medial side of the flexor hallucis longus tunnel. It is superficial to the corresponding tibial plantar hallucal artery.

On the dorsal aspect of the big toe, the dorsal veins and superficial nerve branches are located within or under a superficial fascia. The dorsomedial vein of the big toe joins the medial arm of the dorsal venous arcade and contributes to the formation of the greater saphenous vein.

The distal dorsal arterial supply of the big toe is provided by a branch of the first dorsal metatarsal artery or, predominantly, by a branch from the plantar medial hallucal artery.

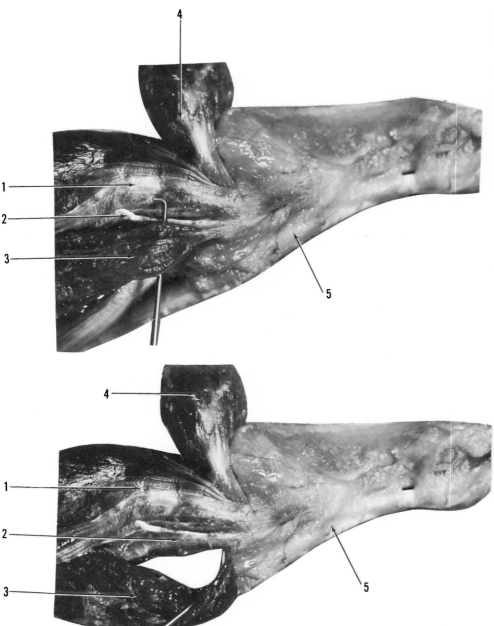

Fig. 9-37. Lateral aspect of the big toe. The first metatarsal is removed, and the proximal phalanx is preserved. (1–3, Three components of adductor hallucis oblique head—lateral [*1*], central [*2*], medial [*3*]; 4, transverse component of adductor hallucis; 5, flexor hallucis longus tendon within its tunnel.)

Details of variations are presented in Chapter 7.

In the first web space the first dorsal metatarsal artery dives plantarward and is accompanied by the perforating veins leading to the dorsal venous arcade.

The dorsomedial nerve of the big toe is provided by the medial branch of the medial dorsal cutaneous nerve of the foot. The dorsolateral aspect of the big toe is innervated by the medial division branch of the deep peroneal nerve and may receive contribution from the medial dorsal cutaneous branch of the superficial peroneal nerve.

Reflection of the superficial fascia and of the neurovas-cular structures exposes the extensor aponeurosis anchoring the extensor hallucis longus tendon to the lateral and medial aspects of the plantar plate and to the sides of the proximal phalanx. A supplementary slip of the extensor hallucis longus is found on the medial side of the tendon in an average of 50%; this slip inserts on the proximal phalanx. The extensor hallucis brevis tendon is located on the peroneal side of the extensor hallucis longus tendon, under the extensor aponeurosis. The possible variations concerning the supplementary tendinous slip to the dorsum of the big toe are presented in Chapter 5.

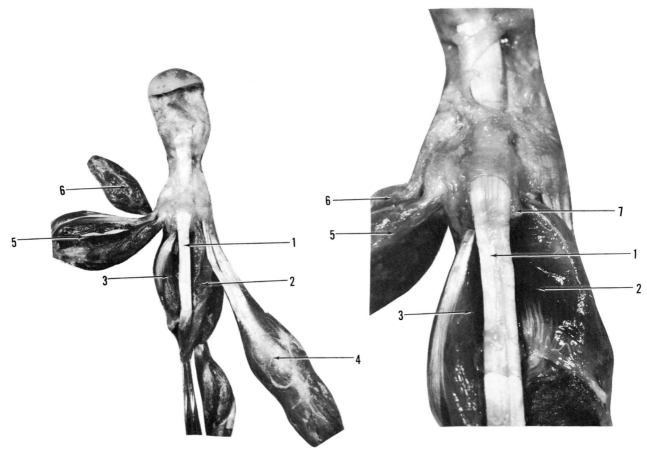

Fig. 9-38.   Plantar aspect of the big toe. (1, Flexor hallucis longus tendon; 2, flexor hallucis brevis muscle, medial head; 3, flexor hallucis brevis muscle, lateral head; 4, abductor hallucis muscle; 5, adductor hallucis muscle, oblique head; 6, adductor hallucis muscle, transverse head; 7, proximal border of plantar plate.)

REFERENCES

1. Testut L, Jacob O: Traité d' Anatomie Topographique avec Applications Médico—Chirurgicales, 2nd ed, Vol II, pp 1022–1114, 1075. Paris, Doin, 1909
2. Winckler G: Les veines du pied. Arch Anat Histol Embryol 37: 175, 1954–1955
3. Horwitz MT: Normal anatomy and variations of the peripheral nerves of the leg and foot. Arch Surg 36: 626, 1938
4. Bellocq P, Meyer P: Contribution a l'étude de l'aponeurose dorsale du pied (Fascia dorsalis pedis, P.N.A.). Acta Anat 30: 67, 1957
5. Huber JF: The arterial network supplying the dorsum of the foot. Anat Rec 80: 737, 1941
6. Rouvière J, Canela Lazaro M: Le ligament péronéo-astragalo-calcaneén. Ann Anat Pathol Anat Normal 9: 745, 1932
7. Henry AK: Extensile Exposure, 2nd ed, pp 268–271, 300–308. Baltimore, Williams & Wilkins, 1957
8. Bellocq P, Meyer P: Le ligament annulaire interne du cou-de-pied. Arch Anat Histol Embryol 37: 23, 1954
9. Baumann J: La région de passage de la loge postérieure de la jambe à la plante du pied. Ann Anat Pathol Anat Normal, 7: 201, 1930
10. Bellocq P, Meyer P: Contribution a l'étude du canal calcaneén. Comptes Rendus Assoc Anat 89: 292, 1956
11. Hovelacque A: Anatomie des Nerfs Craniens et Rachidiens et du Système Grand Sympathique Chez l'Homme, 2nd ed, pp 627–635. Paris, Doin, 1927
12. Adachi B: Das Arteriensystem der Japaner, pp 215–291. Kyoto, Maruzen, 1928
13. Mulfinger GL, Trueta J: The blood supply of the talus. J Bone Joint Surg [Br] 52, No. 1: 160, 1970
14. Delorme: Ligature des artères de la paume de la main et de la plante du pied. Mem Acad Med 1882. Cited in Testut L, Jacob O: Traité d'Anatomie Topographique avec Applications Médico–Chirurgicales, 2nd ed, Vol II, p 1084. Paris, Doin, 1909
15. Grodinsky M: A study of the fascial spaces of the foot and their bearing on infections. Surg Obst Gynecol 49, No. 6: 737, 1929
16. Hallopeau P: Note sur le nerf de l'adducteur oblique du gros orteil. Bull Mem Soc Anat Paris 75: 1078, 1900
17. Bojsen-Møller F, Flagstad KE: Plantar aponeurosis and internal architecture of the ball of the foot. J Anat 121, No 3: 599, 1976

10

Functional Anatomy of the Foot and Ankle

Field of Motion

The functional capacity of the foot and ankle is expressed by the contour and dimensions of its field of motion (Fig. 10-1).[1] The dimensions of the field of motion include all the possible spatial displacements of the forefoot with the distal leg remaining stationary. The field of motion of the foot and ankle is oval in contour. The vertical segment of the field is determined mainly by the talocrural joint and the transverse segment by the talocalcaneonavicular and the midtarsal joints. The functional capacity of the foot and ankle is age-dependent. The functional field is the largest in the newborn, and with aging it gradually constricts, more in the transverse segment than in the vertical. At age 2 to 6 years, the field is transversely oval; at age 40 years it is converted to a high oval; and by age 70 years, it is narrow, limited mainly to the vertical segment. In terms of functional capacity the foot at age 70 years can dorsiflex and plantar flex but has more limited capacity to adapt to walking on uneven ground. During the functional performance the ankle, the hindfoot, and the forefoot are highly integrated. Horizontal rotations induced by the pelvis and hip reach the ankle and are transmitted to the talocalcaneonavicular joint, which converts then, in the weight-bearing situation, into complex hindfoot–forefoot motions resulting in high or low arch anatomic positions.

Axis of Motion and Terminology of Motion

The axis of motion is the imaginary line around which motion occurs (Fig. 10-2). The plane of motion is perpen-

dicular to the direction of the axis. An obliquely oriented axis may be considered as the resultant of three axial components: transverse, vertical, and anteroposterior.

The transverse axis generates the motion of flexion–extension. The vertical axis generates the motion of abduction–adduction when the moving part is the foot or of mediolateral rotation when the moving part is the leg. The anteroposterior axis generates the motion of supination–pronation. Facing the right foot and ankle, pronation is the clockwise rotation and supination is the counterclockwise rotation; the reverse holds for left foot and ankle.

The sagittal plane of flexion–extension is perpendicular to the transverse axis. The horizontal plane of abduction–adduction is perpendicular to the vertical axis. The frontal plane of supination–pronation is perpendicular to the anteroposterior axis. An oblique axis generates simultaneous motion around its vectorial components or secondary axes.

The foot–ankle motion may be defined in the non–weight-bearing positions and weight-bearing positions.

In non–weight-bearing position the following motions are present:

Active
Inversion of the foot: sole faces medially
Eversion of the foot: sole faces laterally
Extension and flexion at the ankle with the foot in neutral position, in eversion, or in inversion
Circumduction of the foot, which encompasses the combination of the above motions. This is representative of the field of motion and reflects the total functional capability of the foot–ankle complex.
Toe flexion—extension and abduction, adduction to a limited degree

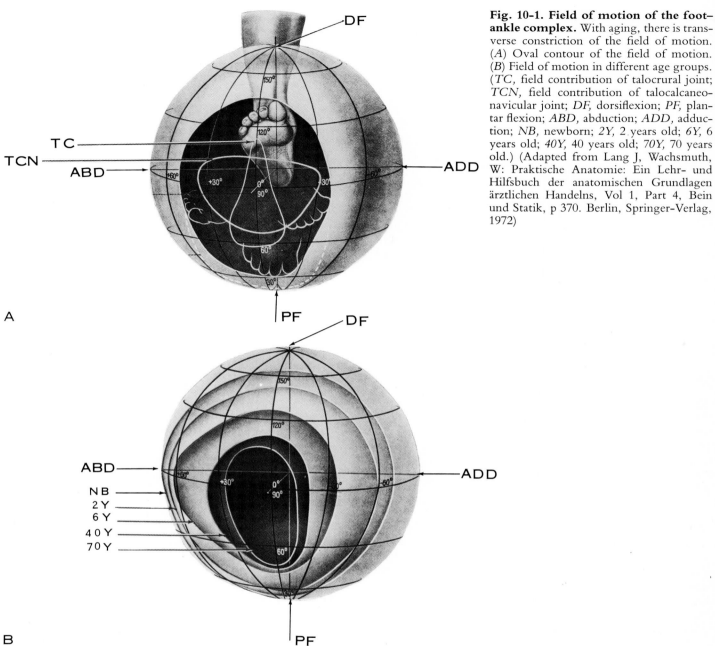

Fig. 10-1. Field of motion of the foot–ankle complex. With aging, there is transverse constriction of the field of motion. (*A*) Oval contour of the field of motion. (*B*) Field of motion in different age groups. (*TC*, field contribution of talocrural joint; *TCN*, field contribution of talocalcaneonavicular joint; *DF*, dorsiflexion; *PF*, plantar flexion; *ABD*, abduction; *ADD*, adduction; *NB*, newborn; *2Y*, 2 years old; *6Y*, 6 years old; *40Y*, 40 years old; *70Y*, 70 years old.) (Adapted from Lang J, Wachsmuth, W: Praktische Anatomie: Ein Lehr- und Hilfsbuch der anatomischen Grundlagen ärztlichen Handelns, Vol 1, Part 4, Bein und Statik, p 370. Berlin, Springer-Verlag, 1972)

Passive

All the above motions are present and can be assessed.

Hindfoot inversion (varus) or eversion (valgus)

Abduction and adduction of the forefoot after blocking the hindfoot motion

Supination and pronation twist of the forefoot after blocking the hindfoot motion

Flexion and extension at the tarsometatarsal joints

Flexion and extension at the digital joints

In weight-bearing position the motion can be assessed by the following:

Flexion and extension of the leg at the ankle

Tiptoe standing involving maximum ankle–midfoot plantar flexion, pronation of the forefoot, and inversion of the hindfoot

Heel standing, assessing the dorsiflexion at the ankle and the tension of the Achilles tendon

External rotation of the leg producing a high arch in the foot (Fig. 10-3)

Internal rotation of the leg producing a low arch in the foot (Fig. 10-3)

The last two motions involve hindfoot–forefoot disso-

Fig. 10-2. Axes of motion. The plane of motion is perpendicular to the axis of motion. Dorsiflexion–plantar flexion occurs around the transverse axis. Abduction–adduction occurs around the vertical axis. Supination–pronation occurs around the longitudinal axis. An oblique axis generates *simultaneously* motion around its vectorial components that act as secondary axes. (*X*, transverse axis; *Y*, longitudinal Axis; *Z*, vertical Axis; *DF*, dorsiflexion; *PF*, plantar flexion; *ABD*, abduction; *ADD*, adduction; *S*, supination; *P*, pronation.)

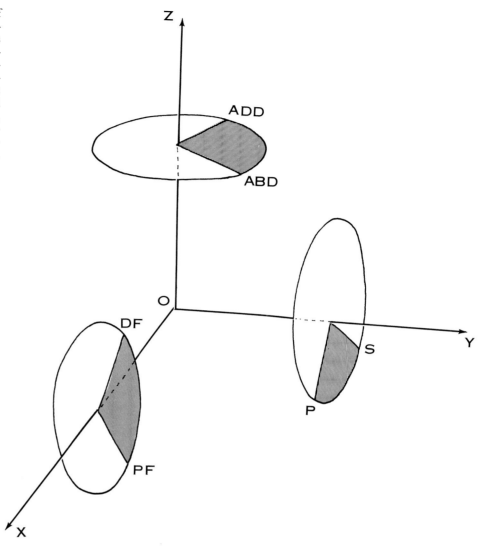

Ankle Motion

AXIS OF MOTION

The empirical axis of the ankle joint passes slightly distal to the tips of the malleoli at 5 mm ± 3 mm (range, 0–11 mm) distal to the tip of the medial malleolus, 3 mm ± 2 mm (range, 0 to 12 mm) distal to and 8 mm ± 5 mm anterior to the tip of the lateral malleolus.[2] The axis is inclined downward and laterally in the frontal plane (Fig. 10-4) and is rotated posterolaterally in the horizontal or transverse plane. In the frontal plane the angle between the empirical axis of the ankle and the midline of the tibia is 82.7° ± 3.7° with a range of 74° to 94° (Fig. 10-5).[2] In the transverse plane the angle of the ankle axis with the transverse axis of the knee is 20° to 30°.[3] The major motion occurring at the ankle joint is that of flexion–extension. The minor accompanying motions are lateral deviation or abduction and pronation in dorsiflexion and medial deviation or adduction and supination in plantar flexion (Fig. 10-6).

The minor and minimal motions are generated by the obliquity of the axis in two planes. In the frontal plane the oblique axis has a transverse component that generates the motion of flexion–extension and a vertical component that generates the motion of abduction–adduction. In the transverse plane the oblique axis has a transverse and a longitudinal component; the latter is responsible for the pronation–supination (Fig. 10-7).

(Text continues on p. 380.)

ciation, which will be analyzed subsequently. In flexion-extension the hindfoot and forefoot also move in opposite directions. In the non–weight-bearing position during inversion or eversion, the hindfoot and the forefoot move in unison in the same direction.

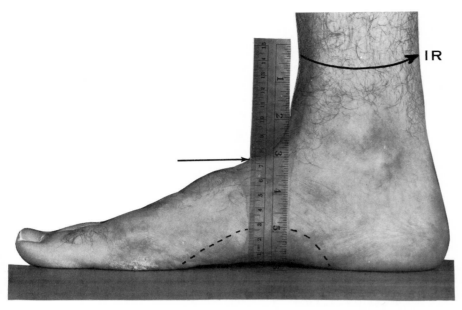

Fig. 10-3. In the weight-bearing position, the external rotation of the leg produces a high arch on the medial aspect of the foot and the internal rotation produces a low arch. From internal rotation to external rotation, the midfoot height increased in this case 1 cm. (*IR,* internal rotation of leg; *ER,* external rotation of leg.)

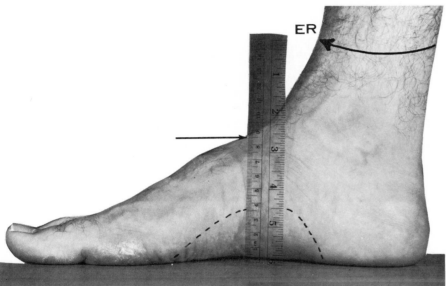

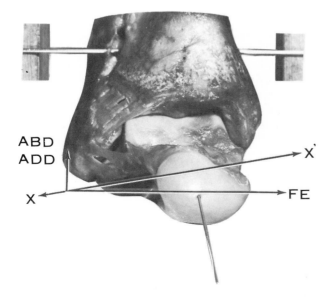

Fig. 10-4. Axis of the ankle joint. The axis of the ankle joint *XX'* is inclined as indicated and has two vectorial components: the major transverse component, which generates the motion of flexion–extension (*FE*), and the lesser vertical component, which generates the motion of abduction–adduction (*ABD–ADD*).

Fig. 10-5. Variations in the angle between the midline of the tibia and the empirical axis of the ankle. This histogram reveals a considerable spread of individual values. (From Inman TV: The Joints of the Ankle, 27. Baltimore, Williams & Wilkins, 1976)

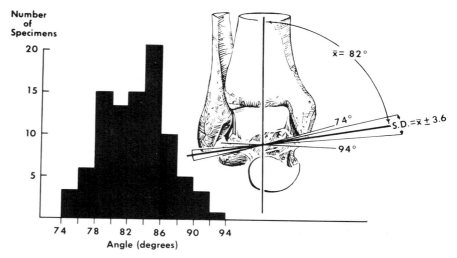

Fig. 10-6. Ankle specimen with K wires passed through the distal tibial (X) and the talar neck (Y). (*A*) The talus is dorsiflexed (*DF*). (*B*) The talus is plantar flexed (*PF*). In the plantar flexion the K wires diverge, indicating the adduction component of the motion.

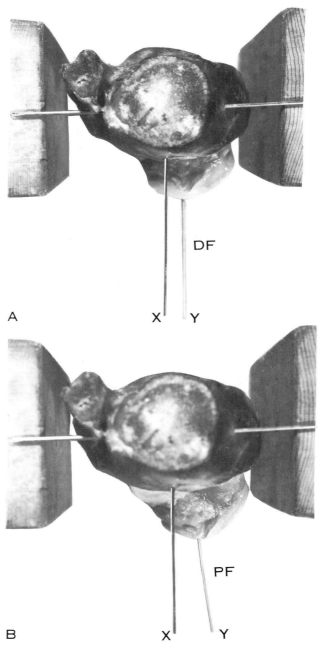

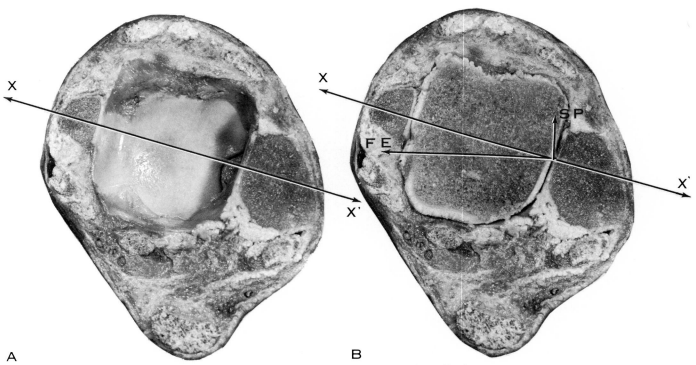

Fig. 10-7. Cross section of the ankle 2 cm above the tip of the medial malleolus, indicating the oblique orientation of the axis of motion of *XX'* of the ankle in the transverse plane. The axis *XX'* has a major transverse component for flexion–extension (*FE*) and a minor longitudinal component for supination–pronation (*SP*). (*A*) Cross section demonstrating the two malleoli and the tibial plafond. (*B*) Cross section with the dome of the talus lodged in the ankle mortise.

Barnett and Napier and Hicks recognize two axes to the ankle joint: a dorsiflexion axis inclined downward and laterally and a plantar flexion axis inclined downward and medially (Figs. 10-8 and 10-9).[4,5] The changeover occurs within a few degrees of the neutral position of the talus (Fig. 10-10). Barnett and Napier based their conclusions on the determination of the curvatures of the lateral and medial marginal profiles of the talar trochlea. The center of the curvature being the axis of motion, the lateral profile is "almost always an arc of a true circle, and in all positions of the talus the axis of rotation must pass through the center of this circle."[4] The medial profile is formed of the arcs of two circles with different radii: The arc of a small circle, occupying the anterior one third of the medial profile, corresponds to the dorsiflexion arc; the center of the circle is high in location. The arc of a large circle, occupying the posterior two thirds of the medial profile, corresponds to the plantar flexion arc; the center of the circle is low in location.

Close and Inman made transverse saw marks across the trochlear surface, along the frontal plane of the distal tibia throughout the range of plantar flexion and dorsiflexion.[6] The markings were not parallel and converged toward a point 4 or 5 inches medial to the ankle joint. The conclusions were, therefore, that the trochlea is not cylindrical but approximately conical with a medial apex and represents a truncated cone, and that transverse rotation occurs as exter-

nal rotation or abduction of the talus in dorsiflexion and as medial rotation or adduction of the talus in plantar flexion.

Inman, in a study of 86 tali, determined the conical angle of the frustum as being 24° ± 6° (range 10°–40°).[2] By considering the trochlear surface as a truncated cone it becomes apparent that the minor abduction or adduction of the talus is "built in" and is determined by the geometry of the surface, and that the talus offers at any time to the bimalleolar fork a transverse dimension that is nearly constant and represents a segment of the generating lines of the truncated cone (Fig. 10-11).

The mid trochlear arc measures approximately 120° and is covered in its two thirds by the tibial arc, which averages 70° to 80°. In full plantar flexion the talar trochlea has its posterior two thirds under the tibial plafond and between the malleoli and is stable (Fig. 10-12). The wedge shape of its posterolateral aspect is not a factor of instability. In full dorsiflexion, when the anterior part of the talus is lodged in the mortise, the intermalleolar distance increases only minimally. As measured by Close, when the ankle moves from full plantar flexion to full dorsiflexion, the fibula moves laterally 1.5 mm and turns laterally on its long axis 2.5°.[7]

It is apparent that the "give" at the tibiofibular syndesmosis is minimal. When reconstructing the tibiofibular syndesmosis at the ankle, it is safer, however, before applying the internal fixation devise, to bring the talus into full dorsiflexed position.

(Text continues on p. 385.)

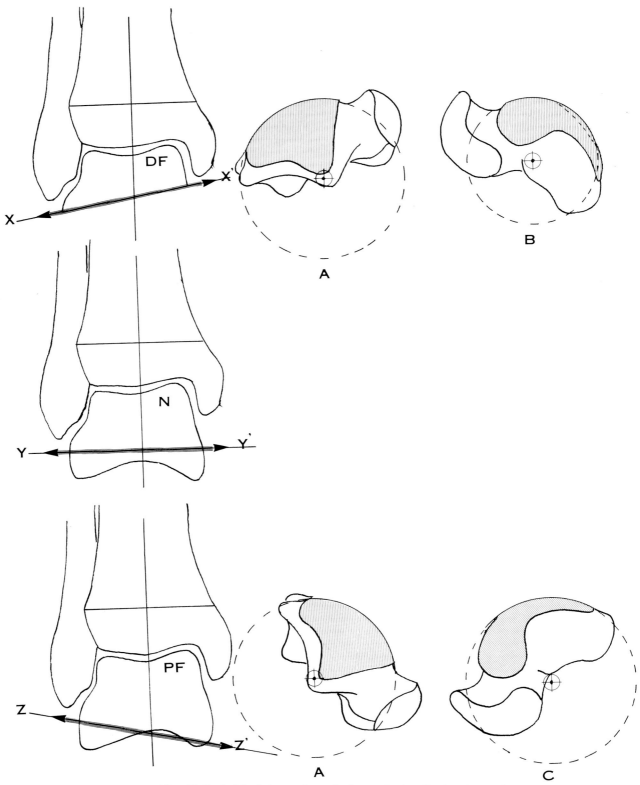

Fig. 10-8. Ankle joint axis variation.   In dorsiflexion (*DF*), the axis of motion *XX'* is inclined downward and laterally. In plantar flexion (*PF*), the axis of motion *ZZ'* is inclined downward and medially. Near neutral (*N*), the axis of motion *YY'* is almost horizontal. The lateral trochlear contour (*A*) is an arc of a true circle. The medial trochlear contour is more complex. Its anterior third or dorsiflexion arc (*B*) belongs to a smaller circle as compared with the posterior two thirds or plantar flexion arc (*C*), which belongs to a large circle. (Adapted from Barnett CJ, Napier JR: The axis of rotation at the ankle joint in man: Its influence upon the form of the talus and the mobility of the fibula. J Anat 86:1, 1952)

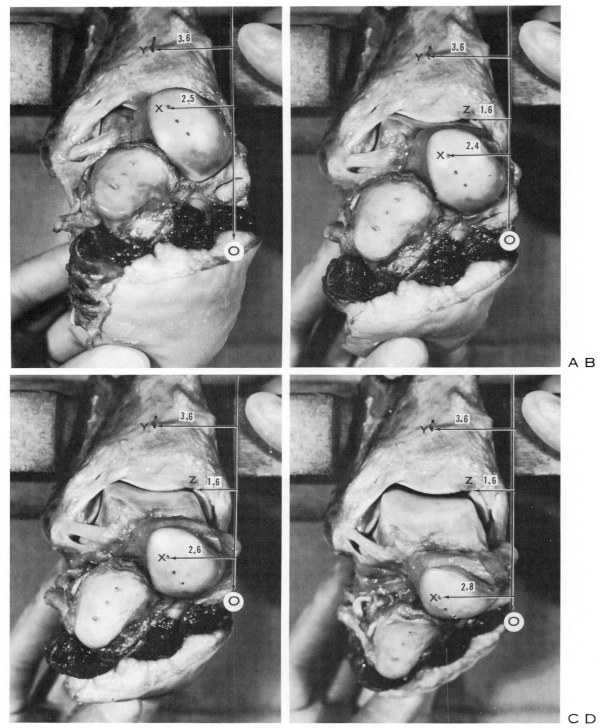

Fig. 10-9. Ankle and hindfoot specimen transfixed through the tibia. The talus is
carried from dorsiflexion (*A*) to neutral (*B*) and plantar flexion (*C* and *D*.) A vertical reference
line *O* is traced. The distance of the tibial reference points *Y* and *Z* from the line *O* remains
constant (3.6 cm and 1.6 cm). A drill point *X* is taken as a reference point on the talar head.
The distance from point *X* to the vertical reference line *O* is measured in all four positions:
dorsiflexion distance, 2.5 cm; neutral distance, 2.4 cm; plantar flexion distance, 2.6 cm;
maximum plantar flexion distance, 2.8 cm. The data indicate that in this specimen, during
dorsiflexion the talus is displaced upward and laterally around an oblique axis inclined
downward and laterally. In neutral the axis is transverse, whereas in plantar flexion the axis
is inclined downward and medially as the talar reference point is displaced downward and
laterally.

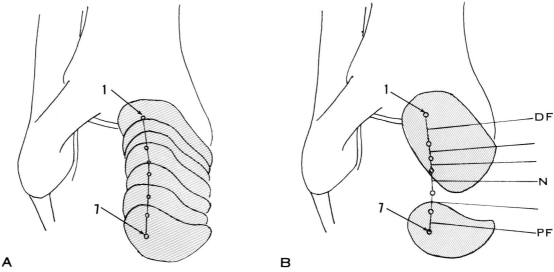

A   **B**

Fig. 10-10. (*A*) **Tracings of the displacements of the talar head reference point from dorsiflexion (*1*) to plantar flexion (*7*).** (*B*) **Motion axes drawn, perpendicular to the displacement lines.** The axis is inclined laterally and downward in dorsiflexion and medially and downward in plantar flexion. The changeover in direction occurs very close to the neutral position of the ankle. (*DF,* dorsiflexion; *N,* neutral; *PF,* plantar flexion.)

Fig. 10-11. The trochlear surface of the talus is a truncated cone. The talus is carried from full dorsiflexion to full plantar flexion, and at each interval a saw cut is made on the trochlear surface along the anterior tibial articular margin. The serial saw cuts are not parallel but converge to the apex *O* of the cone, as demonstrated in the three tali. (From Inman TV: The Joints of the Ankle, 21. Baltimore, Williams & Wilkins 1976)

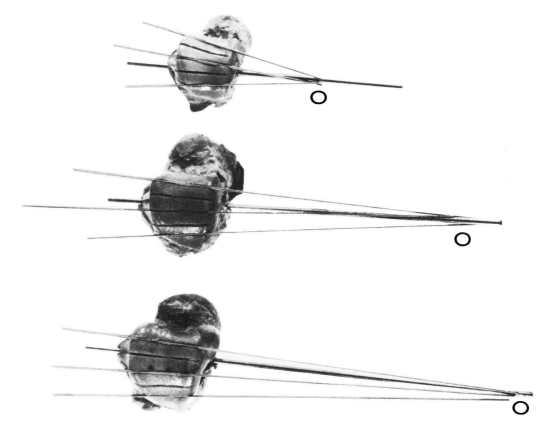

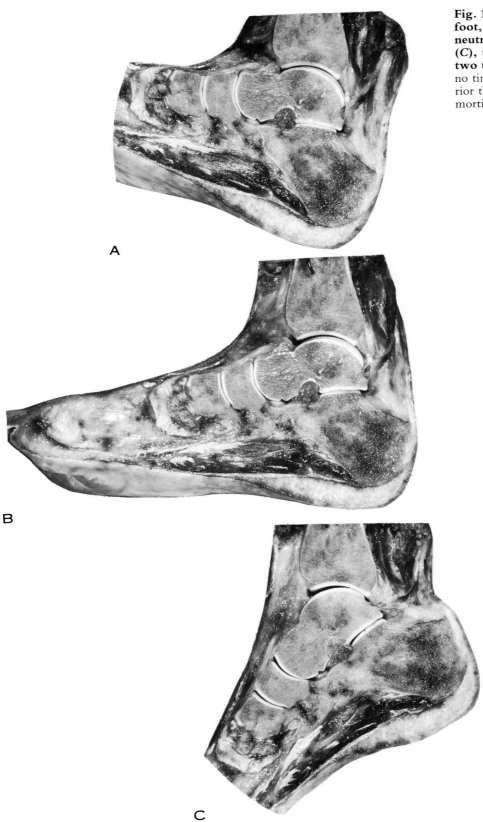

A

B

C

Fig. 10-12. Sagittal cross section of the hind-foot, indicating that in full dorsiflexion (*A*), neutral position (*B*), and full plantar flexion (*C*), the articular surface of the tibia covers two thirds of the talar articular surface. At no time in plantar flexion is the narrower posterior third of the talus occupying the entire ankle mortise.

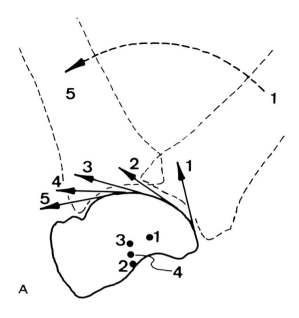

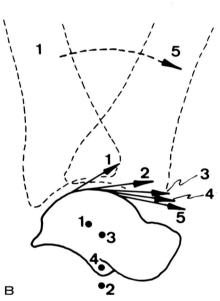

Fig. 10-13. Instant centers of rotation and surface velocities from plantar flexion (1) to dorsiflexion (5) in the ankle. (*A*) Nonweight-bearing: the instant centers of rotation are located in the talus. The surface velocities indicate joint distraction at the beginning of motion, followed by sliding. (*B*) Weight-bearing. An instant center of rotation may be located below the talus. The surface velocities indicate also distraction, followed by sliding. Compression or jamming may occur in maximum dorsiflexion. (From Sammarco JG, Burstein AH, Frankel VH: Biomechanics of the ankle: A kinematic study. Orthop Clin North Am 4, No. 1:75, 1973)

Table 10-1 Reported Normal Ranges of Ankle Joint Motion

Author	Range of motion	
	Dorsiflexion (extension)	Plantar flexion
AAOS[10]	18° (20°)	48° (50°)
Bonnin[11]	10°–20°	25°–35°
Weseley and co-workers[12]	0–10° (maximum 23°)	26°–35° (Minimum 10°, Maximum 51°)
Sammareo and co-workers[18]		
Weight bearing	21° ± 7.21°	23° ± 8°
Non–weight-bearing	23° ± 7.5°	23° ± 9°
Boone and Azen[13] (clinical goniometric measurements)	12.6° ± 4.4°	56.2° ± 6.1°

The total range of external rotation of the talus in the ankle mortise from a position of full plantar flexion to full dorsiflexion is 4°.[7] Most of the rotation (3.25°) takes place from the neutral position of the ankle to full dorsiflexion.

Sammarco and co-workers studied the instant centers of rotation and surface velocities at the point of contact in 24 normal weight-bearing ankles and 6 normal non–weight-bearing ankles.[8] In the weight-bearing group the location of the instant center of rotation was as follows: 12 ankles—within the body of the talus; 8 ankles—one or two centers below the body of the talus; 2 ankles—above the joint surface; 2 ankles—on the joint surface. In the 6 non–weight-bearing ankles, there was also scattered distribution of the centers of rotation. The motion pattern from plantar flexion to dorsiflexion was distraction of the joint surfaces at the beginning, sliding throughout the arc of motion, and jamming of the joint surfaces at the end of the motion (Fig. 10-13).[9]

RANGE OF MOTION

The range of ankle flexion–extension is variable. The methodology used—clinical, roentgenographic, anatomical (cadaveric)—accounts for some of the reported discrepancies. In the clinical measurement, great care is to be taken not to include in the assessment the contribution of the midtarsal and tarsometatarsal joints.

The reported normal ranges of motion at the ankle joint are shown in Table 10-1.

During the stance phase of gait the ankle motion, as reported by Stauffer and co-workers, is 24.4° in average (range 20°–31°) in total; 10.2° dorsiflexion in average (range 6°–16°); and 14.2° plantar flexion in average (range 13°–17°).[14]

"NORMAL" TALAR TILT ANGLE AND ANTERIOR DRAWER SIGN

The talar tilt is a potential degree of inversion (supination–flexion–medial rotation) of the talus at the ankle joint. It is demonstrated with inversion stress applied to the hindfoot and measured roentgenographically by the opening angle between the articular surface of the distal tibia and the transverse trochlear line of the talus. The average "physiologic" degree of talar tilt is reported to range from 0 to 23°, with the variations shown in Table 10-2.[15]

The anterior drawer sign is the forward displacement of the talus at the ankle joint when the leg is pressed and stabilized backward and the heel is brought forward. It is expressed by measuring the distance between the posterior border of the tibia and the talar trochlea. The normal anterior displacement is reported as shown in Table 10-3.

Table 10-2 Variations in Degree of Normal Talar Tilt

Author and method	Normal talar tilt
With manual force without anesthesia	
Duquennoy and co-workers[16]	5° (0–10°)
Cox and Hewes[17]	0° (90.4 %)
	1°–5° (7.9 %)
	> 5°–17° (1.7 %)
With a device without anesthesia	
Rubin and Witten[18]	0–23°
Sedlin[19]	8° (0–15°)
Laurin and St. Jacques[20]	7° (0–27°)
Quellet and co-workers[21]	5° (0–27°)

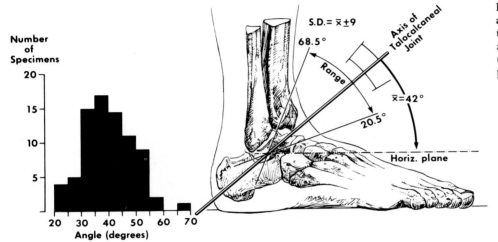

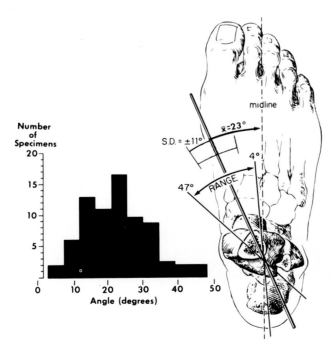

Fig. 10-14. Orientation of subtalar joint axis and variation in the sagittal and transverse planes. Distribution of variations is indicated on the histograms. (From Inman TV: The Joints of the Ankle, p 37. Baltimore, Williams & Wilkins, 1976)

Table 10-3 Normal Anterior Talar Displacement

Author and method	Displacement
With manual force without anesthesia	
Landeros and co-workers [22]	2.5 mm–3 mm
With device without anesthesia	
Castaing and Delaplace[23]	5 mm–8 mm
Laurin and Mathieu[24]	5 mm–7.6 mm

Talocalcaneonavicular Motion

The talocalcaneonavicular joint is formed by two joints but functions as a unit. The posterior talocalcaneal joint is concavoconvex and conoid in contour. The anterior talocalcaneonavicular joint is formed by the acetabulum pedis receiving the convex talar head. The acetabulum pedis has a mosaic pattern and is formed by the articular surfaces of the navicular, the calcaneus, and the inferior and superomedial calcaneonavicular ligaments. The volume of the talar head remains constant, but that of the receiving cup is variable. Motion in one joint is invariably associated with motion in the second joint.

AXIS

The axis of the talocalcaneonavicular joint was studied by Manter, Hicks, Isman and Inman, and Inman.[2, 5, 25, 26] It is oblique, oriented upward, anteriorly, and medially. It penetrates the posterolateral corner of the os calcis, passes perperpendicular to the canalis tarsi, and pierces the superomedial aspect of the talar neck. Manter reported the angulation of the axis to be 42° average (range 29°–47°) inclination in the sagittal plane relative to the horizontal line and 16° average (range 8°–24°) medial deviation in the transverse plane relative to the long axis of the foot passing through the first interdigital space.[25] Inman provided measurements that are very similar: 42° ± 9° of inclination in the sagittal plane and 23° ± 11° of medial deviation in the horizontal plane relative to the axis of the foot passing through the second interdigital space (Fig. 10-14).[2]

MOTION

The oblique axis of the talocalcaneonavicular joint has three vectorial components: transverse, vertical, and longitudinal. Each component generates a basic motion: transverse axis—flexion–extension; vertical axis—abduction–adduction; longitudinal axis—supination–pronation.

Any instantaneous motion is a combination of three simultaneously occurring motions. The axis of the talocalcaneonavicular joint invariably generates two combination patterns of motion: pronation–abduction–extension and supination–adduction–flexion (Figs. 10-15–10-17).[5] No pronation could occur without associated abduction–extension nor any supination without associated adduction–flexion. This basic motion of the hindfoot was clearly demonstrated in our specimens (Fig. 10-18) and in 1889 by Farabeuf on anatomical models.[27] When there is no interference, the hindfoot carries the forefoot in the same direction. Any point of the foot plate is displaced along an arc of a circle of which the plane is perpendicular to the axis of the talocalcaneonavicular joint (Figs. 10-19 and 10-20). The talocalcaneonavicular joint is the major contributor to the transverse component of the field of motion of the foot–ankle complex.

Hicks reports the range of motion at the talocalcaneonavicular joint to be 24°.[5]

Midtarsal or Calcaneocuboid and Talonavicular Motion

The talonavicular joint is an integral part of the talocalcaneonavicular joint complex and moves simultaneously with the talocalcaneal joint. It also has the potential of moving in unison with the calcaneocuboid joint, independent of the subtalar joint.

CALCANEOCUBOID MOTION

The calcaneocuboid joint is a saddle joint. The calcaneal surface is convex transversely and concave vertically. Geometrically, each curvature has a surface-generating axis that is the axis of motion (Fig. 10-21), and the plane of motion is perpendicular to the axis except when the motion is helical in type.

The axis of the convex curvature of the calcaneus, defined by Elftman, is oblique, directed upward, medially, and anteriorly (Fig. 10-22).[28] It passes from the inferolateral segment of the os calcis anteriorly, through the head of the talus. It approximates closely the oblique axis of the midtarsal joint defined by Manter and Hicks (Fig. 10-23).[5,25] The orientation defined by Manter is 52° inclination in the sagittal plane relative to the horizontal and 57° medial deviation in the horizontal plane relative to the axis of the foot passing through the first interdigital space.[25] The oblique axis has three vectorial components—longitudinal, vertical, and transverse—and generates simultaneously occurring motions—supination–adduction–flexion or pronation–abduction–extension.

The axis of the concave curvature of the calcaneus, as defined by Elftman, passes outside the os calcis and through the cuboid and is perpendicular to the previous axis (see Fig. 10-22).[28] It is directed anterolaterally and slightly upward. It generates the motions of flexion–extension, supination–pronation, and, to a much lesser degree, abduction-adduction.

At the calcaneocuboid joint the motion of supination–adduction–flexion is stopped when the inferomedial beak of the cuboid reaches the end of the coronoid fossa of the os calcis. The motion of pronation–abduction–extension is blocked by the overhanging superior lip or beak of the os calcis.

(Text continues on p. 394.)

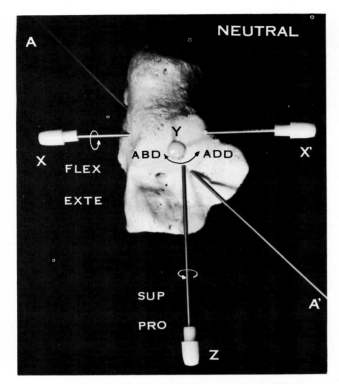

Fig. 10-15. The axis of the talocalcaneonavicular joint *AA'* **as indicated passing through the os calcis in neutral position.**   The axis *AA'* has three components: *XX'*, which generates flexion–extension (*FLEX–EXTE*); *Y*, which generates abduction–adduction (*ABD–ADD*); *Z*, which generates supination–pronation (*SUP–PRO*). In valgus position the anterior aspect of the os calcis is simultaneously extended, abducted, and pronated. In varus position the anterior aspect of the os calcis is simultaneously flexed, adducted, and supinated.

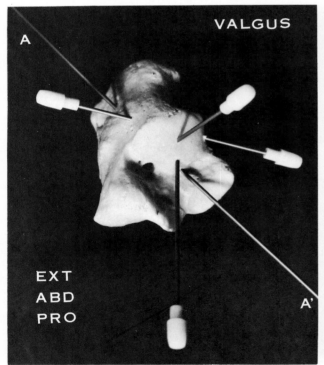

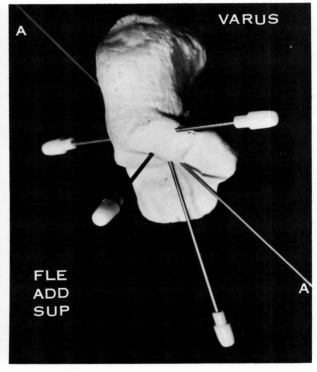

Fig. 10-16. Axis of the talocalcaneonavicular joint *AA'* **seen in lateral view with the secondary axes** *X, Y, Z.* The middle figure indicates the os calcis in varus and demonstrates the flexion (*FLE*) and supination, (*SUP*) components. The bottom figure indicates the os calcis in valgus and demonstrates the components of extension, (*EXT*) and pronation (*PRO*). (*ABD,* abduction; *ADD,* adduction.)

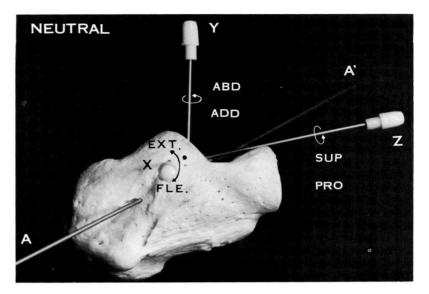

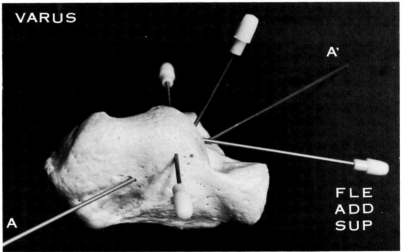

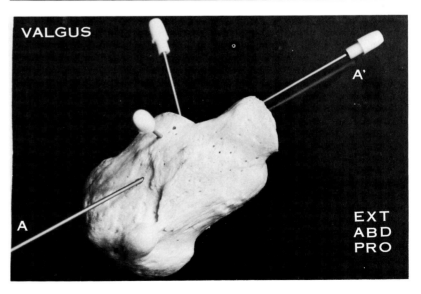

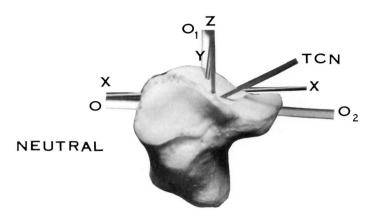

NEUTRAL

Fig. 10-17. Frontal view of the os calcis. In varus of the heel the anterior aspect of the os calcis is flexed (*FLE*), adducted (*ADD*), and supinated (*SUP*). In valgus of the heel the anterior aspect of the os calcis is extended (*EXT*), abducted (*ABD*), and pronated (*PRO*). (*TCN,* talocalcaneonavicular axis; *XX,* transverse axis of flexion–extension; *Y,* vertical axis of abduction–adduction; *Z,* longitudinal axis of supination–pronation; *O, O_1, O_2,* cruciform reference line.)

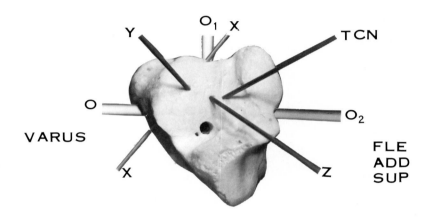

VARUS

FLE
ADD
SUP

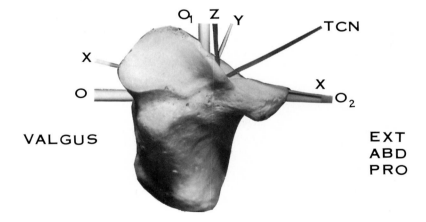

VALGUS

EXT
ABD
PRO

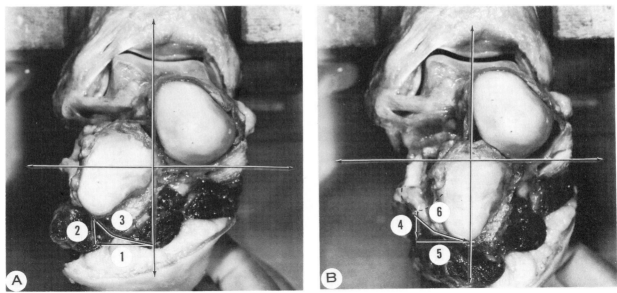

Fig. 10-18. Anatomical model of the hindfoot. (*A*) Valgus position of the os calcis involving (*1*) abduction; (*2*) extension; (*3*) pronation. (*B*) Varus position of the os calcis involving (*4*) flexion, (*5*) adduction, (*6*) supination. The os calcis has moved into valgus from a varus position as in *A* and *vice versa*.

Fig. 10-19. Axes of the talocalcaneonavicular (*TCN*) and ankle (*AN*) joints. The displacement of any point of the foot plate, induced by the motion around the talocalcaneonavicular axis, is an arc of a circle, perpendicular to the same axis. These arcs of circles (*AA', BB', CC'*) are parallel to the circle *1*. The displacement of any point of the foot plate, induced by the motion around the ankle axis, is an arc of a circle perpendicular to this axis and parallel to the circle *2*.

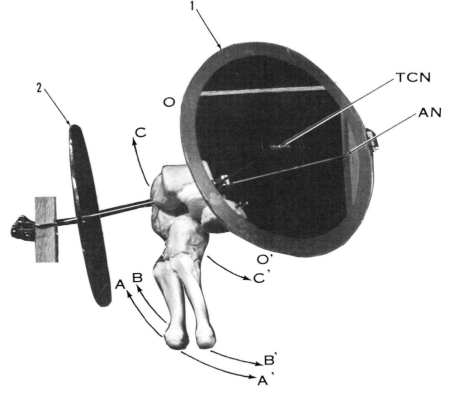

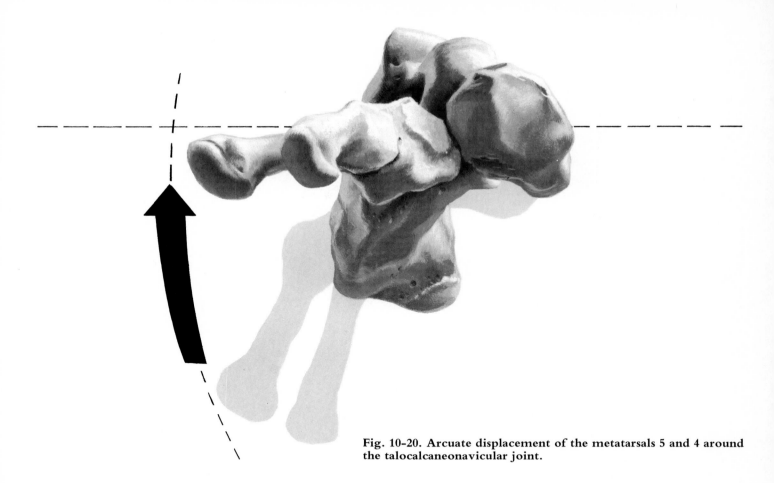

Fig. 10-20. Arcuate displacement of the metatarsals 5 and 4 around the talocalcaneonavicular joint.

Fig. 10-21. The cuboidal surface of the calcaneus (C) is saddle shaped. It is convex transversely and concave vertically. The convexity is determined by the rotating cyclinder O_1 with its generating axis CC_1. The concavity is determined by the circle O_2, turning around its generating axis CC_2 and against the surface of the cylinder O_1. The axes of the geometric surfaces are the axes of motion. They are perpendicular to each other. The perfect matching of the surfaces S and O_2 allows only rotation to occur and there is no sliding, whereas imperfect matching (as indicated in the lower figure) allows rotation and sliding to occur. In the case of a perfect fit of the surfaces, a sliding motion produces jamming of the surfaces at one end and opening at the other end.

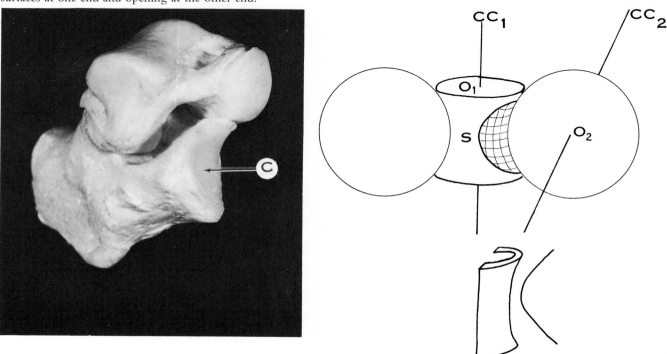

Fig. 10-22. Axes of the transverse tarsal joint in pronation (A) and in supination (B). The axis of the convex curvature of the os calcis CC_1 at the calcaneocuboid joint is located in the os calcis and when projected upward passes through the head of the talus. The axis of the concave curvature of the same surface CC_2 is perpendicular to CC_1 and passes through the cuboid. The axis of the major convexity of the talar head TN_1 at the talonavicular joint and the axis of the lesser convexity of the same surface TN_2 are also perpendicular to each other. The major displacements are perpendicular to the axes CC_1 and TN_1. In full pronation (A) the axes CC_1 and TN_1 coincide, "allowing free movement without involving other axes." The forefoot moves at the midtarsal joint freely without the need of motion between the talus and the os calcis. In supination the CC_1 and TN_1 axes do not coincide and motion is required around the secondary axes CC_2 and TN_2 and around the subtalar joint axis ST, so that the resultant of CC_1 and CC_2 axes is identical to the combined resultant of TN_1–TN_2 and ST axes. In supination the midtarsal joint motion requires associated motion at the subtalar joint between the talus and the os calcis; incongruity of the surfaces may otherwise result. (From Elftman H: The transverse tarsal joint and its control. Clin Orthop 16:41, 1960)

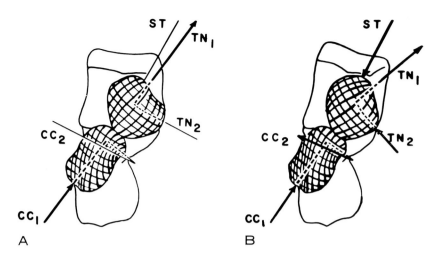

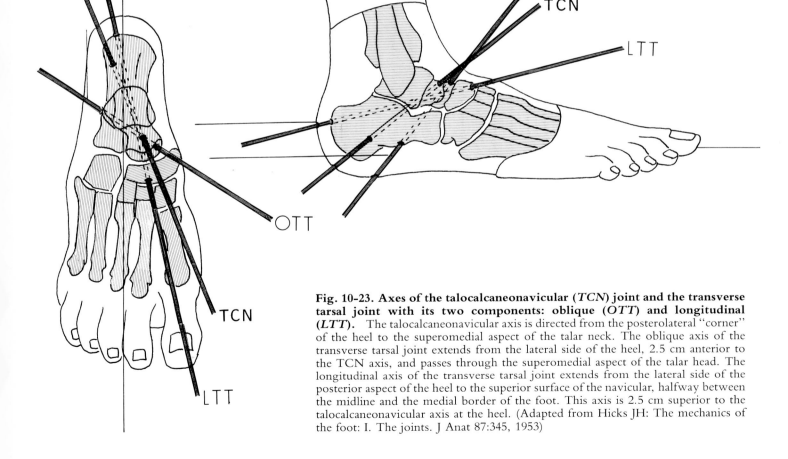

Fig. 10-23. Axes of the talocalcaneonavicular (TCN) joint and the transverse tarsal joint with its two components: oblique (OTT) and longitudinal (LTT). The talocalcaneonavicular axis is directed from the posterolateral "corner" of the heel to the superomedial aspect of the talar neck. The oblique axis of the transverse tarsal joint extends from the lateral side of the heel, 2.5 cm anterior to the TCN axis, and passes through the superomedial aspect of the talar head. The longitudinal axis of the transverse tarsal joint extends from the lateral side of the posterior aspect of the heel to the superior surface of the navicular, halfway between the midline and the medial border of the foot. This axis is 2.5 cm superior to the talocalcaneonavicular axis at the heel. (Adapted from Hicks JH: The mechanics of the foot: I. The joints. J Anat 87:345, 1953)

TALONAVICULAR MOTION

The talar head at the talonavicular joint is condyloid. It is convex in its greater and lesser curvatures.

The axis of the major curvature is oblique, directed upward, medially, and anteriorly, and passes through the talar head (see Fig. 10-22).[28] It is aligned with the axis of the convexity of the calcaneus when the latter is everted. It generates the integrated motions of supination–adduction–flexion or pronation–abduction–extension. This pattern of motion is easily recognized when observing the obliquity—downward and medially—of the talar condylar surface.

The axis of the lesser curvature is perpendicular to the axis of the major curvature and passes through the talar head.

Manter and Hicks have described a longitudinal axis for the midtarsal joint.[5,25] The orientation of this axis is 15° of inclination in the sagittal plane relative to the horizontal and 9° of medial deviation in the horizontal plane relative to the axis of the foot passing through the first interdigital space.[25] The motion generated around this axis is pronation with minimal abduction–extension and supination with minimal adduction–flexion. The midtarsal motion around the

oblique axis is reported by Hicks to be 22° and around the longitudinal axis, limited to 8°.[5]

MIDTARSAL AND TALOCALCANEONAVICULAR RELATIONSHIP

The articular surface of the navicular is smaller than the corresponding talar surface. Similarly, the cuboid surface is slightly smaller than the calcaneal surface of the saddle joint. In a sample measurement the dimensions were as follows: talar head mid axial length along the greater curvature, 4 cm; navicular transverse arc, 2.5 cm; calcaneal convex arc, 2.5 cm; cuboid concave arc, 2 cm.

The maximum linear displacement of the navicular over the talar head is 1.5 cm. The maximum linear displacement of the cuboid over the calcaneal surface is 0.5 cm. Through the subtalar motion, the navicular moves about 1 cm relative to the talus. Further 0.5-cm displacement of the navicular on the talus occurs by the midtarsal joint motion when the cuboid slides 0.5 cm over the calcaneal surface.

When the navicular moves at the midtarsal joint around

Fig. 10-24. (*A*) **The relationship of the talus (*T*), navicular (*N*), cuboid (*CU*), and calcaneus (*C*) in the standing position.** (*B*) **The os calcis is held fixed experimentally and the talus is turned against the calcaneus around the talocalcaneonavicular axis (*TCN*) in pronation combined with abduction and extension.** This is equivalent to a "supination" of the foot. If the navicular and the cuboid are prevented from rotating, a dislocation in the talonavicular joint is observed medially. This is due to the fact that the axis of the talocalcaneonavicular joint and the axis of the revolution of the articular surface of the talar head do not coincide. (*C*) The above dislocation is immediately reduced by the simultaneous motion of the navicular and the cuboid, which undergo an adduction–supination and some degree of flexion. (Diagrams after photographic documentation by Huson A: Een Ontleedkundig-Functioneel Onderzoek van de Voetworte [An Anatomical and Functional Study of the Tarsal Joints], p 134–135. Leiden, Drukkerij, "Luctor er Emergo," 1961)

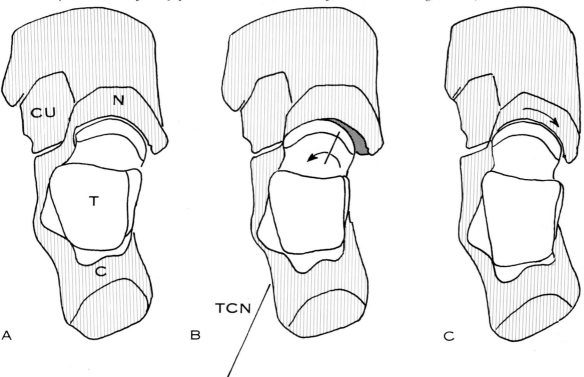

the greater axis of the talar head, the axis of motion and the generating axis coincide and the opposing surfaces remain congruent. But as demonstrated by Huson, when the navicular moves as an integral part of the talocalcaneonavicular joint, around the axis of the latter in supination, the generating axis of the talonavicular joint and the talocalcaneonavicular axis do not coincide.[29] This results in a subluxation of the navicular over the talar head or vice versa as the navicular is forced to rotate around a center that does not correspond to its surface curvature (Fig. 10-24). The talonavicular subluxation with its inferomedial opening is immediately reduced by the midtarsal motion in the form of calcaneocuboid and talonavicular combined motion of adduction–supination–flexion. This phase of the motion utilizes the final inferomedial segment of the talar head articular surface.

The cuboid and the navicular have minor relative movement between them and are considered to move together as the midtarsal joint.[28] The axis of the convex curvature of the cuboidal surface of the calcaneus is at a right angle to the axis of the concavity of the same surface (see Fig. 10-22), and as stated by Elftman, the combined movement about the two calcaneocuboid axes occurs around a resultant axis that passes through a line representing the shortest perpendicular distance between these two axes (Fig. 10-25).[28] In eversion, the axis of the convex curvature of the calcaneous coincides with the axis of the major convex curvature of the talus (see Fig. 10-22), allowing free movement without involving other axes.[28] The forefoot moves freely relative to the hindfoot without movement of the talus in respect to the calcaneus. In inversion "the resultant of both calcaneo-cuboid axes must be identical with the resultant of the two talo-navicular axis and the subtalar axis."[28] The forefoot moves in this instance relative to the hindfoot and with accompanying motion of the talus around the subtalar axis. In passing from the everted position to the inverted position there is a continuous change of the instantaneous transverse tarsal axis.[28]

Tarsometatarsal Motion

The tarsometatarsal joints allow the basic motion of flexion–extension of the metatarsal rays and certain degree of longitudinal axial rotation—supination, pronation—at the marginal rays. The combination results in a supination or a pronation twist of the forefoot as defined by Hicks.[5]

In the supination twist (Fig. 10-26), the first metatarsal is extended and supinated and the fifth metatarsal is flexed and supinated. In the pronation twist (Fig. 10-26), the first metatarsal is flexed and pronated and the fifth metatarsal is extended and pronated.

Hicks reports the ranges of motion as follows: M_1—flexion–pronation, extension–supination 22°; M_5—flexion–supination, extension–pronation 10°.[5]

The axis of the first metatarsocuneiform joint is oblique, directed anterolaterally and slightly inferiorly. It extends from the dorsum of the third metatarsal base to the tuberosity of the navicular. Its three vectorial components have

the potential of generating extension–supination and a minimal degree of abduction or flexion–pronation and a minimal degree of adduction. According to Kelikian, the first metatarsocuneiform joint "allows 10 to 15 degrees of passive up-and-down movement. Side-to-side motion is about half of that range."[30] The second metatarsal with its encased base has limited mobility. The third metatarsal has a range of flexion–extension of only about 10°.[5]

The axis of the fifth cuboideometatarsal joint is oblique, directed posterolaterally and inferiorly. It extends from the $cuneo_1$-$metatarsal_1$ joint to 1.5 cm above and behind the styloid porcess of the fifth metatarsal.[5] Its vectorial components allow the motions of extension–pronation and slight abduction and flexion–supination with slight adduction.

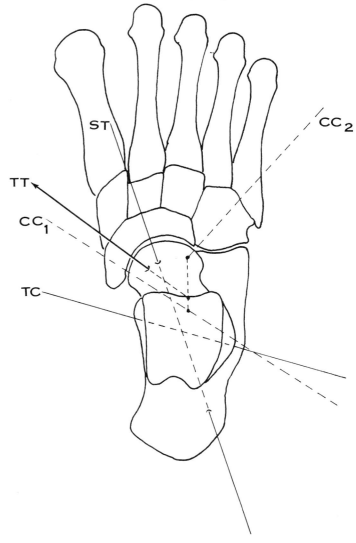

Fig. 10-25. The transverse tarsal joint axis (*TT*) has an instantaneous variable position as the foot passes from a pronated to a supinated position. This *TT* axis passes through a line perpendicular to the major CC_1 and the minor CC_2 axes of the calcaneocuboid joint. (*ST*, subtalar joint axis; *TC*, talocrural joint axis.) (Redrawn from Elfman H: The transverse tarsal joint and its control. Clin Orthop 16:41, 1960)

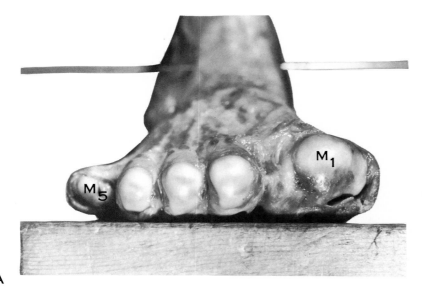

A

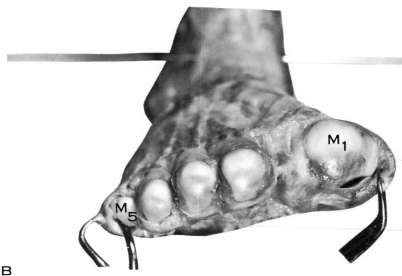

B

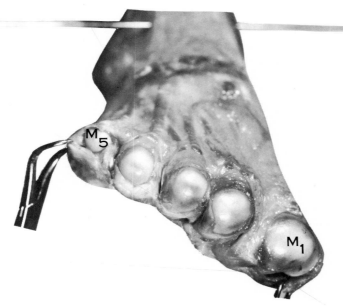

C

Fig. 10-26. Anatomical specimen with a transverse K wire passed through the ankle and parallel to the ground. The ankle, subtalar and the midtarsal joints are transfixed with multiple K wires. (*A*) Neutral position. (*B*) Supination twist. The first metatarsal is extended and supinated and the fifth metatarsal is flexed and supinated. (*C*) Pronation twist. The first metatarsal is flexed and pronated and the fifth metatarsal is extended and pronated.

In the standing position a high arch is produced in the foot through the associated external rotation of the tibia; supination, adduction, flexion at the talocalcaneonavicular joint; supination of the midtarsal joint; and *pronation twist* of the forefoot, which involves flexion–pronation of the first metatarsal and extension–pronation of the fifth metatarsal.[5] This high arch position in standing corresponds to the "pronation" of the lamina pedis as defined by MacConaill.[47] The natural twist of the foot is increased through forefoot pronation and inversion of the heel. This results in a high arch with *flexible* foot defined as a loose pack position of the lamina pedis.

In the standing position a low arch is produced in the foot through the associated internal rotation of the tibia; pronation, abduction, extension at the talocalcaneonavicular joint; pronation of the midtarsal joint; and *supination twist* of the forefoot, which involves extension–supination of the first metatarsal and flexion–supination of the fifth metatarsal.[5] This low arch position in standing corresponds to the "supination" of the lamina pedis as defined by MacConaill.[47] The lamina pedis is untwisted through supination of the forefoot and eversion of the heel. This results in a low arch with a *rigid* foot defined as a close pack position of the lamina pedis.

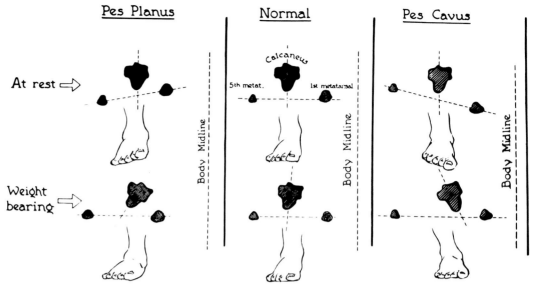

Fig. 10-27. Relationship of the hindfoot and forefoot at rest and in weight bearing in the normal foot, pes cavus, and pes planus. In the normal foot, at rest the heel is in neutral, and the forefoot transmetatarsal headline M_1 to M_5 is perpendicular to the vertical axis of the heel; on weight bearing the same relation of the hindfoot and forefoot is preserved. In pes cavus (flexible type), at rest when the heel is held in neutral, the forefoot is pronated; on weight bearing, the heel moves into varus, carrying the forefoot into a horizontal plantigrade position. In pes planus (flexible type), at rest when the heel is held in neutral, the forefoot is supinated; on weight bearing, the heel moves into valgus, carrying the forefoot into a horizontal plantigrade position. (From McElvenny RT, Caldwell GD: A new operation for correction of cavus foot: Fusion of first metatarso-cuneiform-navicular joints. Clin Orthop 11:85, 1958)

Hindfoot–Midfoot–Forefoot Relationship

The study of the hindfoot–forefoot relationship is essential for the understanding of the functional behavior of the foot and ankle in both the normal and pathologic states. Hicks in an excellent anatomical study, and McElvenny and Caldwell, with a brilliant clinical understanding followed by surgical implications, demonstrated the hindfoot–forefoot relationship in variable conditions (Fig. 10-27).[5,31] More recently, Coleman and Chesnut advocated a test for the assessment of the hindfoot mobility based on the same principles.[32]

HINDFOOT–FOREFOOT RELATIONSHIP IN NON–WEIGHT-BEARING STATUS

When the foot is not bearing weight, the hindfoot and the forefoot move in synchrony in the same direction. With inversion the sole of the foot, including the heel and the forefoot, face medially. Anatomically the contribution of each joint is as follows: talocalcaneonavicular joint—supination–adduction–flexion; midtarsal joint—supination; tarsometatarsal joint—supination twist. With eversion the sole of the foot, including the heel and the forefoot, face laterally. Anatomically the contribution of each joint is as follows:

talocalcaneonavicular joint—pronation–abduction–extension; midtarsal joint—pronation; tarsometatarsal joint—pronation twist.

HINDFOOT–FOREFOOT RELATIONSHIP IN WEIGHT-BEARING POSITION

Heel Neutral and Forefoot Neutral At Rest

A foot in neutral position at rest may bear weight in the same position. The hindfoot–forefoot relationship may change by creation of a high arch or a low arch in the plantigrade foot.

The high arch in a weight-bearing position is brought about by externally rotating the hip and tibia (see Fig. 10-3; Fig. 10-28).[5] The talus turns externally at the talocalcaneonavicular joint, and this is possible only through relative flexion–adduction–supination of the os calcis. The midtarsal joint is also supinated. The forefoot will have a tendency to supinate; however, to remain plantigrade, it is subjected to a pronation twist, which results in the high arch appearance.

The low arch in a weight-bearing position is brought about by internally rotating the hip, tibia, and talus (Figs. 10-3 and 10-29).[5] At the talocalcaneonavicular joint the calcaneus is extended, abducted, and pronated. The midtarsal joint is pronated. The forefoot will have a tendency to

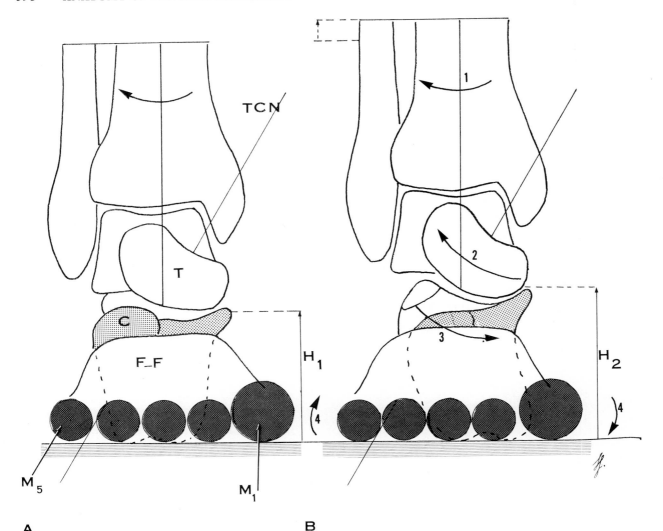

Fig. 10-28. Physiomechanics of the high arch in the standing foot produced by external rotation of the tibia. (*A*) Neutral position. The rotating arrow on the tibia indicates the initiation of external rotation. (*B*) The external rotation of the tibia (*1*) is transmitted to the talus (*2*), which turns laterally around the talocalcaneonavicular axis. This is possible only through a combined talar motion of abduction–extension–pronation at the talocalcaneonavicular joint. Relatively, the calcaneus moves in the reverse direction around the same axis, and the combined motion of the hindfoot is that of supination–flexion–adduction. The heel turns in into varus (*3*). The forefoot is carried into supination by the hindfoot, but to remain plantigrade, a pronation twist (*4*) is applied to the forefoot. The ascension of the talus and the descent and varus of the os calcis combined with the pronation twist of the forefoot result in a high arch with $H_2 > H_1$. (M_1–M_5, metatarsal heads 1 to 5; *FF*, forefoot; *C*, calcaneus; *T*, talus; *TCN*, axis of motion of talocalcaneonavicular joint; H_1, normal height of medial longitudinal arch; H_2, increased height of medial longitudinal arch.)

pronate and raise the lateral border of the foot, but to maintain the plantigrade position, a supination twist is applied to the forefoot, which results in the low arch appearance. In both the high arch and low arch situations in the plantigrade foot, there is a dissociation of the hindfoot and forefoot. When the heel is in varus the forefoot is pronated, and when the heel is in valgus the forefoot is supinated; in both situations the hindfoot dictates the change in the forefoot.

Heel Neutral and Forefoot in Fixed Pronation At Rest

In the weight-bearing position, if the heel maintains its neutral position, the forefoot is not plantigrade, as the lateral border remains elevated (Fig. 10-27).[31] If the heel is turned in through supination–flexion–adduction, the forefoot becomes plantigrade but with a high arch appearance, a variety of cavovarus foot; there is a hindfoot–forefoot dissociation.

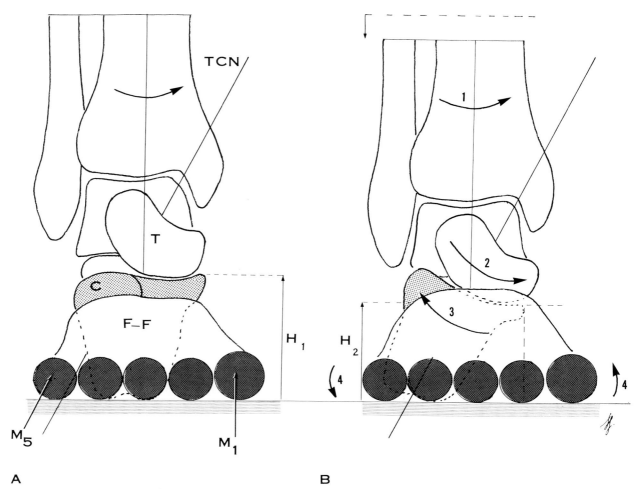

A   B

Fig. 10-29. Physiomechanics of the low arch in the standing foot produced by the internal rotation of the tibia. (*A*) Neutral position. The rotating arrow on the tibia indicates the initiation of internal rotation. (*B*) The internal rotation of the tibia (*1*) is transmitted to the talus (*2*), which turns medially around the talocalcaneonavicular axis. This is possible only through a combined talar motion of adduction–flexion–supination at the talocalcaneonavicular joint. Relatively, the calcaneus moves in the reverse direction around the same axis, and the combined motion of the hindfoot is that of pronation–extension–abduction. The heel turns out (*3*). The forefoot is carried by the hindfoot into pronation, but to remain plantigrade, a supination twist (*4*) is applied to the forefoot. The descent of the talus and the ascent of the os calcis combined with the supination twist of the forefoot results in a low arch with $H_2 < H_1$. The high arch is a loose pack position of the foot, whereas the low arch is a close pack position of the foot, corresponding to the untwisting of the lamina pedis. (M_1–M_5) metatarsal heads 1 to 5; *FF*, forefoot; *C*, calcaneus; *T*, talus; *TCN*, axis of motion of talocalcaneonavicular joint; H_1, normal height of medial longitudinal arch; H_2, decreased height of medial longitudinal arch.)

Heel Neutral and Forefoot in Fixed Supination At Rest

In the weight-bearing position if the heel remains neutral, the medial border of the foot will remain elevated (Fig. 10-27).[31] If the heel is turned out through abduction–extension–pronation at the talocalcaneonavicular joint, the forefoot becomes plantigrade but with a low arch appearance, a variety of flatfoot. There is also dissociation of the hindfoot and forefoot, as they have moved in opposite directions; in both situations the forefoot dictates the position of the hindfoot.

Metatarsophalangeal Motion and Interphalangeal Motion

The articular surfaces of the metatarsal heads are longer in their lateral profile and shorter transversely. They allow flexion–extension and, to a limited degree, abduction–adduction. In general, there is more extension and less flexion at the metatarsophalangeal joints. The big toe hyperextends more at the metatarsophalangeal joint but flexes less than the lesser toes at the same joint.

Joseph, in a study of the range of motion in the big toe of 50 adults, provides the data shown in Table 10-4.[33]

The lesser toes similarly extend more at the metatarsophalangeal joints and flex more at the interphalangeal joints. Sammarco, in the study of flexion–extension at the metatarsophalangeal joint of the big toe, locates the instant velocity centers within the metatarsal head, but in variable positions.[34] The surface instant velocity vectors indicate a sliding motion throughout the arc of motion except at the end of hyperextension, when compression or jamming occurs (Fig. 10-30).

The toes work in unison. During gait, the initial phase of the push-off occurs around an oblique axis passing through the metatarsal heads 2 to 5. This determines the metatarsal break angle, which measures (according to Isman and Inman) 62° in average relative to the mid axis of the foot passing through the second interdigital space (maximum, 72.5°; minimum, 53.5°) (Fig. 10-31).[26] The subsequent phase of the push-off occurs around a transverse axis passing through the metatarsal heads 1 and 2.[35]

Normally a limited degree of abduction–adduction occurs in the metatarsophalangeal joint around a vertical axis, mainly in the big toe. Individual variations are present. This motion is of a sliding variety.[34]

Motor Control and Stabilization of the Foot and Ankle

The action of a muscle is determined by the position of the tendon relative to the axis of motion of the joint. The muscle–tendon unit may act from either end, proximal or distal. With fixation of the distal segment, the muscle contraction results in the displacement of the proximal lever arm, whereas with fixation of the proximal segment, the contraction results in a displacement of the distal segment of the lever arm. Furthermore, in a multisegmented system as in the ankle–foot, all joints crossed by a tendon are submitted to its action.

ANKLE MOTORS AND STABILIZATION

Motors

Plantar Flexors. The tendons located posterior to the talocrural joint axis of motion are the plantar flexors of the ankle. When the foot is fixed on the ground, the same motors rotate the leg posteriorly. During gait the plantar flexors develop four times more energy than the dorsiflexors. The following motors are the plantar flexors with their work capacity in meterkilograms, as presented by Lang and Wachsmuth: triceps surae, 16.4; flexor hallucis longus muscle, 0.9; flexor digitorum longus muscle, 0.4; tibialis posterior muscle, 0.4; peroneus longus muscle, 0.4; peroneus brevis muscle, 0.3 (total, 18.8).[1] Approximately nine tenths of the plantar flexor energy is provided by the triceps surae.

Dorsiflexors. The tendons located anterior to the talocrural joint axis are the dorsiflexors of the ankle. With the

Table 10-4 Range of Motion in Big Toe of 50 Adults

	Metatarsophalangeal Joint	Interphalangeal Joint
Normal standing angle	16° extension (from 5° flexion to 45° extension)	12° extension (from 35° flexion to 4° extension)
Active flexion	23° (3°–43°)	46° (0°–86°)
Active extension	51°	12°
Total extension (Active + passive)	74° (40°–100°)	31° (6°–73°)

Data from Joseph J: Range of movement of the great toe in men. J Bone Joint Surg [Br] 36:450, 1954

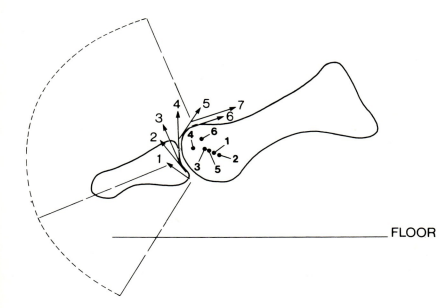

FLOOR

Fig. 10-30. Instant center of motion and surface velocity at the metatarsophalangeal joint of the big toe in the sagittal plane. The numbered dots represent the instant centers and the numbered arrows represent the corresponding surface velocities. The motion is of the sliding type except in the last stages of hyperextension, when compression occurs. (From Sammarco JG: Biomechanics of the foot. In Frankel VH, Nordin M (eds): Basic Biomechanics of the Skeletal System, p 203. Philadelphia, Lea & Febiger, 1980)

Fig. 10-31. Metatarsal break angle (H) or angle between the line connecting the heads of the second and fifth metatarsals and the midline of the foot. This line represents also the oblique axis of the take-off in walking. (From Isman RE, Inman VT: Anthropometric studies of the human foot and ankle. Biomechanics Laboratory, University of California, Berkeley, Technical Report, p 26. May, 1968)

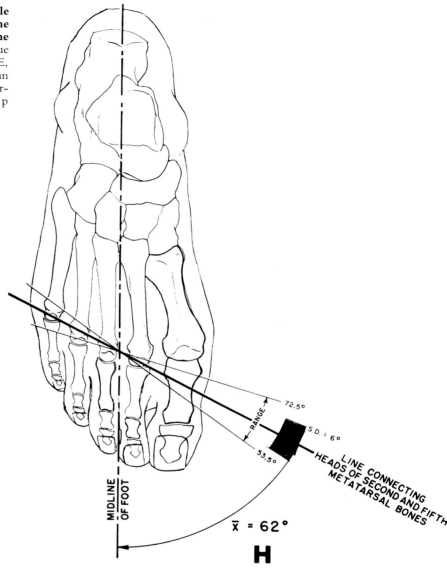

foot fixed on the ground, they rotate the leg forward. The following muscle units are the dorsiflexors with their work capacity in meterkilograms: tibialis anterior muscle, 2.5; extensor digitorum longus muscle, 0.8; extensor hallucis longus muscle, 0.4; peroneus tertius muscle, 0.5 (total, 4.2).[1]

Stability of the Ankle

The stability of the ankle is determined by the integrity of the lateral collateral ligaments, the deltoid ligament, and the inferior tibiofibular syndesmosis.

The maximum bony surface contact and fit occur in the dorsiflexed position, which is the close pack or maximally stable position of the ankle. The side-to-side stability of the ankle is provided by the malleoli and their ligaments, whereas the stability in the sagittal plane is ligament dependent. Posterolaterally and posteromedially, the peronei ten-

dons, the tibialis posterior tendon, the flexor digitorum longus tendon, the flexor hallucis longus tendon, and their sheaths contribute to stability.

With regard to the lateral collateral ligaments, Inman mentions that as they arise from the fibula close to the axis of ankle joint motion, "the normal flexion and extension movements of the ankle lead to little or no changes in tension of these structures."[2] The average location of the axis of motion on the lateral side is 3 mm ± 2 mm distal and 8 mm ± 5 mm anterior to the tip of the lateral malleolus. The anterior location of the axis does introduce appreciable differential tension in the ligaments unless the axis is specifically very close to the tip of the lateral malleolus.

The anterior talofibular ligament is taut in plantar flexion and relaxed in dorsiflexion (Fig. 10-32). It is a major ligament determining the anterior stability in tiptoe standing. In the acutely plantar flexed position, the ligament braces the talus and makes a marked turn around the anterolateral

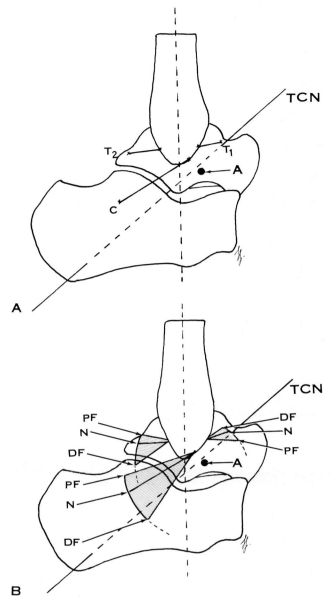

corner of the talar body. It is also contributory in resisting the lateral talar tilt and the medial rotation of the talus. The ligament limits the posterior displacement of the leg and transmits its external rotation force to the talus. According to De Vogel, when the anterior talofibular ligament is formed by two bands, the upper band is taut in plantar flexion but the lower band remains taut in all positions.[36]

The posterior talofibular ligament has increased tension in dorsiflexion and relaxes in plantar flexion (Fig. 10-32). It braces the talus posteriorly. It limits the dorsiflexion of the foot and the anterior displacement of the leg. Anatomically the anterior fibers of the ligament are shorter than the posterior fibers. According to De Vogel, the anterior fibers remain taut throughout the entire arc of motion while the posterior fibers are tense in dorsiflexion.[36] This ligament is contributory in resisting the external rotation of the talus in the mortise and helps to transmit the internal rotation force of the leg to the talus.

The calcaneofibular ligament is the ligament of the ankle joint and of the talocalcaneonavicular joint. The tension in the ligament is affected by both joints. The ligament is taut in dorsiflexion and relaxed in plantar flexion (Fig. 10-32). However, in some specimens the ligament is taut in plantar flexion and less tense in dorsiflexion (Fig. 10-33), while in others the tension in the ligament remains constant in all positions.

At first glance when the tension in the calcaneofibular ligament during the motion of the talocalcaneonavicular joint is being assessed, the results are not only variable but seem contradictory. In most of the specimens, in the valgus position of the heel, the tension in the calcaneofibular ligament is increased and in the varus position it is decreased (Figs. 10-34–10-36); it is the reverse in other specimens. For a clear understanding of the functional behavior of the ligament, it is of importance to refer to the insertional variations of this ligament. As demonstrated by Ruth, the ligament may be oblique, horizontal, vertical (Fig. 10-37), or fan shaped.[37] This has a direct bearing on the tension developed by the ligament during motion. Any point of the foot turning around the oblique axis of the talocalcaneonavicular joint traces an arc belonging to a circle perpendicular to this axis. When the calcaneofibular ligament is nearly horizontal, in valgus position of the heel, the distance between the origin and the insertion increases; the distance decreases in varus (Fig. 10-38). The ligament is taut in valgus and less tense in varus. When the ligament is vertical in neutral, the distance between the origin and the insertion is increased in varus and decreased in valgus. The ligament is taut in varus and less tense in valgus. When the ligament has an intermediary obliquity or when the direction of the ligament intersects the talocalcaneonavicular axis, the ligament tension remains unchanged throughout the motion.

Inman stressed the coupling effect of the calcaneofibular and the anterior talofibular ligament in preventing the talar tilt on the lateral side.[2] In dorsiflexion the calcaneofibular ligament approaches the vertical position, acts as a true collateral ligament of the ankle joint, and prevents the talar tilt of the talus. In plantar flexion the anterior talofibular ligament is vertical and functions as a collateral ligament

(Text continues on p. 406.)

Fig. 10-32. *(A)* Insertion of the anterior talofibular ligament *T_1*, the posterior talofibular ligament *T_2*, and the calcaneofibular ligament *C* relative to axis *A* of the ankle joint and to the axis of the talocalcaneonavicular joint (*TCN*). *(B)* Length of the three above-mentioned ligaments in neutral *(N)*, dorsiflexion *(DF)*, and plantar flexion *(PF)*. The displacements of the insertions of each ligament take place along an arc of a circle perpendicular to the ankle joint axis. The anterior talofibular ligament is shorter or relaxed in dorsiflexion and longer or taut in plantar flexion. The posterior talofibular ligament is shorter or relaxed in plantar flexion and longer or taut in dorsiflexion. The calcaneofibular ligament, starting from the indicated neutral position, is shorter and relaxed in plantar flexion and longer and taut in dorsiflexion.

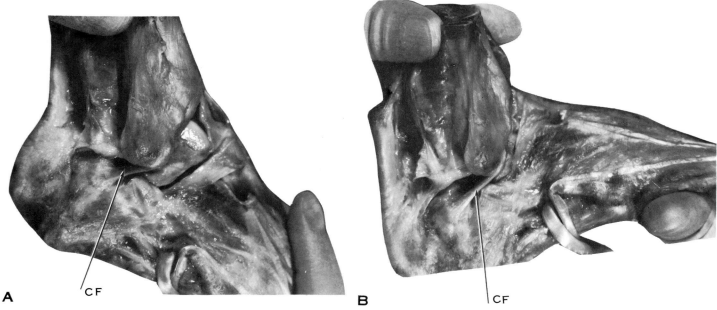

A   CF

B   CF

Fig. 10-33. In this anatomical specimen of the ankle, the calcaneofibular ligament (*CF*) is taut in plantar flexion (*A*) and less tense in dorsiflexion (*B*).

Fig. 10-34. Hindfoot specimen, lateral view.   The ankle is held in neutral position (*N*) and the os calcis is moved into varus (*VR*) or valgus (*VG*). In varus the calcaneofibular ligament is relaxed and the cervical ligament is vertical and tense. In valgus the calcaneofibular ligament is taut and the cervical ligament is oblique or horizontal but still tense. (*CF*, calcaneofibular ligament; *CL*, cervical ligament.)

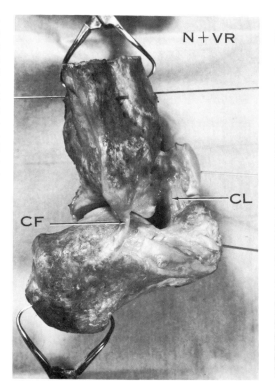

N + VR

CF

CL

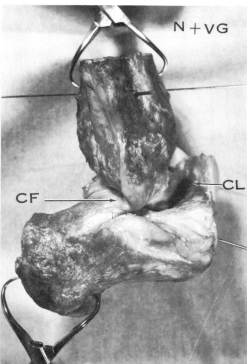

N + VG

CF

CL

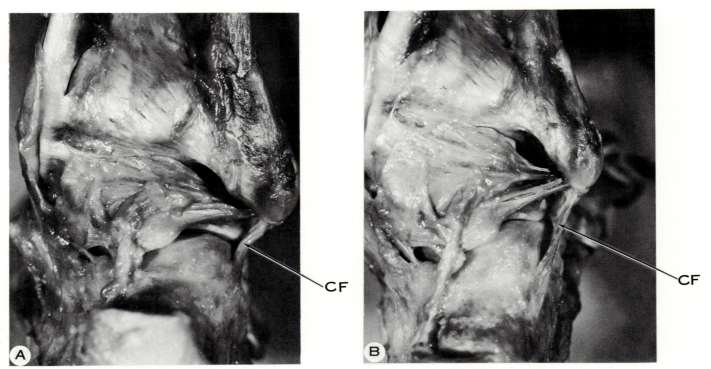

Fig. 10-35. Hindfoot specimen, posterolateral view. The ankle is held in neutral. (*A*) The heel is in varus and the calcaneofibular ligament (*CF*) is relaxed. (*B*) The heel is in valgus and the calcaneofibular ligament is taut.

Fig. 10-36. Hindfoot specimen, lateral view, in dorsiflexion (*DF*) and plantar flexion (*PF*) combined with varus (*VR*) or valgus (*VG*) of the os calcis. The dorsiflexion and plantar flexion are indicated by the K wires implanted in the talus and the os calcis. The valgus and varus are recognized by the relative position of the talus and os calcis: in varus the lateral talar process is away from the posterolateral corner of the sinus tarsi, whereas in valgus the same process strikes or is very close to the sinus tarsi of the os calcis. (*A*) Combination of dorsiflexion and varus. (*B*) Combination of dorsiflexion and valgus. In *A* and *B* the calcaneofibular ligament is taut, more so in valgus. (*C*) Combination of plantar flexion and varus. (*D*) Combination of plantar flexion and valgus. In *C* and *D* the calcaneofibular ligament is less taut than in *A* and *B*, yet slightly more tension is present in the ligament in valgus. The cervical ligament (*CL*) is nearly vertical and parallel to the calcaneofibular ligament in dorsiflexion of the ankle and varus of the heel. The cervical ligament is taut both in valgus and varus.

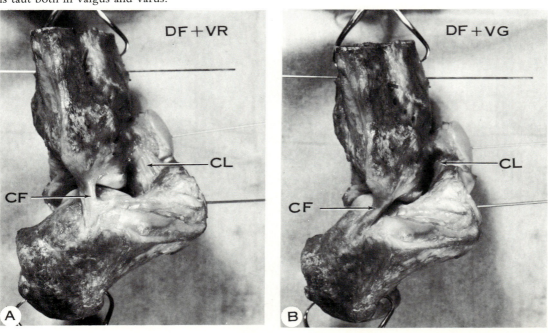

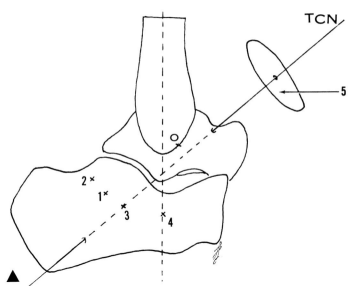

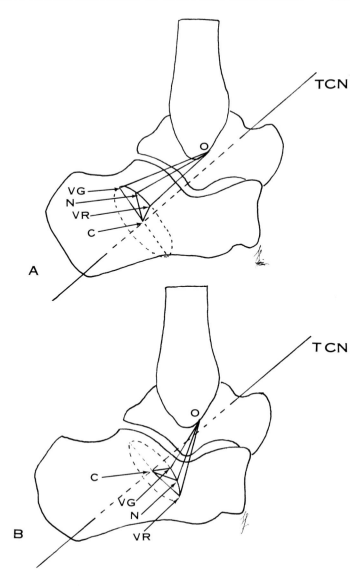

Fig. 10-37. Hindfoot, lateral view. *O* indicates the origin of the calcaneofibular ligament and the numbers *1* to *4* the calcaneal insertion of the same ligament. The variable insertion determines the obliquity of the ligament: *1*, common insertion, oblique ligament; *2*, horizontal ligament; *3*, ligament located along the projection of the talocalcaneonavicular axis (*TCN*); *4*, vertical ligament. The displacement of the insertional points *1* to *4* is along arcs of circles parallel to the circle *5*, which is perpendicular to the talocalcaneonavicular axis.

Fig. 10-38. Calcaneofibular ligament with common insertion. (*A*) *O* indicates the origin of the ligament and *N* the insertional position in neutral. In valgus (*VG*) and varus (*VR*) the displacements occur along the circle *C*, which is perpendicular to the talocalcaneonavicular axis (*TCN*). In valgus the distance from the origin to the insertion is longer and the calcaneofibular ligament is taut. In varus the distance is shorter and the ligament is more relaxed. (*B*) In the vertical type of calcaneofibular ligament, the distance between the origin of the ligament and its insertion is greater in varus and less in valgus. The ligament is taut in varus and relaxed in valgus.

Fig. 10-36. (continued)

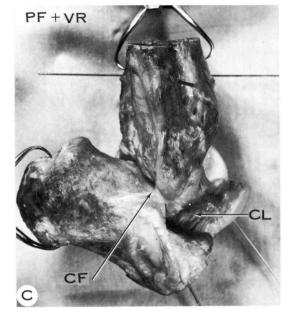

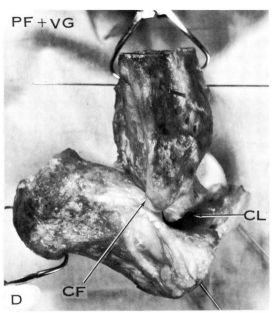

stabilizing the talus laterally. The average angle between the two ligaments, measured in their projection on the sagittal plane, was 105° ± 24°.[2] The reciprocal arrangement of the two ligaments is efficient if the angle between the two ligaments is 90°. A horizontal calcaneofibular ligament does not provide the same stability.

The peroneotalocalcaneal ligament of Rouvière and Canela Lazaro is taut in dorsiflexion and relaxed in plantar flexion. It limits also the anterior displacement of the leg. Both authors have demonstrated that the section of the ligament appreciably increases the anterior displacement of the leg when the foot is stabilized on a table and weight is applied to the anteriorly rotating leg.

The inferior tibiofibular syndesmosis is secured by the anterior and posterior tibiofibular ligaments, the interosseous ligament, and the posterior transverse tibiofibular ligament. The anterior tibiofibular ligament and the interosseous ligaments limit the external rotation, the posterior displacement, and the lateral displacement of the lateral malleolus. The sectioning of the three ligaments, including that of the interosseous membrane, increases only slightly the intermalleolar space. However, when the foot and the talus are rotated laterally, marked posterior displacement of the lateral malleolus, amounting to 4 mm to 5 mm, accompanies the external rotation. As demonstrated by Close, the medial clear space between the talus and the medial malleolus does not increase more than 2 mm unless there is a sectioning of the deep layer of the deltoid ligament.[7]

The tibionavicular ligament and the anterior tibiotalar ligament limit the plantar flexion of the foot and ankle. The anterior tibiotalar ligament limits the external rotation of the talus in the mortise and contributes to transmission of the internal rotation of the tibia to the talus. The segment of the deltoid ligament inserting on the calcaneonavicular ligament provides the suspensory support to the ligament against gravity and against the dynamic pressure exerted inferomedially by the talar head. The plantar segment of the tibialis posterior tendon supplements this support. The talocalcaneal ligament limits the eversion at the talocalcaneonavicular joint and contributes to the medial stability of the talus. The posterior talotibial ligament is the strongest and most important component of the deltoid ligament in stabilizing the talus medially. It prevents the lateral displacement of the talus even when the lateral malleolar buttress yields. It limits the dorsiflexion of the foot and ankle and the anterior rotation of the leg when the foot is stabilized. This ligament contributes to the transmission of the external rotation of the tibia to the talus.

TALOCALCANEONAVICULAR JOINT AND MIDTARSAL JOINT MOTORS AND STABILIZATION

Motors

The axis of the talocalcaneonavicular joint and the oblique axis of the midtarsal joint are very close in orientation. The motor units located on the medial aspect of the talocalcaneonavicular axis of motion are the invertors, whereas the

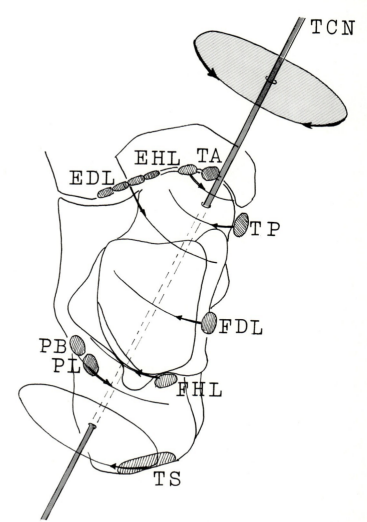

Fig. 10-39. Evertors and invertors of the foot. (*TCN*, talocalcaneonavicular axis; **evertors:** *PL*, peroneus longus; *PB*, peroneus brevis; *EDL*, extensor digitorum longus; *EHL*, extensor hallucis longus; *TA*, tibialis anterior; **invertors:** *TS*, triceps surae; *TP*, tibialis posterior; *FDL*, flexor digitorum longus; *FHL*, flexor hallucis longus; *TA*, tibialis anterior.)

motor units located on the lateral aspect of the same axis are the evertors (Fig. 10-39). With the foot fixed on the ground, the evertors internally rotate the leg and the invertors rotate the leg externally.

Invertors. The following motor units are the invertors and their work capacity in meterkilograms, as presented by Lang and Wachsmuth: triceps surae, 4.8; tibialis posterior muscle, 1.8; flexor digitorum longus muscle, 0.8; flexor hallucis longus muscle, 0.8; tibialis anterior muscle, 1.0 (total, 8.2).[1]

Evertors. The following motor units are the evertors with their work capacity in meterkilograms: peroneus longus muscle, 1.7; peroneus brevis muscle, 1.3; extensor digitorum longus muscle, 0.8; peroneus tertius muscle, 0.6;

extensor hallucis longus muscle, 0.1; tibialis anterior muscle, 0.3 (total, 4.8).[1]

Stabilization

Talocalcaneonavicular Joint.   The stability of talocalcaneonavicular joint is determined by the tension of the ligaments, the medial and lateral bony blocks, and the viscoelastic tension developed by the surrounding tendons in association with the lengthening contraction of the muscles.

The talus moves relative to the oblique motion axis of the talocalcaneonavicular joint. The motions of the talus of extension–abduction–pronation or flexion–adduction–supination can be translated as rotational motions around the innermost and short fibers of the talocalcaneal interosseous ligament of the canalis tarsi, which act as a pivot (Fig. 10-40). The fibers of this interosseous ligament are oriented upward and medially. The lateral fibers are longer and have a longer excursion laterally, whereas the shorter fibers on the inner side have a shorter excursion medially. This arrangement promotes (as qualified by Huson), a "swinging motion," with a center of movement located along the short medial fibers of the ligament of the canalis tarsi.[29] The rotational motion of the talus over the os calcis or vice versa was clearly demonstrated by Farabeuf in 1889.[27] He described the rotational center located in the innermost part of the canalis tarsi and the talus rotating along this axis in "tourniquet" fashion; he stated clearly that the fibers of the interosseous ligament do not allow a gliding of the opposed articular surfaces but allow a rotation of the surfaces through a twisting of the fibers of the interosseous ligament.

As mentioned by Huson, the surfaces of the posterior talocalcaneal joint do not move along the long axis of the joint but rotate relative to each other to decrease the incongruity of the opposed surfaces.[29] This incongruity results from the fact that the axis of motion and the axes that generated the contour of the complex surface do not coincide.

The interosseous ligament of the canalis tarsi is the strongest ligament connecting the talus to the os calcis. It is the guide to the talocalcaneonavicular motion. The inversion at the talocalcaneonavicular joint is limited by the cervical ligament, which is nearly vertical in this position, the calcaneofibular ligament of the vertical type, the lateral talocalcaneal ligament, the peroneus longus and peroneus brevis, and the sustentaculum tali striking the posteromedial talar tubercle. The eversion at the talocalcaneonavicular joint is limited by the cervical ligament, which is nearly horizontal and tense, the calcaneofibular ligament of the horizontal type, the lateral talar process striking the sinus tarsi surface of the calcaneus, similar to a wedge, the tibiocalcaneal fascicle of the deltoid ligament, the medial talocalcaneal ligament extending from the posterior border of the sustentaculum tali to the posteromedial talar tubercle, the tibialis posterior tendon–muscle, and the flexor digitorum longus tendon–muscle.

Midtarsal Joint.   The talar head fits the acetabulum pedis. As described previously, the latter has a mosaic struc-

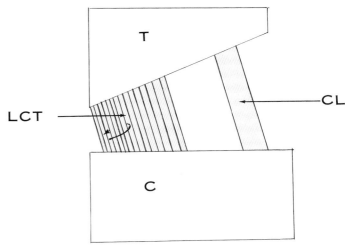

Fig. 10-40. Ligament of the canalis tarsi (*LCT*) and the cervical ligament (*CL*).   The rotational motion of the talus around the os calcis or *vice versa* occurs around the innermost and short fibers of the ligament of the canalis tarsi which act as a pivot. The outer and longer ligamentous fibers have more arcuate excursion, and the inner, short ligamentous fibers have less excursion. (*T,* talus; *C,* calcaneus.)

ture and is formed by the navicular articular surface, the inferior and superomedial calcaneonavicular ligaments, and the superior surface of the sustentaculum tali. In the weight-bearing position, when the tibia rotates medially, the talus turns also medially through the combined motion of flexion–adduction–supination occuring around the talocalcaneonavicular axis. The downward and medial pressure of the talar head stretches the inferior and superomedial calcaneonavicular ligaments, and the talar head is in a compressive fit in the acetabulum pedis. As mentioned by MacConaill and Basmajian, "this screws the talar head into close-pack with the acetabulum pedis."[38] The forefoot is in a supination twist position and rigid. The combination of compressive fit of the talar head into the acetabulum pedis and the supination of the forefoot converts the foot into a rigid mass of bones. The rigidity of the foot is produced by the internal rotation of the tibia–talus or the external rotation of the subtalar skeleton or lamina pedis. In this position, as defined by MacConaill, the foot is in supination with the heel in valgus and the forefoot supinated and all plantar ligaments are taut. The combination of supination and external rotation of the foot is a common mechanism of fracture of the ankle.

The talonavicular joint is in close pack position in pronation. Similarly, the calcaneocuboid joint, as demonstrated by Bojsen–Møller, is in close pack position in pronation.[39] In pronation, the cuboidal surface, pivoting around the beak of the cuboid slides upward and is stopped by the dorsal, overhanging border of the calcaneus. The upward displacement and rotation in pronation tightens the plantar, lateral, and dorsal calcaneocuboid ligaments. The congruency of the joint surfaces in pronation and the tightening of the ligaments creates a close pack fit of the cuboid at the calcaneocuboid joint. In full supination, the same joint is locked "but not in a close-packed position, as the articulating surfaces only oppose each other partly."[39] The calcaneocuboid ligaments are taut again. In this position the medial calcaneal tubercle is closer to the first metatarsophalangeal joint, and this contributes to the relaxation of the plantar aponeurosis.[39]

TOE MOTORS AND FUNCTION

The toes participate in weight bearing, in giving hold against the ground, and in tensing the plantar aponeurosis and the plantar skin during the push-off phase of the walking cycle. The last two functions are more effective with the first and second toes. The long flexors of the toes also act as plantar flexors of the ankle and invertors of the talocalcaneonavicular joint, whereas the long extensors of the toes act as dorsiflexors of the ankle and evertors of the talocalcaneonavicular joint.

In 1889 Ellis stated that "the principal function of the toes is to give good foot-hold by active pressure against the ground, so as to supplement the passive pressure of the body's weight. This is effected by the same means as that which, when the toes are free to move, moves them."[40] The long toe flexors act from their distal anatomical insertions, and as such they act as joint-stabilizing muscles.[41]

During the walking cycle the long toe flexors are in concentric contraction when the metatarsophalangeal joints are extending (30%–55% of the cycle) and act as stabilizers of the toes, invertors of the hindfoot, and plantar flexors of the ankle. The long toe extensors are in concentric contraction during the swing phase of gait and act as extensors of the metatarsophalangeal joints, evertors of the hindfoot, and dorsiflexors of the ankle.

Big Toe Motors

In the big toe in the non–weight-bearing position, the distal joint is extended by the extensor hallucis longus tendon through its wide insertion on the dorsum of the distal phalanx. The proximal phalanx is extended by the extensor digitorum brevis and by the transverse lamina of the extensor aponeurosis activated by the proximal pull of the extensor hallucis longus. This is the sling mechanism of extension described by Sarrafian and Topouzian.[42]

The centralization of the extensor hallucis longus tendon relative to the vertical axis passing through the metatarsal head is of prime importance. If the tendon shifts lateral to this axis—as in hallux valgus—it will act as an adductor of the hallux and will exert a medially directed force on the first metatarsal head, which may result in a varus deformity of the first metatarsal bone.

In the non–weight-bearing position, the distal phalanx is flexed by the flexor hallucis longus.

The flexion of the metatarsophalangeal joint is provided by the lateral head of the flexor hallucis brevis, the medial head of the flexor hallucis brevis, the adductor hallucis, the abductor hallucis, and the flexor hallucis longus.

It is apparent that the flexor or "pressor" power of the metatarsophalangeal joint is greater than the extensor power. Furthermore, the action of a tendon–muscle unit over a joint is measured by the moment developed by the motor unit relative to the axis of motion at the joint. The moment is measured by the product of the acting force and its perpendicular distance from the axis of rotation. The sesamoids in this sense not only have a weight-bearing function but also increase the perpendicular distance of the plantar intrinsic muscles from the axis of flexion–extension of the metatarsophalangeal joint and augment the flexor moment of the intrinsic muscles. Excision of the sesamoids will result in decrease of the flexor moment or flexor power so essential at this joint.

The abductor of the big toe is the abductor hallucis, and the adductor hallucis provides the adduction. Balance between these two deviators is necessary to maintain the big toe in neutral position. In a hallux valgus deformity the abductor hallucis shifts laterally and its abductor component is more in a plantar position. The muscle loses its abductor power and acts mainly as a flexor. The side motion is overtaken by the adductor hallucis.

In the plantigrade position the proximal phalanx of the big toe is normally extended. The flexion of the distal phalanx is possible only if the proximal phalanx is further extended to create the necessary "room" for the flexion to occur. However, this is prevented by the powerful flexion-pressor pull of the intrinsic muscles, and as stated by Ellis, the flexor hallucis longus "exerts all its influence on a straight great toe."[40] Excision of the sesamoids may result in a cock-up deformity of the big toe through weakening of the intrinsic muscles. Occasionally the same deformity may be seen as a complication of a Keller excisional arthroplasty as the flexion power of the intrinsics is lessened by excision of the proximal third of the proximal phalanx.

Lesser Toe Motors

In the non–weight-bearing position the proximal phalanx of the lesser toes is extended by the sling traction exerted by the long extensor on the transverse lamina (Fig. 10-41).[42] The proximal interphalangeal joint is extended by the middle slip of the long extensor and the insertion of the extensor digitorum brevis. The distal joint is extended by the terminal tendon of the long extensor tendon.

The distal joint is flexed by the flexor digitorum longus and the middle joint by the flexor digitorum brevis. The plantar and dorsal interossei are inserted on the deep transverse metatarsal ligaments, the lateral capsule and the glenoid ligament of the metatarsophalangeal joint, the plantar plate of the metatarsophalangeal joint, the deep surface of the transverse lamina, and the base of the proximal phalanx. They function as the flexor–pressors of the proximal phalanx. The dorsal interossei abduct and the plantar interossei adduct the lesser toes. The abductor digiti quinti and the flexor digiti quinti are also flexors of the metatarsophalangeal joint of the fifth toe, and the former is also its abductor. The lumbrical is a very small muscle and may contribute to the extension of the interphalangeal joints and the flexion of the proximal phalanx. In the plantigrade position the pull of the intrinsic muscle cannot prevent some degree of further extension at the metatarsophalangeal joint secondary

Fig. 10-41. Sling mechanism of extension of the metatarsophalangeal joint of the lesser toe. The pull of the extensor digitorum longus *A* is transmitted as a traction to the transverse lamina *B* which acts as a sling and lifts the proximal phalanx into extension. (Redrawn after Sarrafian SK, Topouzian LK: Anatomy and physiology of the extensor apparatus of the toes. J Bone Joint Surg [Am] 51, No. 4:669, 1969)

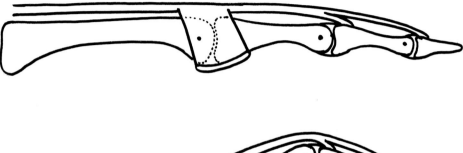

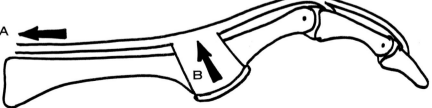

Fig. 10-42. The "windlass." The drum of the windlass is the head of the metatarsal, the handle is the proximal phalanx, and the cable wound onto the drum is the plantar aponeurosis through its attachment to the plantar pad of the metatarsophalangeal joint. The dorsiflexion of the toe winds the plantar aponeurosis around the metatarsal head. The initial length L_1 of the foot diminishes to L_2, and the initial height of the arch H_1 increases to H_2. (From Hicks JH: The three weight-bearing mechanisms of the foot. In Evans FG [ed]: In Biomechanical Studies of the Musculo-Skeletal System, p 176. Springfield, Charles C Thomas, 1961)

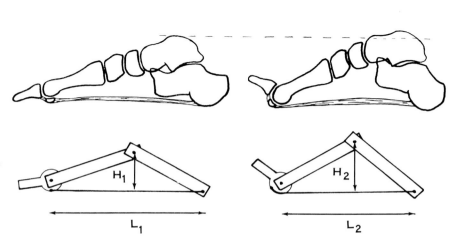

to the flexion of the middle phalanx by the flexor digitorum brevis. The distal phalanx is hyperextended and pressed down by the long flexor. By this mechanism, as stated by Ellis, the lesser toes "grip the ground . . . by pressure of the under surfaces of the tips against the ground."[40] In the absence of the intrinsic power, the hyperextension of the proximal phalanx is increased, resulting in flexion of the interphalangeal joints; this produces clawing of the toes.

Toes as Tensors of the Plantar Aponeurosis and of the Skin

The plantar aponeurosis of the foot is attached posteriorly to the os calcis and anteriorly to the proximal phalanges of the toes through the longitudinal septa (in the big toe the septa are attached to the lateral and medial sesamoids) and to the skin of the ball of the foot through the vertical fibers and through the transverse lamellae of the natatory ligament farther distally.

As described by Hicks, hyperextension of the toes at the metatarsophalangeal joints tenses the plantar aponeurosis, raises the longitudinal arch of the foot, inverts the hindfoot, and externally rotates the leg.[43]

When the toe is extended at the metatarsophalangeal joint, the plantar aponeurosis attached to the proximal phalanges is wound around the metatarsal head, acting as the drum of a windlass; it then tenses (Fig. 10-42). The handle that does the winding is the proximal phalanx and the cable that is wound on the drum is the plantar aponeurosis. The calcaneus remains fixed, the forefoot flexes about 1 cm, and the longitudinal arch becomes shorter but higher. The first metatarsal head is larger in diameter than the lesser metatarsal heads, and the big toe sesamoids further increase the diameter of the first metatarsal drum. As a result, the excess tensing of the big toe plantar aponeurosis results in more flexion of the first ray and a pronation twist of the forefoot. This, combined with the inversion of the hindfoot, creates a high arch pattern, as described previously. The first ray flexes an average of 10° and the lateral rays, 5°. The movement occurs at the cuneonavicular and metatarsocuneiform joints. The displacement of the plantar aponeurosis is reported by Bojsen-Møller to be an average of 15 mm in the big toe and 8 mm in the third toe.[39] The windlass mechanism is passive and depends entirely on the bony and ligamentous integrity.

Extension of the metatarsophalangeal joints of the toes also affects the skin of the ball of the foot, which is transformed (as described by Bojsen-Møller and Lamoreux) from a soft pliable ball "into a firm pad that can resist tangential, or shear forces," and the skin mobility is greatly reduced.[44]

Arches of the Foot, Lamina Pedis, Load Transmission

The definition and the existence of the arches of the foot have been controversial. From a practical, clinical point of view, in the standing position, in the anteroposterior direction, it is evident that there is no clear space between the ground and the lateral border of the foot, and thus there is no evidence of an arch, and that there is usually a clear space with a variable height between the medial border of the foot and the ground, and thus there is a medial longitudinal arch.

In the transverse direction an arch or a niche is found in the mid segment of the foot. Distally all five metatarsal heads bear weight, and a transverse arch is inexistent. Structurally, in the sagittal plane, the foot skeleton is arranged in an arcuate fashion, taking support posteriorly through the os calcis, anteriorly through the metatarsal heads, and spanning the mid segment of the foot; the spanning is high medially and very low laterally. The arcuate units are five in number, fused posteriorly at the level of the os calcis, and separated anteriorly through the corresponding metatarsal bones. Structurally, a weight–bearing arcuate structure may behave as an arch, a truss, or a curved beam.

An *arch* is a multisegmented arcuate structure, usually with a central wedge-shaped keystone and two "flanks" leading down from each side of the keystone, the flanks supported by fixed segments such as two columns or embankments. Without the fixed support at both ends, the arch collapses.

A *truss* is a variant of the arch (Fig. 10-43). The separation of both ends is prevented by a tie-rod at the base. The truss

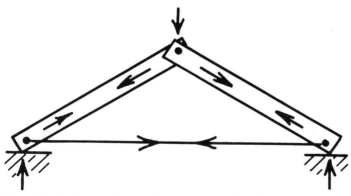

Fig. 10-43. A truss is a variant of an arch. The two struts are connected at the base by a tie. When load is applied at the apex, the struts are under compression and the tie-rod under tension. Bending is eliminated. The three weight-bearing mechanisms of the foot. (From Hicks JH: In Evans FG [ed.]: Biomechanical Studies of the Musculo-Skeletal System. Springfield, Charles C Thomas, 1961. After Lapidus PW: Kinesiology and mechanical anatomy of the tarsal joints. Clin Orthop Rel Res 30:22, 1963)

is triangular in arrangement, with the sides formed by two struts and the base by the tie-rod. When load is applied at the apex, the struts are under compression and the tie-rod under tension; bending is eliminated. A tie-rod mechanism is provided to the foot by the plantar aponeurosis.

A *curved beam* is unisegmental. When loaded vertically in its mid segment, it generates compressive forces on the convex surface and tensile forces on the concave surface. An arch may behave as a convex beam if the multiple segments are bound together on the concave surface by connecting elements such as the strong ligaments seen in the foot (Fig. 10-44).

Lapidus considers the foot as a truss, with the talus and os calcis forming the posterior strut and the forefoot up to the metatarsal heads forming the anterior strut.[45] Both are subjected to compression. The plantar structures, mainly the plantar aponeurosis, are the tie-rod "taking up the tension and eliminating bending."[45]

Hicks, in an experimental study, demonstrated that under weight-bearing conditions in the plantigrade position, the foot reacts as a truss and a beam.[46] The load on the foot tends to force the ends apart, and "the tension in the tie therefore provides a measure of the arch-flattening effect."[46] In the plantigrade standing position, the flattening effect is resisted by both the truss and the beam mechanism. In the toe-standing position or the corresponding phase of walking, the truss mechanism takes over from the beam mechanism; this is caused by the windlass mechanism tightening the plantar aponeurosis. The bending strain on the beam diminishes, and in the extreme heel—raised position, the truss mechanism assumes the entire load.

From a quantitiative point of view, Hicks expresses the tension in the tie or the arch-flattening effect as

$$t = W \frac{l}{L} \cdot \frac{P}{Q},$$

where t = tension in the tie or plantar aponeurosis, W = body weight, L = length of foot from heel to ball, l = distance of line of weight anterior to the heel, P and Q = constants related to the shape of the individual arch (height) (Fig. 10-45).[46]

It is apparent that the arch-flattening effect of the body weight is variable and is nil when W passes through the heel ($l = 0$, $t = 0$) and maximum when W passes through the ball of the foot (l = max., t = max.). In other words, when one leans forward on the plantigrade foot and transfers the weight-bearing line anteriorly, there is more tendency to flatten the longitudinal arch, and subsequently more strain is exerted on the plantar structures and the plantar aponeurosis.

In the average foot the ratio P/Q is 1.8. When W passes through the ball of the foot, l/L is equal to 1 and the flattening effect on the foot is 1.8 W or nearly the double of the body weight. In the high arch foot, Q is increased P/Q decreased and the flattening strain is less on the foot, whereas in the flatfoot, Q is decreased and P/Q is increased, resulting in increased strain on the weight-bearing foot.

MacConaill considers the foot, excluding the toes, as a twisted plate termed the *lamina pedis* (Fig. 10-46).[47] Structurally, the lamina pedis is formed by the entire foot skeleton

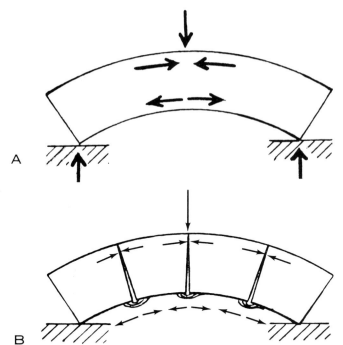

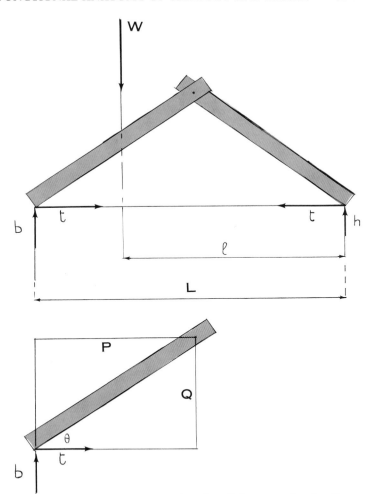

Fig. 10-44. A curved beam (*A*), when loaded vertically in its mid segment, generates compressive forces on the convex surface and tensile forces on the concave surface. An arch (*B*) may behave as a convex beam if the segmental components are bound on the concave surface by connecting elements such as strong ligaments, as seen on the plantar aspect of the foot. The ligaments are under tension. (After Hicks JH: The three weight-bearing mechanisms of the foot. In Evans FG [ed]: Biomechanical Studies of the Musculo-Skeletal System. Springfield, Charles C Thomas, 1961)

Fig. 10-45. The tension in the tie of the truss in the foot. The tension *t* represents the arch-flattening effect. When the load *W* is applied, the sum of the moments at point h is as follows:

$$\Sigma \, M_h = Wl - bL = O$$
$$bL = Wl \qquad (1)$$

$$\text{Tan } \theta = \frac{b}{t}$$
$$b = t \, \text{Tan } \theta \qquad (2)$$
Replacing *b* in (1)
$$t \, \text{Tan } \theta \cdot L = Wl$$
$$t = W \cdot \frac{l}{L} \cdot \frac{1}{\text{Tan } \theta}$$
$$t = W \cdot \frac{l}{L} \, \text{Cotan } \theta$$
$$t = W \cdot \frac{l}{L} \cdot \frac{P}{Q}$$

Q is the height of the arch of the foot. The higher the arch, the greater is *Q* and the lesser the tension *t* or flattening action. The lower the arch, the lesser is *Q* and the greater the tension *t* or flattening action. Obesity increases *W* and the tension *t*. (*t*, tension in tie; *W*, body weight; *h*, upward thrust from ground on the heel; *b*, upward thrust from ground on the ball of the foot; *L*, length of foot from heel to ball; *l*, distance of line of weight anterior to heel [varies from 0 to *L*]; *P*, *Q*, constants related to shape of individual arch [high or low arch]; θ, the inclination angle of the anterior strut of the foot.) (Diagram and equations after Hicks JH: The foot as a support. Acta Anat 25:34, 1955)

and supportive ligaments, minus the talus. The twisted lamina pedis is flattened from above downward at the level of the metatarsal heads and flattened side to side at the level of the os calcis. The twisted plate is flexible. MacConaill defines supination of the foot as the untwisting of the foot plate, and this involves a supination twist of the forefoot associated with eversion or valgus of the hindfoot.[47] Pronation is defined as an increase in the normal twist of the foot plate; this involves an association of pronation twist of the forefoot and inversion or varus of the hindfoot. When an anatomical foot model of the lamina pedis or a living foot is held at both ends and twisted in pronation followed by a push and a pull motion as if playing an accordion, intersegmental movement can be demonstrated and the foot is in loose pack position. When the lamina pedis of the living foot is untwisted into supination—combination of supination twist of the forefoot and eversion of the hindfoot—it is impossible to push and pull, as the bony segments are united into a temporary single rigid mass and the foot is in close pack position. In supination, as defined above, all the plantar ligaments, capsular and extracapsular, including the long plantar and the calcaneonavicular ligaments, are tense.

The twist of the foot plate generates the medial longitudinal arch and the transverse arch of the midfoot. The height of the medial arch is increased with pronation of the

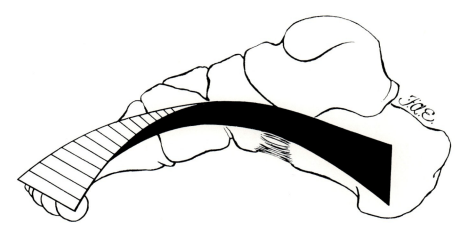

Fig. 10-46. The lamina pedis. (From Mac-Conaill MS, Basmajian JV: Muscles and Movements: A Basis for Human Kinesiology, p 246. Baltimore, Williams & Wilkins, 1969)

lamina pedis, and this is seen when the feet are side by side or crossed on the ground. The height of the same arch is decreased with supination of the lamina pedis, and this is seen when the feet are wide apart and standing (combination of supination twist of the forefoot and eversion of the hind-foot).[38]

In the standing plantigrade position the external rotation of the leg produces a loose pack situation (MacConaill's pronation or a combination of inversion of the heel and pronation twist of the forefoot), whereas the internal rotation of the leg produces a close pack situation (MacConaill's supination or a combination of eversion of the heel and supination of the forefoot). The ankle is in a close pack rigid position in dorsiflexion.[38] When this is combined with the supination of the lamina pedis, the leg–ankle–lamina pedis is converted into a rigid mass of bone, unyielding, liable to fracture if excess force is applied.[38] This may be considered the basis of the supination–external rotation fractures of the ankle.

The role of the muscles in the arch support was investigated electromyographically by Basmajian and Stecko.[48] They demonstrated that in the normal foot, standing at ease position, the muscles are inactive and do not participate in the arch support mechanism. With loads of 45.35 kg (100 pounds) to 90.70 kg (200 pounds) applied to the foot, the skeletal element and their ligaments provide the necessary support. With a 181.40 kg (400 pounds) load the muscles come into play. During activity "the muscles would appear to contribute to the normal maintenance of the longitudinal arches."[48]

In the standing plantigrade position, the body weight is transmitted to the foot skeleton, and as defined by Morton, the load is equally divided between the heel and the fore-foot.[49] At the level of the metatarsal heads, the ratio of weight distribution is 2:1:1:1:1, the first metatarsal through its two sesamoids carrying a double load (Fig. 10-47).[49] Jones demonstrated that the load distribution "is readily changed by a number of factors."[50] In the standing position, eversion brought about by abduction of the leg increases the load on metatarsals 2 to 5, whereas inversion brought about by adduction of the leg increases the load on the first metatarsal head.[50] Dorsiflexion of the ankle increases the load on the first metatarsal head, and plantar flexion of the ankle shifts more weight onto metatarsals 2 to 5.[50]

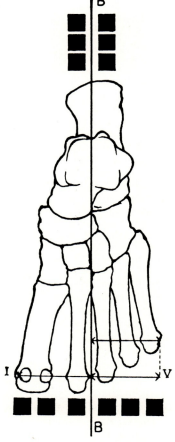

Fig. 10-47. Distribution of weight in the standing position. The load is equally divided between the heel and the forefoot. Each square represents a weight unit. Each lesser metatarsal head carries one unit of weight. The big toe, through its two sesamoids, carries a double load. (From Morton DJ: Biomechanics of the Human Foot in Reconstruction of the Foot: Course No. IV, p 94. American Academy of Orthopedic Surgeons. Instructional Courses, January 1944)

As mentioned previously, Hicks has quantitated the increased load on the ball of the foot and consequently on the metatarsal heads with anterior flexion of the leg at the ankle or relative dorsiflexion of the foot.[46] Hutton and co-workers, in their investigation of the body weight distribution on the standing foot, found the heel and the forefoot to carry almost entirely the body weight and the midfoot to carry "very little load."[51] The distribution of the load between the heel and the forefoot was found "to be quite widely variable and a variety of comfortable stances could be achieved with the heel carrying between one and three times the load on the forefoot."[51] In the standing position

Fig. 10-48. Intraosseous trabecular patterns of the ankle and foot. The anterior tibial trabecular pattern (*1*) is concave posteriorly and continues into the talus, forming the calcaneal thalamic system (*3*). The posterior tibial trabecular pattern (*2*) is concave anteriorly and continues through the talar body, neck, and head (*9*), the navicular, the cuneiforms, and the metatarsals 3 to 1. The calcaneal anterior apophyseal system (*4*) extends from the sinus tarsi to the cuboidal surface. The posterior (*5*) and anterior (*6*) plantar calcaneal systems delineate with the thalamic and anterior apophyseal systems a neutral zone (*8*) void of trabeculae and form a pseudocavity. The dense posterior calcaneal trabeculae (*7*) correspond to the insertion of the Achilles tendon. The anterior plantar calcaneal trabeculae continue through the cuboid and the metatarsals 4, 5. Midtarsal transverse trabeculae (*10*) cross the longintudinal systems.

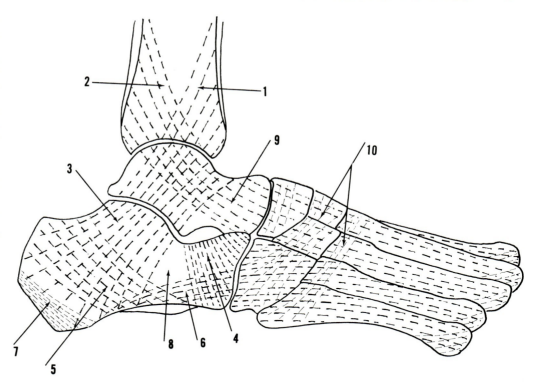

the toes carry 5% to 10% of the forefoot load, and the digital load increases as more weight is transferred anteriorly onto the forefoot.[51]

Within the pedal skeletal framework, the transmission of the forces orients the bony trabeculae. The orientation of the trabeculae is not affected nor interrupted by the presence of an articular interval, and a linear continuity is maintained throughout the skeletal frame. Two curved trabecular systems are initiated from the distal tibia (Fig. 10-48).[1,52] The anterior tibial trabecular system has a posterior concavity and is directed downward and posteriorly. It passes through the talus and terminates in the posterior segment of the os calcis in a fan-shaped pattern. The posterior tibial trabecular system is concave anteriorly, directed downward and anteriorly. It passes through the talus, the navicular, and the medial three metatarsals.

Within the os calcis, four trabecular systems are recognized: thalamic, anterior apophyseal, and plantar, posterior and anterior. The thalamic trabecular system is the continuation within the os calcis of the anterior tibial and talar trabecular system, as described above. The anterior apophyseal system is more or less vertical in direction. It originates from the floor of the sinus tarsi and terminates on the cuboid surface of the os calcis and the anterior segment of the plantar surface. The posterior plantar trabecular arrangement originates from the dorsal and posterior surfaces of the os calcis; the trabeculae are directed downward and anteriorly with an anterior concavity and terminate on the mid plantar aspect of the os calcis. The anterior plantar trabecular system originates from the inferior surface of the cuboidal surface of the os calcis; the trabeculae are directed downward and posteriorly with a plantar concavity and terminate also on the mid plantar segment of the bone. A

fifth trabecular pattern may be recognized, corresponding to the insertion of the Achilles tendon. The four major calcaneal trabecular patterns delineate a triangular intertrabecular zone, located under the lateral angle of the sinus tarsi and the anterolateral aspect of the posterior calcaneal surface.[53] This is the weaker segment of the os calcis, void of trabeculae, and forms a medullary pseudocavity. It yields easily and fractures under the pressure exerted by the lateral wedge-shaped process of the talus (Figs. 10-49 and 10-50).[53,54] The plantar calcaneal trabecular system continues through the cuboid and the lateral two metatarsals. A transverse trabecular system is present in the midfoot and forms a cross pattern with the longitudinally oriented trabeculae.[1]

Foot and Ankle in Walking

WALKING CYCLE

The walking cycle is conventionally divided into two phases: weight-bearing or stance phase and non–weight-bearing or swing phase (Figs. 10-51 and 10-52).[55–59] The stance phase comprises 60% and the swing phase 40% of the cycle.

Stance Phase

The stance phase begins with the heel strike when the decelerating foot comes down and the heel cushion strikes the ground. The big toe is dorsiflexed 20° to 30°.[44] The foot descends rapidly, and its lateral border establishes contact with the ground, followed by the contact of the lateral aspect of the ball of the foot. The forefoot is in supination

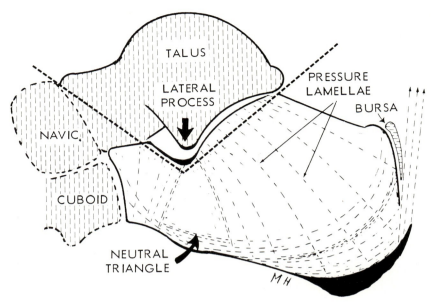

Fig. 10-49. The neutral triangle of the os calcis. (From Harty M: Anatomic considerations in injuries of the calcaneus. Orthop Clin North Am 4, No. 1:179, 1973)

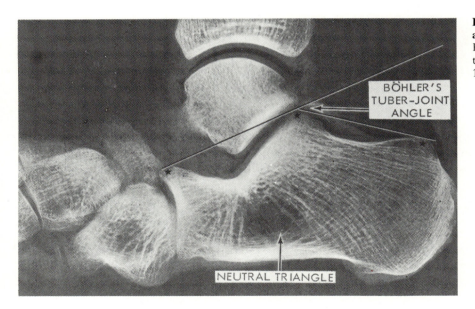

Fig. 10-50. Intracalcaneal trabecular pattern and the neutral vascular triangle. (From Harty M: Anatomic considerations in injuries of the calcaneus. Orthop Clin North Am 4, No. 1: 179, 1973)

twist. The tibia internally rotates, and the subtalar and midtarsal joints evert from the initial slightly inverted position. The pronation component locks the calcaneocuboid joint.[39] The combination of eversion of the hindfoot and midfoot with a supination twist of the forefoot converts the lamina pedis into a rigid mass, and the foot is in a close pack status. The ball of the foot increases its surface contact with the ground progressively from the lateral to the medial side, and the toe contact occurs to all five toes at the same time or "by the first and fifth toes together with the ball, followed by a delayed contact of the second, third and fourth toes."[39] The foot is now in the plantigrade or foot-flat position, which occurs at 15% of the walking cycle. The leg flexes anteriorly, corresponding to a dorsiflexion at the ankle, and turns laterally. The hindfoot and the midfoot invert and the forefoot is pronated; this combination converts the

foot into a more flexible bony mass in loose pack position. Stability is now added through the truss mechanism initiated by the plantar aponeurosis and the plantar supportive structures. Further, the multisegmented foot arch behaves as a curved beam, acquiring rigidity through the compression of its convexity and the tension on its concave side. The tension is determined by the integrity of the plantar ligaments. The metatarsophalangeal joint of the big toe is now in neutral position. At mid stance the leg is perpendicular to the foot. The forward momentum of the leg continues, and the heel comes off the ground at 30% of the walking cycle and the push-off phase is initiated. The tibia continues its external rotation. The hindfoot and midfoot are inverting, and the forefoot has increased its pronation twist. The foot is in a loose pack status. The heel, through its inversion, is closer to the first metatarsophalangeal joint,

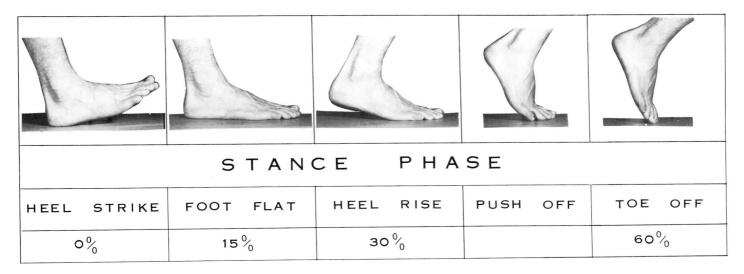

S T A N C E		P H A S E		
HEEL STRIKE	FOOT FLAT	HEEL RISE	PUSH OFF	TOE OFF
0%	15%	30%		60%

S W I N G		P H A S E	
ACCELERATION	TOE CLEARANCE	DECELARATION	HEEL STRIKE

Fig. 10-51. Walking cycle.   100%

and this will have a tendency to relax the supporting plantar aponeurosis.[39] However, through the dorsiflexion at the metatarsophalangeal joints, the windlass mechanism of Hicks comes into play, which restores and increases the tension in the plantar aponeurosis; the foot as a lever arm maintains its rigidity.

As described by Bojsen-Møller, the push-off takes place initially along the oblique axis passing through the metatarsal heads 5 to 2 and subsequently along a transverse axis passing through the metatarsal heads 1 to 2 (Fig. 10-53).[35,44] The windlass mechanism is more effective with the transverse axis of motion, as the plantar aponeurosis is wound around the first metatarsal head, which acts as a larger drum, particularly with the presence of the two sesamoids. When the foot rises along the oblique or transverse axes at the metatarsophalangeal joints, the hindfoot and midfoot move around the talocrural and subtalar axes, with a resultant axis of motion that is parallel to the oblique or transverse metatarsophalangeal axes of motion. During the push-off, along the oblique metatarsal 2–metatarsal 5 axis, the resistance arm offered to the triceps surae is shorter as compared with the resistance arm offered during the push-off around the transverse axis metatarsal 1–metatarsal 2.

Bojsen-Møller characterizes the motion around the oblique metatarsal 2–metatarsal 5 axis as being a low gear motion and the motion around the transverse metatarsal 1–metatarsal 2 axis as being a high gear motion, with a mean ratio of 5:6 between the gears.[35] The resistance lever arm is further increased in the final stage of the push-off when the axis of motion passes through the tip of the great toe.[39] The two-speed construction allows the high gear to be used for sprinting and the low gear for uphill walking with heavy loads and in the first step of a sprint.[35]

The tightening of the plantar aponeurosis converts the foot to a truss, and the acting forces are of the compressive type. The foot continues its plantar flexion at the ankle. The metatarsophalangeal joint of the big toe reaches a maximum dorsiflexion of 58° (50°–60°) between 45% and 50% of the walking cycle.[44] From there on, the extension of the metatarsophalangeal joint diminishes to reach 0 and the big toe is off the ground at 60% of the walking cycle.

The skin of the sole of the foot is mobile during 30% of the walking cycle. The gradual dorsiflexion of the big toe at the metatarsophalangeal joint limits the mobility of the skin of the ball of the foot. The fixed skin now transmits the shear forces to the deeper structures.[44]

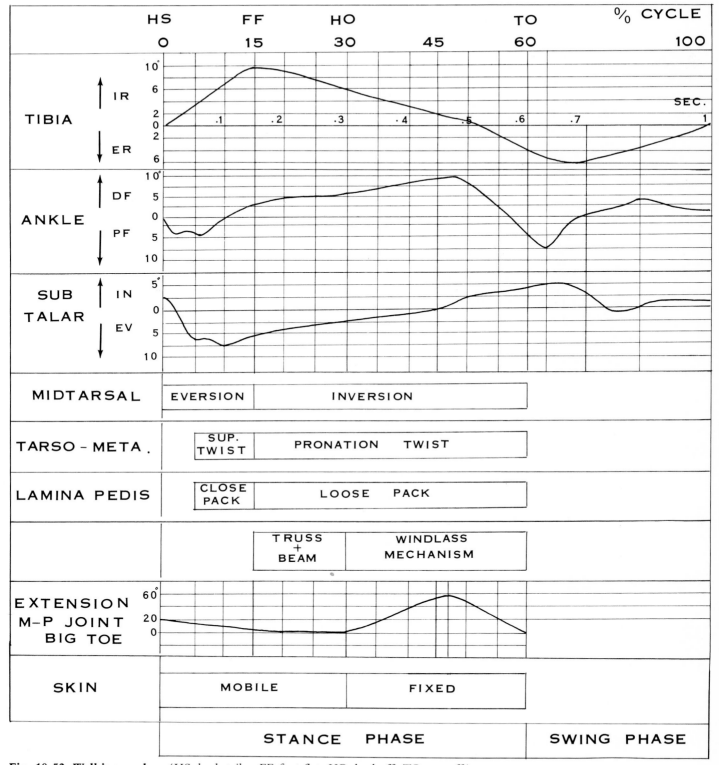

Fig. 10-52. Walking cycle. (*HS,* heel strike; *FF,* foot flat; *HO,* heel off; *TO,* toe off.)

Fig. 10-53. Axes of the push-off.   The push-off is initiated along the oblique axis B_{obl} passing through the metatarsal heads 2 to 5 and continuing along the transverse axis B_{tr} passing through the metatarsal heads 1 and 2 and terminating along the distal transverse axis A_{tr} passing through the tip of the big toe. The dorsiflexion of the toes is accompanied by a motion of the ankle complex involving the axes of the talocrural (tc) and subtalar (st) joints, resulting in a secondary axis C_{obl} or C_{tr} that is parellel to the primary axes B_{obl}, B_{tr}, or A_{tr}. The push-off along the oblique axis B_{obl} acts as a low-gear mechanism, whereas the push-off along the transverse axis B_{tr} acts as a high-gear mechanism of take-off. (From Bojsen-Møller F, Lamoreux L: Significance of free dorsiflexion of the toes in walking. Acta Orthop Scand 50, No. 4:471, 1979)

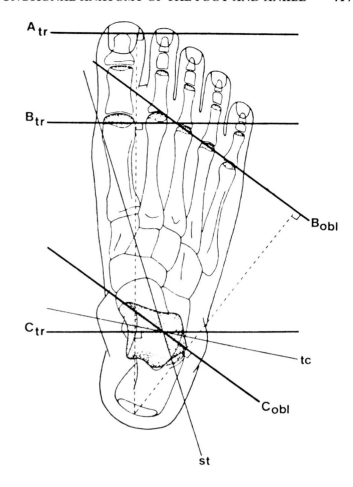

Swing Phase

During the swing phase the foot is off the ground. Initially the foot is accelerated and plantar flexed. In mid swing phase the foot is gradually dorsiflexed and everted and the toes clear the ground. The ankle is at a right angle and the foot is still accelerated forward. In the last stage of the swing phase, the foot is decelerated. The leg is turned in and the heel inverts. The foot descends and strikes the ground with the ankle at a right angle and the heel in minimal inversion; the walking cycle is completed.

The stride is the linear distance from heel–strike to heel–strike of the same foot (Fig. 10-54). The step is the distance between successive points of foot-to-floor contact of alternate feet.[55] There are two steps in a stride (Fig. 10-55). The average duration of the walking cycle is nearly 1 second with 60 strides (or 120 steps) in a minute. The mean measurements of a stride are length, 156.5 cm ± 11.4 cm;

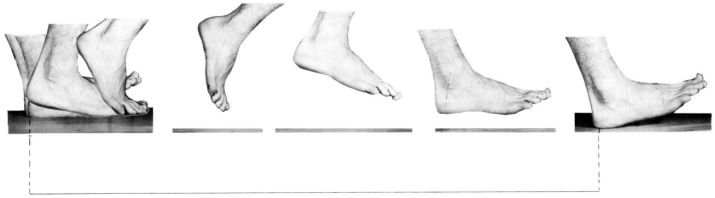

STRIDE LENGTH

Fig. 10-54. The stride is the linear distance from heel-strike to heel-strike of the same foot.

Fig. 10-55. The step is the distance between successive points of foot-to-floor contact of alternate feet.   There are two steps in a stride. (From Murray MP, Drought AB, Kroy RC: Walking patterns of norman men. J Bone Joint Surg [Am] 46, No. 2:335, 1964)

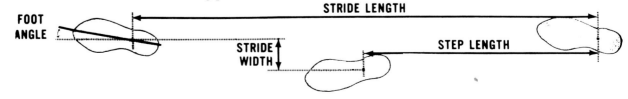

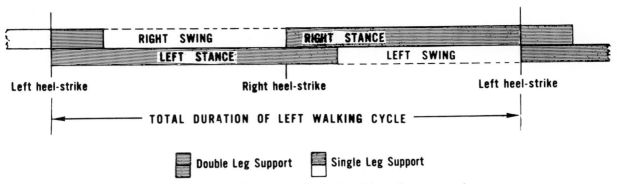

Fig. 10-56. Left walking cycle, showing the temporal relationships of stance, swing, double limb support, and single limb support. (From Murray MP, Drought AB, Kory RC: Walking patterns of norman men. J Bone Joint Surg [Am] 46, No. 2:335, 1964)

width, 8 cm ± 3.5 cm, with mean out-toeing of the feet at 6.8° ± 5.6°.

During the walking cycle, double limb support occurs twice: at the beginning and at the end of the stance phase (Fig. 10-56). Each double support period lasts about 10% of the walking cycle.

Forces

The forces exerted under the foot during gait are measured as vertical forces, fore and aft shear, medial and lateral shear, and torque (Fig. 10-57).

Vertical Forces

As the heel strikes the ground, the vertical force exerted on the ground is approximately 70% to 85% of the body weight (Fig. 10-58).[60-62] The body center of gravity is at a low point and is accelerated upward. This corresponds with the initial spike of the vertical force exerted by the foot at about 12% of the cycle and reaches a magnitude exceeding the body weight by 10% to 15%. The force gradually diminishes to about 80% of body weight, and then a second peak 15% to 20% greater than the body weight occurs, followed by a rapid decline of the vertical force, which disappears at toe off.

Fore and Aft Shear

Fore and aft shear have a lesser magnitude than the vertical forces with two maximums on the order of 10% of the body weight. (Fig. 10-58).[60-62] The first spike occurs at heel strike in the fore direction; the second peak occurs in the aft direction at 50% of the cycle and drops to 0 at toe off.

Medial and Lateral Shear

Medial and lateral shear are also of a lesser magnitude than the vertical force, on the order of 10% of the body weight (Fig. 10-58).[60-62] At heel strike, a medially directed shear force is present, followed by a lateral shear force, which remains until toe off.

Torque

Torque, created in response to the rotation of the tibia and measured in the horizontal plane against the ground, is internally directed at heel strike and continues as an external torque until 50% of the cycle, at which point it gradually diminishes to reach 0 at toe off (Fig. 10-58).[60-62] The torque has a magnitude of 20 inch-pounds.

Stauffer and co-workers have analyzed the compressive and tangential forces created in the stance phase at the level of the ankle joint.[14] The weight-bearing surface of the ankle joint is 11 cm² to 13 cm², and the fibula bears and transmits to the talus one sixth of the load.[14,63] From heel strike to foot flat, the compressive forces exerted on the ankle increase gradually and reach a magnitude of about three times the body weight. A plateau level is reached until heel off, followed by a second peak of compressive forces at 40% of the walking cycle, reaching nearly five times the body weight (Fig. 10-59).[14] The tangential forces created at the level of the ankle joint are biphasic: they are acting in the aft direction from heel strike to foot flat and in the fore direction during the push-off of the gait cycle.

The magnitude of the aft force is nearly 0.7% of the body weight and occurs between 35% and 40% of the walking cycle. The fore tangential force is of lesser magnitude, 0.3% of the body weight, and occurs between 50% and 55% of the walking cycle (Fig. 10-60).

The distribution pattern of the forces acting under the foot while walking has been investigated by many authors (Fig. 10-61).[51, 64-67] As described by Hutton and co-workers, at heel strike and up to 10% of the walking cycle, the load is concentrated on the heel cushion.[51] The center of the load progresses in a linear fashion axially, passing slightly on the medial aspect of the heel (Figs. 10-62 and 10-63). At foot flat (15% of the cycle) and with the gradual flexion of the tibia or relative plantar flexion of the foot, the load is shifted from the heel cushion to the ball of the foot in an increasing fashion. The midfoot does not participate in sharing the load. The center of the load passes on the medial aspect of the sole of the foot. The initial load transmission is rapid. At heel off (30% of the cycle), the entire load is

(Text continues on p. 422.)

Fig. 10-57. Forces during the stand phase of gait. (*A*) At heel-strike the force exerted on the ground F_R has a vertical component F_V and a horizontal component F_H directed anteriorly. The ground reactions are opposite in direction. (*B*) At heel-strike, seen anteriorly, the force exerted has a medially directed shear, horizontal component F_H associated with a medially directed torque T_M. (*C*) At push-off the force exerted on the ground F_R has a vertical component F_V and a horizontal component F_H directed posteriorly. (*D*) At push-off, seen anteriorly, the force exerted has a laterally directed shear, horizontal component F_H associated with lateral torque T_L.

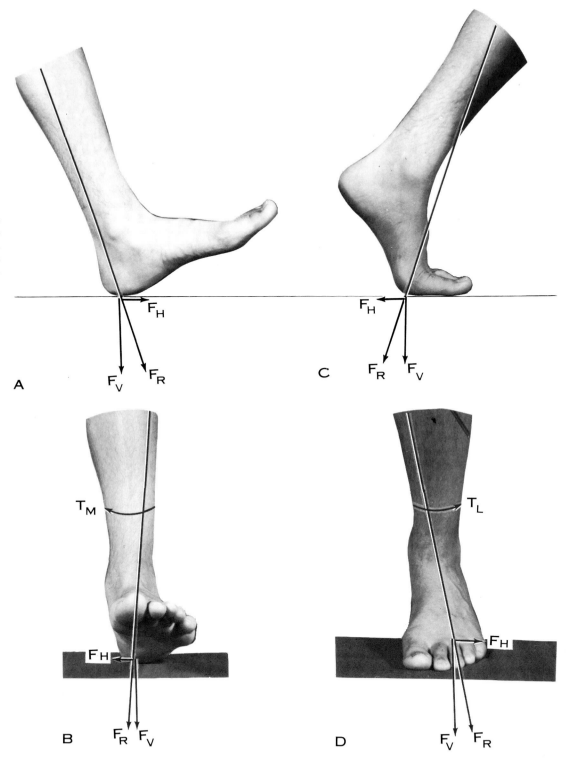

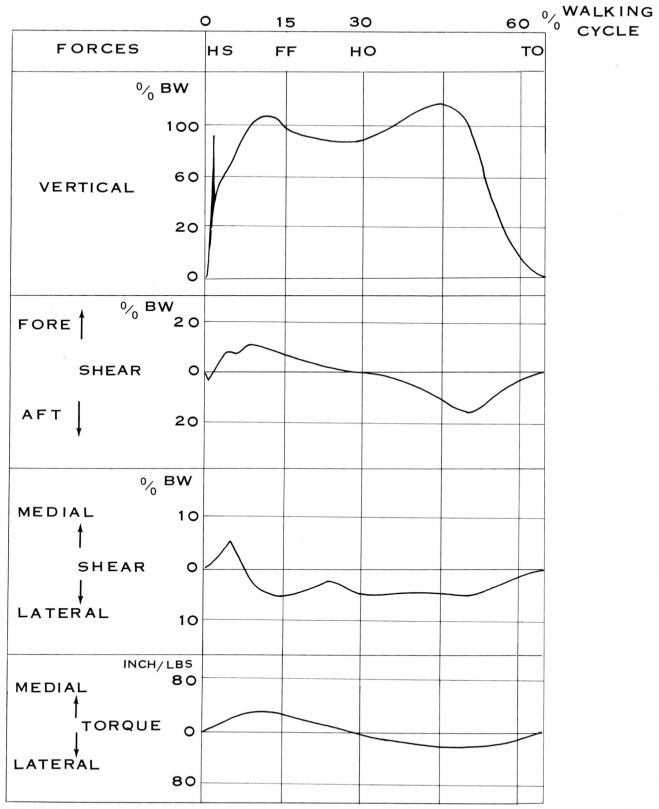

Fig. 10-58. Forces acting during the walking cycle. (Adapted from Mann RA: Biomechanics. In Jahss M [ed]: Disorders of the Foot, Vol 1, pp 47, 49. Philadelphia, WB Saunders, 1982)

Fig. 10-59. Mean patterns of compressive forces at the ankle during the stance phase of the walking cycle. The compressive forces across the ankle are 3 times the body weight at 20% to 30% of the stance phase and 4.5 to 5.5 times the body weight at 60% to 70% of the stance phase. (From Stauffer RN, Chao EYS, Brewster RC: Force and motion analysis of the normal, diseased and prosthetic ankle joint. Clin Orthop 127:189, 1977)

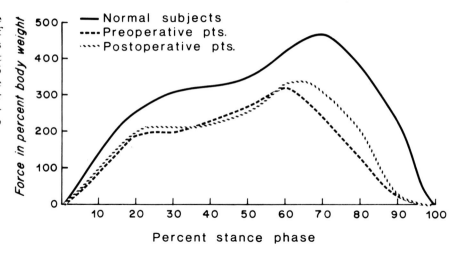

Fig. 10-60. Mean patterns of tangential forces at the ankle during the stance phase of the walking cycle. The tangential forces are biphasic, directed in the aft direction during the heelstrike and foot-flat portions of the cycle and in the fore direction during the push-off. (From Stauffer, RN, Chao EYS, Brewster RC: Force and motion analysis of the normal, diseased and prosthetic ankle joint. Clin Orthop 127: 189, 1977)

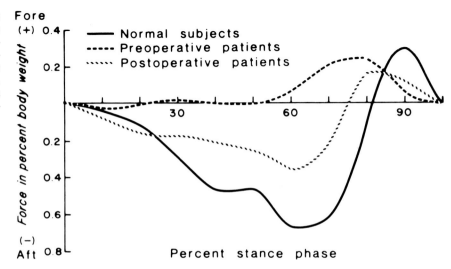

Fig. 10-61. Distribution, magnitude and direction of the forces under the foot in the stance phase of the walking cycle. The point of application of the force is seen passing through the heel and the medial border of the foot. It reaches the ball of the foot at the level of the second metatarsal head, shifts medially toward the first metatarsal head, and progresses rapidly to the big toe. The curve of the magnitude of the forces is bimodal. As indicated, during the heel-strike, the forces are directed downward and anteriorly, become progressively vertical at mid stance, and are directed downward and posteriorly at push-off. (From Elftman H: Forces and energy changes in the leg during walking. Am Physiol 125:339, 1939)

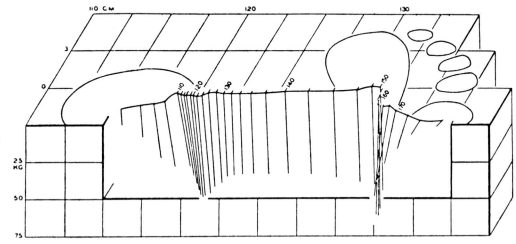

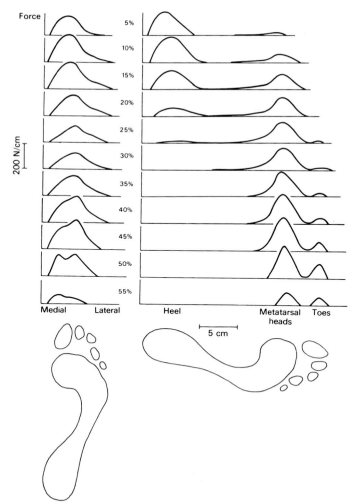

Fig. 10-62. Distribution of load on a normal foot during walking. At heel-strike the load is carried by the medial aspect of the heel. At 15% the load is carried by the heel and the forefoot; the midfoot carries insignificant load. At 30% the load is over the ball of the foot, with participation of the toes. The forefoot load reaches a peak at 45% and gradually diminishes as the load is transferred more to the toes. (From Hutton WC, Stott JRR, Stokes IAF: The mechanics of the foot. In Klenerman L [ed]: The Foot and Its Disorders, p 40. Oxford, Blackwell Scientific Publications, 1976)

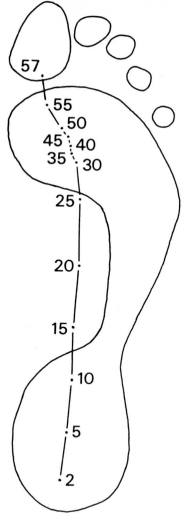

Fig. 10-63. Progression of the center of load during the walking cycle. From heel-strike to heel-off the progression of the center of load is rapid. It passes slightly on the medial aspect of the heel, along the medial border of the foot, and at 30% of the cycle it is over the medial aspect of the ball of the foot. From 30% to 50% the progression slows and shifts farther medially toward the first metatarsal head and then progresses rapidly along the plantar aspect of the big toe. (From Hutton WC, Stott JRR, Stokes JAF: The mechanics of the foot. In Klenerman L [ed]: The Foot and Its Disorders, p 41. Oxford, Blackwell Scientific Publications, 1976)

transferred to the ball of the foot and the center of the load is located more on the medial aspect of the ball of the foot. From 30% to 50% of the cycle, two definite changes occur: the load transmission line shifts medially, and the forward transmission of the load centers slows down; this results in clustering of the pressure centers on the medial aspect of the ball of the foot, and the latter may carry a total load in the order of three times that of the heel.[68]

From 50% to 57% of the walking cycle, the load line passes between the metatarsal heads of the first and second toes and terminates at the level of the big toe. The toes bear a significant amount of the load, sometimes reaching 50% of body weight in the push-off phase of walking.[51]

ELECTROMYOGRAPHIC ACTIVITIES DURING THE WALKING CYCLE

Electromyographically, the muscles acting on the foot–ankle complex may be grouped as follows (Fig. 10-64):[3, 56, 61, 69, 70]

Anterior Muscles: tibialis anterior, extensor digitorum longus, extensor hallucis longus

Posterior muscles: triceps surae, tibialis posterior, flexor digitorum longus, flexor hallucis longus, peroneus. longus, peroneus brevis

Intrinsic muscles: extensor digitorum brevis, flexor digitorum brevis, abductor hallucis, flexor hallucis brevis, abductor digiti minimi, interossei

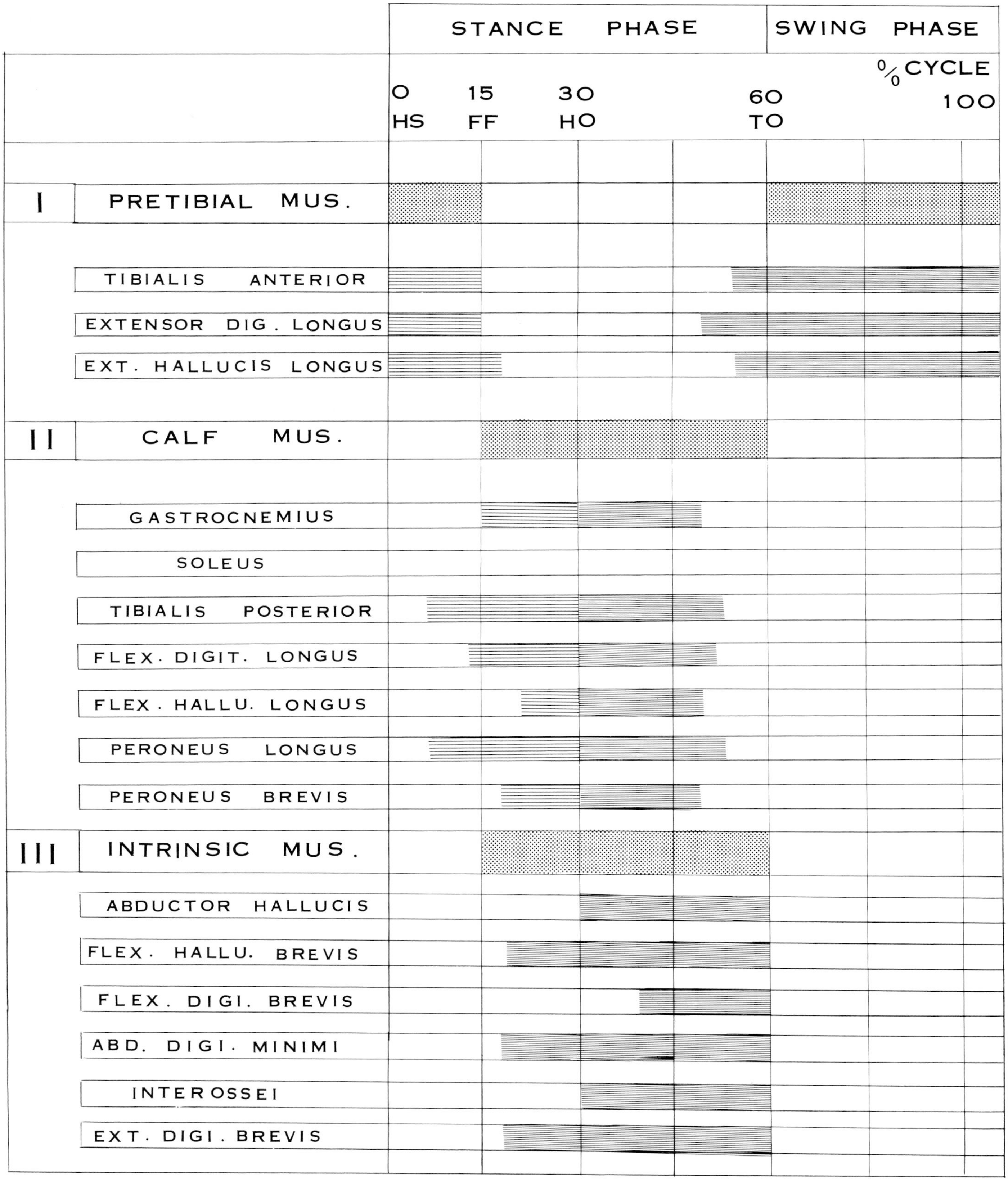

		STANCE PHASE				SWING PHASE	
							% CYCLE
		O	15	30	60		100
		HS	FF	HO	TO		
I	PRETIBIAL MUS.						
	TIBIALIS ANTERIOR						
	EXTENSOR DIG. LONGUS						
	EXT. HALLUCIS LONGUS						
II	CALF MUS.						
	GASTROCNEMIUS						
	SOLEUS						
	TIBIALIS POSTERIOR						
	FLEX. DIGIT. LONGUS						
	FLEX. HALLU. LONGUS						
	PERONEUS LONGUS						
	PERONEUS BREVIS						
III	INTRINSIC MUS.						
	ABDUCTOR HALLUCIS						
	FLEX. HALLU. BREVIS						
	FLEX. DIGI. BREVIS						
	ABD. DIGI. MINIMI						
	INTEROSSEI						
	EXT. DIGI. BREVIS						

Fig. 10-64. Electromyography of the leg and foot muscle during the gait cycle. Wider parallel lines indicate lengthening or eccentric contraction. Narrower parallel lines indicate shortening or concentric contraction. (*HS,* heel-strike; *FF,* foot flat; *HO,* heel off; *TO,* toe off.) (Adapted from Bowker JH, Hall CB: Normal human gait. In American Academy of Orthopedic Surgeons: Atlas of Orthotics: Biomechanical Principles and Application, p 141 St. Louis, CV Mosby, 1975; and from Mann R, Inman VT: Phasic activity of intrinsic muscles of the foot. J Bone Joint Surg [Am] 46, No. 3:469, 1964

The stance phase of the gait cycle may be divided into a single limb support and double limb support. The latter occurs initially until 12% of the cycle and at the end of the support phase from 50% to 62%. The single support phase extends from 12% to 50% of the cycle.[55,61] The anterior muscle group is electrically active during the double support phases and the swing phase of the gait cycle. The posterior muscle group is electrically active during the single stance phase of the cycle.

The intrinsic muscles are inactive during the initial double support phase and early single support phase. They gradually increase their activity during the single support phase and remain active in the second double support phase.[71] More specifically, the anterior muscle group is active during the initial double support phase to control the plantar flexion, decelerate the foot, and prevent the foot from slapping the ground. The muscles undergo a lengthening or eccentric contraction. The second peak of activity of these muscles is related to the dorsiflexion of the foot to clear the toes from the ground. During the swing phase the tibialis anterior muscle is responsible for the dorsiflexion of the accelerated foot. It undergoes a period of electric silence at mid swing as the foot is everting to allow adequate clearance; it increases its activity at deceleration and inverts the foot.[70] The contraction is of the concentric type.

The posterior muscle group is silent during the second double support phase of the cycle and the toe off. During the first half of the single limb stance phase, the demands of propulsion and stability are minimum and the posterior muscle group activity is minimum. During the second half of the single limb stance phase, there is increasing forward velocity and precarious stability "created by the forward position of the body's center of gravity and the opposing swinging limb."[72] The posterior muscle group is active to restrain the forward movement of the tibia. This provides dynamic stability and "allows the body to lean farther forward beyond its base of support" to take a longer stride.[73] The contraction of the posterior muscles is initially of the lengthening type, followed by concentric contraction. It becomes apparent that it is the body forward momentum that causes the push-off or rolling phase, and the posterior muscles are not actively responsible for this phase of the gait cycle. The peroneus longus works in concert with the tibialis posterior and prevents excessive inversion of the foot and contributes to the maintenance of appropriate contact with the ground.[72]

The intrinsic muscles of the foot are considered to be invertors of the foot acting on the subtalar joint and contribute to the stabilization of the foot during propulsion. Their activity ceases at toe off.[71]

REFERENCES

1. Lang J, Wachsmuth W: Praktische Anatomie: Ein Lehr- und Hilfsbuch der anatomischen Grundlagen ärztlichen Handelns, Vol 1, Part 4, Bein und Statik, pp 370–376, 388–390. Berlin, Springer-Verlag, 1972
2. Inman TV: The Joints of the Ankle, pp 19, 26–27, 31, 37, 70–73. Baltimore, Williams & Wilkins, 1976
3. Mann RA: Biomechanics of the foot. In American Academy of Orthopedic Surgeons: Atlas of Orthotics—Biomechanical Principles and Application, pp 257–266. St Louis, Mosby, 1975
4. Barnett CH, Napier JR: The axis of rotation at the ankle joint in man: Its influece upon the form of the talus and the mobility of the fibula. Anat 86:1, 1952
5. Hicks JH: The mechanics of the foot: I. The joints. Anat 87:345, 1953
6. Close JR, Inman VT: The action of the ankle joint: Prosthetic devices research project. Institute of Engineering Research, University of California, Berkeley, Series II, Issue 22, p 5, 1952
7. Close JR: Some applications of the functional anatomy of the ankle joint. J Bone Joint Surg [Am] 38, No. 1:761, 1956
8. Sammarco GJ, Burstein AH, Frankel VH: Biomechanics of the ankle: A kinematic study. Orthop Clin North Am 4, No. 1:75, 1973
9. Frankel VH, Nordin M: Biomechanics of the ankle. In Basic Biomechanics of the Skeletal System, p 183. Philadelphia, Lea & Febiger, 1980
10. American Academy of Orthopedic Surgeons: Joint Motion—Method of Measuring and Recording, pp 68–69, 85. Chicago, AAOS, 1965
11. Bonnin JG: Injuries to the Ankle 1st ed, pp 47–48. London, Heinemann, 1950
12. Weseley MS, Koval R, Kleiger B: Roentgen measurement of ankle flexion–extension motion. Clin Orthop 65:167, 1969
13. Boone DC, Azen SP: Normal range of motion of joints in male subjects. J Bone Joint Surg [Am] 61, No. 5:756, 1979
14. Stauffer RN, Chao EYS, Brewster RC: Force and motion analysis of the normal, diseased and prosthetic ankle joint. Clin Orthop 127:189, 1977
15. Prins JG: Diagnosis and treatment of injury to the lateral ligament of the ankle: A comparative clinical study. Acta Chir Scand [Suppl] 486: 41, 1978
16. Duquennoy A, Lisélélé D, Torabi DJ: Eléments radiographiques du diagnostic et gravité de l'entorse. Rev Chir Orthop 61 (Suppl 2):134, 1975
17. Cox JS, Hewes TF: "Normal" talar tilt angle. Clin Orthop 140:37, 1979
18. Rubin G, Witten M: The talar tilt angle and the fibular collateral ligaments. J Bone Joint Surg [Am] 42:311, 1960
19. Sedlin ED: A device for stress inversion or eversion roentgenograms of the ankle. J Bone Joint Surg [Am] 42:1184, 1960
20. Laurin CA, St. Jacques R: L'investigation radiologique des entorses, récentes et récidivantes de la cheville: Etude expérimentale. Union Med Can 94:737, 1965
21. Quellet R, St. Jacques R, Laurin CA: Laxité ligamentaire de la cheville. Union Med Can 97:861, 1968
22. Landeros O, Frost HM, Higgens CC: Post-traumatic anterior ankle instability. Clin Orthop 56:169, 1968
23. Castaing J, Delaplace J: Entorse de la cheville: Intérêt de l'étude de la stabilité dans le plan sagittal pour le diagnostic de gravité: Recherche radiographique du tiroir astragalien anterieur. Rev Chir Orthop 58: 51, 1972
24. Laurin C, Mathieu J: Sagittal mobility of the normal ankle. Clin Orthop 108:99, 1975
25. Manter JT: Movements of the subtalar and transverse tarsal joints. Anat Rec 80:397, 1941
26. Isman RE, Inman VT: Anthropometric studies of the human foot and ankle. Biomechanics Laboratory, University of California, Berkeley. Technical Report, May, 1968
27. Farabeuf LH: Précis de Manuel Opératoire, pp 836–847. Paris, Masson, 1889
28. Elftman H: The transverse tarsal joint and its control. Clin Orthop 16:41, 1960
29. Huson A: Een Ontleedkundig-Functioneel Onderzoek van de Voetworte (An Anatomical and Functional Study of the Tarsal Joints, pp 133–142. Leiden, Drukkerij, "Luctor et Emergo," 1961
30. Kelikian H: Hallux Valgus, Allied Deformities of the Forefoot and Metatarsalgia, pp 31–33. Philadelphia, Saunders, 1965
31. McElvenny RT, Caldwell GD: A new operation for correction of cavus foot: Fusion of first metatarso–cuneiform–navicular joints. Clin Orthop 11:85, 1958
32. Coleman SS, Chesnut WJ: A simple test for hindfoot flexibility in the cavovarus foot. Clin Orthop 123:60, 1977
33. Joseph J: Range of movement of the great toe in men. J Bone Joint Surg [Br] 36:450, 1954
34. Sammarco JG: Biochemics of the foot. In Frankel VH, Nordin M (eds): Basic Biomechanics of the Skeletal System, pp 202–204, Philadelphia, Lea & Febiger, 1980

35. Bojsen-Møller F: The human foot—a new speed construction. In Asmussen E, Jørgensen K (eds): International Series of Biomechanics, Vol 2-A, pp 261–266. Baltimore, University Park Press, 1978

36. De Vogel PL: Enige functioneel-anatomische aspecten van ket bovenste spronggewricht. Thesis, Leiden, 1970

37. Ruth CJ: Surgical treatment of injuries of the fibular collateral ligament of the ankle. J Bone Joint Surg 43:229, 1961

38. MacConaill MA, Basmajian JV: Muscles and Movements: A Basis for Human Kinesiology, pp 74–84. Baltimore, Williams & Wilkins, 1969

39. Bojsen-Møller F: Calcaneo-cuboid joint and stability of the longitudinal arch of the foot at high and low gear push off. J Anat 129:165, 1979

40. Ellis TS: The Human Foot, Its Form and Structure, Functions and Clothing, pp 1–113. London, Churchill, 1889

41. MacConaill MA: Some anatomical factors affecting the stabilizing functions of muscles. Ir J Med Sci 6:160, 1946

42. Sarrafian SK, Topouzian LK: Anatomy and physiology of the extensor apparatus of the toes. J Bone Joint Surg [Am] 51, No. 4:669, 1969

43. Hicks JH: The mechanics of the foot: II. The plantar aponeurosis and the arch. J Anat 88:25, 1954

44. Bojsen-Møller F, Lamoreux L: Significance of free dorsiflexion of the toes in walking. Acta Orthop Scand 50, No. 4:471, 1979

45. Lapidus PW: Kinesiology and mechanical anatomy of the tarsal joints. Clin Orthop 30:20, 1963

46. Hicks JH: The foot as a support. Acta Anat 25:34, 1955

47. MacConaill MA: The postural mechanism of the human foot. Proc R Ir Acad 50, No. 14:265, 1945

48. Basmajian JV, Stecko G: The role of muscles in arch support of the foot: An electromyographic study. J Bone Joint Surg [Am] 45, No. 5:1184, 1963

49. Morton DJ: The Human Foot: Its Evolution, Physiology and Functional Disorders, p 109. New York, Columbia University Press, 1935

50. Jones RL: The human foot: An experimental study of its mechanics, and the role of its muscles and ligaments in the support of the arch. Am J Anat 68:1, 1941

51. Hutton WC, Stott JRR, Stokes IAF: The mechanics of the foot. In Klenerman L (ed): The Foot and Its Disorders, pp 30–48. Oxford, Blackwell Scientific Publications, 1976

52. Testut L, Jacob O: Traité d'Anatomie Topographique avec Applications Médico-chirurgicales, Vol 2, pp 1110–1113. Paris, Octave Doin, 1909

53. Paturet GL: Traité d'Anatomie Humaine, Vol II, Membres Supérieur et Inférieur, pp 603–605. Paris, Masson, 1951

54. Harty M: Anatomic considerations in injuries of the calcaneus. Orthop Clin North Am 4, No. 1:179, 1973

55. Murray MP, Drought AB, Kory RC: Walking patterns of normal men. J Bone Joint Surg [Am] 46, No. 2:335, 1964

56. Bowker HJ, Hall CB: Normal humain gait. In American Academy of Orthopedic Surgeons: Atlas of Orthotics—Biomechanical Principles and Application, pp 133–143. St Louis, Mosby, 1975

57. Fryer C: Normal Human Locomotion in Prosthetic–Orthotic Course. Northwestern University Medical School, 1979

58. Wright DG, Desai SM, Henderson WH: Action of the subtalar and ankle–joint complex during the stance phase of walking. J Bone Joint Surg [Am] 46, No. 2:361, 1964

59. Inman V, Ralston HJ, Todd F: Human Walking, pp 1–61, Baltimore, Willians & Wilkins, 1981

60. Mann RA, Hagy JL: Running, jogging and walking: A comparative electromyographic and biomechanical study. In Bateman JE, Trott AW (eds): The Foot and Ankle, pp 167–175. Stuttgart, Decker, 1980

61. Mann RA, Baxter DE, Lutter LD: Running symposium. Foot Ankle 1, No. 4:190, 1981

62. Mann RA: Biomechanics. In Jahss M (ed): Disorders of the Foot, Vol 1, pp 37–67. Philadelphia, WB Saunders, 1982

63. Lambert KL: The weight bearing function of the fibula: A strain gauge study. J Bone Joint Surg [Am] 53, No. 3:507, 1971

64. Elftman H: Forces and energy changes in the leg during walking. Am J Physiol 125:339, 1939

65. Elftman H, Manter JT: The axis of the human foot. Science 80:484, 1934

66. Bauman JH, Brand PW: Measurement of pressure between foot and shoe. Lancet 1:629, 1963

67. Stott JRR, Hutton WC, Stokes IAF: Forces under the foot. J Bone Joint Surg [Br] 55, 335, 1973

68. Grundy M, Tosh PA, McLeish RD, Smidt L: An investigation of the centers of pressure under the foot while walking. J Bone Joint Surg [Br] 57, No. 1:98, 1975

69. Eberhart JD, Inman VT, Bresler B: The principal elements in human locomotion. In Klopsteg PE, Wilson PD (ed.): Human Limbs and Their Substitutes, pp 437–471. New York, Hafner Publishing, 1968

70. Gray EG, Basmajian JV: Electromyography and cinematography of leg and foot ("normal" and flat) during walking. Anat Rec 161:1, 1968

71. Mann R, Inman VT: Phasic activity of intrinsic muscles of the foot. J Bone Joint Surg [Am] 46, No. 3:469, 1964

72. Simon SR, Mann RA, Hagy JL, Larsen LJ: Role of the posterior calf muscles in normal gait. J Bone Joint Surg [Am] 60, No. 4:465, 1978

Index

An *f* following a page number represents a figure;
a *t* indicates tabular material.

Dr. T. Derek V. Cooke
La Salle Building
146 Stuart Street
Kingston, Ont. K7L 3N6
Tel: 549-6414